WORLD HISTORY OF
PSYCHIATRY

World History of Psychiatry

Edited by

JOHN G. HOWELLS, M.D.,
F.R.C.PSYCH., D.P.M.

Director, The Institute of Family Psychiatry
The Ipswich Hospital, Ipswich, England

BRUNNER/MAZEL, *Publishers*   New York

Contents

INTRODUCTION

BY

THE EDITOR

History strongly links medicine and psychiatry and it is natural to ask how appropriate this is. There is a fallacious assumption that the term "medicine" covers a discipline concerned with physical phenomena only. It is a commonly held fallacy. In fact, as any authoritative dictionary will show, medicine is a discipline concerned with pathology (disease, literally to be "ill at ease"). Pathology arises out of psychic and physical trauma, has repercussions on the psychic as well as on the organic self, and leads to psychic as well as organic symptoms. For instance, emotional anguish and physical pain are both abnormal and equally significant as pathological phenomena.

Psychiatry is the discipline concerned with the healing of the psyche. But ignorance of pathology and psychopathology has led to unclear differentiation of psychic and somatic syndromes—particularly when the latter have given rise to states not always easy to differentiate from psychic states, e.g., the excitement of delirium and the agitation of acute anxiety. Hippocrates made this essential error in seeing insanity and emotional illness as both arising from the brain and affected by the equilibrium of the humours. The confusion is as well marked today in medicine as it was in antiquity. "Madness" was, and is, a term loosely employed to cover any state of abnormal behaviour of psychic or somatic origin. In these states of abnormal behaviour there are two main groups: those pathological states due to brain dysfunction, and those due to psychic dysfunction. The safest course is for this history of psychiatry to embrace consideration of the former, neuro-psychiatry, and of the latter, true psychiatry.

However, that there was confusion in the past did not mean that psychic states were overlooked, or that due consideration was not given to psychonosis (neurosis). Indeed there were times when more

vii

emphasis was given to it than in many countries today, where neuro-psychiatry often passes for psychiatry. Too often the history of psy-chiatry is assumed to be the history of the care of the insane; that is largely the history of neuro-psychiatry. That true psychiatry with its consideration of psychic states was well recognized throughout the history of medicine can be demonstrated by a brief review of the relevant content of this book.

Before Christianity, the attention given to psychic phenomena and syndromes was manifest in a medicine that was holistic in intent and much concerned with the interaction between soma and psyche. This is demonstrated as far back as the 16th century B.C. in ancient Egyp-tian medicine, as exemplified, for instance, by the contents of the Ebers papyrus. Even this is probably predated by the ancient Chinese medical literature, which can be dated, with some uncertainty, possibly from 26-27th century B.C. onwards, and exemplified by the *Yellow Emperor's Classic of Internal Medicine*. Abundant expression is seen early in Graeco-Roman medicine as exemplified by the "four passions" and later in the works of that interpreter of Greek medicine, Galen.

The emphasis on psychic matters continued during the first ten centuries A.D. and gained support in other quarters, notably in Arab medicine, especially following the influence of Mohammed (570-632) and exemplified by the works of Rhazes (860-932) and of Avicenna (978-1036). Psychic awareness is found in the 1st-2nd century A.D. in India, in the works of Caraka, the eminent physician of the Ayurveda, the ancient system of Indian medicine. Again, it is found in the Nordic sagas.

From the 10th to the 16th century, there is a strong emphasis in the works of physicians on a medicine that takes full account of psychic events. A few outstanding exponents from a number of coun-tries are Constantinus Africanus (c. 1020-1087), Petrus Hispanus (1200-1277), Girolamo Fracastoro (1478-1553) and Paolo Zacchia (1584-1659), all of whom worked in Italy; Hildegard of Bingen (1098-1179) in Germany; Maimonides (1113-1205) in Cordova, Spain, and Cairo, Egypt; the great Vives (1492-1541) in Belgium; Dona Oliva Sabuco de Nantes, in Spain, in 1587, with her views on the passions and the use of speech in therapy; in England, Bartholomeus Anglicus (fl. 1230-1250), Andrew Boorde (1490-1549) and Timothy Bright (1551-1615), the first psychiatrist writer in the English language.

As we enter the somatic era, medicine gives overwhelming emphasis to pathology and organic syndromes. Interest in psychic phenomena is kept alive by a thinly scattered, but nevertheless distinguished group of practitioners. They carry the torch through the dark ages. In England, we have Jorden, Sydenham, Cheyne, Dendy and Prichard; in Switzerland we find Tissot, Zimmermann and Dubois; in France there are Moreau de Tours, Liébeault, and Bernheim; in Poland, Szokalski and Biernacki; in the U.S.A., Thomas Trotter, Morton Prince and Austen Riggs; John Quier in Jamaica; Lenhossék in Hungary; in Germany/Austria are Reil and Langermann and the pre-Freudian group of Benedikt, Struempell, Moebius and Breuer. The 20th century opens with the promise of Freud, Jung, Adler and the undervalued Janet, and the impetus grows to meet the needs of the emotional wrecks of the First Great War. That the workers of the early part of this century opened a new road, but that it led in the wrong direction, may be the evaluation of history.

Viewing the development of world psychiatry, it is possible to discern a series of eras, each dominated by a theme. There is world wide movement through the eras in a predictable direction. This movement has direction, but cannot necessarily be claimed to be uniformly progressive if one defines progress to be increasing knowledge and improving practice. There can be regression and recession. It may be useful to bring this pattern to relief, perhaps overstark relief, as it may offer the reader a guide in his appreciation of the psychiatric history of a particular region or of the whole.

The first era can be termed *primitive*. Other terms associated with it might be folk medicine, irrational practices, magic, myth, animism. The individual is assumed to be affected by spirits, demons, goblins, gods, goddesses, supernatural influences, etc. They can effect good or evil. They may be associated with natural forces, such as sea, wind, sun, rain, storm, and thunder. They may be found in the natural environment, in woods, mountains, streams, lakes, wells, etc. They may have links with the astral bodies. These forces could be used, antagonised, propitiated—by gifts, the wearing of ornaments and amulets, ceremony, and concoctions. Healing practices were simple, unsystematized, irrational, often containing a heavy overlay of suggestion. There was no lack of wisdom, but it was not organized. This stage could in the past be found in all areas of the world, e.g., it applied in ancient India, in the pre-Islamic period in Arab countries, and in Europe; it can still be found in many areas, e.g., in modern India, parts of Europe, regions of South America; in a few areas there has been no significant movement away from it, e.g., in underdeveloped parts of the world.

The second stage could be termed *rational*. Associated terms might be systematisation, organisation of knowledge, a cultured approach, civilised. An attempt is made to base practice on theory. Practices are advanced and organised. Practitioners are as educated and knowledgeable as it was then possible. Both theory and practice may be in tune with the best of today. In some fields they may be more advanced than today; this is especially true insomuch as a holistic attitude, combining the somatic and the psychic, is usually adopted in medical practice. Somatic and psychic medicines are one—psychosomatiatria. This era is strikingly brought out in this book. In at least four regions of the world this stage had reached advanced points of development. These areas are ancient Egypt, which predates the next, the Graeco-Roman civilisation, the post-Vedic period in India from the 6th century B.C. to the 2nd century A.D., and, probably predating the others, ancient China from the time of the Yellow Emperor (possibly 2600 B.C. onwards). Each development may have been reached independently, but each could still influence the other, even incorporate another, and also sustain another as did post-Islamic Arab medicine which protected and handed on the contributions of Graeco-Roman medicine. Each was greatly concerned with interaction of soma and psyche and each had constructed a physiology of sorts; humoral theory was an aspect of this and exerted a major influence in the Graeco-Roman and in the Indian medicine. Often there were ideas on personality, the range of the emotions and the linking of the emotions with somatic areas. Practices in psychiatry embraced almost all the procedures used today and were based on theory which may have been true or false, but not inferior to our efforts today. This stage invariably coexisted with the primitive stage. This stage suffers from not being well documented or from being recorded in a form difficult to interpret. Much research is yet required here.

Religious describes the third stage. Associated terms might be deistic, demonological, humanitarian, monastic. A religion influenced both theory and practice. This stage is well illustrated by faiths such as the Christian, Moslem, and Buddhist after its introduction to China in the 5th century A.D. At its best, there was emphasis on brotherly love and care of the weak and poor. Sometimes, as in the Christian and Moslem faiths, it produced movements inspired by saints, which led to the care of the mentally ill in religious houses, and later to cells in pauper or general hospitals, and later still, as in Arab countries and in Spain, in Valencia, to mental hospitals. At its worst, in this stage there could be repressive measures due to puritanism. A belief in devil possession dictated treatment by exorcism; an over-assiduous search for heretics could cause ill-treatment of the mentally ill mistaken for them. This stage could coexist with the two previous stages and be influenced by them.

Somatic describes the fourth stage. Associated terms might be technological, industrial, urban, secular institutionalization. From the 16th century onwards, progress in anatomy, physiology and technology in many countries led to real and exciting progress in somatic medicine; the physician followed the paths opened by technology. This was not balanced by real progress in psychic medicine; indeed it led to neglect, except where neurology impinged on psychiatry. Increase in population, urbanization, advances in treatment led to the foundation of large general hospitals and mental hospitals. The care of those suffering from neuro-psychiatric disorders was organized and its control legalized. The care of those suffering from emotional disorders barely survived. A major liability was abandoning the holistic and adopting a dualistic approach to the sick, based on the somatic and the psychic. This stage could coexist with the previous stages, but the second, the rational stage, became of less importance and was largely lost.

The fifth and last stage could be termed a stage of *harmonization*. Associated terms are re-balance, resolution, international, and contemporary. The attempt is made to rekindle the almost extinguished emphasis on the psyche. Inevitably, progress is unpredictable due to the absence of substantial knowledge. At times, extreme measures and movements hold sway. An example is psychoanalysis, Freudian analysis, that extraordinary, speculative and fanciful approach more remarkable as a phenomenon for being than for its contribution. The hold of psychoanalysis may be explained by the fascination of its highly developed imagination, its sexual content, which appeared in an era of puritanism, its studied appeal for general support and thus for support from the inexperienced and the uncritical, and its tendency for its practitioners to lack experience of patients in institutions. But the most significant explanation for its hold is the absence of a rational psychopathology to which it could be compared. Again, there is existential psychiatry, which only being only being can be. Strands of non-sense appear in the fabric. Dualism is exaggerated as the psychic field rebels from the somatic, and the somatic ignores the psychic. An exhausting, troubled, erratic course may end, perhaps guided by rediscovered truths from the second stage, in a final holistic approach. We are in its midst.

It must be emphasized that the pattern outlined above must be re-evaluated and adjusted for a particular area. Some regions, e.g., Europe, have passed through all five stages. A stage might be missed here and there: Scandinavian psychiatry did not feel the second stage impact of Graeco-Roman psychiatry as much as the southern European countries, and the same would apply more markedly in the West Indies, which moved from the primitive to the religious stage, as indeed also occurred in Mid, Central and West Africa. The rational stage passed South America by, except inasmuch as its own civilisations contributed to it.

Each stage would be flavoured by cultural, economic, geographical, political and ecological factors. Colonisation by another people could bring rapid, harsh, and sometimes harmful changes, e.g., the Spanish influence in South America. Imported ideas could stultify progress, e.g., Meyer's psychobiological approach has been accorded a proper but not dominant place in American psychiatry, but its dominance in British psychiatry has retarded progress.

There could be regression at any point in the movement, e.g., after the Graeco-Roman influence had abated, there was a return to the primitive in Jewish medicine. In Arab countries, after the high period of ancient Egyptian medicine in the second stage, there was a return to the first and primitive phase, before a resurgence of progress with the post-Islamic era.

All the stages, as has been said, could coexist and remnants of all can be found today. Like a rope, strands could be added or a strand be worn out and disappear. Each era is well documented in this volume with illustrations from a number of regions.

This book counteracts giving excessive weight to "modern" knowledge. In the absence of a sense of history, too much importance can be given to contemporary progress. The word "modern" is often empty of meaning, as is frequently the term "research" in psychiatry, which today often amounts to nothing more than utilizing technological aids to explore concepts that lack originality. Systematic investigation based on careful observation, creative speculations and planned experiment can be demonstrated throughout history and are not "modern." While technology leads to real progress in the material fields, it assists very little in the psychic field. Technological advances, it seems, add but little to man's well-being, the state of being at ease psychically, being happy, as the man in the street would say. This still eludes us. At the same time, spectacular advances in the material field have attracted resources and the best minds. The result is that psychiatry today can claim little advance, and sometimes only regression, compared with other periods in history. Particularly at the rational stage knowledge and practice compare well with psychiatry today. It is difficult to pinpoint any area where a significant new departure has been made. If we take a few elements in psychiatric practice, we can well be surprised at its lack of innovation when we trace its course in history.

Humane or "moral" treatment of the insane has often been at a high level in the past, and there are frequent allusions to a gentle approach being more effective. It was an essential part of the ancient psychiatry of China, India, Egypt and Greece. It was a special feature of Arab psychiatry in the post-Islamic era as the mad were believed to have a special affinity with the Deity. It appertained even during the Inquisition. The heretics, not the insane, were its target. Confusion could occur, but when the diagnosis was clear, keen witch hunters such as James I could be delighted at making the differentiation. Inhumanity reached its highest peak in the overlarge mental institutions from the 18th century onwards. It created the reaction initiated by the work of Chiarugi in Italy, Tuke in England, and Pinel in France, antedated by the enlightened approaches of Valsalva and Daquin. The same institutions today still threaten humanity and call for a large number of contrived humanizing procedures. But milieu therapy was known to Aurelianus and Soranus before 500 A.D.

Mental hospitals have been with us for a long time. Institutional care was probably first practiced by the Arabs and, it would seem, in association with general hospitals, e.g., in the 8th century A.D. at Damascus and again in the 10th century at Basra. Others followed. There is mention of a mental hospital, which may be the first built for this purpose alone, at Mandu (Behar), in India, about 1000 A.D. The Turks had hospitals admitting mental patients in Anatolia: in Kayseri in 1205, Sivas in 1217, Kastamonu in 1272 and Amasya in 1308. There was an out-patient clinic for mental patients in Istanbul in the middle ages. In Europe, St. John's Home in Ghent admitted the insane, as well as vagrants and paupers, in 1191. At first, in Europe, the insane were admitted with the physically sick into shelters or hospitals, e.g., into a general hospital at Elbing, Germany, in 1326, and into a shelter at Bergamo, Italy, in 1352. Many other general hospitals, e.g., St. Bartholomews in London, admitted mental patients. Yet today, in Europe, it is regarded as "enlightened" to accept mental patients in general hospitals, and integration tends to be tenuous. In Europe, the first hospital opened exclusively for mental patients was in Valencia, Spain, in 1409. In retrospect, this could be regarded as a retrogressive form of care and a step in the alienation of the insane.

All the treatments practiced today are echoed from the past. Electrical therapy was practiced in Italy before Cerletti, at Aversa in the early 18th century; a little later it was practiced by the evangelist Westley in England, but much earlier Scribonius Largus, in 46 A.D., used the shock of electric eels for intractable headache. Our artificial drugs are predated by the hallucinogens of the indigenous peoples of America, and by herbal remedies that are still with us today; the physician Ibn El Baitar lists 1400 drugs in his pharmacopeia, the "Jami." Sleep therapy goes back at least to Imhotep, in 2080 B.C., and was a prominent feature of the ancient psychiatries of the rational era. Neuro-surgery had its antecedents in the trephaning of the American Indians and the peoples of Africa.

The use of speech in treatment is as old as man and was formulated by the ancient Egyptians, as shown by the Ebers Papyrus, in the 16th century B.C.; by the Thracians and the ancient Greeks; by Caraka in the 1st century A.D.; and by Pietro d'Abano in Italy in the 13th century. The Mayas, Aztecs and Incas of South America practiced group therapy, as did Asclepiades in Greece and Celsus in Rome. Dona Oliva Sabuco de Nantes advocated psychotherapy in Spain, in 1587, and the same approach was advocated by Perzyna in 1793 and Jakubowski in 1831 in Poland, and by Reil in Germany in the late 18th century. Miraglia practiced psychodrama in Naples in the early 19th century, but Aristotle, Asclepiades and Celsus predated him. Again in the 18th century, Castiglioni utilized occupational therapy in Senavra, Italy, but he too was predated—by the ancient Egyptians who had advocated it centuries earlier. Music therapy was known to the Greeks and the Turks and Ambroise Paré employed it to hasten healing after surgery, in Paris in the 16th century.

Throughout history, legislation to care for and treat the insane, to control their admission to hospital, to protect their property, to judge their testamentary capacity and to decide whether they were responsible for their actions has been influenced by the legal enactments of the past. The Romans started with their "Twelve Tables," in the 5th century B.C., defined criminal responsibility in their Corpus Juris Civilis, and elaborated legal codification with Justinian. Hywel Dda, the Celt King of Wales, codified practice in *The Laws of Hywel Dda*. The Danes upheld humane practices in their Zealand Laws, in force since the 13th century.

A fundamental question that arises out of this book is "Does the history of psychiatry suggest any means by which we can make progress?" This book emphasizes the same messages as would the history of any subject. Advance depends on knowledge, knowledge on careful observation, observation leads to worthwhile theories, theories need to be proved by systematic enquiry (much more than just statistically orientated "modern" research; the obvious barely require statistical verification). Humility is a valued ingredient in an investigation and this book will not enhance any mistaken arrogance in what is "modern." Humility leads to a mood of learning; it is wasteful to ignore lessons learnt and knowledge already acquired. Thus we can profit by a careful appraisal of psychiatric history, especially in the rational era.

When champagne was developed in the 17th century, it was called the "Devil's Wine." This was because it was not known from whence the bubbles came and they were assumed to be the work of the Devil. Fermentation within the bottle had yet to be understood. Without knowledge, speculation flourishes. In psychiatry, without clearly understood pathology and psychopathology it is impossible to delineate syndromes with accuracy. Thus the nosology of psychiatry throughout history is confused and complex.

Nosology must be based on pathology. Devising rational psychopathology is an immediate task; from this will spring effective therapy on its own account. Now we rush to treat with no precise knowledge of what is to be put right. The public properly presses for relief. The therapist of the psyche, psychiatrist, has encouraged all to participate in his field, sometimes from a selfish desire to share out his work. Everyone is an expert on the psyche today, as in the past everyone treated the physically ill. No one has assessed the damage done by this misdirected enthusiasm, for it is hidden under the cloak of ignorance.

When making cross comparisons between regions of the world, the reader must be struck by the fact that so many views and practices are held in common. It raises the question of what factors account for these similarities, for example the humoral theory as held in ancient India and in ancient Greece. There are similar remedies in many regions, similar rituals, etc.

It could be postulated that it is a matter of common origin. As man moved from equatorial Africa to other parts of the world, he carried his primitive psychiatry with him. Should it be shown that man developed at a number of centres, some differences in the cultural practices of each inheritance would be expected. However, another explanation is readily available. In general, man, wherever he is placed on the globe, meets the same essential psychic situations, usually the most significant being those in relation to his immediate family and close acquaintainces. Given the same knowledge, endowment, and situation, he will perforce handle them in the same way. Even so, the environment must influence the situation. For example, while many cultures introject gods into natural phenomena, these can vary according to climatic conditions: for instance, in a hot dry country the prime deity may be associated with the rain rather than with the sun.

The most ready explanation for similarity lies in direct communication. Conquering peoples carry their mores with them and even impose them on the conquered, particularly if they improve on the native practice. There are many examples of the spread of knowledge in this fashion—for example, the Greeks, through direct expansion of territory, and later the Romans, who acted as host for Greek knowledge and thus spread Greek medicine far and wide. The Arabs nurtured the Graeco-Roman inheritance and passed it back to Europe. More recently, British medicine and psychiatry made a significant impression through Britain's imperial connections. But there are more pervasive spreaders of knowledge; in Europe, the first universities marshalled knowledge, helped by Latin being the common language, and students came from far and wide. These centres have their counterpart today. We pride ourselves on rapid transportation, but we fail to comprehend that a determined traveller at a steady pace of five miles per hour could encompass the earth on foot in less than two years. We may have underestimated the spread of knowledge by travellers in pre-recorded history. Man was as avid for self-improvement then as now and learned wherever he went.

Faced with its immensity, one approach to information on the history of psychiatry is, as it were, to sink shafts at various points on the crust of knowledge. Thus, in this book a number of contributors tap for information at many points; in all, 90% of the geographical area is represented, and at many points the shafts sink deep through ancient civilizations. It is hoped that seeking separately, in detachment from the next contributor, not all will make the same mistakes at the same point in time. Comparisons of the areas sampled may reveal a pattern of knowledge that will stand for all time, although it sometimes will reveal areas of ignorance.

Our global history of psychiatry must start at some point in time. To start at the beginning of the scientific era, or with a new dynasty, or at the beginning of the Christian calendar would result in artificial breaks in the thread of time. But to speculate about the distant reaches of time would be unprofitable. Thus, to start with recorded history is most apposite and has been the method employed by most contributors. Exceptionally, there have been good reasons for starting at some point later in time.

That the material here concerns a sphere makes for special difficulty in its order. At what point do we start, and do we proceed eastward or westward or north or south? The editor felt it best to follow established practice. The text is divided according to the continents. Pivoting on Europe we proceed westward to America and then eastward to Africa. Asia leads us to Australasia.

The contributors have suffered the same limitations as all historians. Of man's history of at least two million years, the records extend for barely five thousand years. Thus, this book must largely be a history of recent psychiatry. Only by the study of recently discovered small isolated enclaves of very primitive peoples is it possible to surmise the nature of pre-recorded history. Faced with the same essential, everpresent emotional vicissitudes, how far had man proceeded in the understanding of himself? He certainly must have sought relief before recorded history and the so-called scientific period of the last three hundred years.

To add to the historian's difficulties, it is apparent that progress is uneven over time. There are recessions. For instance, in man's physical environment the changing size of the ice cap affected his material development. Equally, his psychic environment ebbed and flowed over time, determined by the growth and decline of civilisations. This book poses one clear question on the state of psychiatry—are we advancing or receding? Our position in the present may prejudice the answer.

Each contributor, in the necessarily limited space given to him, has unearthed in his "dig" a considerable amount of material about the history of psychiatry in the region studied. Sometimes the contributions are unique in that they break new ground. Especially noteworthy and of great interest is the coverage given to indigenous populations in America and Africa. The major ancient civilisations are covered in depth. By good fortune, where a region might have called ideally for greater coverage, this is available in comparable regions elsewhere. As exciting as to sample in depth the history of a geographical region is to take one moment in history and compare the state of psychiatry in all regions. In such a way many viewpoints are strengthened, some appear in a new light, a few prove contradictory. It can also be seen how psychiatry is forced to respond to the pressures of a particular time.

The contributors cannot be free of the biases of history and of historians. Data on history are but a shadow of history. The shadow is not reality, it can only reflect it. The shadow gains in substance when it is possible to go back to primary sources; if these are vivid enough to make it possible to relive an episode, the approximation to reality is great. But primary sources are rare and are often forced to accept the interpretations of a series of commentators on commentators. Each commentator interprets the data according to his biases. It could also be true of our commentators today and thus of our contributors. Especially must one guard against the biases of the extreme viewpoints—psychoanalysis, prone to fantasy, on one hand, and neuro-psychiatry, lacking in imagination, on the other. What is popular, or the mode, can be wrong. Too cryptic assessments in history can also distort by oversimplifying. Assumptions can be carried from authority to authority, from book to book. It is hoped that many biases are corrected by an appeal to the facts rather than to opinion, by relying on the original material, by cross checking from a number of sources, by making allowances for known biases, and by expertise in the area covered. In addition here we rely on multiple authorship, multiple approaches, and multiple sampling. The reader must be the final arbiter.

This book paints on a broad canvas—that of the globe itself. All its material is original. It could not aim at being complete, large as it is. It provides the reader with information about his own region, sometimes for the first time. It encourages him to add to its understanding. The great figures of psychiatry march through its pages, sometimes with enhanced reputations. Perhaps a few are deflated as they are re-evaluated against the background of the massive whole. Conspicuous advances stand out and they are often repeated in history; seldom is there a decisive reorientation, a breakthrough. We can learn from the failures, sudden and eye-catching developments, that prove to be as puffs of smoke. Lessons emerge from the cross comparison of regions.

It would be pleasant if the book helped more readers toward a sense of history. By knowing the past we are better orientated to judge the present. Perspective is deepened. The real issues stand out against the detail; the recurring themes make these clear. As we cull more from history, we get closer to a mood of spontaneous generation, to the need to shed a skin and be refreshed in a new movement. The happiest thought for the present generation of psychiatrists is the extent of the undiscovered. If we had arrived, we would die. Our age is yet to come. And as Shakespeare said, "Things won are done: joy's soul lies in the doing" (*Troilus and Cressida*, I, ii, 313).

CONTRIBUTORS

TAHA BAASHER, M.D., Former Senior Psychiatrist, Democratic Republic of the Sudan

P. BANNISTER, M.D., The West Indies

M. H. BEAUBRUN, M.D., Professor of Psychiatry, Department of Psychiatry, University of the West Indies, Kingston, Jamaica, West Indies

T. BILIKIEWICZ, M.D., Ph.D., Professor of Psychiatry, Clinic for Mental Diseases, Gdańsk Medical Academy, Debinki, Poland

D. CHRISTODORESCU, M.D., Research Worker in Psychiatry, Institute of Neurology and Psychiatry, The Academy of Medical Sciences, Bucharest, Rumania

CHRISTO CHRISTOZOV, M.D., Professor, Department of Psychiatry, Medical Academy, Sofia, Bulgaria

E. CUNNINGHAM DAX, F.R.C.P., F.A.N.C.P., Coordinator in Community Health Services, Mental Health Services Commission, Hobart, Tasmania, Australia

OSKAR DIETHELM, M.D., Professor Emeritus of Psychiatry, Cornell University Medical College, New York, New York, U.S.A.

CHARLES DUCEY, M.A., Department of Psychology and Social Relations, Harvard University, Cambridge, Massachusetts, U.S.A.

ESTHER FISCHER-HOMBERGER, M.D., Privatdozent of Medical History, Institute of History of Medicine, University of Zurich, Switzerland

A. G. GALACH'YAN

NANDOR HORANSZKY, M.D., Emeritus Chief Physician, Outpatient Department for Mental Care of the Buda Area, Budapest, Hungary

JOHN G. HOWELLS, M.D., F.R.C. Psych., D.P.M., Director, The Institute of Family Psychiatry, The Ipswich Hospital, Ipswich, England

LEWIS A. HURST, M.D., Ph.D., F.R.C. Psych., Professor of Psychological Medicine, University of Witwatersrand, Johannesburg, South Africa

T. ADEOYE LAMBO, O.B.E., M.D., Deputy Director-General, World Health Organization, Geneva, Switzerland

CARLOS A. LEON, M.D., M.S., Professor and Chairman, Department of Psychiatry, Universdad del Valle Medical School, Cali, Colombia

L. F. E. LEWIS, The West Indies

J. J. LOPEZ IBOR, M.D., Professor of Psychiatry, Department of Psychiatry and Clinical Psychology, University of Madrid, Spain

MARY B. LUCAS, Assistant Librarian-in-charge, Witwatersrand Medical Library, University of Witwatersrand, Johannesburg, South Africa

M. LYSKANOWSKI, M.D., Assistant Professor of History of Medicine, Institute of Social Medicine, Warsaw Medical Academy, Warsaw, Poland

G. MAHY, The West Indies

EDWARD L. MARGETTS, M.D., Professor of Psychiatry and Lecturer in the History of Medicine, University of British Columbia, Vancouver, British Columbia, Canada

LOUIS MILLER, M.D., Ch.B., Chief National Psychiatrist, Mental Health Services, Ministry of Health, Jerusalem, Israel

GEORGE MORA, M.D., Research Associate, Department of History of Science and Medicine, Yale University, New Haven, Connecticut, U.S.A.

M. LIVIA OSBORN, Research Officer, The Institute of Family Psychiatry, The Ipswich Hospital, Ipswich, England

YVES PELICIER, M.D., Professor of Psychiatry, Paris, France

R. PIERLOOT, M.D., Professor of Psychiatry, University of Leuven, Belgium

V. PREDESCU, M.D., Professor of Psychiatry, Dr. Gh. Marinescu Hospital, Bucharest, Rumania

K. C. ROYES, The West Indies

NILS RETTERSTOL, M.D., Professor of Psychiatry, University of Oslo, Oslo, Norway

HUMBERTO ROSSELLI, M.D., President, Colombian Psychiatric Association, Bogotá, Colombia

PHON SANGSINGKEO, M.D., Special Consultant to the Director, SEATO Medical Research Laboratory, Bangkok, Thailand

JEROME M. SCHNECK, M.D., Attending Psychiatrist, Division of Psychiatric Training and Education, St. Vincent's Hospital and Medical Center, New York, New York, U.S.A.

BENNETT SIMON, M.D., Department of Psychiatry, Harvard Medical School at The Cambridge Hospital, Cambridge, Massachusetts, U.S.A.

P. SMITH, The West Indies

F. C. STAM, M.D., Professor of Psychiatry, Free University, Amsterdam, The Netherlands

ILZA VEITH, Ph.D., Professor and Vice-Chairman, Department of the History of Health Sciences, University of California, San Francisco, California, U.S.A.

EUGEN VENCOVSKY, M.D., Head of the Psychiatric Clinic, Faculty of Medicine, Plzen, Czechoslovakia

A. VENKOBA RAO, M.D., Ph.D., D.P.M., F.R.C. Psych., Professor of Psychiatry, Madurai Medical College, Department of Psychiatry, Erskine Hospital, Madurai, India

VAMIK D. VOLKAN, M.D., Professor of Psychiatry, University of Virginia School of Medicine, Charlottesville, Virginia, U.S.A.

Z. WISINGER, The West Indies

JOSEPH WORTIS, M.D., Professor of Psychiatry, Department of Psychiatry, Health Sciences Center, School of Medicine, State University of New York at Stony Brook, New York, U.S.A.

ACKNOWLEDGEMENTS

I must thank many for their assistance in the preparation of this book. The contributors have been enthusiastic in their co-operation. Introduction to some contributors came as a result of the willing assistance of Dr. Dennis Leigh, Hon. Secretary of the World Psychiatric Association. The complexities of many languages, distance, and customs have added to the task of dealing with the immense amount of historical material and that this was accomplished is in considerable measure due to the efficient, informed and enthusiastic help of my Research Assistant, Mrs. M. Livia Osborn. Mrs. Osborn is also responsible for the index.

Grateful acknowledgement is also made to the following:

1. ANCIENT GREECE AND ROME. PLATE I is reproduced by the courtesy of the British Museum; PLATE II, courtesy of the Museum of Fine Arts, Boston, H. L. Pierce Fund; PLATE III, courtesy of the Museum of Fine Arts, Boston, Bequest of Mrs. Martin Brimmer.

2. ITALY. PLATE V is reproduced from the book by Pietro Piperno, *Della superstiziosa noce di Benevento,* Napoli, 1640.

6. THE NETHERLANDS. PLATES XXII and XXVI are reproduced by the courtesy of the Rijksmuseum, Amsterdam.

7. GREAT BRITAIN. PLATES XXVIII, XXIX and XXXII are reproduced by the courtesy of the Wellcome Institute of the History of Medicine; PLATE XXX, courtesy of the Archivist of Bethlem Hospital.

8. SCANDINAVIA AND FINLAND. Special acknowledgement for furnishing information and valuable pictures is made by the Author to the following distinguished representatives of Finnish, Danish and Swedish psychiatry: Kalle Achté, Professor of Psychiatry, Helsingfors Universitetscentralsjukhus, Psykiatriska kliniken, Helsingfors, Finland; Erling Dein, Associate Professor, Rigshospitalet, Copenhagen, Denmark; and Gunnar Holmberg, Associate Professor, Psykiatriska kliniken, Danderyds sjukhus, Danderyd, Sweden. PLATE XXXIII is reproduced by the courtesy of Snorres Kongesagaer, Gyldendal, Oslo; PLATES XXXIV, XXXV, XLI, XLV and XLVI, courtesy of Medicinhistoriska Museet, Stockholm; PLATE XXXVI, courtesy of Helsingfors Universitets Medicinhistoriska Museums Samlinger; PLATES XXXVII, XXXVIII and XLVIII are from Gaustad sykehus gjennom 100 år, Oslo, 1954; PLATE XL is reproduced from Helweg, *Sindssygevaesenets udvikling i Danmark,* Jacob

Lund Medicinsk Boghandel, Copenhagen, 1915; PLATE XLVII was procured by Assistant Professor Erling Dein, Copenhagen.

11. HUNGARY. The Author gratefully acknowledges the help of I. Herman, M.D., who gave him valuable verbal information concerning psychoanalysis in Hungary.

12. UNION OF SOVIET SOCIALIST REPUBLICS. The Editor is grateful to Science House for permission to reproduce, for the chapter on U.S.S.R., part of the chapter on Soviet Psychiatry by A. G. Galach'yan from *Psychiatry in the Communist World,* edited by A. Kiev, and to Williams & Wilkins Co. for permission to reproduce a section of *Soviet Psychiatry* by Joseph Wortis. PLATES LX, LXI, LXII, LXIII and LXV are reproduced with the kind permission of the Archive of Bekhterev Museum.

18. CANADA. Many individuals and organizations have been generous with their time and advice. Financial assistance for library work has been provided the author over three decades of historical research by Ciba, McGill University Hiram N. Vineberg fund, Social Service Research Council of Canada, and the Medical Research Council of Canada. All this support has been much appreciated by the Author. PLATE LXXXVI is reproduced from Boas (1907), plate x, p. 511; PLATES LXXXVII and LXXXVIII are reproduced by courtesy of Mrs. K. Desrochers, Photo Librarian, 1972, National Museums of Canada, Ottawa; PLATES LXXXIX, XC and XCI, courtesy of Mr. Robert Drake, Curator, 1964. City Museum, Vancouver—photos, Department of Medical Illustration, University of British Columbia, 1964; PLATES XCII and XCIII, courtesy of Mme. Louise Minh, archiviste, 1972, Archives Nationale du Québec; PLATE XCIV is reproduced from a photograph of a multi-colored architect's drawing by Argo Rangus, 1972, by the courtesy of Dr. Ihsan A. Kapkin, one-time Medical Director of the Provincial Hospital (different site), Dr. Nural Alam, present Director, 1972, and Dr. Ernest Cahill Menzies, 1950, super-intendent at that time.

19. UNITED STATES OF AMERICA. PLATE XCV is reproduced by the courtesy of Pennsylvania Hospital, Philadelphia; PLATES XCVI and XCVII, courtesy of the National Association for Mental Health; PLATE XCVIII, courtesy of Little, Brown and Company, Publishers, Boston; PLATE XCIX is reproduced from a photograph in *A History of Medical Psychology* by Gregory Zilboorg and George W. Henry, by the courtesy of W. W. Norton & Co., Inc., New York.

21. THE WEST INDIES. PLATE C is reproduced by the kind permission of W. H. Allen & Co. Ltd., London and New York, from *A Jamaican Plantation* by M. Craton and J. Walvin, 1970.

22. ISRAEL AND THE JEWS. PLATE CII is reproduced from the *Encyclopaedia Judaica,* Photo Archives. The sections on Mental Health in the Bible, Talmud, Mediaeval and Modern Periods are reprinted from: L. Miller, "Psychiatry," in *Encyclopaedia Judaica,* Jerusalem. The sections on the First Decade and the Second Decade of the State of Israel are a revision of that portion, written by L. Miller, of a chapter, "Psychiatric and Mental Health Services," in *Health Services in Israel,* Th. Grushka (ed.), 1968, Ministry of Health, Jerusalem, Israel.

25. SOUTH AFRICA. Special acknowledgements are due to Dr. Max Minde to whose work entitled *Mental Health Services in South Africa, 1652-1952* frequent reference has been made. PLATES CXIII and CXIV are reproduced by permission of the Cape Archives Depot.

26. INDIA. The Author expresses his grateful thanks to Dr. S. A. Kabir, M.B.B.S., D.A. (Lond.), F.F.A.R.C.S. (Eng.), Dean, Madurai Medical College, and Dr. N. R. Ratnakannan, M.D., Director of Medical Education, Madras, for the encourage-

ment and permission offered for the preparation of this chapter. Thanks are due to Dr. M. D. Nair of Ciba (India) Ltd., Bombay, for supplying the reference to Rawolfia Serpentina. He would also like to acknowledge with thanks that PLATE CXVIII has been taken from the book *Pictorial History of Psychology and Psychiatry*, by A. A. Roback and Thomas Kiernan, Vision Press Ltd., London, 1969; and PLATES CXIX and CXX are taken from the book *The History of Suicide in India*, by U. Thakur, published by Munshi Ram Manoharlal, Delhi-6.

29. AUSTRALIA. The historial material could only be collected with many peoples' generous assistance. The Author has especially to thank Mrs. Roma Emmerson, Mrs. Mary Marshall, Mrs. Anne Rood, Professor John Cawte and Doctors W. A. Dibden, S. A. Ellis, L. Gluckman, S. W. P. Mirams, and Mr. H. T. Kaye. The Author is grateful to the Trustees of the Mervyn Archdall Medical Monograph Fund for permission to use much material from Bostock's book. Brothers' and Tucker's books have been most valuable as have other works and documents, some of which appear in the Bibliography.

1

ANCIENT
GREECE AND ROME

CHARLES DUCEY, M.A.

Department of Psychology and Social Relations
Harvard University

AND

BENNETT SIMON, M.D.

Department of Psychiatry, Harvard Medical School at
The Cambridge Hospital, Cambridge,
Massachusetts, U.S.A.

1

INTRODUCTION AND SCOPE OF THIS SURVEY

The history of ancient Greek and Roman psychiatry encompasses a period of 12 centuries, from the time of Homer (ca. 700 B.C.) to the age of the later Graeco-Roman physicians and encyclopedists (ca. 500-600 A.D.). Apart from its intrinsic interest, there are two main reasons for studying the history of psychiatry during this span. First, the final legacy of antiquity in this area—the writings of Galen (2nd cent. A.D.) and of summarizers such as Caelius Aurelianus (5th cent. A.D.) and Alexander of Tralles (6th cent. A.D.)—provided the basic framework of medical psychiatric thought and practice that endured through the Middle Ages of Europe and into the Renaissance and, in short, persisted as the "paradigm" for psychiatry well into the 19th century (29, 30, 46). Second, classical antiquity has defined for us in

1

large measure our sense of the nature of man, of what is accurate, realistic, and vivid in the portrayal of human life. To the degree that we wish to understand notions of sickness and healing in other cultures, as well as the array of subcultures within our own, we must get a clearer understanding of those assumptions about man and his psyche that derive from antiquity but underlie and inform our contemporary theories and practices.

The study of clinical psychiatry in antiquity is problematical, since this field scarcely existed as a defined area of inquiry or as a category of knowledge. Textbooks, specialists in the field, and even a technical term for psychiatry were lacking. The infrequent, brief, and anecdotal medical accounts that do exist could not be termed case histories, i.e., documents detailing both present illness and significant or extended portions of the patient's previous life. Undoubtedly, much accumulated knowledge was transmitted via oral traditions of medical practice, and extensive written case records of medical practice were probably not kept.

The rough-hewn diagnostic categories emphasized primarily the distinction between mental disturbances that were obviously accompanied by physical illness, and those that were not. No institutions devoted to the care of the "mentally ill" existed. The family seems to have been primarily responsible for the care and, if necessary, confinement of deranged family members. A harmless madman without a family could wander freely, though at times the object of fear and ridicule, but seriously unmanageable people were undoubtedly put to death or exiled (54). A few drugs were widely used; some had sedative properties, but probably the major ones (such as the emetic and cathartic *hellebores*) helped by means of their symbolic significance and by placebo effects (65).

Casual and disorganized as the official definitions and treatments of mental disorder might have been, we find the Greek and, to a lesser degree, the Roman literature of every genre replete with portrayals of madness and madmen, explorations of the interconnections between madness and human conflict, and attempts to understand and master the sometimes awesome phenomena of madness. Thus, any aspect of Greek and Roman civilization could be studied fruitfully for its bearing on madness and related issues. Accordingly, we shall discuss in detail several selected and representative topics rather than attempt a comprehensive survey. We refer the interested reader to a number of works that, among them, would provide the equivalent of such a survey. (See in particular Mora (42) and Rosen (54); see also 3A, 9, 13, 22, 30, 31, 35, 37, 44.)

Our presentation focuses on two major topics: 1) the major models of mind and madness in Greek and Roman thought, and 2) the relationship between the illnesses described and the social-psychological stresses and strains in Greek and Roman civilization. The choice of these topics is in part governed by our definition of the major issues and controversies in contemporary psychiatry with respect to determination, etiology, and treatment of mental illness. Especially relevant is the notion of the various "models of madness" (e.g., medical, social-causation, psychodynamic; cf. 58, 59, 60, 61, 67) and the closely related problems of the social and psychological context of mental illness.

2

MODELS OF MIND IN ANCIENT GREEK CULTURE

Four models of mind, mental disturbance, and therapy may be distinguished within the context of classical Greek literature: Homeric (epic), tragic, Platonic (philosophical), and Hippocratic (medical).

Homeric

As Book 20 of the *Odyssey* begins, Odysseus, disguised as a beggar, has returned home to Ithaka and encountered the insolent suitors, bent on taking away his wife and possessions. His son, his old nurse, and the faithful swineherd know his true identity, but the suitors, all the other servants, and his wife Penelope do not. The scene portrays Odysseus trying to fall asleep and the attendant emotional turmoil within him. He hears the laughter of his own servant girls, who are going off to sleep with the suitors, and can barely restrain his rage:

> And his spirit was stirred up inside his own dear chest. And he pondered many things in his "mind" and in his spirit, whether he should rush upon them and deliver death unto each one of them, or for one last and final time let them lie with the arrogant suitors. And the heart within him barked. As when a dog, standing firm to guard her tender pups, barks at a man she does not recognize and is prepared to fight, so the heart within him barked, as he raged at their evil deeds. Striking his chest, he addressed his heart with this story.
>
> "Bear up, oh my heart. Even something worse than this you had to suffer on that day when Cyclops and his invincible strength ate up my brave comrades. And you endured, until guile got you out of that cave where you had thought to die."
>
> Thus he spoke, addressing his dear heart in his chest.

Thus, his heart stood firm, bearing up, persuaded, but he himself tossed back and forth. As when a man turns a sausage over a
roaring fire, bursting with fat and blood, and it strains to be cooked
quickly, so Odysseus rolled this way and that, pondering how he,
one against many, might slay the shameless suitors. And then
Athena came near to him—she had come down from the heavens—
in the form of a woman. She stood above his head and addressed
him:
"Why do you lie there sleepless, most unhappy of all men? This
is your house and your wife in this house, and your son, a son
any man would wish for." (27, XX:9-35; translation modified after
Lattimore.)

Here Odysseus tells Athena of his perplexity over how to proceed
against the suitors, and Athena reassures him that together they cannot
fail, no matter how great the numbers against them.

This passage illustrates some salient features of the representation
of mental life, disturbances in the mental life, and the methods of
relieving such disturbances as they are found in the Homeric poems
(8, 18, 20, 35, 38, 40, 45, 55, 60).

1. Mental activity is depicted as a "personified interchange" between
the person and his parts, between different parts of the person, or
between the person and some outside agent. (His heart barks, and he
speaks to his heart.)

2. A thought, feeling, or impulse is typically portrayed as coming
upon the person, who is in a passive recipient position. Mental processes
and the stimuli for them are portrayed as originating from the outside.

3. There is no sharp "mind-body" distinction; the "mental" and
"physiological" vocabulary are both quite concrete and not distinguished from each other.

4. The thrust of the language is to render public and observable
processes which we might represent as idiosyncratic and private. The
similes in this passage help render visible processes inside Odysseus.

5. The disturbance and turmoil of Odysseus are not regarded as
bizarre or unusual, but rather as completely intelligible in the context
of the story. They are not caused by a "melancholic humor," for example. Though no actual representations of frank psychosis occur in
Homer, such as can be readily found in Greek tragedy, there are allusions to people being "touched," "out of their heads," "sick in the
head," etc. (8) .

6. Odysseus's conflict is not defined along the lines of reason versus
impulse but has more the tone of "kill 'em now, or kill 'em later."
Ultimately the tension must be relieved by action.

7. From our perspective, there are no precise boundaries between

what is inside and what is outside the person: e.g., is Athena a dream or a real entity? In Homer, dreams are represented as coming down to the person; the dream itself is personified and is represented as a dialogue between two people. But even in this brief passage one can see that the divine interventions are quite consistent with the character of the hero. The gods can be viewed, from our perspective, as projections of self-representations (or as projections of self-other interactions).

8. One form of verbal interchange (which serves, *inter alia,* the function of allowing the hero to delay his action and get temporary relief) is that of telling a story. Odysseus tells his heart a tale that is actually a piece of the *Odyssey,* the adventure in the Cyclops cave. This is an example of a pervasive theme in the poems: the power of the epic tale to stir up emotions and then to relieve a character of distressing emotions.

The chief form of mental disturbance in these poems is not out-and-out madness (as depicted in the tragedies), but rather irrational but intelligible behavior under the pressure of conflicts and competing demands: e.g., the stubborn arrogance of Achilles, vengefully nursing his wounded pride; the stupidity of Agamemnon in placing his own "honor" ahead of the needs of the army he commands; and the self-deception of the reckless suitors in the *Odyssey.*

Dodds, in his now classic work, *The Greeks and the Irrational,* has demonstrated how the notion of *ate,* a divinely sent "madness" or "infatuation," serves as a culturally syntonic explanation of the kinds of irrationality mentioned above. Thus, Agamemnon's explanation that *ate* made him act irrationally adamant is accepted easily both by himself and Achilles, whom he has wronged. No one doubts his explanation, nor, on the other hand, does anyone think that Agamemnon is still not responsible to make considerable material restitution to Achilles. Dodds's view, that the pressures of a shame culture (the aristocratic culture depicted in the epics) are handled by externalizing responsibility for socially disapproved behavior, has considerable merit. We must expand it, however, by noting that externalization in the moral sphere is part and parcel of the general Homeric mode of rendering all mental events as if caused by the action of some external agent. Thus, although phrases such as "rage can make even a wise man foolish" may have their equivalent in post-Homeric discourse (as well as in our own everyday speech), they are the dominant mode in Homer.

Therapy for mental distress similarly comes from outside of the person and takes place as if in an interaction between the external agent and the person. Food, wine, and certain marvelous drugs like *nepenthe,* "no-pain," administered by Helen (*Odyssey,* IV:221), may relieve or abolish mental anguish. "Words" in the form of dialogue, storytelling, or prayer are the most significant instruments of relief of emotional suffering. Characteristically, words structured in the form of a brief illustrative tale or a heroic myth serve to relieve distress by offering to the suffering person a noble example or cultural model of how to deal with his problem. Thus, Achilles does not merely urge Priam to eat (knowing what it means for Priam to accept food from his son's murderer) but reminds him of the tale of Niobe, who ate after Apollo had slain all her children (*Iliad,* XXIV: 602-620). Indeed, the bard who sings the epic tales performs precisely this function. His healing power, implicit but pervasive in the Homeric epics, is made explicit by Hesiod:

> For though a man have sorrow and grief in his newly troubled soul, and live in dread because his heart is distressed, yet when a singer, the servant of the Muses, chants the glorious deeds of men of old, and the blessed gods who inhabit Olympus, at once he forgets his heaviness and remembers not his sorrows at all (23, ll. 98 ff.; cf. Havelock [20]).

The researches and formulations of a number of scholars of oral epic poetry have allowed us to reach a clearer understanding of the therapeutic power of the epic word (35, 55, 60). First, the mode of composition and performance of these poems is relevant. The bard composes the tales from a stock of traditional formulaic phrases, traditional thematic and metrical building blocks, and fashions the work out of these in front of his audience. He does not memorize poems and then recite them. As such, he is quite responsive to the emotional needs and desires of his audience. A poem of epic scope encourages and allows each member of the audience, young or old, noble or plebeian, to identify with one or more characters in the work. This technique creates and utilizes a mood of symbiotic closeness that facilitates vicarious experience and relief of distress through several kinds of identifications:

(1) with the characters in the mythohistorical tales, divine or human, who experience conflict and pain but eventually find relief and resolution;

(2) alternating or shifting identifications with several facets of a character, such as with the female aspect of a male hero, a masculine side of a woman, or a childlike side of an adult;

(3) with other members of the audience, including imagined past audiences of these tales and future audiences as well;

(4) with the bard himself, who is in contact with the source of divine assistance, the Muse.

The individual is thereby reintegrated into the ongoing, continuous life of the tribal group, a group that is perceived as coeval with the gods and with the universe. This reintegration is achieved by means of a number of psychological regressions and progressions that establish a new equilibrium. The sickness thereby becomes socially defined and the pathway of resolution as well (55, 60).

Thus, these notions of mind, mental distress, and therapy for distress are highly appropriate for and adaptive in the close-knit, "tribal" culture portrayed in the Homeric epics. With the transition in Greek culture over the next few centuries to a new notion of "tribe" and a new sense of "the individual" we see different models of mind and mental disturbance developing. The portrayal of mental life and of madness in Greek tragedy reflects this changing definition of the individual and provides a transition to the new conceptions of the person and his mind in philosophy.

Tragic

The following excerpt is from Euripides's *Orestes* (17, ll. 385-415). Menelaus, having just heard first of the murder of his brother Agamemnon by Agamemnon's wife (Clytemnestra) and her lover and then of the murder of Clytemnestra by her son, Orestes, now encounters Orestes, driven mad by the Furies (Plate I).

Men: Gods in heaven, is this some corpse I see?
Orestes: More dead than living, I admit. Still alive, but dead of my despair.
Men: And that wild, matted hair—how horrible you look!
Or: It is my crimes, not my looks, that torture me.
Men: That awful stare—and those dry, cold eyes . . .
Or: My body is dead. I am the name it had.
Men: But I did not expect this—alteration.
Or: I am a murderer. I murdered my mother. . . .
Men: What is your sickness?
Or: I call it conscience. The certain knowledge of wrong, the conviction of crime. . . . I mean remorse. I am sick with remorse.
Men: A harsh goddess, I know. But there are cures.
Or: And madness too. The vengeance of my mother's blood.
Men: When did this madness start? . . .
Or: The very day we built her tomb. My poor mother's tomb. . . .
Men: But these phantoms. Can you describe them?
Or: I seemed to see three women, black as night.
Men: Say no more. I know the spirits you mean. I refuse to speak their name. . . .

Men: And these women, you say, hound you with madness for
    killing your mother?
Or: If you knew the torture, knew how they hounded me!
Men: That criminals should suffer is hardly strange.
Or: There is one recourse left.
Men: Suicide, you mean? Most unwise. . . .

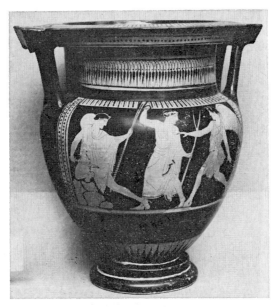

PLATE I. Orestes at Delphi. Left to right: Orestes,
Apollo, a Fury.

1. The most vivid and dramatic portraits of madness are in tragedy.
Euripides's surviving plays offer the largest number of examples but
Aeschylus and Sophocles also portray heroes gone mad (44). The
medical literature, by contrast, presents scarcely any detailed portrayal.

2. In many if not all respects, the portraits are extremely accurate
by modern clinical standards. Though not so obvious in this passage,
a rich vocabulary of madness and emotional states exists, even if it is
not a fixed or technical one.

3. The madness is set in a context of unbearable conflict that leads
to a breakdown of reality testing and/or social judgment; here the
torments of conscience are responsible for internal upheaval. Madness
is also regarded as a sickness, with the possibility of cure, though this
may be partially metaphorical. That the tragic view is a transitional

model between the Homeric and the Platonic is shown by the presence of a divine apparatus, here the Furies; but this apparatus enhances rather than detracts from the vividness of the hero's individual conflicts and personal sense of impasse.

4. The madman is regarded with fear and awe. He is both cursed and considered a wrongdoer who deserves punishment. (The Furies and their variants are expressions of the popular notion of madness

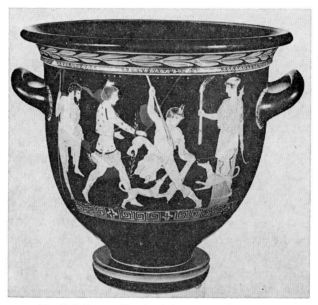

PLATE II. Bell Krater. Death of Actaeon. Left to right: Lussa (Raving Madness or Frenzy, with dog's head), Actaeon (becoming a stag), Artemis. Attic Red-figured.

as a revenge. These variants include *Mania*—"madness"—and *Lussa* —"she who loosens" or "unhinges"—the latter figure appearing in a famous speech in Euripides' *Heracles* and in a lost play of Aeschylus dealing with the myth of Actaeon. Plate II depicts the scene of *Lussa,* with a dog's head, watching Artemis wreak her vengeance by turning Actaeon into a stag to be devoured by his own hounds (19A, 57, 70).

5. Throughout the dramas dialogue is intense and is used to reveal character and motivation. Dialogue also serves as a way of relieving pain, of restoring sanity, and of helping the hero come to terms with the consequences of his madness, particularly in Euripides (7B).

6. Typically, there is a contrast between the socially held values of moderation ("nothing in excess," "beware of *hubris*") and the actions of the protagonists, which go beyond "reasonable" boundaries. This conflict provides much of the dramatic power and seems to be the matrix out of which the madness arises.

7. The frequent representation of madness in these dramas, which were so popular and so important in Greek culture, suggests that it must have been somewhat familiar and intelligible to the audience. Since most of the actions involve terrible conflicts within a family, we can surmise that the themes of familial tensions in the dramas must have meaningfully resonated within families in that culture (62).

8. That the plays have therapeutic value is implied in Aristotle's discussion of catharsis. In fact, in later Graeco-Roman medical literature drama was prescribed as part of the treatment for overtly psychotic patients.

Aristotle's notion of *catharsis* seems to include the notion that tragedy stirs up certain emotions and then provides a "cleaning out" of them, as of distressing foreign bodies. Some interaction between the emotional and intellectual aspects of the play seems necessary for the proper kind of catharsis (35). The plays, as public performances, partake of the quality of the performances of the Homeric epics and tend to foster similar kinds of identifications. It does seem, however, that with the more vivid portrayal of madness (and other horrors) in tragedy the artist must provide means by which the audience can distance itself from the action within the play. The chorus seems to be one such device, as it simultaneously empathizes with the characters and tries to protect itself with pleas such as "may such a fate never befall us."

9. Music, dance, poetic language, and rhythms all enhance the effect of the dialogues and contribute to the therapeutic and cathartic effects. *Pari passu* with the realizations and self-discoveries that the characters experience through dialogue and through action, the audience must experience some kind of "working through" of conflicts. The dual themes of knowledge and self-knowledge are central to many of the plays, most explicitly *Oedipus Rex*, which deals with the issues of too much or too little knowledge and of its proper use (Plate III). In general, the plays have generated a notion of *insight* that seems to combine knowledge with intense emotional experience.

10. Finally, it can be said that a new definition of the individual emerges from Greek tragedy, in connection with the experience of suffering and the acquisition of tragic knowledge. Both the language of mental life and the behavior of the heroes suggest that the person is

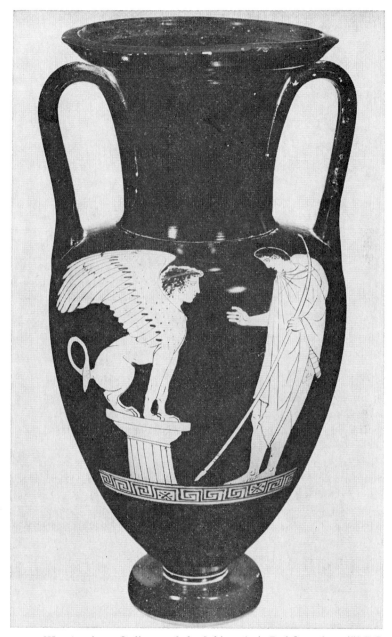

PLATE III. Amphora. Oedipus and the Sphinx. Attic Red-figured ca. 450 B.C.

viewed as an active agent, whose mind is the active part of his ego and of his self. Madness is, in effect, the birth pangs of this new individual.

Platonic

Plato (429-347 B.C.), justly regarded as a philosopher of mind, largely defines for subsequent Western thought the implications of the terms "mind" and "mental." He is also the philosopher of mind-gone-awry and of irrationality; indeed his discussions and definitions of mind and madness are interdependent (61). The following passage illustrates a number of important features of Plato's views of mental disturbance:

> Such is the manner in which diseases of the body arise; those of the psyche, which depend upon the body, originate as follows. We agree that disease of the psyche represents a lack of intellectual function and of this there are two kinds: namely, madness and ignorance. In whatever state a man experiences either of them, that state may be called disease; and excessive pains and pleasures are justly to be regarded as the greatest diseases to which the psyche is liable. For a man who is in great joy or in great pain, in his unseasonable eagerness to attain the one and avoid the other, is not able to see or hear anything correctly; but he raves and is at the time utterly incapable of any participation in reason (48, *Timaeus*, 86b; translation modified after Jowett).

1. Madness is a species of disease, to be taken either metaphorically or by analogy to diseases of the body. But passages such as this one indicate a more intrinsic connection between body and mind. There is a mind-body split in Plato, unlike in Homer, but it is not quite a definitive or absolute split.

2. Psyche, a term with rich connotations from Homer on, in Plato becomes gradually equated with the *rational* in man, especially the abstracting and generalizing functions of the mind (20, 21). A division exists between the rational functions and the irrational, appetitive, or somatic ones. This division is usually presented as between portions of the psyche (e.g., *Republic, Timaeus*) but may also be conceptualized as the split between psyche and soma (*Phaedo*; cf. 53).

3. Madness becomes equated with the dominance of the impulsive, appetitive functions of man, and sanity with the dominance of the rational, calculative, abstracting, and categorizing functions. Variants of this contrast portray madness as ignorance (*Timaeus*, 86), as vice and discord (*Sophist*, 227), as unbridled lust for power, sexual gratification, and excess emotion (*Republic*, 571-573), while sanity is viewed as harmony and health (*Republic*, throughout, especially 444) and as

justice (*ibid.*). Each different part of the psyche seems to have its own characteristic way of "thinking." The descriptions of the functioning of the baser parts of the mind convey the sense of flux, impermanence, illusion, dreams, pictures, and shadows, while the higher part functions with permanence and fixity, employs ideas and propositions, and represents true knowledge. This is the same fundamental classification of forms of thinking as is in Freud's distinction between "primary process" and "secondary process" (61). Plato extends then current terms for madness (especially *mania*) to create a notion of sanity as the highest form of reasoning and of insanity as overlapping with much of the thinking that characterizes the ordinary life of men. (Note that Plato's term for ordinary thinking, *doxa*, "seeming," is used in drama, and later in medicine, for hallucination (39)).

4. "Heal my psyche, for you will do me much greater good by putting an end to ignorance of my psyche than if you put an end to an affliction of my body" (*Hippias Minor*, 372-373; see also 35, 61 for a fuller discussion of "therapy" in Plato). Plato contends that the ideal therapy is philosophy. Philosophy in the earlier dialogues seems to mean "Socrates philosophizing" or Socrates in dialogue. Philosophy comes eventually to mean "using the method of dialectic," a form of verbal interchange which only superficially resembles dialogue (64). Dialogue involves all the emotions of ordinary human interchanges—persuasion, seduction, threats, appeal to emotions, etc.—while dialectic is aimed at the active process of dissecting, defining, gaining truth through clear demonstration, arriving at fixity, and not wallowing in flux. To arrive at truth means to put away ignorance; ignorance is not accidental but is motivated and maintained by vested interests within the person. Dialectic, therefore, meets with great resistance. Nevertheless, dialectic is what the true philosopher must be trained to do, either with another or with himself. In studying the transition from dialogue to dialectic within Plato we begin to see the establishment of a set of ideals for effective verbal "therapy," involving people and the spoken word, yet in a sense impersonal; the goal is to seek truth, independent of the self-deceptions, personalities, or temperaments of the participants.

A series of implied equations thus gradually emerges. The rational part of the mind is equivalent to the philosopher, or dialectician; the baser parts of the mind are equivalent to those who stop at dialogue, or worse (bad rhetoric, poetry, or drama). Both in political and in intellectual terms, the most rational part of the mind is seen as the ruler of the rest of the mind, just as the philosopher king is the ruler of the true Republic.

Through the notion of the dialectic as the method of attaining truth, Plato has broadened the meaning of knowledge and self-knowledge (insight); the phrase "know thyself" has for him the meaning of rational insight, along with its traditional meaning of "know your relations to the gods and to mortal men." The ideal type of individual that emerges from this picture is rational man, whose major ties are to ideal forms of truth and goodness that are eternal and exist beyond parochial social definition. This view may in fact be an analogue, if not a precursor, to the ideals of "analytic" (as opposed to "therapeutic") treatment (the distinction drawn by Rieff (52) in *The Triumph of the Therapeutic*). It can be shown that Plato rejects as dangerous to his rational mode of therapy precisely those features of poetry and drama which in our scheme account for their therapeutic power (see Havelock (20) on Plato's rejection of Homer and of *mimesis*—"imitation" or "identification"). Furthermore, perhaps with the rejection of the Homeric ethos of "tribal" coherence, Plato feels a need to establish a new community—a community of those who live by dialectic (the utopian vision of the *Republic* and the actual foundation of the Academy).

5. Dialectic is for the few (*cf.* Dodds). For the masses, myths, contrived fairy tales, and "noble lies" will sugarcoat the use of force. Plato feels that the masses of men are unwilling and/or unable to seek the higher forms of truth. Included in Plato's notions of remedies for the forms of incorrect thinking that he tends to equate with madness is an institution called the *sophronesterion*—"house of moderation" or "house of sanity" (43). To this place, people who out of ignorance (not malice) persist in incorrect thinking are sentenced for up to five years, and are subject to repeated conversations and discussions. If their ideas are then corrected, they are freed, but if not, they are executed (*Laws,* 908c, *ff.*). One can point to this development (*cf.* Popper, *The Open Society and Its Enemies* (51)) as the prototype of the use of a mental hospital as an instrument of political oppression. In the totalitarian state, madness equals open dissent. One can view these two facets of Plato, the truth-seeking and the coercive, as a corollary of the Platonic split between reason and impulse, or between psychic motives and somatic motives. Having split these Plato tried to devise (but did not succeed) the ideal solution of how the two could live together and cooperate.

What we see in Plato, then, is a vision of something that seems to lie on the borderlands of education, psychotherapy and political reform. Plato does not have a theory, let alone a system, of psychotherapy. Some implicit principles in Plato, however, become more focused as psychotherapy in the works of some of the Hellenistic philosophers (35, 37, 47).

Medical

Hippocrates, in *Sacred Disease* (25, XVII), commented,

> Men ought to know that from the brain and from the brain only arise our pleasures, joys, laughter and jests, as well as our sorrows, pains, griefs and tears. . . . It is the same thing [the brain] which makes us mad or delirious, inspires us with dread and fear, whether by night or by day, brings sleeplessness, inopportune mistakes, aimless anxieties, absentmindedness, acts that are contrary to habit. . . . Madness comes from moistness. . . . The corruption of the brain is caused not only by phlegm but by bile. You may distinguish them thus. Those who are mad through phlegm are quiet, and neither shout nor make a disturbance; those maddened through bile are noisy, evildoers, and restless, always doing something inopportune. These are the causes of continued madness. But if terrors and fears attack they are due to a change in the brain.

1. In Hippocrates (in the second half of 5th century B.C.) human mental functioning, including emotional states, originates from the brain. Madness arises from a disturbance of the brain (not from a disturbance of passions or from an inner conflict, for example).

2. The functioning of the brain (as is true in Greek medicine for all somatic functioning) depends on the right admixture of various material elements (e.g., the humors, such as bile and phlegm) and on various qualities (such as "moist," "hot"). Health is the proper balance, while sickness is an imbalance.

3. Different diseases and different temperaments are associated with the predominance of one or another of the humors.

4. The brain functions as an "interpreter" or "translator" (analogous contemporary terms would be "transformer" or "transducer of experience") of incoming sensation and/or of the effects of various elements and qualities. The brain is not a completely passive organ; its only activity is that of a "translator." It serves the body but is subject to powerful physical and physiological influences.

5. There is a remarkable congruence between the descriptions of the activities and functions of the brain vis-à-vis the rest of the body and those of the physician vis-à-vis the patient and the illness. The brain "diagnoses," just as the physician does (*Sacred Disease,* XIX); the brain is subject to many influences and has a limited scope of power, just

as the physician, the "servant of his craft," is subject to many limitations:

> The medical craft has to consider three factors, the disease, the patient, and the physician. The physician is the servant of his craft, and the patient must cooperate with the doctor in combatting the disease. (24, *Epidemics,* I:11.)

In all, the physician can be considered the "brains of the organization" in the fight against the disease, subject to the same constraints as the brain in the body.

6. One cause for disturbances (mental or somatic) may be the patient's poor regimen of life, sometimes based on ignorance of proper regimen (e.g., not knowing that one has a bilious disease and eating foods that would generate bile).

7. Treatment, then, consists of trying to restore the proper balance, with drugs, regimen, or both. Another important feature of treatment, however, is to remove the ignorance of the patient. This involves explaining and interpreting to the patient the facts of his disease. This is the limit of the major verbal activity of the physician. There is no hint of verbal psychotherapy. The treatment for some forms of madness, for example, would be *hellebore,* a powerful cathartic, combined with explaining the illness to the patient (65). The idea of the use of words by physicians to combat madness expands into later Hellenistic and Graeco-Roman medicine, but never evolves into a therapeutic dialogue (35).

8. Undoubtedly these Hippocratic notions are based on *bona fide* scientific and clinical observations about madness with obvious concurrent physical disease. Descriptions of conditions involving delirium with acute febrile illnesses (e.g., malaria associated with toxic brain states, typhoid, dysenteries, and perhaps even *delirium tremens*) are the most vivid in the Hippocratic *corpus;* probably mental disturbances with head injury were carefully observed. It is understandable, then, why the physician should be prone to ascribe all madness to physical and physiological causes. Furthermore, we have evidence that the Hippocratic physicians saw physiological and physical etiologies as the only alternative to rank superstition and mindless flailing about (see the opening of *Sacred Disease*).

9. The Hippocratic ideas about hysteria are quite important and characteristic of this medical model. Hysteria, regarded as a disease of the *hystera* (womb), is particularly caused by the propensity of the womb to wander. A variety of conditions are ascribed to the movements of the uterus: shortness of breath, pain in the chest, a lump in

the throat, pain in the groin and legs, and some forms of syncope and seizure. Hysteria is a woman's disease that occurs most commonly in virgins and widows; it is sometimes alleviated by medicines applied inside the vagina as if to coax the uterus to return to its place and rest, while marriage, intercourse, and child-bearing frequently help (35, 71). (See below for Plato's description of hysteria and suggestion of its psychogenic origin.)

Thus, the propensity of the medical model is to "physiologize" rather than "mythologize" its explanation of mental disturbance. This is clear, for example, from the contrast between Hippocrates's (*Air, Waters, and Places,* XXI-XXII) and Herodotus's (*Histories,* I:105), discussions of effeminacy and impotence among the Scythians. This contrast should not, however, obscure the realization that in one sense we have with Hippocrates returned full circle to the Homeric model of madness: insofar as the imbalance of the bodily humors is outside one's own control, responsibility for mental disorder has been assigned to forces external to the individual. (For further details on Hippocrates, see 10, 11, 12,, 14, 15, 16, 24, 25, 33, 44.)

3

THE PSYCHOSOCIAL BACKGROUND OF GREEK MADNESS

The following table summarizes the directions of change in notions about mind and madness from Homer to Plato (8th-4th century B.C.):

HOMER	PLATO AND TRAGEDIANS
1. Mental life is externally caused, interactional, and accessible to public view.	1. Mental life originates from within and is private.
2. The person is submerged within family tradition.	2. The individual is recognized in his own right.
3. Thought and affect are not differentiated from one another, nor are mind and body.	3. There are splits between thought and affect and between mind and body, with thinking more highly valued.
4. Social rewards and sanctions focus on the dimension of public honor and loss of face; hence, shame imagery is extensive.	4. Social rewards and sanctions shift to a moral dimension; imagery of guilt is employed, and virtue is the goal.

HOMER	PLATO AND TRAGEDIANS
5. Disturbance and conflict are caused by external events or forces.	5. Disturbance arises from inner conflict among structures within the self.
6. Disturbance is relieved by attempts to reintegrate individual to tribe; the model of the therapist is the bard with his poetry.	6. Therapy, as ideal, is new knowledge and new inner experience; "insight" is the crucial goal.

The societal changes during these centuries have been the object of much study by students of classical antiquity. The works of Dodds, Glotz, Havelock, Jaeger, Misch, and Snell (8, 19A, 30A, 41A, 63) are most important, and synoptic essays by Barbu (3) and De Saussure (7A) focus on how these changes relate to notions of personality and individualism. The main trends are the following:

1. The breakup of the tribe or extended clan in the face of colonization, the rise of city-states, with attendant bureaucratization, and the displacement of land by commerce and coined money as the basis of wealth;

2. The weakening of the absolute authority of the father; legal safeguards for each individual, even against other family members; new stresses between generations and between the sexes;

3. A new sense of the relative nature of morals and laws, now viewed as human and not divine in origin; new sense of individual responsibility;

4. The rise of widespread alphabetic literacy; the break-up of the timeless authority of oral tradition and the elders who transmit it (sons can read when their fathers cannot); and finally,

5. The spread of abstract, rational, and scientific thinking and the preference for "physiological" (natural science) rather than "mythological" thinking.

In brief, these changes are the causes, concomitants, and consequences of a new sense of the individual and his relations to the social nexus. Though by 20th-century standards a 5th-century Athenian was still very much embedded in an extended family network, in comparison with his counterpart several centuries earlier he has become a much more autonomous individual. It is our contention that these changes, which have usually been discussed in the context of Greek creativity and "the Greek miracle," are also the context for viewing the representation of mental conflict and of madness. The individual, possessing new freedom and new possibilities, becomes prey to new sources of anxiety and distress. The portrayals of conflict and madness in tragedy, then, convey a poetic truth about the plight of the individual striving for a new kind of individualism and a new balance between himself and the collectives in his life. The "fear of freedom" (Dodds) is echoed in the choruses of the tragedies (especially Euripides) and is a central, unspoken issue in Plato. We would further suggest that the Hippocratic model of mental illness and of its treatment may have provided an important source of relief of anxiety, guilt, and responsibility, by translating inner conflicts and dissonances into physiological and physicalistic terms.

We shall illustrate this last point in our discussion of hysteria. Several authors, most notably Dodds (8) and Slater (62) (a sociologist), have argued that with the emergence of this new sense of the individual there must have been new sources of stress and conflict within the family. Dodds, for example, argues that the weakening of absolute paternal authority is accompanied by an increase in the themes of guilt and in representations of oedipal conflicts in poetry, philosophy, and law (e.g., the opening of Plato's *Euthyphro,* with a son bringing his father to court, and Aristophanes's *Clouds,* in which the son's thrashing of the father is used to portray "modern times"). Slater's formulations emphasize the strains in the mother-son relationship, as evidenced by the popularity of such mythological themes as Orestes's murder of his mother, and Medea's slaying her sons. He argues that by the 5th century B.C. the Greek male unconsciously viewed the female as a powerful, pre-oedipal (i.e., before sexual love for the mother holds sway), devouring, and castrating creature. (This imagery sharply contrasts with Homer's portrayal of women; the Archaic period, 6th century B.C., is the turning point.) In the tragedies, heroes are mostly driven mad by goddesses. "Bogey-women" are more prominent in the nursery than are "bogey-men," and creatures such as sphinxes, harpies, the Gorgon-Medusa, the Empusae, and the Furies abound in art and myth. Women seek the liberation of Bacchic ritual and frenzy, where, as depicted by Euripides, themes of cannibalistic incorporation of men and children are symbolically (and occasionally literally) enacted (see Dodds's "Maenadism," 8, pp. 270-282). The social correlate of these fantasies is the relative suppression of women in a culture that unabashedly encourages phallic worship. Male children are preferred and have greater economic and civil rights; for both its real and its symbolic implications, female children are not fed as well. The prototypical—though we do not know whether statistically the most common—marriage is that of a man in his late 20's to a much younger girl (15-18) who has never left her mother. The man has seen something of the world and has a life that is rich outside the home (34). He is remote from early child-rearing and derives most of his social pleasures from activities that exclude the wife. There is a vicious cycle, leading to generational repetition and reinforcement of these strains. Women are envious of and angry at men; they are left alone to bring up little boys, who become the unsuspecting objects of the intense ambivalence that their mothers feel toward their own distant fathers and husbands. The boy is then the narcissistic enlargement of the mother, her phallic pride, and as a consequence of this traumatic treatment he becomes frightened of mature female sexuality. Greek homosexuality, both the institutionalized and non-institutionalized variants, are related to this fear of female sexuality (62).

Overall, propositions such as these put forth by Dodds and Slater may be a bit overstated, but they offer rich possibilities for understanding the forms of conflict and madness that find expression in classical Greece. Using these propositions in combination with what we know psychodynamically and cross-culturally about conversion hysteria (especially in women), we can see that hysteria is a disorder paradigmatic for Greek culture. Note, for example, Plato's version of the Hippocratic notion of the wandering uterus as the cause of various diseases:

> . . . And in women . . . whenever the matrix, or womb, as it is called—which is an indwelling creature desirous of child-bearing —remains without fruits long beyond the due season, it is vexed and takes it ill; and by straying all ways through the body and blocking up the passages of the breath and preventing the respiration it casts the body into the uttermost distress, and causes, moreover, all kinds of maladies until the desire and love of the two sexes unite them. (49, *Timaeus,* 916-c; Bury translation)

Thus, hysteria is a channel available for expressing some of the same tensions in male-female relationships that are presented in the tragedies. It is the disease of women whose social and psychic equilibrium has been disturbed by the failure to get (temporarily) the penis or (permanently) a child. It is simultaneously a way of controlling and expressing sexual impulses and of venting rage upon males. In a culture where the courtyard of a typical house has a statue of Hermes with a prominent erection, the woman may be in a precarious position without some phallic equivalent. At the same time, hysteria is the disease *par excellence* of repression; the emotional knowledge of disturbed and frustrated sexuality is present but must be ignored and denied. The medical formulation gives social sanction to this repression, but the more anthropomorphic ("gynecomorphic") version of

Plato reveals the truth. Within the woman there is a wild, animalistic, Bacchantic, frenzied creature, who must be gratified, or else she goes berserk.

It is striking that issues of knowledge and of ignorance permeate the literature of the 5th and 4th century B.C. Purposeful ignorance and the significance of knowledge are of course the central themes of Sophocles's *Oedipus Rex,* which outlines the typical fantasy involved in the repressive style in hysteria. The principle of knowing oneself and the obstacles to self-knowledge are Socrates's major concern. For Plato, knowledge is power, and ignorance, though a common state, is detestable. Madness is a species of ignorance. But certain socially fostered forms of ignorance are necessary for the smooth functioning of the body politic. Thus, it is striking to find that Plato's "noble lie" is cut from the same cloth as the fantasies of hysterics who need to remain ignorant of the facts of sexuality and its relation to childbirth. Thus, in the *Republic* (414 ff.), the work dealing most explicitly with gradations of knowledge and ignorance, we find the following myth to be told to the masses: children are not born from women by means of sexual intercourse, but are molded and reared inside the earth's womb and delivered when their bodies and minds have been completely formed. (It is notable that the Greek theories about conception centered around the notion that the father has the seed, and mother is merely the soil or vessel.) Thus, we find in philosophy fantasy themes similar to those that play a role in the pathogenesis of conversion hysteria. Plato, then, detects and tries to regulate in his own way the ongoing tensions between men and women and between parents and children. Plato and Hippocrates provide complementary defensive fantasies.

We should recall that these themes that we have presented from the perspective of conflict and symptom also provide the background for the creative discoveries of the Greeks. Concerns over knowledge and ignorance also reflect the fact that the Greeks were engaged in active discovery and were attempting to come to grips with a rapidly expanding knowledge of the universe; their curiosity, which served intrapsychic functions, had awesome intellectual results. Although confusions of sexual differentiation and of bisexuality may have been an index of conflicts in the culture, the ability to see and live with bisexuality suggests a tolerance for ambibuity and complexity in the world (2). It could be argued, then, that the unique weaknesses of Greek culture may have also been related to the greatest sources of strength and creative invention.

4

MADNESS IN ROMAN CIVILIZATION

The difficulties inherent in the study of madness in past cultures are compounded when one examines ancient Rome. Unusual mental states did not capture the Roman imagination as they did the Greek, in part for psychological reasons which will be elaborated below. Moreover, the Romans, lacking the introspective and inquisitive spirit that forms the foundation of Greek thought, were generally content to rely upon Greek models of understanding puzzling phenomena. Hence, although sensitive descriptions and subtle explanations can be found in the literature and will be discussed, in general one searches in vain for organized approaches to pathological thinking and behavior. As in the Greek section, we shall first examine the Romans' intellectual comprehension of the subject and then make inferences about the psychology of the ancient Romans from their writings and deeds, relying on the structural consistency of psychosocial-familial influences on normal and abnormal behavior.

Six basic approaches, organized in roughly chronological fashion, may be identified in understanding madness: legal, comic, tragic, philosophical, poetic, and historical.

Legal

The earliest mention of madmen in Rome occurs in the *Twelve Tables,* the Roman codification into law of traditional customs and practices. They date from about 450 B.C. In *Table Five,*

> If a man is raving mad, rightful authority over his person and chattels shall belong to his agnates (blood relatives through father's line) or to his clansmen. (72, p. 451)

It is quite remarkable that this basic law remained virtually the only legal principle applied to madmen throughout the following nine centuries or more. Lunacy (*furor,* stronger than *insania*) seems to have been considered curable and therefore was no bar to full legal rights during "lucid intervals" (5). No legal definition of a *furiosus* ever existed, so that a determination of sanity had to be made separately in each individual case (56; for Greek law see 34, p. 125).

Comic

Roman comedy by Plautus and Terence (3rd and late 2nd century B.C.) should give indications of the popular views of madness, as this passage, in which Tyndarus tries to convince Hegio that Aristophontes is mad (though he is actually not), will illustrate:

A. I can't control myself any longer.

T. Hey, did you hear what he said? Shouldn't we get out of here? In a second he'll be pelting us with rocks unless you have him arrested.

A. I can't bear this!

T. His eyes are burning; you must, Hegio! Do you see his whole body splotched with those ghastly yellow blotches? Black bile has the man in its grasp.

A. If this old man had any sense, black pitch would have you in *its* grasp at the executioner's block and would be blazing on your head.

T. Now he's speaking deliriously, the spirits (*larvae*) are driving the poor man.

H. What if I were to order him arrested?

T. You'd be much the wiser.

A. What I can't bear is not having a stone so that I could beat this scoundrel's head in; he's driving me insane with his drivel.

T. Hear that? He's looking for a stone. (50, ll. 592-602; our translation)

1. In the popular mind, the madman's major characteristic is proneness to violence, which must be met with coercion or reciprocal violence.

2. Two explanations of madness are offered side by side without contradiction, a physiological and a demonic one. For the comic writers, *atra bilis,* black bile (Greek *melancholia*), is the first popular explanation at hand in accounting for peculiar behavior classified as mad, but, like many of our medical folk principles, is not intended as a serious or rigorous one. It could just as easily be caused by *larvae* (later "ghosts," but at this time merely vague supernatural forces who possess their victim). In other words, these "explanations" are little more than empty terms designed to perpetuate the *illusion* of understanding the unknown.

3. All behavior exhibited normally by a sane person, like justifiable anger, may be used as evidence of madness. The glaring eyes, flushed skin, and angry outbursts are used to support Tyndarus's "diagnosis." Aristophontes's behavior reinforces Tyndarus's feigned fear of violence.

4. Although charges of madness and feigned madness abound in the comedies, no real madness ever occurs; it is a device whose purpose is to satirize and deflate man's pretensions for comic effect (44).

Tragic

The fragments of Roman tragedy from the same period, largely derived from Greek drama, concern mantic inspiration, bacchic madness, and the fury-driven matricide, as in Ennius's *Alcumeo*.

a. For me inner feeling does not completely coincide with my wild-eyed look.
b. Where did this burning come from? They're coming, they're coming; they're here, attacking me! Help me, drive this plague from me, this fiery assault tormenting me! They're coming, wreathed with dark snakes, they're surrounding me with burning torches. (44; our translation)

The former passage is spoken in a "lucid interval," the latter a transcript of his delusion.

1. Despite his madness Alcumeo can in periods of sanity recognize his delusions as delusions. Madness is not a mere comic pose, but a terrifying and painfully real "illness."

2. An internal, private world is clearly demarcated from one's external behavior, unlike in Homer. On recovering his sanity, Alcumeo recognizes that what in madness he had accepted as true external perceptions are only *visa* ("hallucinations"). The gap, however, between attribution of madness to purely external causation and the recognition of internal generation of ideas has not been completely bridged within this model; for the completion of that development we must await the abstract formulations of the philosophers.

Philosophical

As in Greek thought, the most sensitive, complex, "modern," and psychologically oriented explanation of madness in Roman thought may be found in the philosophical literature, especially in Lucretius, poet-philosopher of the 1st century B.C., who stated in *De Rerum Natura*:

People can so clearly feel a burden upon their minds that depresses them with its weight; if only they could also recognize the causes from which the depression arises and the origin of such a heavy mass of misery that lies upon their hearts, they would not at all lead their lives in the way we see so commonly now, with everyone not knowing what he really wants and always seeking a way of altering his present position, as if he could thereby throw off this load. Time and again a man who is bored sick of being at home leaves his great dwelling, only to return at once, since he feels the situation to be no better outside. Driving on his Gallic steeds, he flies at full speed to his country home, as though pressing ahead to bring aid to a house on fire. He starts yawning the moment he touches the doorstep of his country home, or else he drifts off deep into sleep and seeks oblivion thus, or else he makes for the city again and revisits it at top speed. In this way, each individual is running away from himself, whom it is of course not possible to escape, as is natural; he clings to this "self" against his will and hates it, because as a sick man he does not grasp the cause of his illness.

. . . What is this harmful yet powerful lust for life that compels us to tremble in the face of dangers of such uncertain outcome? An irrevocable limit to life in fact awaits mortals, and it is impossible for us to avoid meeting our death. Besides, we spin round and round in the same place and stay there until the end, and no new form of pleasure is forged merely by living. But as long as what we crave is out of reach, it seems to surpass everything else in importance; once we get it we crave something else, and an unquenchable thirst for life keeps us forever gaping in frustration. (41, III:1053-1070, 1076-1084; our translation.)

1. Mental disorder is fully recognized as an "illness," different from normal behavior and analogous to physical sickness. Despite this fact, his portrayal is intended to remind us of ourselves, since everyone manifests this neurotic behavior to some extent. This particular form of madness is intrinsic to the human condition.

2. A sharp dichotomy between external causation of behavior and individual motivation for it is clearly demarcated. No longer is man merely a string that reverberates only in response to the movement of other strings in an interactional web or network, as the Homeric model of mind implies; he may behave as an individual totally in isolation from other people, gods, and other external agents.

3. More explicitly than ever before, an internal, psychologically based model of mental disorder is offered here. Man acts in the neurotic fashion depicted because he is trying to avoid the full force of depression that arises from the unconscious fear of death. Thus Lucretius recognizes not only a sharp break between internal and external causation of behavior, but also a sharp *intrapsychic* dichotomy between conscious and unconscious motivation. The etiology of mental disturbance is entirely intrapsychic: a man does not know what he wants and runs away from a disavowed part of himself. This disavowal invariably involves the denial of the fear of death or the denial of death as absolute non-existence. All the projects in which mankind invests so much energy and to which he assigns such great significance stem from the flight from death: internecine struggles for political power, grand displays of military strength, the heaping up of wealth

(II:1-61), and even the undefinable bitterness of love that results in unconscious impulses to hurt the beloved (IV: 1079-1136). Bland, self-satisfied rationalism provides merely temporary and superficial protection against the underlying pervasive fear, since,

> In severe circumstances they turn their minds all the more severely to superstition. Hence it is the more appropriate to appraise a man when he is in the midst of critical dangers and to get to know what sort of a person he is under adverse conditions. For then and only then are the true expressions of his feelings conjured up from the depths of his heart, and the mask is ripped off: the reality remains. (41, III:53-58; our translation).

4. If Lucretius has shown that the fear of death inevitably motivates and pollutes all our grand and elaborate defenses against it, how do we undertake to cure our madness? Only by recognizing, he says, the pervasive role of this fear in our lives, by realizing that belief in an afterlife is an unrealistic, hallucinatory wish fulfillment, and by devoting ourselves to a rationalistic, dispassionate study of the universe according to Epicurean principles can we accept the inevitability of death and nonexistence. If we live our lives without the comfort of illusions about ourselves and the world, we will cease to base them on unfulfillable cravings for things that are designed to protect us from the fear of death; then we will be capable of resigning ourselves to the fact of death whenever it should overtake us.

5. Lucretius anticipates to a surprising degree the theories and outlook of Freud and modern psychoanalysis. Expressed in the latter's terminology, areas of overlap or parallel would include the universality of neurotic defenses, the differentiation of external causes and internal motives, intrapsychic disavowal and repression, unconscious anxieties and impulses, the defensive function of cultural institutions, and understanding and disillusionment as therapeutic.

6. Of greater historical importance, in his role as transmitter of Greek thought (especially Stoic and Academic philosophy), is Cicero, philosopher of the 1st century B.C. Besides expanding and enriching the vocabulary of the emotions (36), he makes a distinction between *insania* and *furor,* both usually translated as "madness." *Furor* is more serious and can befall even a wise man; it apparently involves delusion, as it may be illustrated by Ajax, who slew sheep in the belief they were Greek generals, or by the case mentioned by Aretaeus of the man who thought he was a brick and was afraid of being broken. *Insania* may be translated as "folly," as it concerns worldly values, like miserliness and lack of good sense (6, III, v). *Hellebore* may help the

former but would be pointless in the latter. Lucretius, if confronted with this dualism, would probably negate its basic premise; insofar as they believe in an afterlife, those afflicted with only *insania,* but not *furor,* are laboring under just as much of a delusion as a *furiosus,* an outright madman.

An interesting contrast is provided by Horace, poet of the 1st century B.C. He mentions a case of circumscribed delusion: a man who was otherwise sane (good husband, neighbor, host, and master) had the quirk of sitting and applauding in an empty theater. He was, in other words, *furiosus* but not *insanus.* When his relatives took it upon themselves to "cure" him with *hellebore,* successfully by their definition, he told them, "Truly you've killed, not saved me, friends, as you've wrenched out of me my pleasure by forcibly taking away my most agreeable delusion" (28, II, ii:128-140; our translation). For Lucretius culture perpetuates mass delusion *(furor)* under the aegis of religious and political institutions; for Horace, people become "civilized" through a substitution of common human illusions *(insania)* for exotic private delusions *(furor).*

7. In regard to the external-internal dichotomy, O'Brien-Moore makes the following point:

> Cicero distinguishes exterior object, presentation, and judgement, and recognizes the productive imagination. Hence presentations in any way falsely judged (or *falsa visa* [hallucinations"] accepted by the *animi adsensus* ["acceptance of perceptual evidence by the mind"]) would build up an internal structure not corresponding, but believed to be corresponding, to an exterior reality, and that would be madness (44, p. 158).

Thus, by Cicero's time the explicit recognition of the possibility of internal ideas not corresponding to external reality has been firmly achieved.

Poetic

In contrast to Roman philosophy, Roman poetry generally treats madness in a stylized and static fashion; madness seems unmotivated, intrusive, and inconsistent with the character in whom it appears. The poets by and large have lost sight of its human reality. Even in the work of the most honored Roman poet, Vergil, a younger contemporary of Lucretius, the theme of madness is employed more as a convenient (because arbitrary) way of advancing the plot than as a necessary outcome attributable to the inexorable internal forces within

the character. Thus, the madness of Amata in the *Aeneid* (VII), caused
by one of the Furies, is appropriate to the poem and to the poet's historical context (44, pp. 162-179), but virtually useless for advancing the
psychological comprehension of madness. After Vergil this "Fury model
of madness" becomes a mere tired literary convention, as in Ovid.

Historical

The emperor Tiberius supposedly addresses the Senate in a letter,
on the issues of luxury, excess, gluttony, and dissipation, as follows:

> As even bodily disorders of long standing and growth can be
> checked only by sharp and painful treatment, so the fever of a
> diseased mind, itself polluted and a pollution to others, can be
> quenched only by remedies as strong as the passions which inflame
> it. Of the many laws devised by our ancestors, of the many passed
> by the Divine Augustus, the first have been forgotten, while his
> (all the more to our disgrace) have become obsolete through con-
> tempt, and this has made luxury bolder than ever. The truth is,
> that when one craves something not yet forbidden, there is a fear
> that it may be forbidden; but when people once transgress pro-
> hibitions with impunity, there is no longer any fear or any shame.
> Why then in old times was economy in the ascendant? Because
> everyone practised self-control; because we were all members of
> one city. (68, III:54.)

1. Roman history is first and foremost moral history, especially in
the works of Livy (1st century B.C.) and Tacitus (1st and early 2nd
century A.D.). The former is in the position of watching the Roman
Republic crumble: his theme is the moral fiber of Republican ancestors, perhaps as an intellectual call to arms or at least a reminder
to present Romans of what Rome had been and could once again be
like. Tacitus, by contrast, writes from the perspective of a man enjoying some freedom under a benign despotism; his intent is to remind
the Romans of the evil the state had experienced under the first few
emperors in the hope that analysis would help prevent their falling
into the trap of tyranny again. (Needless to say, he failed.) Hence,
both historians idealize the Republic and long for its restoration.
2. The implications of Lucretius's notion that we all could be mad
are carried to their logical extreme by Tacitus, who demonstrates that
the whole age of the early emperors *was* mad. The madness of the
emperors was a microcosmic representation of the madness of the
entire society.
3. The major cause of this madness is the excess of unchecked pas-

sions. Rome's political, economic, and military successes led to a "silver-platter" attitude: the upper classes had come to regard luxuries as necessities since from infancy they had experienced automatic fulfillment of their wishes (66). Frustration is unbearable to those not accustomed to it; thus violence becomes a more viable way of reaching power and prestige than good service, patriotism, or even family position. Furthermore, once one has experienced automatic wish-fulfillment for a large portion of his life, he will sacrifice almost anything to maintain it. Thus, past laws and other restraints become meaningless since they block this eternity of gratification.

Megalomania best characterizes this attitude and is one version of the paradigmatic mental disturbance for the Roman Empire. This tendency is beautifully illustrated in the behavior of the Roman emperors, who at first were deified after death but gradually came to expect deification while still alive. Thus, Vespasian's facetious, deathbed remark—"I think I'm turning into a god" (65A)— sounds ridiculous only to someone who does not know that other emperors declared themselves gods during their lifetime. (Cf. similar trends in the Hellenistic period (3)).

4. Tiberius, no saint himself, recognizes with horror (at least as Tacitus represents him) that he has no real way of stopping these excesses. He calls for as radical a treatment for the disorder as the disorder itself; but if the defining characteristic of this disorder is its tendency to make the patient ignore all prohibitions, even the most radical suppression would be ineffectual, especially if the enforcer of the prohibitions were enjoying and benefitting from the excesses. If one cannot instill fear or shame in people by means of external prohibition, he can only appeal to self-control or internal prohibitions. But if the capacity for self-control does not already exist, appeal to a "more moral" historical past avails nothing.

5

THE PSYCHOSOCIAL BACKGROUND OF
ROMAN MADNESS

Roman history may be divided into three epochs according to the state's political orientation: Kingdom (about 250 years), Republic (500 years, interspersed with emergency dictatorships), and Empire (500 years). Especially during the first two periods the Romans' orientation toward external action and conquest rather than toward thought and introspection found expression in the uninterrupted expansion of their power over the Mediterranean world. The Romans were extroverted, intensely practical, and down-to-earth, with little use for examination of internal motives. The Roman value system was heavily paternalistic and emphasized the sense of duty and responsibility. The word *virtus* clearly conveys the Roman ideal: originally derived from *vir* (a "real man," a "hero," superior to the common man, *homo*), it means "manhood, strength, courage, excellence, virtue, worth." Several specific "virtues" that the Romans prized give some indication of their ideal character type. A man's most important trait is *pietas,* "sense of duty," including duty to parents or filial affection, duty to country or patriotism, and duty to the gods or piety. *Gravitas,* "severity, seriousness, unruffled dignity," consists primarily in the holding in of one's feelings. This is related to *constantia,* "self-possession, firmness, constancy." Finally, there is the significant term that contains its own antithesis (19) by including both injunction and the intrapsychic punishment for its violation: *pudor,* "sense of shame, modesty, sense of honor" and "shame, disgrace." *Pudor* regulates one's behavior by keeping him conscious of the above listed virtues. The outlines of a particular character style emerge here, with its emphasis on a masculine, paternal, hardheaded, unemotional, duty-bound, and conservative orientation.

These characteristics are consistent with the Romans' child-rearing techniques. The extended families, the *gentes,* were ruled by a patriarch as the king ruled early Rome, and in each nuclear family the father, *paterfamilias,* had absolute power, including the power of life and death over children. The Romans called their senate (originally composed of the heads of *gentes*) the "fathers," *patres conscripti,* and under the Republic they selected their two annual ruling officials, the consuls, from this august body. Every Roman youth entered the military for a period of training and left it for a political career (1). Hence, the Roman family was the mirror image of the Roman state; their influence intertwined and perpetuated each other, predicated on their emphasis upon "masculine" and paternal values.

Women internalized this same value system and appear to have been largely satisfied with it. The Roman matron had more freedom and respect than her Greek counterpart and does not appear to manifest that complex of penis envy, omnipotent control of children, and angry resentment discussed previously. The Romans paid tribute to her esteemed position in the family. Although women lacked political power, they seem to have had economic power. Furthermore, since Roman men customarily married, at age 30, women half their age, it is likely that the many widows who had outlived their husbands attained great actual, if not nominal, power and prestige, either on their own account, or through honor bestowed on their deceased husbands, or because of their coveted position as wealthy marriageable widows. From our perspective they seem stately, cold, and haughty, a result of identification with their own similar mothers and with Roman paternal and masculine values. Patriotic women died for Rome just as men did in the tales of the Roman past. Unlike Greek women, Roman women seem successfully to have identified with fathers as well as mothers, so that they were not compelled to covet the unobtainable phallus as the former did.

Although on the outside Roman men and women seem hard, cold, unemotional, and distant, probably sufficient emotional warmth existed in marriages and in child rearing so that the child grew up with a sense of stability and strength derived from early "good-object" internalizations. Men did not marry until they had come home from the army and then took an active role in child rearing, so that they were not distant, unreal figures. That mothers supplied more affection to children than their brittle surfaces would indicate is beautifully illustrated in the story of Cornelia, mother of the Gracchi and most admired of Roman matrons, who refused marriage with the Egyptian king since it would draw her away from her children, her "jewels." The combination of mother-child closeness and the early and strong training in the paternalistic values mentioned resulted in competent, capable, outer-directed people whose talents for organization and mastery were unsurpassed in antiquity.

The interweaving of this character style and the propensity for externalizing behavior brought about the peculiarly Roman solution to the conflicts of life: aggressive domination of the world became a moral duty. They externalized or "lived out" their intrapsychic conflicts in the arenas of politics and military conquest. They could with impunity direct their aggression outward in military domination; the Roman dream of narcissistic completeness and perfection was embodied in their "swallowing up" and controlling the whole world. They could justify this aggressiveness as behavior required by their sense of duty to parents, gods, and country.

The Roman *malaise* consisted precisely in the realization that they could not attain peace of mind through subjugating the external world or accumulating power and wealth. From earliest Roman literature on, one of the major themes of the culture is the fantasy of an earlier, better time, when corruption and immorality did not exist. This idealization of the past is evident in every author, whether historian, poet, philosopher, or politician. Vergil created a timeless, perfect "Arcadian landscape," far removed from the growing urbanization, expansion, and conflict of his world (63), and celebrated Rome's glorious origins. Livy tries to escape his own strife-filled era by recounting the deeds of past Roman heroes, while Tacitus envies Livy for the nobility of his subject matter, in contrast to the degrading nature of his own. Lucretius vividly portrays the inevitable disgust and disillusionment attendant upon the realization that absolute power, excessive wealth, and world domination cannot fill up the yawning emptiness of men's present lives; he contrasts his contemporaries with primitive men who, while they too had their problems, at least did not devote their lives to satisfying superfluous needs and did not perish in pursuit of their fulfillment.

From a psychological viewpoint, this idealized past is a cultural version of the individual's earliest relationship with his mother, before external demands and unnecessary desires arose to destroy this matrix. A culture that demands independence training for children quite early, as Roman culture did, encourages a residue of lifelong nostalgia for the lost utopia of the mother-child bond. We must concur with Lucretius's assessment that the mental problem that is paradigmatic for Roman culture is the restless flight from and manic denial of depression, manifest in its attempt to coerce the world into satisfying its wishes and meeting its demands so as to re-create an illusory narcissistic perfection that disappeared with the loss of the mother. Again, as with the Greeks, we are stigmatizing as psychopathological some characteristics that make Roman culture unique in its orientation to the environment; Rome could never have conquered such a vast area of the world and organized it unless its denizens could deny and externalize internal conflicts. Nevertheless, the work of Lucretius shows that such behavior is maladaptive if carried to extremes and can easily lead to a life driven by dissatisfaction.

Before proceeding to an examination of the Empire phase of Roman history that differs so markedly on the surface but is so fundamentally similar underneath to the Roman psyche of the Regal and Republican eras, we should take note of how the Romans viewed madness in general. Madness to the Roman mind is the behavioral manifestation of frenzied emotional turmoil, as exemplified in the Eastern religions that so fascinated and repelled the Romans. They continually wavered between incorporating and expelling these religions until they were firmly established under the Empire. The worship of Cybele, the "Great Mother"—significant, of course, for the Roman psyche—was formally instituted in 204 B.C.; bacchic rites were banned in 186 B.C.

because of excessive popularity and contradiction of traditional Roman values and were reinstituted by Caesar just before the Empire replaced the Republic (4, 7, 44). Almost all literary madness was caused by the Furies, whose name, replacing the Greek Eumenides, signifies "raving madness" (*furor*), always depicted as uninhibited emotional frenzy. The Romans of the Republic feared that if they let down their guard against carefully and rigidly controlled emotions, they would fall prey to overwhelming and irredeemable madness.

The Roman psyche under the Empire *appears* radically different from that of the Republic. In a sense the Roman dreams of narcissistic grandeur became a present reality rather than an idealized past attainable only in the distant future. Rome had devoured and gained control of the world; now Augustus, the first emperor, could institute worldwide peace, the *Pax Romana,* after a history of war and domination. After Augustus, the emperor became a symbol of the Empire: he was the grand, exalted, narcissistic, and megalomanic baby whose every desire was gratified by servants and whose perfection and godliness were continually reaffirmed by hired or ambitious sycophants. Gradually the emperor's divinity came to be self-declared during his life rather than an honor voted him after death, and he became a veritable god on earth. Furthermore, he was the idealized mirror image (32) of the pampered masses whose favor he curried through gratuitous doles so that they would remain dependent upon and in love with him.

Clearly the old paternalistic Roman values have by this time passed away from the official state version of morality, and with their passing the importance of the family's influence on the individual diminished markedly. Indeed, Augustus, the first emperor, whose temperament remained relatively republican in his concern for the preservation of the state and some degree of individual liberty, had to institute artificial rewards for marriage and family, so that the radical decline in the Roman birth rate would not result in the dying out of the Empire at its very inception (66, 68). This remarkable fact supports our contention that the Romans were no longer obsessed with past and future but only with an eternal present, as befits a narcissistic civilization that shows little concern with extending itself into the future through children. But not everyone had forgotten the Republic and its values. Throughout the first century of the Empire several unsuccessful plots to overthrow the emperor were formulated and crushed; at this time they were invariably planned by the *patres,* the "fathers" or senators, or by nobles from patrician families, never by the lower classes who were usually political allies of the emperor or, more often, indifferent and powerless onlookers. In other words, it is as if the fathers with their old paternalistic Roman values plotted against the exalted narcissistic baby, who reacted to every attempt to shake his omnipotence with paranoid suspiciousness of everyone and sadistic fury against found or suspected conspirators.

The aggression that Rome once directed against foreign powers was now turned inward upon the Roman State and its citizens. Personal safety and mutual trust and trustworthiness disappeared from the Roman world that had once so highly valued solidarity among Roman citizens. Rome became safe for no one: the emperor was always in danger of being murdered by a jealous aspirant to his position of perfection, while everyone else in government could at any time be accused of conspiracy by a jealous rival or the (somewhat justifiably) paranoid emperor, and put to death. Lower-class citizens still lived as precarious an existence as ever, either waiting near subsistence level for the emperor's handouts or dying in the many border wars, now waged for protection rather than conquest. They were entertained by the emperor's gladiatorial games and other spectacles: the ancient power of life and death which the father exercised over the child was here distorted into a sadistic version of the primal scene, with the parents omnipotently controlled by the narcissistic baby embodied in emperor and populace. This device served as well to kill off rivals and pretenders to the throne of narcissistic perfection held by the emperor. Here again the transvaluation of all Republican values is apparent: the child controls the parents in the upside-down world of the Empire.

Concomitant with this "transvaluation of values" was the relaxation of Republican inhibitions; the Imperial Romans seem to be trying to make up for opportunities for gratification lost by Republican Romans. Moralists with Republican sympathies, like the historian Tacitus and the satirist Juvenal, cannot restrain their glee over Imperial dissoluteness, profligacy, excess, and dissipation, and their depiction is supported in outline even by writers sympathetic to the emperors or discreetly non-opinionated ones. Romans seem to have in part lost that "sense of shame" (*pudor*) that once restrained them, not to mention the other Republican "virtues."

But even if Roman character structure had altered due in part to laxity of Imperial child-rearing techniques, had the Roman hierarchy of desires and avoidance of emotional expression actually changed? Clearly, the answer is no. The Romans were no less power-oriented than ever; they simply did not have the discipline of character or the appropriate external circumstances required for competent control, except in a few instances. As the historians make clear, children were trained to value and seek to gain power as much as ever, often now by their mothers, but power now derived from deviousness and indifference to suffering rather than from compulsive scrupulousness and strength of character.

The same applies to the important emotional configuration we have identified in Roman culture: the manic and now megalomanic denial of depression and the powerful but unconscious wish to return to the mother. As is clear from the widespread gratuitous killing, plotting, and suspiciousness so characteristic of the Empire, narcissistic perfection and omnipotence are unattainable in reality; hence, emperor, senators, people, and culture distorted reality and lived in part in a world of fantasy. This fact may simply be inferred from the peculiar practices of the age that seem to have more in common with childhood fantasy than adult adaptation of and to the environment: emperor worship, mystery religions, palace plots, gladiatorial games, the voracious search for new pleasures, deviant sexual practices, and so on. We can, however, go further in specifying the sources of such behavior. Its connection with the denial of depression and loss of the mother seems even more obvious here than when Lucretius made the same connection for Republican Romans, perhaps because Imperial Romans carried implicit Republican patterns to their logical extreme.

Imperial Rome illustrates perhaps better than any other culture (with the exception of ours?) the operation of the "manic defense against depression," the "reassurance through reality against death inside" (73, p. 131). Roman streets were gay and bustling with activity during the daytime, but at night they became the sinister domain of thieves and murderers, against whom wealthy citizens could protect themselves only with the help of many slaves and many torches to light the way, if they dared to go outside at all.

The extreme popularity of the mystical mother religions from the East (7) clearly reflects the emotional abandon of the Empire, the manic flight to exciting new experiences because of the boredom and deadness of everyday life, and the fantasy of a return to and salvation by an idealized mother, as a compensation for the insecurity and depression that ensue from loss of a secure relationship with the real mother. Indeed, all the peculiar practices of the Empire listed above seem to have the function of intensifying experience so that people can convince themselves that they are still alive. Plots and executions make interesting an otherwise boring, because absolutist, regime. Games and spectacles were displayed on an ever vaster scale by the emperors to curry popular favor, as if people could thereby attain some ultimate and sublime pleasure. The ever more exotic sexual pleasures, including eating, succeeded neither in facilitating greater emotional contact among people nor in filling up the emptiness or enlivening the deadness within. Lucretius, who first identified this panicked flight from inner deadness, described it best:

> As long as what we crave is out of reach, it seems to surpass everything else in importance; once we get it we crave something else, and an unquenchable thirst for life keeps us forever gaping in frustration. (4, III:1082-1084.)

REFERENCES

1. ABBOTT, F. F. (n.d.): *Roman Political Institutions*. Boston: Ginn and Co.
2. ABRAHAM, K. (1913): Restrictions and transformations of scoptophilia in psycho-neurotics. In: *Selected Papers on Psycho-Analysis*. London: Hogarth Press, (1927) pp. 169-234.
3. BARBU, Z. (1960): The emergence of personality in the Greek world. In: *Problems of Historical Psychology*. New York: Grove Press, pp. 69-144.
3A. BRETT, G. S. (1962): *Brett's History of Psychology*, R. S. Peters, ed. Cambridge, Mass.: MIT Press.
4. BRUNS, C. G., ed. (1909): *Fontes Juris Romani Antiqui*. 7th ed. Tübingen: O. Gradenwitz.
5. BUCKLAND, W. W. (1932): *A Textbook of Roman Law from Augustus to Justinian*. 2nd ed. Cambridge: Cambridge Univ. Press.
6. CICERO, M. T. (1960): *Cicero's Tusculan Disputations*, J. King, ed. Loeb Classical Library. London: Heinemann.
7. CUMONT, F. (1909): *Oriental Religions in Roman Paganism*. New York: Dover (1956).
7A. DE SAUSSURE, R. (1938): Le miracle grec. *Rev. Franc. de Psychoanal*, 10, 87-148; 323-377; 471-536.
7B. DEVEREUX, G. (1970): The psychotherapy scene in Euripides' *Bacchae*. *J. Hellenic Studies*, 90; 35-48.
8. DODDS, E. R. (1956): *The Greeks and the Irrational*. Berkeley: Univ. of California Press.
9. DRABKIN, I. E. (1955): Remarks on ancient psychopathology. *Isis*, 46, 223-234.
10. EDELSTEIN, L. (1937): Greek medicine and its relation to religion and magic. *Bull. Hist. Med.*, 5, 201-246.
11. EDELSTEIN, L. (1939): The genuine works of Hippocrates. *Bull. Hist. Med.*, 7, 236-248.
12. EDELSTEIN, L. (1943): *The Hippocratic Oath*. Baltimore: Johns Hopkins Press.
13. EDELSTEIN, E. J. & L. (1945): *Aesclepius: A Collection and Interpretation of the Testimonies*, 2 vols. Baltimore: Johns Hopkins Press.
14. EDELSTEIN, L. (1945): The role of Eryximachus in Plato's *Symposium*. *Trans. Amer. Philol. Assoc.*, 76, 97 sq.
15. EDELSTEIN, L. (1952): The relation of ancient philosophy to medicine. *Bull. Hist. Med.*, 26, 299-316.
16. EDELSTEIN, L. (1956): The professional ethics of the Greek physician. *Bull. Hist. Med.*, 30, 394-419.
17. EURIPIDES (1959): *Orestes*. In: *The Complete Greek Tragedies*, Vol. IV, ed. D. Grene and R. Lattimore. Chicago: Univ. of Chicago Press.
18. FRÄNKEL, H. (1962): *Dichtung und Philosophie des Frühen Griechentums*, 2nd ed. München.
19. FREUD, S. (1910): The antithetical meaning of primal words. *Standard Edition*, 11, 153-161. London: Hogarth Press, 1957.

19A. GLOTZ, G. (1930): *The Greek City and Its Institutions*, trans. N. Mallinson. New York: Knopf.

19B. HARRISON, J. E. (1922): *Prolegomena to the Study of Greek Religion*, 3rd ed. New York: Meridian Books, 1955.

20. HAVELOCK, E. A. (1962): *Preface to Plato*. Cambridge: Harvard University Press.

21. HAVELOCK, E. A. (1970): The Socratic self as it is parodied in Aristophanes' *Clouds*. *Yale Classical Studies*, 22.

22. HEIBERG, J. L. (1927): Geisteskrankheiten im klassischen Altertum. *Allgemeine Zeitschrift für Psychiatrie*, 86, 1-44.

23. HESIOD (1950): *Theogony*, In: *Hesiod, The Homeric Hymns and Homerica*, trans. H. G. Evelyn-White. Loeb Classical Library. Cambridge, Mass: Harvard University Press.

24. HIPPOCRATES (1849): *Oeuvres Complètes*, E. Littré, ed. Tomes 1-10. Paris.

25. HIPPOCRATES (1931): trans. W. H. S. Jones. Loeb Classical Library. Vol. I-IV. London: Heinemann.

26. HOMER (1951): *The Iliad*, trans. R. Lattimore. Chicago: Univ of Chicago Press.

27. HOMER (1965): *The Odyssey*, trans. R. Lattimore. New York: Harper and Row.

28. HORACE (1901): *Epistulae*, In: *Q. Horati Flacci Opera*, E. C. Wickham, ed. Oxford: Clarendon Press.

29. JACKSON, S. W. (1969): Galen on mental disorders. *J. Hist. Behav. Sci.*, 5, 365-384.

30. JACKSON, S. W. (1972): Unusual mental states in medieval Europe. I. Medical syndromes of mental disorder: 400-1100 A.D. *J. Hist. Med. Allied Sci.* 27, 262-297.

30A. JAEGER, W. (1945): *Paideia: The Ideals of Greek Culture*. New York: Oxford Univ. Press.

31. KAUFMAN, M. R. (1966): The Greeks had some words for it: Early Greek concepts on mind and "insanity." *Psychiatric Quarterly*, 1-33.

32. KOHUT, H. (1971): *The Analysis of the Self*. New York: International Universities Press.

33. KUDLIEN, F. (1967): *Der Beginn des Medizinischen Denkens bei den Griechen von Homer bis Hippocrates*. Zurich: Artemis Verlag.

34. LACEY, W. K. (1968): *The Family in Classical Greece*. Ithaca: Cornell Univ. Press.

35. LAIN-ENTRALGO, P. (1970): *The Therapy of the Word in Classical Antiquity*, trans. L. J. Rather and J. M. Sharp. New Haven: Yale Univ. Press.

36. LANG, F. R. (1972): Psychological terminology in the Tusculans. *J. Hist. Behav. Sciences*, 8, 419-436.

37. LEIBBRAND, W. & WETTLEY, A. (1961): *Der Wahnsinn: Geschichte der Abendländischen Psychopathologie*. Freiburg/München: Verlag Karl Alber.

38. LESKY, ALBIN (1961): *Göttliche und Menschliche Motivation im Homerischen Epos*. (Sitz, der Heidelberger Akad. der Wiss., Phil-Hist. Kl. 1961, 4). Heidelberg.

39. LIDDELL, H. G., SCOTT, R. & JONES, H. S. (1940): *A Greek-English Lexicon*, 9th ed. Oxford: Clarendon Press.

40. LORD, A. (1960): *The Singer of Tales*. Cambridge, Mass.: Harvard University Press.

41. LUCRETIUS, T. (1942): *De Rerum Natura*, W. E. Leonard and F. B. Smith, eds. Madison: Univ. of Wisconsin Press.

41A. MISCH, G. (1950): *A History of Autobiography in Antiquity*. Cambridge, Mass.: Harvard Univ. Press.

42. MORA, G. (1967): The history of psychiatry. In: *Comprehensive Textbook of Psychiatry*, A. Freedman and H. Kaplan, eds. Baltimore: Williams and Wilkins.

43. NORTH, H. (1966): *Sophrosyne: Self-Knowledge and Self-Restraint in Greek Literature*. Ithaca: Cornell Univ. Press.

44. O'BRIEN-MOORE, A. (1924): *Madness in Ancient Literature*. Weimar: Wagner.
45. PARRY, M. (1971): *The Making of Homeric Verse. The Collected Papers of Milman Parry*, A. Parry, ed. Oxford: Clarendon Press.
46. PINEL, P. (1806): *Treatise on Insanity*, trans. D. D. Davis. Sheffield.
47. PIVNICKI, D. (1969): The origins of psychotherapy. *J. Hist. Behav. Sciences*, 5, 238-247.
48. PLATO (1937): *The Dialogues of Plato*, trans. B. Jowett. New York: Random House.
49. PLATO (1904): *Timaeus*, trans. R. G. Bury. Loeb Classical Library. Cambridge: Harvard Univ. Press.
50. PLAUTUS (1904): *Captivi*. In: *Plauti Comoediae*, Vol. I, W. M. Lindsay, ed. Oxford: Clarendon Press.
51. POPPER, K. (1963): *The Open Society and Its Enemies. I. The Spell of Plato*. New York: Harper Torchbooks.
52. RIEFF, P. (1966): *The Triumph of the Therapeutic*. New York: Harper and Row.
53. ROBINSON, T. M. (1970): *Plato's Psychology*. Toronto: Univ. of Toronto Press.
54. ROSEN, G. (1969): *Madness in Society*. New York: Harper and Row.
55. RUSSO, J. & SIMON, B. (1968): Homeric psychology and the oral epic tradition. *J. Hist. Ideas*, 29, 483-498.
56. SCHULZ, F. (1951): *Classical Roman Law*. Oxford: Clarendon Press.
57. SECHAN, L. (1926): *Etudes sur la Tragédie Grecque dans ses Rapports avec la Céramique*. Paris.
58. SIEGLER, M. & OSMOND, H. (1966): Models of madness. *Brit. J. Psychiatry*, 112, 1193-1203.
59. SIEGLER, M., OSMOND, H. & MANN, H. (1971): Laing's models of madness. In: *R. D. Laing and Anti-Psychiatry*, R. Boyers and R. Orrill, eds. New York: Harper and Row (Perennial), pp. 119-150.
60. SIMON, B. & WEINER, H. (1966): Models of mind and mental illness in ancient Greece: I. The Homeric model of mind. *J. Hist. Behav. Sci.*, 2, 303-314.
61. SIMON, B. (1972 & 1973): Models of mind and mental illness in ancient Greece: II. The Platonic model. *J. Hist. Behav. Sci.*, 8, 389-404; 9, 3-17.
62. SLATER, P. E. (1968): *The Glory of Hera*. Boston: Beacon Press.
63. SNELL, B. (1953): *The Discovery of the Mind*. Cambridge: Harvard University Press.
64. STANNARD, J. (1959): Socratic eros and Platonic dialectic. *Phronesis*, 4, 126-134.
65. STANNARD, J. (1961): Hippocratic pharmacology. *Bull. Hist. of Medicine*, 36, 497-518
65A. SUETONIUS, G. (1931): *The Lives of the Twelve Caesars*. J. Gavorse, ed. New York: Random House.
66. SYME, R. (1952): *The Roman Revolution*. Oxford: Oxford Univ. Press.
67. SZASZ, THOMAS (1961): *The Myth of Mental Illness*. New York: Delta.
68. TACITUS, P. C. (1942): *Annals*. In: *Complete Works of Tacitus*, trans. A. J. Church and W. J. Brodribb. New York: Random House.
69. TEMKIN, O. (1949): *The Falling Sickness*. Baltimore: Johns Hopkins Univ. Press.
70. TRENDALL, A. D. & WEBSTER, T. B. L. (1971): *Illustration of Greek Vases*. London: Phaidon Press.
71. VEITH, I. (1965): *Hysteria: The History of a Disease*. Chicago: Univ. of Chicago Press.
72. WARMINGTON, E. H. (1938): *Remains of Old Latin*, vol. III. Loeb Classical Library. Cambridge, Mass.: Harvard Univ. Press.
73. WINNICOTT, D. W. (1935): The manic defense. In: *Collected Papers*, London: Tavistock, pp. 129-144.

2

ITALY

George Mora, M.D.

*Research Associate, Department of History of Science and Medicine,
Yale University, New Haven, Connecticut, U.S.A.*

1

INTRODUCTION

A history of psychiatry of any Western country can be presented from two essentially different viewpoints: as the development of psychiatry as a specific field of medicine in the last century and a half; or as the development of attitudes toward the mentally ill by individuals and groups in the context of cultural and religious backgrounds from early times onwards. This chapter is written from a perspective which combines these two viewpoints, inasmuch as it deals in more detail with the events of the last 150 years, while not disregarding the importance of attitudes toward mental illness which, incidentally, are evident even during the period of "scientific" psychiatry.

A word is also needed about the boundaries of the present chapter. Italy as an independent nation is little more than a century old. However, from the geographical, historical and cultural perspective, Italy has been traditionally considered as a nation since the fall of the Roman empire around the fourth century A.D. This presentation follows this latter view. Moreover, in view of the many and extensive invasions that the various Italian regions underwent throughout history, it is particularly difficult to identify and to separate the develop-

---

A considerable amount of material for this study was gathered with the support of Grant #M-5758 by the National Institute of Mental Health.

ments relative to psychiatry which took place in Italy from those of foreign origin.

Regardless of this question, the pervasive participation of religious orders in the care of the mentally ill, especially up to the establishment of Italy as an independent political nation, has to be kept constantly in mind. Since the unification of Italy a number of events, such as the foundation of state-supported mental hospitals, the passing of legislation for the mentally ill, the organization of training of personnel to work with mental patients, and others, point to a decreased involvement of the Church in the care of the mentally ill.

Finally, up to the present, no history of psychiatry in Italy has been written. The available literature consists of very short historical notes (168, 188, 190, 236, 239), biographies of psychiatrists (77), and chronicles of mental institutions (2, 238). The Italian school of history of medicine, though quite imposing, has never been particularly interested in the developments of psychiatry; the notable exception is the work of Gustavo Tanfani (229-232). Among the psychiatrists, Emilio Padovani (181-183) and Carlo Ferrio (86) have written on several aspects of Italian psychiatry. Much of the material relating to the cultural attitudes toward the mentally ill is scattered in many publications from the fields of history, religion, philosophy, literature and art, aside from medicine, of course. In the limits of the present volume, this chapter intends to be a short comprehensive presentation of the subject, which perhaps may be of incentive to someone else to prepare a thorough study.

2

GREEK AND ROMAN BACKGROUND

It is well known that in history there is a continuity of tradition rather than a break between one culture and another, as well as between one period and another. To understand the initial period of the history of Italy, spanning several centuries, it is essential to take into account this continuity. In retrospect, it is impossible to separate the beginning from the later phase of the Roman civilization. Even the rise of Christianity, which constitutes the traditional landmark between antiquity and the Middle Ages, runs imperceptively from one era to the other. In view of this, a critical presentation of the cultural attitudes and practices toward mental diseases and the people affected by them must necessarily begin with a discussion of the Roman background and the Greek antecedents. In fact, not only Roman medicine, but religion, philosophy, and literature as well represent a continuation of the Greek civilization. Only in regard to practical aspects of life, such as architecture, economics, and jurisprudence, did the Roman civilization produce innovations which lasted for centuries. Of these various aspects, the last one is particularly relevant for psychiatry.

Cultural attitudes and practices toward mental diseases and the mentally ill in the Greek and Roman cultures are seen today as complex phenomena, resulting from the interplay of many factors. Pragmatically, they can be divided into popular concepts, medical concepts, and philosophical-literary concepts.

Of the three, the popular conception of "madness" is particularly pervasive and has many common elements with the preceding primitive—or better, non-literate—cultures. Central to this concept is the belief that madness is caused and healed by supernatural agents, personified by particular gods or goddesses who act toward mortals in an anthropomorphic way in a state of anger, or, conversely, of favorable disposition. Without entering into the dynamic of this belief (essentially based on the ambivalent feelings of men toward their ancestors personified in supernatural beings), the fact remains that the main expressions of these practices are the ones traditionally described in the history of magic and superstition, often in the context of religious systems; these include powerful action of particular verbal formulas and objects operating at a distance and reflecting the wish of an individual or a group, which can be counteracted only through particular ceremonies. Students of religions, and especially of folklore, have investigated this aspect, exemplified by a variety of natural objects (talismans, amulets, fetishes, etc.) and of human expressions, such as magic utterances and religious ceremonies of all sorts, which have continued uninterrupted since the classical period. Among the Italian contributions to the study of the former, mention should be made of the writings by Giuseppe Pitré and his school of folklore (47), Arturo Castiglioni (40), Giuseppe Cocchiara (48, 49), Alberto Pazzini (189, 191), and others (89). The study of the latter are very much part of the religious tradition and especially of the rituals which Christianity took over from the original Hebrew and Greek sources. Paramount among human expressions related to psychiatry are the value attributed to dreams and the healing practices employed in places of worship. As far as dreams are concerned, the importance attributed to them in antiquity has been well illustrated in the scholarly monographs by Oppenheim (180) and, for the Greek, by Dodds (71). It is clear that, in the course of the progressive evolving of the classical civilization, the in-

terpretation of dreams (which bears many similarities with the Freudian technique, except for the emphasis on the future rather than on
the past of the dreamer) slowly degenerated from a "pure," flexible,
and personalized form (as in the dreams reported in the Egyptian
and Hebrew cultures) into the "popular" conception focused on the
rigid meaning of stereotyped dreams (typically as in Artemidorous
Daldianus). Early in the classical civilization healing practices like the
shamanistic seances (which have continued uninterrupted to our days
in non-literate cultures) evolved into the more structured techniques
of incubation, on which an extensive literature is available (including
at least one attempt to explain them in Jungian terms) (147). It is
interesting that, according to legend, on the occasion of a severe
epidemic of plague in the year 293 B.C., a delegation of Roman citizens was sent to Greece, to the temple of Asclepios, the god of medicine, to ask for leniency. While there a snake, the traditional symbol
of Asclepios, entered the boat and, on the return journey, it disem-
barked at the Tiberine Island, near Rome. A temple was erected
there and incubation techniques, allegedly resulting also in the cure
of mental patients, flourished for a considerable time (144) (Plate IV).

Similarly, the medical concepts of the Roman culture, which persisted for centuries, were essentially a continuation of Greek medicine,
even in regard to mental disorders (254): Hippocrates' emphasis on
the brain, as the seat of mental diseases, and the four humors as the
basis of the four temperaments (sanguine, choleric, melancholic, and
phlegmatic) were the forerunners of modern constitutional theories;
the methodological school of Asclepiades (who differentiated between
illusions and hallucinations) was based on Democritus' athomic hypothesis; the empirical school was based on practice rather than on
theoretical assumptions; and the pneumatic school was founded on the
principle that "pneuma" is the basis of health. Incidentally, among
the medical theories, mention should be made of that of Alcmaeon
(5th century B.C.), a physician and pupil of Pythagoras—both au-
thochtonus from Southern Italy—who asserted that the seat of senses
and the center of intellectual life should be sought in the brain and
not in the heart as it had been hitherto asserted (205).

Regardless of the subtle differences among these various schools,
what is important here is the enlightened treatment of the mentally
ill recommended by their most illustrious representatives, Asclepiades
and Celsus, the author of the classic De re Medica (both 1st century
B.C.); both recommended isolation of the mentally ill from excessive
stimuli in quiet surroundings, use of music, reading in groups and dramatic performance. In his treatise On Acute and Chronic Diseases (34)

Caelius Aurelianus (1st century A.D.) reported the views of the contemporaries Aretaeus of Cappadocia (who described forms of melancholia which terminated in mania) and Soranus; both recommended
humanitarian principles in the management of the mentally ill: they
had to be kept in quiet rooms and away from relatives, cared for by
sympathetic personnel, subjected to the minimal degree of physical

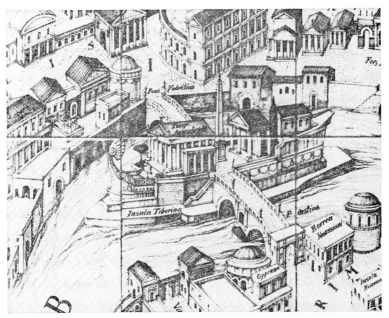

PLATE IV. The Tiberine Island in Rome, where an Asclepeion was erected
in the 3rd century B.C. (from an old map, showing the reconstruction of
the temple to Asclepios and its medical facilities).

restrictions, and occupied in various intellectual activities. Undoubtedly, however, the greatest Roman physician was Galen (ca. 130-
200 A.D.), whose theory of the natural, vital and animal spirits of
Platonic origin (essentially based on the notion of a progressive purification of the essence of life from the abdomen through the heart to
the brain) persisted until the 17th century. Less known is that in his
treatise on the passions, he stressed their role in the causation of
mental disorders (98). Strictly, medical treatment of mental diseases
consisted in the use of vapors, baths, diet and, more specifically, emetics
and cathartics (mainly black hellebore), which, in their intrinsic mean-

ing of purification from pollution ("miasma") through purification ("catharsis"), also continued for centuries.

The issue of passions leads to the philosophical-literary concepts which also stemmed from the Greek tradition of Plato and Aristotle (both 4th century B.C.). Also in regard to their view of mental illness, Plato's metaphysical psychology (based on a triadic division of rational, i.e., immortal, passional, and instinctual soul) stands in contrast to Aristotle's biological psychology (based on a triadic division of mortal soul into vegetative, sensitive, and intellectual). While for Plato madness in very broad terms is seen as a spontaneous or provoked state of unusual excitement, for Aristotle the passions constitute the initial stage of emotional disorder which can lead eventually to mental illness. Mental illness in turn can be treated through the use of passions elicited in various ways, mainly through music by Plato, or through drama by Aristotle. The power of the word in the treatment of mental disturbances was, thus, clearly established in Greek antiquity, as thoroughly demonstrated in the recent volume by Lain Entralgo (122).

These three main approaches to mental illness, the popular, the medical, and the philosophical-literary, can be followed throughout the Roman civilization and, from there, to the medieval era. Hence, the pagan religious ceremonies of incubation were slowly, and not without contrasts, transformed into the Christian ceremonies of worship of saints in the Tiberine Island and elsewhere (110). In philosophy, Cicero (106-43 B.C.) described the four main passions as discomfort, fear, joy, and violent desire (i.e., "libido," this being the first time that this term was used in its psychological sense). The fundamental concepts of the stoic school, to which Cicero belonged, have been seen as anticipating the tenets of modern psychotherapy (126). In literature the representation of the madman as living in an unreal, rather than a supernatural, world in Sophocles (5th century B.C.), and as showing visible signs of insanity in Euripides (5th century B.C.), was substituted in the Roman theater by a stereotyped representation of madness reaching frenzied paroxysms in Virgil (1st century B.C.) and anticipating (through the use of hell broth, magic philters, and love potions) the typical themes of the medieval world in Ovid (1st century A.D.) (179). In medicine, the theoretical systems of the Greek physicians continued well into the medieval era, while the practical approach toward the mentally ill, mentioned above, already revealed the influence of the Christian spirit of brotherhood. Unfortunately, this enlightened attitude was of short duration and was followed by a very long period, up to the 18th century, of widespread unconcern by physicians (with few exceptions) toward the mentally ill. In practice, however, it is likely that the mentally ill were either taken care of and sheltered by their own families, or were abandoned to themselves and left wandering through the country, when not directly abused and persecuted.

In the legal aspects of mental disorders the Romans have exercised an influence which persists to our days. Already in the 5th century B.C., according to the *Twelve Tables,* the mentally ill were deprived of freedom of action and were declared legally incompetent. For centuries the judicial position of the insane was continuously refined and reached the highest possible systematization in the *Corpus Juris Civilis* during the late period of the Roman Empire. Specific norms were issued for establishing the criminal responsibility of the alleged mentally ill and persons temporarily incapacitated by the influence of drunkenness, by unusual passions, and so on, and for deciding—by judges, not by physicians!—on the ability on the part of the mentally ill to contract marriage, to be divorced, to dispose of his possessions, to leave a will, and to testify (217). Under the Emperor Justinian (483-565 A.D.) this legislation was codified in the definite form which persisted for centuries in the history of jurisprudence.

3

THE MIDDLE AGES

There is no definite agreement among historians on the beginning of the Middle Ages. What is certain is that new political, social, and cultural configurations slowly emerged from the ruins of the Roman empire. To be sure, such an empire did not come to an end overnight. For one thing, its secular organization provided the substratum for the spread of the Christian message. Moreover, only the Western part of the empire, which is of interest here, collapsed and was taken over around the end of the 5th century by younger civilizations coming from the North, resulting in the medieval culture, expression of the reciprocal interplay of the old Roman and the new "barbarian" forces.

The Eastern empire, which embodied more directly the heritage of the Greek civilization, survived another thousand years. In it, the joint endeavor of a very spiritual church and of a solid political organization made possible the extended network of Byzantine philanthropy and social welfare, on which a recent thorough monograph has thrown much needed light (52). On the wave of the tradition of the temples devoted to Asclepios, where incubation was practiced, and of the Christian doctrine of charity, a variety of institutions for the poor, the foreigners, the aged, the orphans, and the sick flourished in the Eastern empire from the 5th to the 12th century under the joint auspices of religious and political authorities. Only in one case, however, in the Pantocrator in today's Istanbul, is there evidence that a psychiatric clinic was in operation. The influence of this charitable trend on other countries, notably Italy, appears to have been insignificant.

Italy was heavily influenced in the early Middle Ages by the teaching of the Church fathers and, notably, St. Augustine (354-430), who spent part of his life in Milan and in Rome. Today, Augustine is recognized as the greatest introspective mind before Freud, for the depth and boldness which he displayed in his *Confessions,* a psychological document thus far unmatched. There is mounting evidence, however, that his personal conflicts, mainly in regard to the control of his ebullient sexuality, led to his repressive and puritanic views which, through his tremendous influence on the Church, have persisted to our days.

The spirituality of the Western world, not supported by a social structure, had to turn toward an inner search rather than toward the charitable endeavors of the Eastern empire. Today, under the condition of sorrow and melancholia, the so-called "acedia," which afflicted many monks, and was thoroughly described by John Cassian (360-435), one perceives the dimensions of an existential conflict (1, 253). Spiritual guidance, remarkably outlined by Gregory the Great (540-604) in his treatise on *Pastoral Care,* obviously covered also many aspects of today's psychotherapeutic relationship (46).

But these were still expressions of that small elite of enlightened religious people who, working in isolated monasteries, perpetuated the memory of the classical world. For all the others, the period between the fall of the Roman empire and the so-called early Renaissance of the 13th century represented in Italy a long era of invasions, migrations, famines, plagues, and wars. It is difficult to obtain an idea of the attitudes toward the mentally ill at that time. Some analogies between the lepers and the mentally ill have been put forward, as both were ostracized by society. However, it is possible that from a theocentric conception of the world, where man's position had significance only in relation to his creator, the mentally ill may have enjoyed a certain degree of tolerance, if not of sympathy. We know for sure that, like the paupers, the cripples, and the other outcasts of society, the mentally ill were often left begging and wandering in the country and in places of worship, or abandoned in ships to an unknown destiny, as later immortalized in Sebastian Brandt's *The Ship of Fools* (1494). It is also possible, though not proven, that in the Middle Ages episodes of collective psychopathology took place in Italy on a small scale, similar to the great epidemics of St. Vitus' dance, of flagellantism, of lycanthropy, often under the influence of peculiar religious sects and of superstitious beliefs.

Because of the reciprocal animosity between Christian and Moslem countries, the contribution of the Arabs to the understanding and treatment of the mentally ill has come to the fore only recently. It has been pointed out that the Arabs, although lacking originality, were able to continue the tradition inherited from Greek medical science and from the enlightened Byzantine administration (68). They revived the scientific tradition of the school of Alexandria, which, in the 3rd century B.C., with Erasistratus and Herophilus, had opened the way to the study of the human nervous system; they translated many Greek texts and founded their own medical schools. Between the 8th and the 13th centuries, a number of asylums exclusively for the mentally ill were founded in Baghdad, Damascus, Aleppo, Cairo, Fez, and elsewhere. Reports by later travelers indicated that the methods of treatment employed in these very attractive and tranquil institutions were quite enlightened, and consisted of special diets, baths, drugs, perfumes and concerts (225). Perhaps not foreign to this permissive attitude was the Moslem belief, stated by the Prophet, that the insane person enjoys a particular relationship with God and that he is chosen by Him to tell the truth (213).

The relevance of the Arabian approach to mental illness in relation to Italy lies in the fact that the Arabian culture influenced Italy through many channels, notably Spain and Sicily, before the end of the millennium. In particular, the medical school of Salerno, near Naples, which acquired great renown in the late Middle Ages, resulted from the confluence of Greek, Roman, Hebrew, and Arabian traditions. It was here that Constantinus Africanus (ca. 1020-1087), generally considered as the founder of this school, composed his treatise *De Melancholia* (54). More than for the humoral etiology of mental disorders which was attributed to excess of bile, according to the classical tradition, this work is important for the attribution of the seat of melancholia either to the brain or to the stomach, which became important again in the 18th and 19th centuries. It was especially valuable for its description of psychiatric symptoms: sadness (loss of the loved object), fear (of the unknown), withdrawal (staring into space), delusions related to siblings and parents (based on ambivalent motives), and intense guilt in religious people (10, 56).

In contrast to other countries in the Western hemisphere, in Italy the 13th century brought about an early Renaissance, typically expressed in the works of Dante and of Giotto. Although a new emphasis was placed on the meaning of man in the universe in relation to God, that was the century of the greatest theological systems which have persisted to our days, particularly represented by the work of St. Thomas Aquinas (1225-1274). Born from a noble family near Naples and influenced by the Aristotelian and the Arabian traditions, Thomas was a pupil of the German Albert the Great (1193-1280), a pioneer of biology, who anticipated the modern theory of psychological temperaments (116). Regardless of his theological formulations, which are at the basis of his concept of the soul as the form of the body, hierarchically divided into anima vegetativa (physiological functions), anima sensitiva (external and internal perception, influenced by aggressive and lustful tendencies), and anima intellectiva (reasoning), Thomas gave some indications of his psychopathological concepts. Central to them was his conviction that the soul, being of divine origin, cannot become sick; consequently, mental diseases were related to organic factors. This fundamental postulate, which combines the Platonic and Christian beliefs with those of Hippocrates, has remained a pervasive feature in the history of Italian psychiatry (257), which explains its resistance to the acceptance of a psychodynamic theory of personality, until very recently. In accordance with it, mental disorders were attributed by Thomas to deficient use of reason, caused by insane passions, or to a faulty "physical apparatus" (i.e., when dreaming or in a state of intoxication). Aside from melancholia, mania, organic psychosis, and epilepsy, he described *stultitia, hebetudo,* and *ignorantia,* corresponding, respectively, to current concepts of psychopathic personality, mental deficiency, and social retardation (117, 118, 208).

Like his contemporaries, Thomas believed in astrological influences on the human personality (45). In this respect, perhaps more enlightened is the little-known contribution of Petrus Hispanus (1200-1277), who later in life became Pope John XXI (the only "psychologist" to achieve this honor); he considered passions, midway between soma and psyche, as leading to emotional disturbances, thus anticipating modern psychosomatic medicine (214). Unfortunately, because of his condemnation as a heretic, the figure of Pietro D'Abano (ca. 1250-1316), a follower of the Arabian philosopher Averroes and a teacher of medicine, philosophy, and astrology in Padua, has remained virtually unknown in psychiatry. Yet in his *Conciliator Differentiarum,* published posthumously in 1476, he held that suggestion (*praecantatio*), when practised by a kind and, at the same time, authoritative personality, had definite effects on mentally disturbed people well disposed toward this method of treatment; moreover, he advocated that dreams should be explained according to the personality and the moral characteristics of the individual (232).

No matter how enlightening and pioneering these views were, they were an expression of a limited cultural elite. The great majority of the population was still subjected to all sorts of abuses on the part of the rulers, as well as physical and emotional hardship related to the various social factors mentioned above. There is also evidence, however, that there was plenty of warmth and mutual support in the context of the feudal world, where roles and functions were rigidly imposed at birth and transmitted to the offspring. It is likely that a number of mentally ill who were not tolerated as "characters" in their own towns found a socially acceptable escape from the strictures of that world into crusades, pilgrimages, wars, or in a religious retreat.

4

RENAISSANCE

With the advent of the Renaissance in Italy, and then elsewhere in the 15th century and later, the gap widened between the persistence of medieval social institutions and the unlimited horizons open to man's newly achieved intellectual freedom. In attempting to explain this contrasting phenomenon, cultural and medical historians have delved into the pervasive economic and social depression related to extenuating wars, migrations of entire populations, religious fights and, even worse, collapse of centuries-old ideals (207).

Italy was by no means immune to all this; during the Renaissance it underwent tremendous social upheavals, certainly more than France and England where the monarchic rulers provided a minimum of social structure. Also, Italy was not immune to religious heresies, such as the one initiated by Joachin of Floris in the 12th century, though the most widespread heretic movements of the Albigenses, of the Cathars, and of the Waldenses took place in other countries. It was essentially to counteract the threat posed by these movements that the Church, in the 13th century, established the Inquisition, which, by putting alleged witches on trial, contributed to the dissemination of the witchcraft mania.

Witchcraft, on which a large and varied literature has accumulated in the last four centuries, is of interest here only in regard to psychopathology. Its distant origins can be found in the art and literature of the Middle East, including the Bible. Many references to practices of black magic in the late Roman civilization were described by Horatius, Petronius, Apuleius, and others. Even during most of the Middle Ages, there was relatively little concern for those acused of magic practices, except in the form of religious sanctions, as defined by the canonic laws crystallized in Gratian's *Decretum* in the 12th century. Only in the 14th and, especially, the 15th century, at the time of the greatest social unrest, did witchcraft acquire the proportions of an epidemic. By that time, the temporal role of the Church had become quite strong, leading to the repression of the sexual instincts on the wave of the Augustinian tradition, while aggressive instincts found socially acceptable expression in the Crusades and other frequent religiously motivated wars. The role of the woman came to be increasingly split, on the one side, into that of the metaphysical ideal of the French troubadours and of the German *Minnesängers,* in Italy immortalized in Beatrice in the *Divine Comedy;* on the other side, into that of the inferior and corrupted creature of the Biblical tradition aiming at man's perdition. What has been described in a scholarly book (78) on witchcraft by an Italian philosopher as the "horror diabolicus" appears to be related to the unconscious need to find permissible expressions of sexuality, under religious or secular disguise, on the part of oppressed populations (51, 123).

Regardless of its location, the issue of the mental status of the alleged witches is far from being solved. Zilboorg (263, 264) and others after him (33, 111), have taken almost for granted that these people were mentally sick, affected by hallucinations, sexual perversions, or frank psychoses; others, notably Szasz (226), consider them scapegoats of the joint repressive forces of the Church and of the state. In between these two extremes, the notion that these unfortunate beings were in a state of psychological imbalance due to fear, torture, reciprocal suggestions, social malaise and, possibly, influence of drugs is perhaps the most likely (113).

In Italy witchcraft has played a less significant role than in central European nations and in the British Isles, as already stated by Burckhardt more than a century ago (32). Not only is the Italian literature on witchcraft very limited, but themes related to demonology and to witchcraft rituals are very rare in the immense artistic production of the Italian Renaissance. There is virtual agreement on this point in all the histories of witchcraft, including the only two published in Italy by S. A. Nulli (177) and G. Bonomo (27): the first is inclined to view it in the narrow context of a Church-related phenomenon; the second, instead, aims at its broad comprehension in the ethnological perspective, on the basis of a thorough knowledge of the literature.

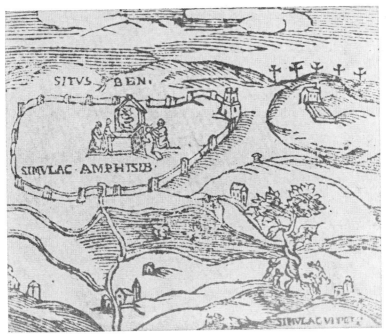

PLATE V. Seventeenth-century illustration showing the famous walnut of Benevento, near Naples, where alleged witches used to congregate.

The main episodes of witchcraft occurred in Italy in isolated Alpine valleys in the 15th, 16th and 17th centuries, with the exception of the well-known episode of the walnut of Benevento, near Naples, in the 15th century (50) (Plate V). Italy produced, on the one side, some of the outstanding believers in the reality of witchcraft, beginning with the Genoese Pope Innocent VII, author of the famous 1484 *Bulla* advocating the persecution of alleged witches and, on the other side, some of the most courageous and outspoken advocates of a serene and rational approach to the issue of witchcraft, such as the lawyers Alciatus and Ponzinibio and the humanists Cardano, Pomponazzi, and Porta, whose arguments were often quoted by Wier in his book *De Praestigiis Daemonum* (1563) against the belief in witchcraft. From the psycho-pathological perspective, of interest also was the issue regarding the alleged presence of individuals interested in disseminating the conta-gion of plague in Lombardy in the 17th century, which resulted in a famous trial and a controversy immortalized in Manzoni's historical novel *The Betrothed* (1825-1827) (176, 196, 201).

Physicians were notoriously absent from the many aspects related to witchcraft, which were considered the realm of ecclesiastic and secular arms. They were not interested in the care of the mentally ill, which was considered the realm of private charity. Most of the 16th century medical literature relevant to psychiatry dealt with the notion of melancholia, a then widely used term which included most of today's psychopathology, from hysteria to schizophrenia (231). In contrast to the advance made in many fields of medicine in the 16th century—i.e., in anatomy by Vesalius, in surgery by Paré—in psychiatry the medieval themes were pedantically repeated, the only innovation being, perhaps, constituted by the universal use of bloodletting for the treatment of mental diseases. The etiology of these diseases was often ascribed to noxious influences on the brain—for instance, by the Paduan profes-sor Giovanni Battista da Monte (1498-1551), or by the Venetian Pros-pero Alpino (1553-1616). The latter, together with Vittorio Trincavelli (1479-1568) and others, stressed the therapeutic value of hydrotherapy. Girolamo Mercuriale (1530-1606), well-known for his various contri-butions to medicine, in line with the Aristotelian tradition, attributed melancholia to a disturbance of imagination localized in the heart rather than in the brain, and described the role of lascivious passions in the causation of mental disorders, whose prognosis he considered favorable in many cases. Girolamo Capivacca (1479-1568), like the professor at Padua, then the leading medical school in the world, focused on the signs which often precede the occurrence of mental diseases: sleep disturbances, nightmares, feelings of fatigue, and visual blurring. Above all these physicians towers the figure of the humanist Gerolano Fracastoro (1478-1553), mostly known for his poem on syphi-lis. Very little known, instead, is his booklet on *The Sympathy and Antipathy of Things* (1546) in which, under the apparent attempt to find harmony among various things in the world and an explanation for obscure material phenomena (a theme central to the pantheistic view of Renaissance man), he dealt extensively with many aspects of human psychology (relation between senses and imagination, sadness and hate, fear, ecstasy, wrath, shame), anticipating later notions of mesmerism and of dynamic psychology (94). Finally, among the physicians, mention should be made of the learned Marsilio Ficino (1433-1490), the main representative of Florentine Platonism (175). In his book on the regime for scholars (*De Studiosorum Sanitate Tuenda* 1482) (143), which includes autobiographical observations, he offered a series of suggestions for people dedicated to intellectual pursuits, which anticipated by three centuries a similar volume, *Sur la santé des gens de lettres* (1766), by the Swiss Simon André Tissot.

However, three Italian humanists outside of the academic world left a permanent contribution to psychopathology: Leonardo da Vinci, Girolamo Cardano, and Giovanni Battista Porta. Leonardo da Vinci (1452-1519), the all-embracing Renaissance genius, was very interested in the study of the human body, as shown in the stupendous anatomical drawings of the nervous system; among his contributions was the exact reproduction of the cerebral ventricles, achieved by injecting cadavers. He investigated the psychophysiology of perception (stereoscopic vision, binomial aspect of colors, persistence of images), the expression of emotions in physiognomy, and the emotional selectivity of memory. He anticipated modern concepts of the functioning of the nervous system (Jackson's motor automatisms), and the Rorschach test by pointing to the individual reaction to the configuration of spots and clouds in his *Treatise on Painting*. He stressed the instinctual component of the mind and hinted at the importance of self-suggestion (hypnotic fascination, especially in women) and of dreams, while shying away from any autobiographical observation (57). This rather detached attitude, reflected in his apparent heterosexual repulsion coupled with his homosexual orientation, became the subject of a famous study by Freud (96), which has stirred up controversies to our day (73, 97, 211).

Girolamo Cardano (1501-1576) represented with his own life the many contradictory attitudes, from superstition to skepticism, of the Italian Renaissance, to the point that he was considered mentally sick (138, 165). In the late 19th century his life was regarded as a typical example of the interplay of genius with insanity (9). Today, it is recognized that some books among his voluminous production contain valuable psychological insight (14, 154). Not only did he oppose the belief in witchcraft by portraying the alleged witches as simple, miserable women, but he recognized the importance of collective suggestion, especially among young women in convents; he hinted at the differentiation between illusions and hallucinations; he advocated liberal educational methods and gave a detailed description of the various temperaments on the basis of a correspondence between physical and psychological traits. As far as dreams are concerned, he wrote that "It is not necessary that dreams correspond perfectly to reality (not unlike the images reflected by mirrors are somewhat different from the real objects), nor that an exact sequence of times occur," thus confirming that quite often men have dreams analogous or quite contrary to their own habits. In dreams, like on a stage, very long series of ideas take place in a short time. Mentally sick people dream a lot, while idiots, like children, have very simple dreams. Even more important than this, for today's psychiatry, is the blunt frankness with which he described himself in his autobiography *The Book of My Life* (35): his nightmares and childhood stuttering, which he ascribed to his father's pathological influence, were later followed by sexual impotence, hallucinations, and grandiose ideas. Under the influence of such an unusual personality, it is no wonder that his own son became disturbed to the point of killing his wife. Probably as an unconscious attempt to justify his son's behavior, Cardano described a type of criminal void of moral judgment, thus anticipating the notion of "moral insanity" of the 19th century (28, 202, 224, 229, 230).

The Neapolitan Giambattista Porta (1535-1615), or Della Porta, also represented a strange combination of scientific inquiry and superstitious beliefs; in his many writings he anticipated several discoveries of optical instruments. In contrast to Cardano, whose life was punctuated by all sorts of adventures, he led an apparently serene life, having achieved early renown with his famous book on *Natural Magic* (1558). In regard to psychiatry, his importance lies in his other book *De Humana Physiognomia* (1586) (195), which gave to physiognomy the role of at least a pseudo-science (5, 21, 29). Physiognomy is based on a syncretistic belief in an inherent correspondence between morphological and psychological traits; men whose heads have certain characteristics present psychological traits similar to the animals they resemble. In support of his thesis, Porta inserted in the book his famous paired pictures of men and corresponding animals. This method of so-called "theriologic physiognomy," given to divination employing such comparison with animals, represents the culmination of a long tradition (128). Initially, in early religions, magic traits were assigned to anthropomorphic gods, then in astrology to the planets and stars, and lastly, in physiognomy, to parts of the human body, mainly the head. Theriologic physiognomy was the favorite approach of the ancient Greeks (Aristotle), then passed to the Arabs, and was later cultivated by many, among whom were the above mentioned Pietro d'Abano, Michael Scott, astrologer to the Emperor Frederick II, and Michael Savonarola, grandfather of the famous religious reformer (62). Following Porta's influence, physiognomy split into two different branches: in art, through Rubens, Le Brun, and others, it turned into the dynamic study of passions typical of the baroque period (11); in science, it anticipated the trend of comparative anatomy cultivated by the humanists Lavater, Goethe, and Carus, as well as Gall's phrenology, which, in turn, led to modern constitutional theories and the doctrine of brain localizations (60).

Although these humanists advanced novel ideas which have many connections with modern psychopathology, they were, like the academicians, also theoreticians, not in direct contact with the mentally ill. To get a lively if not scientific glimpse of the latter, one has to turn to the literary description of insanity. In the medieval French literature, one frequently finds the theme of the hero led by passions of love and jealousy to paranoiac ideations, ideas of grandiosity, and manic attacks (256). The Italian prototype of this genius, the *Orlando Furioso* (1532), a famous poem by Ludovico Ariosto (1474-1533), deals with the fantastic vicissitudes of the protagonist, who is portrayed as the "pure" insane, a completely uninhibited young man, not unlike Wagner's Parsifal. A certain tolerant attitude toward madness was evident here, typified in literature by the ironic position of Erasmus' *Praise of Folly* (1509), and, in real life, by the parody of madness in many popular expressions, such as in the phantasmagoric world of the carnival, culminating in the shrewd imitation of insanity by courtly buffoons, in which Italians have traditionally excelled (125, 252). In the figurative arts, instead, the Italian Renaissance shied away from the grotesque representation of madness of Hieronymus Bosch and other Flemish painters.

The Italian Renaissance did not have any writer of the stature of Shakespeare able to portray the complexity of the human psyche, as in Hamlet, Othello, and King Lear. But Torquato Tasso (1544-1595) personified the drama of mental illness; because of persecutory delusions, he was confined in the hospital of St. Anne, in Ferrara, for seven years, during which he conceived the *Gerusalemme Liberata* (1590), one of the masterpieces of Italian literature. In his letters from St. Anne, Tasso occasionally referred to the atmosphere of unreality and magic of his environment.

A more systematic attempt to present the variety of mental diseases by using the daily experiences of the senses was attempted by the learned Monk Tomaso Garzoni (1549-1589) in several of his writings, but in particular in his *L'Hospidale de' Pazzi Incurabili* (1586) (99), which had the distinction of being translated into English (Plate VI) and, later on, into French. According to the literary fashion of the time, the work was divided into a number of "discourses," each one devoted to a certain kind of mental patient. In succession, thus the author described psychiatric symptoms in primitive cultures, phrenesy, alcoholism, melancholia, imbecility, dementia, psychopathic personalities, delusions of grandiosity, cyclic manic-depressive forms, and

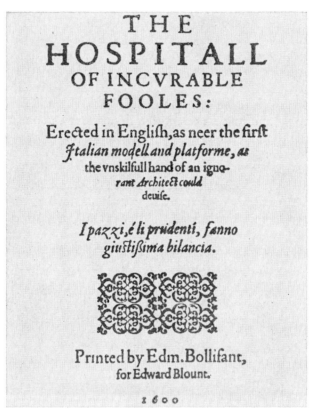

PLATE VI. Title page of *The Hospital of Incurable Fools,* by the learned Italian monk Tomaso Garzoni (1549-1589), which appeared in English translation in 1600.

simulation of insanity. Imbued by the Galenic theory of the spirits, and with the psychological and moral notions of a clergyman, he stood midway between determinism and free will. In his hospital, he did not include people possessed by the demon, who he felt were more in need of exorcism than of treatment. In a later work he subtly distinguished between natural causes and demoniac possessions, and often used subterfuge to escape the anger of the Inquisition. More than for his subdivision of insanity, which in a way already hinted at the classifications of the following centuries, his descriptions of clinical pictures have maintained their freshness to this day. Melancholics, for instance, were described as having very little courage, being replete with fear without knowing the cause of it, being inclined to frequent crying spells, desire of solitude, hate of human intercourse, contempt for amusement, longing for death. It is also worth mentioning his fine description of the state of mind of the individual who would like life and death at the same time, almost an anticipation of the romantic pathos (121, 186, 240).

The literary and artistic representation of insanity was closer, of course, to the popular beliefs regarding mental illness. On the surface the Renaissance presented a mixed attitude of fear, abuse, and disregard for the mentally ill, coupled with the traditional attribution of insanity to unbalanced humors, which needed evacuation from the body through cathartics, emetics, and bloodletting. But, at a deeper level, as shown by Foucault (93), the mentally ill were considered as the expression of the animality of lower beings—not unlike the lepers in the Middle Ages—whose purpose was to bring testimony of divine intervention into human affairs, manifested through the tempting role of the devil. Hence, the most varied and contrasting approaches to mental illness—from exorcism to punishment, from seclusion to abandonment—found justification at that time.

Regardless of this pervasive belief, a new attitude based on a better understanding of human nature slowly manifested itself in the *pietas liberata* of Vives, Thomas More, Erasmus, and others, as pointed out by Zilboorg (264). There is concrete evidence that asylums or shelters for the mentally ill were already in existence in Bergamo, near Milan, since 1352, in Florence since 1387, in Reggio Emilia since 1536, and later in Rome. In terms of historical continuity, it is important to notice that the two gentlemen who opened a shelter for the mentally ill in Rome in 1548 were of Spanish origin. It is in Spain, in fact, perhaps under the influence of both the Judeo-Christian and the Arabian tradition, that the earliest known mental hospitals were opened in the 15th century following the one founded by Father Jofré in Valencia in 1409. In Valencia, St. John of God established the Order of the Brothers of Charity, devoted to the care of the ill. With the help of some private charity, the *Ospedale di Santa Maria della Pietà* was eventually opened in Rome, in 1561, through a Papal Bull. Two years later specific rules were emitted by Cardinal Francesco Barberini, aiming at respecting the dignity of the patients and offering them medical and nursing care; this was in contrast to the careless attitude prevailing at that time (103).

5

THE 17TH AND 18TH CENTURIES

The slow change toward the scientific study of nature, which had been anticipated by Leonardo's work in the Renaissance, became suddenly manifest at the beginning of the 17th century under the impetus of Galileo's and Bacon's writings in Italy and in England, respectively. Because of the universality of the Latin language, scientists from various countries freely interchanged ideas, with the support of the newly established academies of learning. The first academy, the Italian Accademia de' Lincei, was established in 1603, followed by similar ones in France, England, and Germany during the same century. The names of Harvey, Malpighi, Borelli, Van Helmont, Sylvius, Lancisi, Sydenham, and Boyle are the most frequently remembered in connection with the new scientific developments in medicine and science.

Mention should be made here of the substantial contribution to the development of neurology made by some physicians and scientists during these two centuries; the most prominent were G. Baglivi, A. Pacchioni and D. Mistichelli, all three working in Rome under Papal auspices; N. Stensen and F. Fontana, in Florence, under the sponsorship of the Medicis; A. Scarpa, L. Spallanzani and A. Volta, in Pavia; A. Galvani, in Bologna, and D. Cotugno, in Naples (15). Although the controversy over the meeting point of body and mind, initiated in France by Descartes, did not reach a high level in Italy, the relevance of the nervous system to mental disturbances acquired a paramount position in much of the neurological and psychiatric literature of the time.

Undoubtedly, however, the main concern of physicians interested in psychiatry during these two centuries was focused on the issue of classification of mental disorders. The only Italian classifier worth remembering is Paolo Zacchia (1584-1659), the Papal physician, well-known as a founder of legal medicine. In his praised *Questiones Medico-Legales* (Rome, 1621-1650) (258) and, even more, in his Italian monograph on hypochondriac disorders (259) he dealt with many psychiatric aspects. First of all, he insisted that the physician, rather than the theologian or the lawyer, is the only one competent to judge the mental condition of a person on the basis of his behavior, speech, reasoning and emotional state. Nosologically, the clinical pictures were divided by him into: 1) *fatuitas,* or mental deficiency, subdivided into three groups according to its severity; 2) *insania,* including bewitchment, melancholia, organic and—interestingly—emotional conditions;

3) *phrenitis* which, in accordance with the classical tradition, referred to mental conditions accompanied by fever. More than for this classification, however, Zacchia is important for his medico-legal comments (*consilia*) related to psychiatry. According to him imbeciles and idiots are not imputable; patients affected by mania have lucid intervals during which they are partially imputable; marriage can be beneficial for certain emotionally disturbed people; individuals affected by love passions may act irresponsibly; epileptics should wait several years after their apparent recovery before being considered for religious orders; melancholics are inclined to become possessed by the devil (a statement showing the attempt to offer a scientific justification for the religious beliefs of the time); finally, those who simulate insanity are unable to reproduce all the mental symptoms (121, 242).

Zacchia's rational approach to the understanding of mental disorders does not mean that superstitious beliefs and practices did not continue in those two centuries. During that period, several trials for witchcraft took place in Italy, as well as the literary controversy on witchcraft between the learned men Girolamo Tartarotti (235) and Scipione Maffei (140). Even more important are the epidemics of so-called "tarantism," a form of collective psychopathology attributed to the alleged bite of the tarantula and characterized by acute depression and withdrawal, which dramatically improved at the sound of the "tarantella." This disorder, which occurred especially in the very Southern part of Italy in the two centuries under consideration here, was studied by many during that period (220) and later (115). Recently, the phenomenon of tarantism, which has continued to our days on a small scale, has been viewed from the cultural, anthropological, and ethnological perspective and in relation to the tradition of psychotherapy of mental disorders stemming from the Greeks (61, 160).

The mixed attitude of rationalism and irrationalism toward mental diseases affected the methods of care of the mentally ill during those two centuries. In Italy, a great part of this care was undertaken by old or newly established religious orders on the wave of the movement of the Counter-Reformation. This is what Foucault has called "the era of confinement," namely the trend toward institutionalizing all those socially deviant, afflicted by physical handicaps, retardation, delinquency, or mental disease. This attitude, completely opposed to the previous one of considering misery in the realm of the divine conception of the world, carried in itself a puritanical mark and was particularly evident in countries, like France, where the monarchic regime was strong. In Italy, then divided into many states under Papal, French, Spanish, or Austrian auspices, there were great geographical variations in the care of the mentally ill. In some places, the influence of the moral theology of St. Alphonsus de Liguori, which included also a role of counselling, not unlike the Jesuit casuistry, was particularly strong (262).

In Rome, at the Santa Maria della Pietà, the mentally ill were separated from the pilgrims and the paupers and special separate quarters were built for men and women in 1726, when the institution was placed under the auspices of the *Ospedale del Santo Spirito*. In Florence, through the dedication of some clergymen and of a purposely established body, the institute of *Santa Dorotea* was allocated to mental patients and a section of the *Ospedale di Santa Maria Nuova* began to accept mentally ill patients in the 17th century. Around the same time, a home for abandoned and delinquent children was founded there (215). In Reggio Emilia, in 1754, the Duke Francesco III d'Este decided that the *Ospizio di San Lazzaro* be exclusively devoted to the care of the mentally ill (Plate VII). In Turin, King Vittorio Amedeo II opened, in 1727, the *Ospedale dei Pazzerelli*, essentially under the supervision of a group of laymen. In Bologna, a religious body opened a section for mental patients near the *Ospedale di Sant'Orsola*, in 1710. It is here that the anatomist Antonio Maria Valsalva (1666-1723), the teacher of Morgagni, abolished violent coercion and introduced a more lenient attitude in the treatment of the mentally ill (23, 198). An even more enlightened attitude was introduced by Daquin at the mental hospital of Chambéry, in the Alpine region of Savoy, which then belonged to the Kingdom of Sardinia. Joseph Daquin (1733-1815), a graduate of the medical school of Turin, became superintendent of Chambéry Hospital in 1787 and there initiated reforms in the care of the mentally ill which anticipated the so-called moral treatment" of the succeeding century. He illustrated his method of treatment in his *Philosophie de la Folie* (1791) (58) which contains interesting observations mixed with old-fashioned beliefs, like the influence of the moon on mental disorders (87, 178, 218).

The events just mentioned are related to the second half of the 18th century. By that time, the Enlightenment was flourishing in France and in England, as typically represented by the work of Montesquieu and Locke. The Enlightenment was not uniformly acknowledged in Italy, mainly because of the political fragmentation which limited the communication of ideas to small areas (162). Yet, it is well represented by *Scienzia Nuova* by Giambattista Vico (1668-1744), which anticipated many notions of dynamic psychology (72), or by *On Crimes and Punishments* (1764) (13) by Cesaria Beccaria (1739-1794), in which modern ideas against the death penalty were first presented (153). Material more relevant to psychopathology has been found in some of the writings of the historian Ludovico Antonio Muratori (1672-1750). In his book *On the Power of Human Fantasy* (1745) (170) he described fantasy, not unlike Aristotle's *sensorium commune,* as being halfway between external senses and intellect.

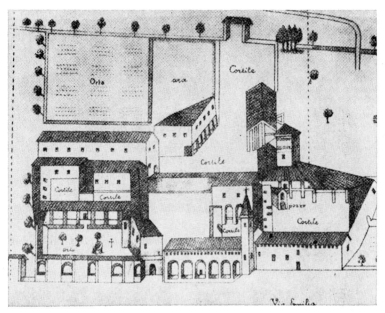

PLATE VII. Sketch representing the Hospice of San Lazzaro, in Reggio Emilia (originally built in 1217 for lepers and epileptics), as it was in the 17th century. At that time, like the "hôpital general" in France, it housed all kinds of social outcasts, such as handicapped, retarded, delinquent, and mentally ill.

During sleep, fantasy is influenced by dreams, which reflect bodily urges, even of genital origin; during waking hours fantasy is likewise influenced by passions. Moreover, in dreams, like in insanity, the individual is not responsible for his own actions. While dreams were still attributed by Muratori to the action of pathological humors, ecstasies and other unusual expressions were viewed purely as psychological phenomena which had to be carefully studied by theologians and physicians to avoid the aberrations of the witchcraft mania (19, 212, 244, 245).

Despite their anticipation of modern concepts, these various works are still somewhat peripheral to the core of psychiatry when compared to the reforms in the treatment of mentally ill which took place in Florence at the end of the 18th century. Such reforms can be understood only in the context of the contemporary Enlightenment sponsored by the Lorraine dynasty in France and the scientific and cultural atmosphere encouraged by the Medicis (53, 148) in Florence. There, since the middle of the 17th century, a small number of mental patients were housed in Santa Dorotea. As a part of the comprehensive program of economic, judicial, political, and educational reforms introduced by the Grand Duke Pietro Leopoldo (1747-1792) (248), the mentally ill were taken into consideration. On January 24, 1774, a pioneering piece of legislation, the "law on the insane," was passed to regulate the procedure for the commitment of mentally sick people to hospital. In 1788, the hospital of Bonifazio, for about 120 patients, was opened and the young physician Vincenzo Chiarugi (1759-1820) (Plate VIII) was appointed superintendent (55). In the *Regulations* of the hospital published the following year (199), he explicitly stated that mental patients should be given humanitarian care, restraint should be kept to a minimum, physicians should visit the wards daily, and a program of recreation and work should be initiated (Plate IX).

In 1793-1794 Chiarugi's three-volume work *On Insanity* appeared (44). In it, he made an attempt to present human psychology as based on Aristotelian-Tomistic and Cartesian views, without disregarding Platonic influences, revealing the shift of emphasis from the philosophical to the scientific characteristic of his time. According to Chiarugi, the *sensorium commune,* which is the point of confluence of the various sensations, is the mediating organ between body and soul; everything experienced by the soul has an emotional undertone; the soul is unalterable in its substance and cannot be affected by disease; insanity, though caused by psychological events such as passions, eventually causes impairment in the physical structure of the brain. Chiarugi accepted William Cullen's division of insanity into three main categories: melancholia (true, false or violent), a "fixation of the mind on one or few distorted ideas, while the other intellectual functions remain untouched"; mania, a "generalized insanity accompanied by violent and impetuous actions"; and dementia, a "general insanity characterized by abnormal actions of both the intellect and the will, performed without any show of emotions." Causes of insanity included congenital and acquired factors and, among the latter, preeminence was given to environmental forces because "through education a man's character is molded, his senses develop, and even his inclinations may be modified." To reach a diagnosis, it is important to consider the "external signs and the general phenomena which accompany insanity"

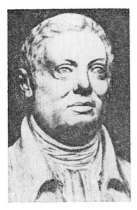

PLATE VIII. Vincenzo Chiarugi (1759-1820), director of the mental hospital of Bonifazio in Florence.

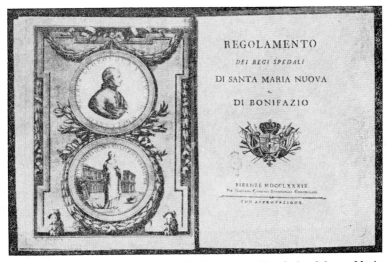

PLATE IX. Title page of the "Regulations of the Hospitals of Santa Maria Nuova and of Bonifazio," 1789, in which Chiarugi introduced a reform in the treatment of mental patients which anticipated the so-called "moral treatment" later developed in France and England.

and to be aware of the cyclical pattern which is often presented by many psychiatric conditions. Conditions due to acute or physical causes have a better prognosis than long-term conditions, especially if these latter are associated with inappropriate education.

Chiarugi's main contribution to psychiatry, however, lies in his reform of the treatment of mental patients. As he put it, "It is a supreme moral duty and medical obligation to respect the insane individual as a person." "It is especially necessary for those who treat the mental patient to gain his confidence and trust. It is best, therefore, to be tactful and understanding and try to lead the patient to the truth and to instill reason in him little by little, in a kind way." "The attitude of nurses and doctors must be authoritative and impressive, but at the same time pleasant and adapted to the impaired mind of the patient. Generally, it is better to follow the patient's inclinations and give him as many comforts as is advisable from a medical and practical standpoint. It is absolutely forbidden to make patients work for the hospital, except by a special prescription of the physician, in cases where certain activities are indicated as a form of therapy or relief." In addition to this, other important points were spelled out in detail in his writings. A detailed history obtained from the patient and his relatives was gathered in each case. High hygienic standards were prescribed for the hospital. The characteristics of the rooms and furniture were conceived of in such a way to offer maximal comfort and protection to the patients. Even more important is the statement that, under no circumstances, could force be used on the patients. The only methods of restriction allowed were straitjackets and strips of reinforced cotton, that would not impair the patient's blood circulation.

Interestingly, Chiarugi—a follower of Morgagni—was convinced that the highest merit of his work rested in the one hundred anatomo-pathological reports of brains of mental patients; today these reports are of little value. He was not aware of the importance of his reform of treatment of the mentally ill, which he described in a very un-assuming way. This explains why, at variance with Pinel's *Traité médico philosophique sur la manie,* published a few years later (1801), he did not include in his book an historical sketch on the development of psychiatry, though he was quite familiar with the previous literature in the field. Moreover, his book, written in the rather difficult Italian of the time, was probably published on a small scale and was a bibliographical rarity. It is even more important that Florence was at that time the capital of one of the many states in which Italy was divided and the reforms occurring there under the influence of the Grand Duke, an expression of the waning enlightened absolutism, were of short and limited nature. This was at variance with Pinel's reforms initiated in Paris, during the highest peak of the Revolution, in a country whose language was then universally known in cultural and scientific circles and whose political ideas led to the foundation of modern democracy. Also, the movement for the kind treatment of mental patients introduced by William Tuke at the *Retreat* in York, England, in 1796, was more fortunate, inasmuch as it was an expression of the Quaker church and it had the support of the stable English regime; from it originated the American tradition of "moral treatment." Because of these and other factors, until recently Chiarugi has not been given proper credit as a pioneer in the reform of the treatment of the mentally ill (155, 158, 181, 243). This has resulted in a controversy, at time acrimonious, between a few Italian psychiatrists and others on whether Chiarugi or Pinel pioneered these reforms (105, 182). Today, from a broad perspective, the reforms initiated by Chiarugi, Pinel, and Tuke can be seen as an expression of the same spirit of the age, although in each the emphasis was different: Chiarugi's work is to be seen against the background of the "ancient regime," Pinel's work in the context of the new democratic society, Tuke's work in the perspective of a religious humanitarian movement.

6

THE 19TH CENTURY

Chiarugi's reforms took place at the very end of the 18th century and were not continued by his followers, even in Florence. In the first part of the 19th century, the unfortunate political situation in Italy contributed to the relatively backward state of psychiatry in comparison with France, England, and the United States: in the north the power was divided between the conservative and mountainous kingdom of Savoy in the west and, in the east, the Austrian province, administratively well organized but, in effect, repressive; in central Italy, except for Tuscany, where the enlightened tradition still persisted, the various regions were poorly administered by the Church; in the south, the Bourbons continued the passive and backward regime initiated by the Spaniards a century before, except for a few isolated groups of intellectuals. The struggle to achieve national autonomy, the *Risorgimento*, exhausted most of the energy of the best people and resulted in revolutions and wars on many fronts. It is no wonder that, in such circumstances, science and medicine, in particular, could hardly progress. Thus Italian psychiatry was left far behind the brilliant clinical French school and the important movement of moral treatment and of legal psychiatry in England and in the United States. Even in Germany, then also divided into many states, the two opposed psychiatric trends respectively based on the psychological and on the anatomopathological etiology of mental diseases anticipated many later concepts. This was not the case in Italy, which was then mainly influenced by the French culture. In medicine, the attention was focused on the great controversy elicited by John Brown's theory of stimulus and counter-stimulus; in psychology, Condillac's sensism prevailed, while mesmerism had a very small following. However, in psychiatry, the reforms instituted in Paris eventually influenced Italy, too; Pinel's book was translated in 1830 and Esquirol's ample treatise in 1846.

As an expression of the Neapolitan Enlightenment, Antonio Sementini (1743-1814), a physician of the *Grande Ospedale degli Incurabili*, wrote on insanity at the age of 21. In his short treatise this disease is attributed to brain pathology, while environmental influences are not disregarded (219). Later, Luigi Ferrarese (1795-1855), active at the mental hospital of Aversa, near Naples, wrote two books on mental diseases in 1830 and 1841 (80, 120). Aversa's hospital had been founded in 1813, during the two years (1813-1815) in which southern Italy was governed by Napoleon's brother-in-law, Gioacchino Murat, who introduced many liberal legal, educational and economic ideas brought to the fore by the French Revolution (204). Giovanni Maria Linguiti (1773-1825), the first lay superintendent of the hospital, published a book on mental diseases in 1812 (130) and introduced humanitarian principles there. Interestingly, the practice of electrotherapy for the mentally ill was used in Naples for several years with apparent success (203). Most of the famous physicians—such as J. P. Frank (95), Esquirol (74), Valentin (241), Brierre de Boismont (30), Guislain (108)—and other well known people who visited the hospital during the early part of the century left very favorable descriptions of it, with the exception of a critical report by Domenico Gualandi, who was then director of the hospital of Saint Orsola in Bologna (106). After a short period of decline, Aversa's hospital was to flourish again during the second part of the 19th century, as described later (37, 197).

During the same period, the mental hospital of Palermo, Sicily, was experiencing a period of enlightened reforms under the leadership of a layman, Baron Pietro Pisani (1760-1837). Already known for his philanthropic work, at the age of 64 (coincidentally, the same age at which William Tuke initiated his reform at York), Baron Pisani opened in Palermo, in 1824, the *Real Casa de Matti*, an institution for the mentally ill. In less than three years, he abolished the systems of restraint then in use and in his *Istruzioni* (1827) (194) outlined the program of reforms which he partially developed in the following years. On admission, each patient underwent a period of observation, during which a history was obtained from him and from his relatives;

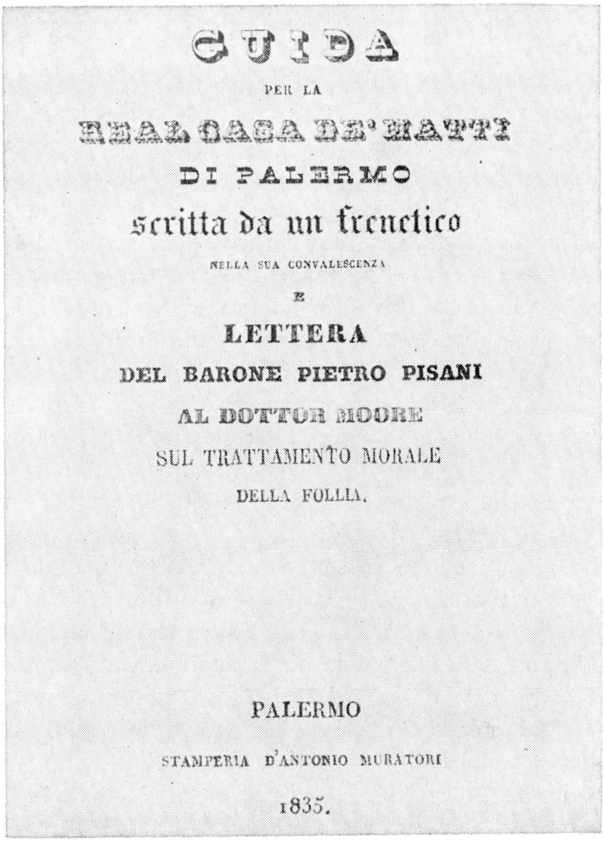

GUIDA

PER LA

REAL CASA DE' MATTI

DI PALERMO

scritta da un frenetico

NELLA SUA CONVALESCENZA

E

LETTERA

DEL BARONE PIETRO PISANI

AL DOTTOR MOORE

SUL TRATTAMENTO MORALE

DELLA FOLLIA.

PALERMO

STAMPERIA D'ANTONIO MURATORI

1835.

PLATE X. Title page of the "Guide to the mental hospital of Palermo written by a convalescent patient," probably a unique case in the 19th century psychiatric literature. That hospital was founded and run by Baron Pietro Pisani (1763-1837), who added in this booklet a description of his method of treatment of mental patients directed to a Dr. Moore of England.

this was followed by a staff conference. The superintendent, assisted by nurses and attendants, was directly responsible for the treatment of each patient. This consisted of a combined program of support and friendship and of manual work in the country, while attempts were made by the personnel to change the patient's thoughts from pathological to normal. Patients had a considerable role in the institution; for instance, a brochure describing its philosophy was prepared by them and distributed to each new patient (107) (Plate X). When an inmate became violent he was firmly tied to a hammock and rocked back and forth until he fell asleep. This very brief description of Pisani's reforms shows that he should have obtained a permanent place in the history of psychiatry. In spite of the very favorable reports left on his institution by Morel (163) and, especially, by the Germans Mandt, Rust (112) and Güntz (109), he was entirely forgotten after his death during the cholera epidemics of 1837 (159).

Coming back to Naples, Biagio Miraglia (1814-1885), a patriot, a literary man, and a psychiatrist, was nominated physician of the mental hospital of Aversa in 1843. In that same year, he founded the first Italian psychiatric periodical (184), followed by a new classification of mental diseases, a project for a model mental hospital (1847) and a treatise on phrenology (1854) (150), a doctrine to which he remained faithful throughout his professional career. Miraglia, in 1860, founded another psychiatric journal, a year later the Italian Psychiatric Association (*Società Frenopatica Italiana*), and three years later the chair of psychiatry at the University of Naples (151, 152, 157). However, Miraglia is most remembered for the first systematic attempt to encourage mental patients to present well-known dramas on the stage (an early anticipation of modern psychodrama); for this he was greatly admired by many contemporaries, including Alexander Dumas, father (156). Another outstanding Italian phrenologist was Giovanni Antonio Fossati (1786-1874), who assisted Gall in Paris for many years and published a handbook of phrenology in Paris in 1845 (92).

While all this was happening in Southern Italy, in the north some progress in the field of psychiatry was being made, both in the Kingdom of Savoy and in the two regions of Milan and Venice, which won independence from Austria in 1859, followed in the next year by the establishment of the Kingdom of Italy under Victor Emmanuel II of Savoy. In Turin, Benedetto Trompeo, before his nomination to superintendent of the newly-built mental hospital, in 1834, had already published (1830) a statistical work on mental diseases, the first of this kind in Italy (237). He was followed, in 1849, by Giovanni Stefano Bonaccossa (1804), who, after having visited many mental hospitals in Europe, introduced progressive reforms in Turin, revised the legislation regarding the commitment of the mentally ill and their imputability in criminal courts and introduced compulsory teaching of psychiatry in the medical school of Turin (the first in Italy) in 1850 (185) (Plate XI).

In Milan, Andrew Verga (1811-1895), whose works were gathered in three ponderous volumes in 1896-1897 (246), introduced reforms in the treatment of the mentally ill at the mental hospital of Senavra (1848-1851) and then at the *Ospedale Maggiore di Milano* (1851-

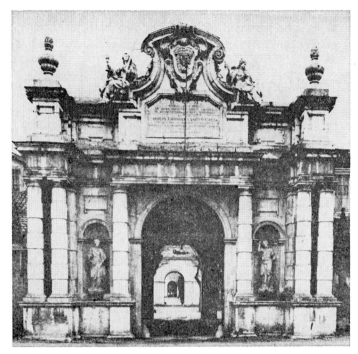

PLATE XI. Main entrance to the mental hospital of Collegno, near Turin. It was built in 1737 from an original drawing made by the famous architect Filippo Juvalta. The construction, called "Certosa" (because it housed monks, "Certosini"), was first occupied by mental patients in 1853.

1864), having served as superintendent in both hospitals. In 1852 he founded a psychiatric appendix to the periodical *Gazzetta Medica Italiana*, which lasted until 1864, when it was superseded by the *Archivio Italiano per le Malattie Nervose* (1864-1891) edited by Verga, Biffi, and Castiglioni. As an independent group branching off from the *Congressi degli Scienziati Italiani* (originated in Pisa, in 1839), Verga founded, in 1873, a national psychiatric organization, the *Società Freniatrica Italiana,* which met for the first time the following year under his presidency. That same year, he organized with Biffi a society in aid of mentally ill paupers (*Società di Patrocinio per i Pazzi Poveri*). Cesare Castiglioni (1808-1873), superintendent of the mental hospital of Senavra from 1851 to 1871, introduced there many improvements, such as occupational therapy, a school of music, and a theater. Serafino Biffi (1822-1899), whose works were published in five imposing volumes in 1902 (22), was superintendent for many years of the private hospital of Saint Celso in Milan; he became well known for the reports he prepared of his visits to mental institutions abroad and especially for his interest in institutions for correction for young men.

Elsewhere, Giuseppe Girolami in Pesaro and then Rome, and Francesco Bonucci in Perugia wrote treatises on mental diseases; many studies were published in the mid-century on the psychiatric aspects of pellagra and on those of cretinism, which were made the object of investigations by especially established commissions. Carlo Livi (1823-1877), superintendent first of the mental hospital of Siena and, then, in the last three years of his life, of that of S. Lazzaro near Reggio Emilia, in central Italy, founded there a valuable library and a laboratory, and in 1874 the *Rivista Sperimentale di Freniatria e di Medicina Legale,* which is still published today.

In the second part of the 19th century, the Italian school of psychiatry became increasingly influenced by German psychiatry, especially in regard to the predominance given by this latter, from Greisinger onward, to anatomo-pathology and histology in the etiology of mental disorders. The great histologist, Nobel prize winner Camillo Golgi (1843-1926), professor in Pavia, is especially remembered for his method of silver staining nervous tissue (1874) which carries his name (81, 193). Among others, A. Corti, A. Ruffini, and L. Luciani in the 20th century are to be remembered as representatives of the flourishing school of neurophysiology and neurohistology. In the same period, a number of textbooks and other important studies in psychiatry were translated into Italian from French, English, and especially German; among them were works by Broussais, Feuchtersleben, Weigandt, Schüle, Maudsley, Leidesdorf, Beard, Krafft-Ebing, Meynert, and others.

The number of mental hospitals had increased from 21, in 1840, to 35 in the 1870's, and to 50 in the 1880's. Of these about ten were private and the others state supported (187, 222). Most of them consisted of old buildings, only a few (Turin, Genoa, Macerata, Imola, Novara, and Mombello in Milan) having been purposely built as mental institutions. They were administered in a variety of ways, either by laymen or by physicians, and were often staffed by religious orders. Around 1865, it was calculated that the total number of institutionalized mentally ill was between 11,000 and 15,000. It was conceivable that there was also a great deal of difference in the methods of treatment from one institution to another. The hospital of Mombello was highly praised by contemporary visitors; the hospital of Reggio Emilia organized a society for the moral and material improvement of former patients; the same hospital and that of Ancona abolished external fences; at Reggio Emilia and at Macerata agricultural colonies were founded in the 1870's. Most of the institutions were located in the most progressive regions of Northern Italy and most of the inmates were in the 20 to 40 age group. The procedure for the commitment of a person consisted of two statements, one by a relative and one by a physician, accompanied by a report of the local authorities. The commitment became effective after a two-week period of observation.

As mentioned before, except for a few men and a few systematic programs of treatment, Italian psychiatry lagged behind that of other nations in the 19th century. Toward the end of that century, however, the movement in criminal anthropology originated in Italy and gave international renown to its adherents. The beginning of this movement was rather modest. At the mental hospital of Aversa, near Naples, Gaspare Virgilio (1836-1908) introduced important innovations when he was nominated superintendent in 1876 (7). In 1889, he opened there a hospital for criminally insane (*Manicomio Criminale*). For this and for his monograph on the pathological nature of crime (247) he was later called by Lombroso "the father of criminal anthropology." In the same period, Antonio Marro (1840-1912), was director of the mental hospital of Turin from 1890 to his death. He is especially known for his ample monograph on puberty (142).

The name most often associated with the movement of criminal anthropology is that of Cesare Lombroso (1836-1909). A prolific writer in the fields of legal medicine, anthropometry, criminality, and psychiatry, he spent most of his academic years in Turin, first as professor of legal medicine (1878), then of psychiatry (1896) and, finally, of criminal anthropology (1905); to this last field he devoted much energy, resulting in the foundation of an important museum. Like many of his contemporaries, he was influenced by the French positivists (Comte), the German materialists (Moleschott) and the English evolutionists (Darwin). Of his many books (131, 132, 133, 135, 136), particularly important are *The Delinquent Man* (1876), *The Female Offender* (1893), *The Legal Psychiatric Evaluation* (1905), in addition to his volumes on *Genius and Insanity* (1866, up to 6th edition in 1894) and *Genius and Degeneration* (1897). Yet, it is not easy to judge his work, for at least two main reasons: the continuous changes that he introduced in his concepts and the controversies and polemics in which he was involved until the end of his life (70, 88, 100, 104, 114, 119, 124, 134, 137, 192, 255, 260, 261). Today, his notions of the atavistic characteristics of the delinquents, of the generative theory of psychiatry, and of the degenerative epileptic-like nature of genius are considered

things of the past, although they bear relationship with modern formulations of creativity (161). Lombroso's main merit is his emphasis on
the study of the individual personality, which gave rise to an interest
in pathographies, a name coined by the German psychiatrist Möbius
to indicate psychopathologically oriented biographies. In Italy, pathographies were written by Roncoroni on Tasso (1896), by Niceforo
on Dante's *Inferno* (1898), by Portigliotti on Savonarola (1902) and
St. Francis (1910), by Mariani on Tolstoi (1903), by Bilancioni on
Luther (1926) and by Lugiato on Shakespeare (1926), Zola (1927),
Manzoni (1930), D'Annunzio (1931), as well as on some characters of
Greek tragedy (1932), and on the *Divine Comedy* (1935).

Lombroso's many pupils and sympathizers (whose writings frequently appeared in the journal *Archivio di Psichiatria, Antropologia
Criminale e Scienze Penali,* founded in 1880 by Lombroso, Garofalo,
and Ferri and published until 1937) constituted the so-called positive
school of criminology (*scuola positiva*), which focused on the biological and anthropological study of the individual delinquent and played
an important role in prevention, education, and rehabilitation, thus
anticipating the study of the individual personality undertaken later
by the psychodynamic schools (209). In opposition to the positive
school was the classical school of criminology, which held that the
greatest happiness of the greatest number was the primary objective
of punishment, and saw deterrence as the means of achieving this
condition. The issue was clouded by the allegiance of the followers of
the classical school to traditional Catholic belief, while the adherents
of the positive school often embraced socialistic ideas. Outstanding
among these was Enrico Ferri (1856-1929), a colorful criminal lawyer
and teacher (84, 210, 216), who wrote many books, among which
his *Criminal Sociology* was translated into English (82-85). In retrospect, it may be said that the Italian school of criminal anthropology
represented an innovating trend in an important area of psychiatry,
although biased by its allegiance to the positivistic school of
philosophy.

7

THE 20TH CENTURY

At the beginning of our century, psychiatry was in a rather complex
situation, which can be simplified in the following terms: a) the
criminal anthropological school, the only area of psychiatry in which

Italian scientists obtained international recognition, was still flourishing in many countries; however, signs of fatigue were already evident in this school, essentially due to the decline of positivism and materialism and to the rise of idealism in scientific and philosophical quarters; b) four decades after the establishment of the Kingdom of Italy in 1860, that country still presented (and the problem is still not solved today) a great deal of variability between different regions which reflected itself in the psychiatric services geared at improving the care of the mentally ill and at the fostering of the anatomo-pathological study of the nervous system; c) there was an initial interest on the part of a few young men in the scientific investigation of the psychological factors in mental disorders, especially after a school of experimental psychology was established by Giuseppe Sergi (1841-1936) in Rome with the opening of a laboratory in 1889 (221); he was preceded by a few others, among whom were Gabriele Buccola (1854-1885) and Ernesto Rignano (1870-1930), founder of the international journal *Scientia* and author of many books (200).

In the school of criminal anthropology, Lombroso's later pupils, such as Ferri, Antonio Labriola (1854-1904), Mario Carrara (1866-1931), Mariano Patrizi (1866-1935) (who succeeded Lombroso in Turin), Scipio Sighele (1868-1913), Guglielmo Ferrero (1871-1942) , and a few others represented the declining stage of this movement. In the first decade of our century, the strong influence of idealism in Italian philosophy, under the influence of Benedetto Croce (1866-1952), and Giovanni Gentile (1875-1944), had the effect of checking the development of criminal anthropology and of challenging even the development of clinical psychiatry, on the assumption that the psyche, being spirit, can never be objectivized, and thus does not belong under the category of science. Because of the political power of the idealistic school—especially as represented by Gentile during the Fascist regime —experimental psychology had a very hard time until the end of World War II. Less than two decades after the 5th International Congress of Psychology, held in Rome in 1905, most of the chairs of experimental psychology were eliminated. The illustrious school of special education founded in Rome by Maria Montessori (1870-1952), while flourishing abroad, met with difficulties in Italy, where it was opposed by the Fascist regime. Only a few laboratories and schools of psychology, with the exception of those in Milan and Rome (discussed later), managed to survive. Those surviving were in Florence under the leadership of Francesco de Sarlo (1864-1937), in Reggio Emilia under Giulio Cesare Ferrari (1868-1932), who founded the *Rivista di Psicologia* (1905-present) and translated James' *Principles of Psychol-*

ogy, and in Turin under Federico Kiesow (1858-1940), a German worker trained by Wundt, who in turn had a number of excellent pupils and founded the *Archivio Italiano di Psicologia* (1920-1942). However, experimental psychology remained isolated from clinical psychiatry (124a, 152a).

The 20th century opened with the passing of new legislation for the mentally ill in 1904, which still aimed at the protection of society rather than at the welfare of the patient. Livi's successor in Reggio Emilia was Augusto Tamburini (1848-1919) (227), who became also professor at the University of Modena and established a very important training center attended by many psychiatric academicians. In 1905, he became professor in Rome and, shortly before his death, he wrote with G. C. Ferrari and G. Antonini a very valuable volume on Italian and foreign psychiatry (228). Another important training center— whose history has been recently recounted by Emilio Padovani in a moving article (183)—was the mental hospital of Ferrara, also in central Italy, reorganized in 1873 by C. Bonfigli, who, in 1874, initiated the publication of an important Bulletin. From 1893 to 1930 the hospital was directed by Ruggero Tambroni (1855-1943) whose pupils—mainly Jacopo Finzi, Alberto Vedrani, Antonio D'Ormea, Marco Levi-Bianchini, Gaetano Boschi, and Emilio Padovani—attempted to introduce in Italy the new psychiatric concepts of Kraepelin, Kretschmer, and others, and founded, in 1902, the *Giornale di Psichiatria e Technica Manicomiale.* A third center notable for psychiatric research and training was that of Florence, where the professor of psychiatry from 1895 to 1931 was Eugenio Tanzi (1856-1934), well-known for his comprehensive treatises on mental diseases (1904) (233) and on forensic psychiatry (234), and for having founded the *Rivista di Patologia Nervosa e Mentale,* which is still published.

Other Italian psychiatrists whose work stretches into the beginning of our century, although belonging to the 19th century tradition, were Leonardo Bianchi (1848-1927), professor in Naples from 1890 to 1923, known for his studies on cerebral localizations in the prefrontal lobes and for his treatise on psychiatry (20); Enrico Morselli (1852-1929), professor in Turin and then Genoa, author of several works on hypnotism (166), psychopathology, anthropology, and clinical psychiatry, and of an important manual of psychiatric diagnosis (167); Giovanni Mingazzini (1859-1929), director of the psychiatric clinic in Rome (1921-1929), the only Italian neuropathologist to achieve international renown; Ernesto Belmondo (1863-1939) who fought for a long time for the passing of the 1904 law on mental hospitals and the mentally ill; Giuseppe Antonini (1864-1938), director for many years (1911-

1931) of the mental hospital of Mombello, near Milan, where he introduced many progressive ideas; finally, Ernesto Lugaro (1870-1940), who directed the psychiatric clinic of Turin from 1911 to his death and contributed to various fields of psychiatry.

As mentioned above, the only two centers where experimental psychology was cultivated, even during the Fascist regime, were in Rome and in Milan. In Rome, Sante de Sanctis (1862-1935), author of an early book on dreams (63), became professor of experimental psychology in 1906 and of neuropsychiatry in 1929. During this time, he published the important volumes on forensic psychiatry (67), on child psychiatry (65), and on experimental psychology (66), showing the fruitfulness of the application of psychology to clinical psychiatry. He established himself as a pioneer in the field of child psychiatry and, in 1908, described *dementia praecocissima,* a form of child schizophrenia (64); he was a remarkable teacher and an internationally recognized scientist (6). Also well known in Italy and abroad for his many studies and for his defence of the Catholic doctrine, first against the positivistic school and then the idealistic, as well as the psychodynamic schools, was the physician Father Augostino Gemelli (1878-1959), who founded the Catholic University of the Sacred Heart in Milan in 1919, where he established a well equipped laboratory of experimental psychology (141) and edited the *Archivio di Psicologia, Neurologia e Psichiatria* (1939-present), as well as a series of monographs on psychology (102, 152b). Particularly important among these latter are the two volumes by C. Fabro on the phenomenology of perception (75) and on perception and thought (76), in which modern psychological notions are discussed on the background of Catholic philosophy. Perusal of the survey of psychology in Italy written in 1940 by Gemelli and Banissoni shows, however, how little relevance this field had for psychiatry (12).

During the two decades of the Fascist regime, the tradition of Italian institutional psychiatry became obsolete. Very few new mental hospitals were built (e.g., that in Varese, near Milan); rather, new clinics were opened in connection with chairs of neuropsychiatry (in Rome, Milan, Genoa, and Bari), in which neurology dominated teaching and training, while psychiatry lost even the little prestige and autonomy acquired at the end of the 19th century. The number of hospitalized patients increased from 60,000 in 1926, to 100,000 in 1940, followed by a precipitous decline during World War II; however, on the positive side, the physician-patient ratio was about 1 to 150 and the ratio of nurses (mainly nuns) to patients was also high. During this period, more than in clinical psychiatry (with exception of the endocrinological-constitutional school, cultivated especially by Nicola Pende and pupils), some advances were made in fields close to psychiatry. Several orthophrenic schools, specifically psycho-pedagogical institutions for defectives and psychotic children (described by S. De Sanctis and G. Corberi), were opened near mental hospitals. In 1936 B. Di Tullio, professor of criminology in Rome, established there the first center for juvenile criminals. The National League for Mental Hygiene, formed in 1924, played a limited role. Undoubtedly, the scientific isolation of Italy during the four years (1914-1918) of World War I and during the 20 years (1923-1944) of Fascism was a major factor in limiting progress in psychiatry. Even the introduction of electric shock treatment by Ugo Cerletti (1877-1963) (Plate XII) and Lucio Bini (1908-1964) in Rome in 1938, soon hailed as a major advance in the therapy of psychoses (42), did not receive proper consideration; a group of 18 papers published in 1940 on the subject passed almost unnoticed (41). This discovery represented the zenith of the Italian trend of biological psychiatry, which received further impetus by the introduction of psychosurgery in Italy, by Fiamberti's "transorbital" techniques in the 1940's.

Psychoanalysis and other psychodynamic schools remained little known in Italy until very recently, as demonstrated in a thorough and well informed volume by Michel David (59). Putting aside the superficial slogans that in Italy—the country of sun, of Mediterranean sensuality, of uninhibited extroversion, and of the worship of the "Great Mother" (79)—deep psychology is not necessary, David has convincingly showed that four main factors can be identified as responsible for the resistance to psychoanalysis: 1) from the philosophical perspective, Lombroso's insistence on the hereditary aspect of the personality on the one side, and the idealists' devaluation of psychology as a science on the other; 2) from the political perspective, Fascism's fear of the possible liberal consequences of psychoanalysis, reinforced by Freud's analysis of dictatorship and by Italy's acceptance in the late 1930's of the Nazi anti-semitic attitude (which, on the other hand, in Italy hardly reached the level of persecution); 3) from the religious perspective, the materialistic and pan-sexualistic views mistakenly attributed to Freud by Catholic circles; 4) from the academic perspective, the violent opposition elicited in neuro-psychiatric departments of medical schools, which were then entirely controlled by the organicists. As David indicated, psychoanalysis was viewed as a Teutonic product during and after World War I (the psychiatrist Lugaro wrote an entire volume against German psychiatry during that war (139)), as a Jewish product during the period of Fascism's compliance to Nazi's anti-semitism and, finally, as an American product after World War II. In fact, for a few years (1908-1915) there was a certain interest in the scientific popularization of the new psychoanalytic concepts.

The next three decades (1915-1945) were characterized by opposition and criticism, as in the monograph published by E. Morselli in 1926 (169), but also by partial success: Vittorio Benussi (1878-1927) attempted to test experimentally psychoanalytic principles at the University of Padua (18); his pupil Cesare Musatti (1897-   ), today a leading Italian psychoanalyst, conducted a thorough study of this

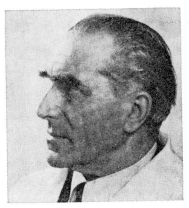

PLATE XII. Ugo Cerletti (1877-1963) who, together with Lucio Bini, introduced electric shock for the treatment of mental disorders in Rome in 1938.

field; Eduardo Weiss (1889-1971), a pupil of Freud and Federn, after a didactic analysis in Vienna (250), practised psychoanalysis first in Trieste and then in Rome, founded the Italian Psychoanalytic Society in 1925, published a compendium of psychoanalysis (249) and the *Rivista Italiana di Psicoanalisi* from 1932 to 1934, and eventually emigrated to the United States and practised in Chicago until his death; Marco Levi Bianchini (1875-1961) was instrumental in preparing some translations of Freud's works in the 1920's and published an almost forgotten, yet valuable, history of hysteria (129); Enzo Bonaventura (1891-1948) wrote an excellent monograph on psychoanalysis (26), praised by Freud himself. In the mid-1930's, it seemed that psychoanalysis had the possibility of some expansion in Italy, as evidenced, for instance, by a commemorative volume published on the occasion of Freud's 80th birthday (251); but World War II and the alignment of Fascism with Nazism in the persecution of the Jews put a quick end to this temporary interest in psychoanalysis.

During the war, Italy lost practically all contacts with the scientific world, in psychiatry as in other fields. The number of hospitalized patients decreased considerably and teaching and research declined, as well. A survey of Italian psychiatry carried out jointly by an American and an Italian in 1949 well depicted the gravity of the situation (127). By that time, however, some signs of a renewed interest in psychiatry were already noticeable, as pointed out in a comprehensive chapter on Italian psychiatry prepared by Cerletti in 1961 (43). Some workers, such as V. M. Buscaino in Naples, M. Gozzano and T. Bazzi in Rome, G. E. Morselli in Novara, as well as L. Longhi, V. Porta, A. Rubino, G. Fattovich, and C. Fazio, acquired a leading position similar to that already achieved by G. Boschi, E. Medea, L. De Lisi, G. B. Belloni, B. Disertori, G. Berlucchi, G. Moruzzi (in the field of neurophysiology), and others. In 1948, the Italian Society for Medico-Pedagogical Assistance to Retarded Minors was founded. Efforts were made to improve the teaching of psychiatry in medical schools (which eventually obtained independent status for neurology, first in Milan with G. L. Cazzullo and then elsewhere) and to establish a three-year postgraduate course in psychiatry (especially well organized in Milan and in Rome). In 1953, there were 85,000 patients in the 63 state-supported hospitals, in addition to 14 hospitals for the criminally insane. Aside from shock therapies, work therapy, and new treatment techniques, such as placement of patients in foster homes, were in use. Statistical data concerning ratio and type of mental diseases in Italy and comparison with the United States have appeared in the American literature (8, 206). The number of members of the Italian Psychiatry Society, which was 300 in 1949, continued to rise steadily and is more than 1,000 today. Regional and national conventions began to be organized regularly and some new journals were founded. Among them are *Medicina Psicosomatica,* edited by F. Antonelli, and *Infanzia Anormale* (which later became *Psichiatria Infantile*), edited by G. Bollea; both are published in Rome, where these two fields are particularly cultivated. Also, a number of psychiatric publications, including some on psychoanalysis and on psychotherapy, were translated into Italian, mainly from English. A comprehensive textbook of psychiatry was published by Bini and Bazzi (25).

The main difficulty, however, was the almost total absence of senior psychoanalysts or psychotherapists available for the training of young people. For a while, before emigrating to the United States, an Austrian-born psychoanalyst, Joachim Flescher, practised in Rome, where he wrote a book (90) and edited a journal. Also in Rome, N. Perrotti, E. Servadio (223) and a few others including the Jungian, E. Bernhard, have been active and have reorganized the Italian Psychoanalytic Society. By the mid-1950's about 20 psychoanalysts, including a number of lay analysts, were in practice in Italy, but the center of this movement slowly switched to Milan, where C. Musatti had gained wide renown for his several publications on Freud's concepts (171, 173, 174), including a thorough treatise of psychoanalysis (172), and for editing the *Rivista di Psicoanalisi* from 1955 on. In spite of the ambivalent attitude toward psychoanalysis maintained by Father Gemelli (101) following the more lenient attitude of Pope Pius XII, in 1952, considerable interest in psychoanalysis has been shown by Catholics in the last decade (3). L. Ancona, who succeeded Gemelli in Milan and who recently moved to the Catholic University in Rome, wrote a highly praised volume favorable to psychoanalysis (4).

By that time, the anthropological-existential trend had developed in Italy (38, 39), too, mainly supported by B. Callieri, F. Barison, and especially D. Cargnello (36), and translations of the relevant literature from the German became available. To this may be added the interest in some of the neo-Freudians and in the left-wing psychoanalysts such as W. Reich (265), as well as in the Pavlovian school, in which A. Massucco Costa (145, 146) showed interest. The most important works of Freudian psychoanalysts and of those of other psychoanalytic schools, which in the 1950's were made available in Italian translations, are now in the process of being presented in a more systematic fashion. Perhaps, more than in the clinical field, application of psychodynamic concepts to political problems (69, 91), to architecture (149), to art (especially films) (16), as well as to ethnology, has been a characteristic feature of the Italian scene. In the early 1960's, a group for the advancement of psychotherapy, *Gruppo Milanese per lo Sviluppo della Psicoterapia,* was founded in Milan, under the leadership of P. F. Galli and with the help of G. Benedetti, an Italian-born Swiss professor of psychiatry, well known for his contribution to the psychotherapy of schizophrenia and for an attempt to create a comprehensive synthesis of neurology and psychology (17). This group has promoted some important meetings, has founded a lively journal, *Psicoterapia e Scienze Umane,* has edited an important series of psychiatric classics, has raised the level of training in psychotherapy, and now aims at introducing dynamic concepts and forms of therapy into mental hospitals. As in other countries, in Italy the population in the mental hospitals has steadily decreased following the introduction of chemotherapy in the mid-1950's (in which the Italian school of psychiatry has shown considerable inteerst, because of its tradition of biological psychiatry) and other events, such as a more up-to-date legislation for hospitalized patients. However, the gap between the progressive university clinics and the old-fashioned state hospital persists to a certain extent. Likewise, a gap—to which P. F. Galli has recently called attention (164)— has been developing between a public increasingly well informed on contemporary psychiatric trends and most of the medical profession, which still adheres to the organic model of mental disturbances. In spite of all this, psychiatry, like any other field of science, is rapidly becoming internationalized under the spread of mass media of communication. This trend is already affecting Italy.

REFERENCES

(Some of the dates in the text do not match the dates in the references because in the text they refer to the first Italian edition, while in the references they refer to the first English translation.)

1. ALPHANDÉRY, P. (1929): De quelques documents médiévaux relatifs à des états psychasténiques. *J. Psychol. Norm. Path.*, 26, 763-787.
2. AMALDI, P. (1926): Vicende di nomi e di istituti manicomiali. *Riv. Storia Sci. Med. Nat.*, 17, 49-71.
3. ANCONA, L. (Ed.), AVTFB)s *Dinamismi normali e patologici* (Atti del Symposium sui rapporti tra psicologia e psichiatria). Milano: Vita e Pensiero.
4. ANCONA, L. (1963): *La psicoanalisi.* Brescia: La Scuola.
5. ANTONINI, G. (1900): *I precursori di Lombroso.* Bocca: Torino.
6. APPICCIAFUOCO, R. (1946): *La psicologia sperimentale di Sante De Sanctis.* Roma: Orsa Maggiore.
7. ARCIERI, G. P. (1952): Gaspare Virgilio. In *Figure della medicina contemporanea italiana.* Milano: Bocca.
8. ARIETI, S. (1959): Some socio-cultural aspects of manic-depressive psychosis and schizophrenia. *In Progress in Psychotherapy.* Vol. IV (Masserman, J. H., Ed.) New York: Grune & Stratton.
9. ASTURARO, A. (1887): Girolamo Cardano e la psicologia patologica. *Riv. Filos. sci.*, 7, 720-742.
10. BAADER, G. (1967): Zur Terminologie des Constantinus Africanus. *Med Hist. J.*, 2, 36-53.
11. BALTRUSAITIS, J. (1957): *Aberrations, Quatre essais sur la légende des formes.* Paris: Perrin.
12. BANISSONI, F. & GEMELLI, A. (1940): Psicologia. In: *Antropologia e psicologia.* Landra, G., Gemelli, A. and Banissoni, F., (Eds.) (Enciclopedia scientifica monografica italiana del ventesimo secolo, Serie II, N. 3). Milano: Bompiani.
13. BECCARIA, C. (1819): *An Essay on Crimes and Punishments.* Eng. Trans. Philadelphia: Nicklin. (Repr. Academic Reprints, Stanford, Cal. 1953).
14. BELLINI, A. (1947): *Gerolamo Cardano e il suo tempo (sec. XVI).* Milano: Hoepli.
15. BELLONI, L. (Ed.), (1963): *Per la storia della neurologia italiana* (Atti del Simposio internazionale di storia della neurologia, Varenna, 30. VIII/I.IX, 1961). Milano: Istituto di Storia della Medicina, (Studi e Testi, 6).

16. BELUFFI, M. (1969): *Cinema d'arte, Alienazione psicoterapia*. Bologna: I Mulino.
17. BENEDETTI, G. (1969): *Neuropsicologia*. Milano: Feltrinelli.
18. BENUSSI, V. (1932): *Suggestione e psicanalisi*. Messina: Principato.
19. BERTOLANI DEL RIO, M. (1951): Fantasia, delirio e pazzia nel concetto di L. A. Muratori. *Miscellanea di Studi Muratoriani*, Modena: Aedes Muratoriana.
20. BIANCHI, L. (1904): *Trattato di psichiatria*. Napoli: Idelson.
21. BIANCHI, Q. (1894-1897): Giambattista Della Porta e l'antropologia criminale nei secoli XVI e XVII. *L'anomalo* (Napoli), 6, 97-116; 209-222; 7, 15-21; 46-54; 83-88.
22. BIFFI, S. (1902): *Opere complete*. 5 vols. Milano: Hoepli.
23. BILANCIONI, G. (1913): Per una rivendicazione italiana. I precursori di Pinel. (Valsalva). *Riv. Stor. Crit. Sci. Med. Nat.*, 2, 75-79.
24. BILLOD, E. (1884): *Les aliénés en Italie*. Paris: Masson.
25. BINI, L. & BAZZI, T. (1963-1967): *Trattato di Psichiatria*, 3 vols. Milano: Vallardi.
26. BONAVENTURA, E. (1938): *La psicoanalisi*. (2nd. ed., 1945). Milano: Mondadori.
27. BONOMO, G. (1959): *Caccia alle streghe. La credenza nelle streghe dal secolo XIII al XIX con particolare riferimento all'Italia*, Palermo: Palumbo.
28. BONUZZI, L. (1969): Dalla follia alla malattia mentale: il contributo psichiatrico di Gerolamo Cardano. *Ann Freniat.*, 82, 7-33.
29. BOUCHET, A. (1957): Jean-Baptiste Porta et la physiognomie aux XVIe et XVIIe siècles. *Cah. Lyon. Hist. Med.*, 4, 13-42.
30. BRIERRE DE BOISMONT, A. (1830): Des établissements d'aliénés en Italie. *J. Compl. Sc. Méd.*, 43, 225-49; 44, 162-82.
31. BUCCOLA, G. (1883): *La legge del tempo nei fenomeni del pensiero*. Milano: Dumoland.
32. BURCKHARDT, J. (1929) *The Civilization of the Renaissance in Italy*. Eng. Trans. New York: Harper.
33. BURSTEIN, S. R. (1949): Aspects of psychopathology of old age revealed in witchcraft cases of the sixteenth and seventeenth centuries. *Brit. Med. J.* 6, 63-72.
34. CAELIUS AURELIANUS (1950): *On Acute Diseases and On Chronic Diseases*. Eng. Tr. Chicago: Univ. Chicago Press.
35. CARDAN, J. (1930): *The Book of My Life*. Eng. Trans. New York: Dutton. (Repr. New York, Dover, n.d.).
36. CARGNELLO, D. (1961): *Dal naturalismo psicoanalitico alla fenomenologia antropologica della Daseinsanalyse. Da Freud a Binswanger*. Roma: Istituto di Studi Filosofici.
37. CASCELLA, F. (1913): *Il R. Manicomio di Aversa nel 1. centenario della fondazione*. Aversa: Noviello.
38. CASTELLI, E. (Ed.), (1952): *Filosofia e psicopatologia*. Milano: Bocca.
39. CASTELLI, E. (Ed.), (1961): *Filosofia della alienazione e analisi esistenziale*. Padova: Cedam.
40. CASTIGLIONI, A. (1946): *Adventures of the Mind*. Eng. Trans. New York: Knopf. (Orig. Italian: *Incantesimo e Magia*. Milano: Mondadori, 1934).
41. CERLETTI, U. (1940): L'elettroshock. *Riv. sper. Freniat.*, 120 ff. (various articles).
42. CERLETTI, U. (1950): Old and new information about electroshock. *Amer. J. Psychiat.*, 107, 87-94.
43. CERLETTI, U. (1961): Italy. In *Contemporary European Psychiatry*. (Bellak, L., Ed.) New York: Grove.
44. CHIARUGI, V. (1793-4): *Della pazzia in genere e in specie trattato medico-analitico*. 3 vols. Firenze: Carlieri; 2nd ed. Firenze: Pagani, 1804 (only 1st vol.); Germ. Trans. *Abhandlung über den Wahnsinn*, Leipzig, 1795 (abridged ed.).

45. CHOISNARD, P. (1926): *Saint Tomas d'Aquin et l'influence des astres*. Paris: Alcan.
46. CLEBSCH, W. A. & JAEKLE, C. R. (1964): *Pastoral Care in Historical Perspective*. Englewood Cliffs: Prentice-Hall.
47. COCCHIARA, G. (1941): *Giuseppe Pitré e le tradizioni popolari*. Palermo: Ciuni.
48. COCCHIARA, G. (1945): *Il diavolo nella tradizione popolare italiana*. Palermo: Palumbo.
49. COCCHIARA, G. (1954): *Storia del folklore in Europa*. Torino: Einaudi.
50. COCCHIARA, G. (1956): *Il paese di cuccagna*. Chap. 6. Torino: Einaudi.
51. COHN, N. (1957): *The Pursuit of the Millennium*. New York: Essential Books.
52. CONSTANTELOS, D. J. (1968): *Byzantine Philanthropy and Social Welfare*. New Brunswick, N. J.: Rutgers Univ. Press.
53. CORSINI, A. (1954): La medicina alla corte di Pietro Leopoldo. *Riv. Ciba*, 8, 1510-1540.
54. COSTANTINO L'AFRICANO, (1959): *Della melancolia*. Roma: Istituto di Storia della Medicina dell 'Universitá.
55. COTURRI, E. (1959): L'ospedale cosi detto "di Bonifazio" in Firenze, *Pagine Storia Med.*, 3, 15-33.
56. CREUTZ, R. U. W. (1932): Die "Melancholie" bei Konstantinus Africanus und seinen Quellen. *Arch. Psychiat. Nervenkr.*, 97, 244-269.
57. DALMA, G. (1956): Leonardo precursore della psicofisiologia e psicologia dinamica moderna. *Nevrasse*, 6, 231-253.
58. DAQUIN, J . (1791): *Philosophie de la folie*. Chambéry.
59. DAVID, M. (1966): *La psicoanalisi nella cultura italiana*. Torino: Boringhieri.
60. DELAUNAY, P. (1928): De la physiognomie à la phrénologie, *Le progrès médical*, No. 29, 1207-1211; No. 30, 1237-1251; No. 31, 1279-1290.
61. DE MARTINO, E. (1961): *La terra del rimorso. Contributo a una storia religiosa del Sud*. Milano: Ill Saggiatore.
62. DENIEUL-CORMIER, A. (1956): La très ancienne physiognomie de Michel Savonarole. *Biol. Med.*, 45 (numéro hors série).
63. DE SANCTIS, S. (1899): *I Sogni. Studi psicologici e clinici*. Torino: Bocca.
64. DE SANCTIS, S. (1906): Sopra alcune varietá della demenza precoce. *Riv. sper. Freniat.*, 32, 141-164 (Eng. trans.: On some varieties of dementia praecox. In *Modern Perspectives in International Child Psychiatry*. Howells, J. G. (ed.) New York: Brunner/Mazel, 1971.
65. DE SANCTIS, S. (1925): *La neuropsichiatria infantile*. Roma: Stock.
66. DE SANCTIS, S. (1929-30): *Psicologia sperimentale*. 2 vols. Roma: Stock.
67. DE SANCTIS, S. & OTTOLENGHI, S. (1909): *Trattato pratico di psicopatologia forense*. Milano: Vallardi.
68. DESRUELLES, M. & BERSOT, H. (1938): L'assistance aux aliénés chez les arabes du VIII aux XII siècles. *Ann. Méd. Psychol.*, 96, 689-709.
69. DI FORTI, F. (1971): *Le radici profonde della mafia*. Milano: Silva.
70. DI TULLIO, B. (1955): Cesare Lombroso, *Sci. Med. Ital.*, 4, 187-192.
71. DODDS, E. R. (1957): *The Greeks and the Irrational*. Berkeley: Univ. of California Press.
72. DOGANA, F. (1970): Il pensiero di G. B. Vico alla luce delle moderne dottrine psicologiche. *Arch. Psicol. Neurol. Psichiat.*, 31, 514-530.
73. EISSLER, K. R. (1961): *Leonardo da Vinci: Psychoanalytic Notes on the Enigma*. New York: Inter. Univ. Press.
74. ESQUIROL, E. D. (1826): Notes sur les aliénations comparées dans le royaume de Naples et les hôpitaux de Paris. *Acad. de Med.*, Sept. 5.
75. FABRO, C. (1941): *La fenomenologia della percezione*. Milano: Vita e Pensiero.
76. FABRO, C. (1941): *Percezione e pensiero*. Milano: Vita e Pensiero.
77. FACHINI, G. (1946): I nomi italiani. In: *Uomini contro la pazzia* Selling, L. S. Ital. Trans. Milano: Mondadori.

78. FAGGIN, G. (1959): *Le streghe.* Milano: Longanesi.
79. FERNANDEZ, D. (1965): *La mère méditerranée.* Paris: Grasset.
80. FERRARESE, L. (1832): *Delle malattie della mente.* Napoli.
81. FERRARO, A. (1953): Camillo Golgi (1843-1926). In: *The Founders of Neurology.* Haymaker, W. (Ed.). Springfield, Ill.: Thomas.
82. FERRI, E. (1917): *Criminal Sociology.* Boston: Little, Brown & Co.
83. FERRI, E. (1925): *L'omicida nella psicologia e psicopatologia criminale,* 5th ed. Torino: Utet.
84. FERRI, E. (1941): *Enrico Ferri maestro della scienza criminologica.* Torino: Scritti vari. Bocca.
85. FERRI, E. (1968): *The Positive School of Criminology. Three Lectures.* Grupp, S. E. (Ed.) Univ. of Pittsburgh Press, Pittsburgh.
86. FERRIO, C. (1948): *La psiche e i nervi. Introduzione storica ad ogni studio di psicologia, neurologia e psichiatria.* Torino: Unione Tipografico-Editrice Torinese.
87. FERRIO, L. JR. (1954): Un pioniere dell assistenza psichiatrica, Giuseppe Daquin. *Riv. Storia Sci. Med. Nat.,* 45.
88. FERRIO, L. (1962): *Antologia Lombrosiana.* Pavia: Societa' Editrice Pavese.
89. FILIPPONE, L. (1955): *Il substrato degli amuleti in Italia.* Napoli: Pironti.
90. FLESCHER, J. (1949): *Psicoanalisi della vita istintiva.* Roma: Scienza moderna.
91. FORNARI, F. (1964): *Psicanalisi della querra atomica.* Milano: Communità.
92. FOSSATI, J. (1845): *Manuel pratique de phrénologie.* Paris: Baillière.
93. FOUCAULT, M. (1965): *Madness and Civilization.* Eng. Trans. New York: Random House. (Abridged edition of *Histoire de la folie.* Paris: Plon, 1961.)
94. FRACASTORO, G. (1968): *La simpatia e l'antipatia della cose,* Ital. Trans. Roma: Cossidente.
95. FRANK, J. P. (1827): *Medizinische Polizei.* Leipzig, Suppl., Vol. III, p. 71.
96. FREUD, S. (1910): Leonardo da Vinci and a Memory of His Childhood. In: *The Complete Psychological Works of Sigmund Freud.* Vol. XI Standard Edition 1964. Strachey, J. et al. (Eds.). London: Hogarth Press and the Institute of Psycho-Analysis.
97. FUMAGALLI, G. (1952): *Eros di Leonardo.* Milano: Garzanti.
98. GALEN (1963): *On the Passions and Errors of the Soul.* Eng. Trans. Columbus, Ohio: Ohio State Univ. Press.
99. GARZONI, T. (1586): *L'hospedale de' pazzi incurabili.* Ferrara: Cagnacini. Eng. Trans. *The Hospital of Incurable Fools.* London: Bollifant 1600. Fr. Tr. *L'hospital des Fols Incurables,* Paris: Julliot 1620. Repr.: Marchionni, T. (Ed.). Lanciano: Carabba 1915; Senise, T. (Ed.). Napoli: Biblioteca de "Il Cerbello", 1953.
100. GEMELLI, A. (1911): *Cesare Lombroso,* 3rd ed. Firenze: Libreria Editrice Fiorentina.
101. GEMELLI, A. (1955): *Psychoanalysis Today.* Eng. Trans. New York: Kenedy.
102. GEMELLI, A. & ZUNINI, G. (1947): *Introduzione alla psicologia.* Milano: Vita e Pensiero.
103. GIANNULI, F. (1924-25): Il manicomio di Santa Maria della Pietà e la scuola neuro-psichiatrica romana. *Arch. Storia Sci.,* 5, 272-283; 6, 214-221; 331-346; 401-427.
104. GOLD, M. (1960): The early psychiatrists on degeneracy and genius. *Psychoanal. Psychoanal. Rev.,* 47, 37-55.
105. GRANGE, K. M. (1963): Pinel or Chiarugi. *Med. Hist.,* 7, 371-380.
106. GUALANDI, D. (1823): *Osservazioni sopra il celebre stabilimento d'Aversa nel Regno di Napoli.* Bologna: Masi.
107. *Guida per la Real Casa de Matti di Palermo scritta da un frenetico nella sua convalescenza.* 1835. Palermo: Muratori.
108. GUISLAIN, J. (1840): *Lettres médicales sur l'Italie.* Gan: Gyselynk.

109. Güntz, E. W. (1878): *Don Pietro Baron Pisani, der Vorläufer John Connollys.* Leipzig: Reklam.
110. Hamilton, M. (1906): *Incubation or the Cure of Diseases in Pagan Temples and Christian Churches.* London: Henderson.
111. Hemphill, R. E. (1966): Historical witchcraft and pychiatric illness in Western Europe. *Proc. roy. Soc. Med.* (Sect. Hist. Med.), 59, 891-901.
112. Hoffman, H. (1935): Ein Beitrag zur Geschichte der Psychiatrie. *Allg. Z. Psychiat.*, 103, 76-127 (On the description of Pisani's mental hospital in Palermo by the physicians M. N. von Mandt and J. N. Rust).
113. Hoffman, H. (1935): *Der Hexen und Besessenglaube des 15 und 16. Jahrhunderts im Spiegel des Psychiaters* (Arbeiten der deutsch-nordischen Gesellschaft für Geschichte der Medizin, N. 12). Greiswald: Universitätsverlag Bamberg.
114. Jeffery, C. R. (1959): The historical development of criminology. *J. Crim. Law. Criminol. & Police Sci.*, 50, 3-19 (Repr. In: *Pioneers in Criminology*, 1960. H. Mannheim (Ed.). Chicago: Quadrangle).
115. Katner, W. (1956): *Das Rätsel des Tarantismus, Eine Aetiologie der Italienischen Tanzkrankheit.* Nova Acta Leopoldina, n.s. 18, no. 124, Leipzig: Barth.
116. Kopp, P. (1933): Psychiatrisches bei der Scholastik. I. *Z. ges. Neurol. Psychiat.*, 147, 50-60.
117. Kopp, P. (1935): Psychiatrisches bei Thomas von Aquin. Beiträge zur Psychiatrie der Scholastik. II *Z. ges Neurol. Psychiat.*, 152, 178-196.
118. Krapf, E. E. (1943): *Tomas de Aquino y la psicopatologia.* Buenos Aires: Index.
119. Kurella, H. (1910): *Cesare Lombroso. A Modern Man of Science.* New York: Reban.
120. Lacava, M. (1890): *Luigi Ferrarese e le sue opere.* Napoli: Morano.
121. Laignel-Lavastine, M. & Vinchon, J. (1930): *Les malades de l'esprit et leurs médecins du XVI aux XIX siècles.* Paris: Maloine.
122. Lain Entralgo, P. (1970): *The Therapy of the Word in Classical Antiquity.* (Eng. Trans.) New Haven, Conn.: Yale Univ. Press.
123. Lanternari, V. (1963): *The Religions of the Oppressed. A Study of Modern Messianic Cults,* Eng. Trans. New York: Knopf.
124. Lattes, L. (1957): Retour à Lombroso. *Rev. Méd. Liège,* 12, 41-56.
124A. Lazzeroni, V. (1972): La psicologia scientifica in Italia. In: *Nuove Questioni di Psicologia.* Ancona, L. (Ed.). Brescia: La Scuola.
125. Lefebvre, J. (1968): *Les fols et la folie. Étude sur les genres de comique et la création littéraire en Allemagne pendant la Renaissance.* Paris: Klincksieck.
126. Leibbrand, W. (1959): Stoische Reliquien im geschichtlichen Gang der Psychopathologie. *Confin. Psychiat.*, 2, 1-18.
127. Lemkau, P. V. & De Sanctis, C. (1950): A survey of Italian psychiatry. *Amer. J. Psychiat.*, 107, 401-408.
128. Lessa, W. A. (1952): Somatomancy: precursor of the science of constitution. *Sci. Mon.*, 75, 355-365.
129. Levi Bianchini, M. (1913): *L'isterismo dalle antiche alle moderne dottrine.* Padova: Drucker.
130. Linguiti, G. M. (1812): *Ricerche sopra le alienazioni della mente umana.* Napoli.
131. Lombroso, C. (1864): *Genio e follia.* Milano: Chiusi.
132. Lombroso, C. (1876): *L'uomo delinquente.* Milano: Hoepli. (5th ed. Torino: Bocca, 1896-1897, 3 vols).
133. Lombroso, C. (1895): *The Female Offender.* London: Unwin.
134. Lombroso, C. (1906): *L'opera di Cesare Lombroso nella scienza e nelle sue applicazioni.* Torino: Bocca.
135. Lombroso, C. (1908): *Genio e degenerazione.* Palermo: Sandron.

136. LOMBROSO, C. (1913): *Crime: Its Cause and Remedies*. Boston: Little, Brown & Co.

137. LOMBROSO, FERRARO G. (1921): *Cesare Lombroso*, 2nd ed. Bologna: Zanichelli.

138. LUCAS-DUBRETON, J. (1954): *Le monde enchanté de la Renaissance. Jérome Cardan l'halluciné*. Paris: Fayard.

139. LUGARO, E. (1916): *La psichiatria tedesca nella storia e nell'attualitá*. Firenze: Topgrafia Galileiana.

140. MAFFEI, S. (1750): *Arte magica dileguata*. Verona: Carattoni.

141. MANOIL, A. (1938): *La psychologie expérimentale en Italie. Ecole de Milan*. Paris: Alcan.

142. MARRO, A. (1898): *La puberta' studiata nell'uomo e nella donna*. Torino: Bocca.

143. MARSILIO, FICINO (1964): *Il "De studiosorum sanitate tuenda."* Ital. Trans. Milano: Quaderni di Castalia N.10.

144. MARTIRE, E. (1934): *L'isola della salute. Dal tempio romano di Esculapio all'Ospedale di S. Giovanni di Dio*. Roma: Rassegna Romana.

145. MASSUCCO, COSTA (1963): *Psicologia sovietica*. Torino: Boringhieri.

146. MASSUCCO, COSTA A. (1968): *Storia della psicologia*. In: *Storia delle Scienze*. Abbagnano, N. (Ed.). Torino: Unione Tipografica Editrice Torinese.

147. MEIER, C. A. (1967): *Ancient Incubation and Modern Psychotherapy*. Eng. Trans. Evanston, Ill.: Northwestern Univ. Press.

148. MICCA, G. (1968): Medici ed organizzazione sanitaria alla Corte del Granducato di Toscana, sotto il governo di Pietro Leopoldo. *Minerva Med.*, 59, 2022-2026.

149. MIOTTO, E. (Ed.) (1966): *Aspetti sociopsicopatologici dell'architettura e dell'urbanistica*. Treviso: Societa'Industrie Tipografiche.

150. MIRAGLIA, B. (1853): *Trattato di frenologia*. 2 vols. Napoli. Ancora.

151. MIRAGLIA, B. JR. (1936): *Un alienista patriota. Biagio Miraglia*. Napoli: Scuola Tipografica Villa Russo.

152. MIRAGLIA, B. JR. (1960): Albori di assistenza psichiatrica nella Campania. *Ann. Neuropsichiat. Psicoanal.*, 7, 512-521.

152A. MISIAK, H. & STAUDT, V. M. (1953): Psychology in Italy. *Psychol. Bull.*, 50, 347-361.

152B. MISIAK, H. & STAUDT, V. M. (1954): Agostino Gemelli. In: *Catholics in Psychology. A Historical Survey*. New York: McGraw-Hill, 1954.

153. MONACHESI, E. (1955): Cesare Beccaria (1738-1894). *J. Crim. Law. Criminol. & Police Sci.*, 46, 439-449. (Repr. In: *Pioneers in Criminology*. 1960. Mannheim, H. (Ed.). Chicago: Quadrangle).

154. MONDINI, A. (1962): *Gerolamo Cardano*. Roma: Edindustria Editoriale.

155. MORA, G. (1954): Vincenzo Chiarugi (1759-1820). His contribution to psychiatry. *Bull. of Isaac Ray Medical Library*. (Butler Hospital, Providence, R. I.), 2, 50-104.

156. MORA, G. (1957): Dramatic presentations by mental patients in the middle of the nineteenth century and A. Dumas' description. *Bull. Hist. Med.*, 31, (260-277.

157. MORA, G. (1958): Biagio Miraglia and the development of psychiatry in Naples in the eighteenth and nineteenth centuries. *J. Hist. Med. Allied Sci.*, 13, 504-523.

158. MORA, G. (1959): Vincenzo Chiarugi (1759-1820) and his psychiatric reform in the late 18th century. *J. Hist. Med. Allied Sci.*, 14, 424-433.

159. MORA, G. (1959): Pietro Pisani and the mental hospital of Palermo in the early 19th century. *Bull. Hist. Med.*, 33, 230-248.

160. MORA, G. (1963): An historical and sociopsychiatric appraisal of tarantism and its importance in the tradition of psychotherapy of mental disorders. *Bull. Hist. Med.*, 37, 417-439.

161. Mora, G. (1964): One hundred years from Lombroso's first essay on "Genius and Insanity." *Amer. J. Psychiat.*, 121, 562-571.
162. Moravia, S. (1969): An outline of the Italian Enlightenment. *Comp. Lit.*, 4, 380-409.
163. Morel, F. (1864): Pathologie mentale en Italie. *Ann. Méd. Psychol.*, 7, 45-83.
164. Moreno, M. (1968): *Breve storia della psicoterapia.* Torino: Edizioni RAI.
165. Morley, H. (1854): *The Life of Girolamo Cardano, of Milan, Physician.* London: Chapman & Hall. 2 vols.
166. Morselli, E. (1886): *Magnetismo animale.* Torino: Roux e Favale.
167. Morselli, E. (1885-94): *Manuale di semeiotica delle malattie mentali,* 2 vols. Milano: Vallardi.
168. Morselli, E. (1920): Per la storia della psichiatria, Cento e piu' anni di conquiste della psichiatria. *Quad. Psichiat.*, 7, 229-236.
169. Morselli, E. (1926): *La psicoanalisi,* 2 vols. (3d. ed., 1944). Torino: Bocca.
170. Muratori, L. A. (1740): *Della forza della fantasia umana.* Venezia: Pasquali.
171. Musatti, C. L. (1949): *Freud.* Firenze: L'Arco.
172. Musatti, C. L. (1950): *Trattato di Psicoanalisi.* 2 vols. Torino: Einaudi.
173. Musatti, C. L. (1959): *Freud.* Torino: Einaudi.
174. Musatti, C. L. (1960): *Psicoanalisi e vita contemporanea.* Torino: Boringhieri.
175. Nardi, M. G. (1952): Marsilio Ficino, medico. *Minerva Med.*, 43, 898-914.
176. Nicolini, F. (1937): *Peste e untori nel "Promessi Sposi" e nella realta' storica.* Bari: Laterza.
177. Nulli, S. A. (1939): *I processi delle streghe.* Torino: Einaudi.
178. Nyffeler, J. R. (1961): *Joseph Daquin und seine "Philosophie de la Folie".* Luzern: Bucher.
179. O'Brien Moore, A. (1924): *Madness in Ancient Literature.* Weimar: Wagner.
180. Oppenheim, A. L. (1956): The interpretation of dreams in the ancient near East. *Trans. Amer. Phil. Soc.*, 46, 179-373.
181. Padovani, E. (1927): Pinel e il rinnovamento dell'assistenza agli alienati. I suoi precursori. I precedenti italiani: Giuseppe Daquin e Vincenzo Chiarugi. *G. Psichiat. Menic.*, 55, 69-124.
182. Padovani, E. (1957): Fortune e sfortune di Vincenzo Chiarugi. *Note Riv. Psichiat.*, 50, 394-397.
183. Padovani, E. (1966): Psichiatria eroica. *Neuropsichiatria*, 22, 1-32.
184. Padovani, G. (1946): *La stampa periodica italiana di neuropsichiatria e scienze affini.* Milano: Noepli.
185. Padovani, G. (1949): Gli inizi dell'insegnamento universitario della psichiatria in Italia e Stefano Bonacossa. *Rass. Studi psichiat.*, 38, 94-105.
186. Padovani, G. (1949): "L'Hospidale de' pazzi incurabili" di Tommaso Garzoni. *Rass. Studi Psichiat.*, 38, 217-299.
187. Pandy, K. (1908): *Irrenfürsorge in Europa. Eine vergleichende Studie.* Berlin: Reimer.
188. Parenti, F. (1966): *Dal mito alla psicanalisi. Storia della psichiatria.* Milano: Silva.
189. Pazzini, A. (1949): *Storia, tradizioni e leggende nella medicina popolare.* Correggio: Laboratorio Farmacologico Recordati.
190. Pazzini, A. (1950): Neuropsychiatry in Italy throughout the centuries. *Sci. Med. Ital.*, 1, 580-596.
191. Pazzini, A. (1951): *Demoni, streghe e guaritori.* Milano: Bompiani.
192. Perrando, G. G. (1943): Antropologia criminale. In: *Dizionario di Criminologia,* vol. I, 53-73. Florian, E., Niceforo, A. and Pende, N. (Eds.). Milano: Vallardi.
193. Pilleri, G. (1959): Camillo Golgi. In: *Grosse Nervenärzte.* Kolle, K. (Ed). Stuttgart: Thieme.
194. Pisani, P. (1827): *Istruzioni per la novella Real Casa de Matti in Palermo,* Palermo. (Germ. Trans., In: Güntz, E. W., Ref. 109 above.)

195. PORTA, G. B. (1586): *De Humana Psysiognomia*. Vico Equense: Cacchio.

196. *Processo Originale degli untori nella peste del 1630*. Milano, 1839.

197. PUCA, A. & ENSELMI, C. (1955): L'ospedale psichiatrico di S. Maria Maddalena (gia' Real Manicomio di Aversa). Cenni storici. *Rass. Neuropsichiat.*, 9, 1-84.

198. RAVANELLI, P. (1966): *A. M. Valsalva (1666-1723)*. *Anatomico, medico, chirurgo, primo psichiatra*. Imola: Galeati.

199. *Regolamento dei Regi Spedali di Santa Maria Nuova e di Bonifazio*. 1789. Firenze: Cambiagi.

200. RIGNANO, E. (1923): *Psychology of Reasoning*. Eng. Trans. New York: Harcourt Brace.

201. RIPAMONTI, G. (1945): *La peste di Milano del 1630*. Ital. Trans. Milano: Muggiani.

202. RIVARI, E. (1906): *La mente di Girolamo Cardano*. Bologna: Zanichelli.

203. ROMANO, A. (1901): L'elettroterapia e l'elettrobiologia nel secolo XVIII a Napoli. *G. Elett. Med.* 2, 251-269.

204. ROMANO, A. (1902): La seconda fase del pensiero psichiatrico nel secolo XVIII a Napoli e le sue conseguenze nella cura e governo dei folli. *Gli Incurabili* (Napoli), 17, 347-371.

205. RONCALI, D. B. (1929): *L'anatomico fisio-patologo crotoniate Alcmeone*. Napoli: Inag.

206. ROSE, A. M. (1964): The prevalence of mental disorders in Italy. *Int. J. Soc. Psychiat.*, 10, 87-100.

207. ROSEN ,G. (1968): *Madness in Society. Chapters in the Historical Sociology of Mental Illness*. Chciago: University of Chicago Press.

208. ROTH, G. (1961): Thomas von Aquin in der neuren und neuersten Psychiatrie. In: *Der Arzt in der Technischen Welt*. (IX Internationaler Kongress Katholischer Aerzte, München). Salzburg: Müller.

209. SANTORO, A. (1943): Scuola positiva. In: *Dizionario di Criminologia*, vol. 2, 893-902. Florian, E., Niceforo, A. and Pende, N, (Eds.). Milano: Vallardi.

210. SANTORO, A. (1943): Enrico Ferri. In: *Dizionario di Criminologia*, Vol. I, 360-367. Florian, E., Niceforo, A. and Pende, N. (Eds). Milano: Vallardi.

211. SCHAPIRO, M. (1956): Leonardo and Freud: An art-historical study. *J. Hist. Ideas*, 17, 147-178.

212. SCHIFF, P. (1947): Père Ludovico Antoine Muratori précurseur de Freud. *Presse Méd.*, 49, 562.

213. SCHIPPERGES, H. (1961): Der Narr und sein Humanum im islamischen Mittelalter.*Gesnerus*, 18, 1-12.

214. SCHIPPERGES, H. (1961): Zur Psychologie und Psychiatrie des Petrus Hispanus. *Confin. Psychiat.*, 4, 137-157.

215. SELLIN, T. (1926): Filippo Franci, a precursor of modern penology. *J. Crim. Law Criminol.*, 17, 104-112.

216. SELLIN, T. (1960): Enrico Ferri. In: *Pioneers in Criminology*. Mannheim, H. (Ed.). Chicago: Quadrangle.

217. SEMELAIGNE, A. (1869): *Études historiques de l'aliénation mentale dans l'antiquité*. Paris: Asselin.

218. SEMELAIGNE, R. (1930): Joseph Daquin. In: *Les pionniers de la psychiatrie française avant et après Pinel*. Vol. I. Paris: Ballière.

219. SEMENTINI, A. (1766): *Breve dilucidazione della natura e varietà della pazzia*. Napoli: Giaccio.

220. SERAO, F. (1750): *Della tarantula ovvero falangio di Puglia*. Napoli.

221. SERGI, G .(1873): *Principi di psicologia*. Messina.

222. SÉRIEUX, P. (1903): *L'assistance des aliénés en France, en Allemagne, en Italie et en Suisse*. Paris: Imprimerie Municipale.

223. SERVADIO, E. (1965): *Psychology Today*. Eng. Trans. New York: Garrett.

224. SIMILI, A. (1968): Il pensiero di Girolamo Cardano nella psichiatria, nell'antropologia criminale e nella sociologia. *Minerva Med.*, 59, 874-884.

225. STAHELIN, J. E. (1957): Zur Geschichte der Psychiatrie des Islams. *Schweiz. Med. Wschr.*, 87, 1152-1156.

226. SZASZ, T. S. (1970): *The Manufacture of Madness.* New York: Harper & Row.

227. TAMBURINI AUGUSTO (1848-1919): *In Memoria* (1920). Roma: Tipografia dell'Unione Editrice.

228. TAMBURINI, A. FERRARI, G. C. & ANTONINI, G. (1918): *L'assistenza degli alienati in Italia e nelle varie nazione.* Torino: Unione Tipografica Editrice Torinese.

229. TANFANI, G. (1931): Gli attributi somato-psichici del carattere anormale secondo Cardano. *Riv. Storia Sci. Med. Nat.*, 22, 433-440.

230. TANFANI, G. (1931): L'eugenetica di Girolamo Cardano. *Ill. Med. Ital.*, 13, 69-71.

231. TANFANI, G. (1948): Il concetto di melancholia nel Cinquecento. *Riv. Storia Sci. Med. Nat.*, 39, 145-170.

232. TANFANI, G. (1934): Le conoscenze neurologiche al tempo di Petro d'Abano (1250-1316). *G. Psichiat. Neuropat.*, 62, 180-196.

233. TANZI, E. (1904): *Trattato delle malattie mentali.* (3d. ed., with Lugaro, E., 1923). Milano: Societa'Editrice Libraria.

234. TANZI, E. (1911): *Psichiatria forense.* Milano: Vallardi.

235. TARTAROTTI, G. (1749): *Del congresso notturno delle lammie.* Rovereto: Pasquali.

236. TONNINI, S. (1892): Historical notes upon the treatment of insane in Italy. In: *A Dictionary of Psychological Medicine,* Vol. II, 715-720. Tuke, D. H. (Ed.). London: Churchill.

237. TROMPEO, B. (1830): *Prospetto statistico del R. Manicomio di Torino,* Torino.

238. UGOLOTTI, F. (1949): Panorama storico dell'assistenza ai malati di mente in Italia. *Note Riv. Psichiat.*, 65, 73-148.

239. UNGERN, STERNBERG, F. (1898): Sviluppo storico della psichiatria in Italia. In: Leidesdorf, M., *Trattato delle malattie mentali,* Ital. Trans. Torino: Loescher.

240. VALDIZAN, H. (1913): *Un psichiatra del secolo XVI (Tommaso Garzoni).* Roma: Vespasiani.

241. VALENTIN, L. (1826): *Voyage en Italie.* Paris: Gabon.

242. VALLON, C. & GENIL-PERRIN, G. (1912): *La psychiatrie médico-légale dans l'oeuvre de Zacchia (1584-1659).* Paris: Doin.

243. VEDRANI, A. (1892): Vincenzo Chiarugi. In: *Gli Scienziati Italiani.* Mieli, A. (Ed.). Roma: Nardecchia.

244. VEDRANI, A. (1922): Il trattato della forza della fantasia umana di L. A. Muratori. *Vita e Pensiero,* 8.

245. VEDRANI, A. (1927): Muratori psicologo e patologo. *Vita e Pensiero,* 13, 721.

246. VERGA, A. (1896-1897): *Studi anatomici sul cranio e sull'encefalo, psicologici e freniatrici,* 3 vols. Milano: Manini-Wiget.

247. VIRGILIO, G. (1874): *Osservazioni sulla natura morbosa del delitto.* Roma: Loescher. (Repr. 1910). Torino: Bocca.

248. WANDRUSKA, A. (1965): *Leopold II.* 2 vols. Wien: Herold. (Unfortunately, there is no mention of Chiarugi's reform in this ample monograph on the Grand Duke Leopold).

249. WEISS, E. (1930): *Elementi di psicoanalisi* (2d ed., 1937). Milano: Hoepli.

250. WEISS, E. (1970): *Sigmund Freud as a Consultant.* New York: Intercontinental Medical Books Corp.

251. WEISS, E. ET AL. (Eds.), (1936): *Saggi di psicoanalisi in onore di Sigmund Freud.* Roma: Cremonese.

252. WELSFORD, E. (1935): *The Fool. His Social and Literary History.* London: Farber & Farber.

253. WENZEL, S. (1967): *The Sin of Sloth: Acedia in Medieval Thought and Literature.* Chapel Hill, N. C.: Univ. of N. C. Press.

254. WHITWELL, J. R. (1936): *Historical Notes on Psychiatry.* London: Lewis.

255. WOLFGANG, M. E. (1960): Cesare Lombroso. In: *Pioneers in Criminology,* Mannheim, H. (Ed.). Chicago: Quadrangle. (Repr. In: *J. Crim. Law Criminol. & Police Sci.,* 1961, 52, 361-391).

256. WRIGHT, E. A. (1939): Medieval attitudes towards mental illness. *Bull. Hist. Med.,* 7, 352-356.

257. WYRSCH, J. (1957): Ueber Geschichte der psychiatrie. In: *Beiträge zur Geschichte der Psychiatrie und Hirnanatomie.* Basel: Karger.

258. ZACCHIA, P. (1621-35): *Quaestiones medico-legales.* Roma

259. ZACCHIA, P. (1635): *De'mali hipocondriaci.* Roma: Facciotti.

260. ZAMBIANCHI, A. (1963): L'opera neurologica di Cesare Lombroso. In: *Per la storia della neurologia.* Belloni, A. (Ed.). Milano: Istituto di Storia della Medicina.

261. ZAMBIANCHI, A. (1963): Cesare Lombroso. In: *Grosse Nervenärzte.* Vol. 3. Kolle, K. (Ed.). Stuttgart: Thieme.

262. ZIERMANN, B. (1947) *Nervöse Seelenleiden und ihre seelsorgliche Behandlung bei Alfons von Liquori.* Heidelberg: Kerle.

263. ZILBOORG G. (1935): *The Medical Man and the Witch during the Renaissance.* Baltimore: Johns Hopkins Univ. Press.

264. ZILBOORG, G. (1941): *A History of Medical Psychology.* New York: Norton.

265. ZOLLA, E. (1960): *La psicanalisi.* Milano: Garzanti.

3

SPAIN AND PORTUGAL

J. J. Lopez Ibor, M.D.

*Professor of Psychiatry, Department of Psychiatry and
Clinical Psychology, University of Madrid, Spain*

1

INTRODUCTION

The history of Spanish psychiatry has been influenced, as have all
aspects of Spanish history, by the fusion of many races, which slowly
and at times painfully have succeeded in forming a common Spanish
tradition. Apart from pre-history and the early Iberians and Celts,
Phoenicians, Carthagenians, Greeks, Romans, northern invaders and
Arabs have left their marks on Spain. This ethnic diversity is one of
the constants of the Spanish peoples, whose history it would be impossible to understand without bearing this in mind. The Inquisition
tried to destroy this multi-racial society in its effort to free Spain of
invaders.

Hispania or Spania were the names the chroniclers used to designate
the whole of the Iberian Peninsula. The expression "al-Andalus"
which goes back to the period of the Arab conquest, and from then,
up to the conquest of Granada, was only meant for that part of the
Peninsula occupied by the Arabs.

2

EARLY PERIOD

Medicine in general, and psychiatry in particular, were first practised
scientifically during the period of Greek and Roman occupation. Greek

and Roman practices were introduced into Spain during different periods; since they are described in this book in the chapter on ancient Greece and Rome, they will receive only brief mention here. In that period the most important Spanish-born philosopher who wrote on medical matters was Lucius Annaeus Seneca, born in Cordova about 4 B.C., but even he moved on to Rome; among other subjects, he wrote on mental disorders. He asserted, for example, that excessive anger produces insanity, for which he recommended hellebore.

Medicine leaned on humoral pathology, and the methods of treatment came mostly from Greece. Apart from hysteria and epilepsy, it seems that no other mental illness was recognized except melancholia in various forms. The tendency to describe and study the various forms of melancholia proves that the physicians of that time did not wish to analyze this disorder symptomatologically, but studied it in its essential aspect merely to distinguish it from health. St. Isidor of Seville (c. 560-636) wrote that he found medicine and philosophy indivisible in medicine, and more so in psychiatry.

The influence of Roman rule in our country can be traced through laws and institutions. A section of the population, for instance, had no legal rights, although they could engage in many occupations. The proclamation of Vespasian and the edict of Domitian gave some protection to the mentally ill. Slaves were considered responsible for their actions, but the mentally ill and children were generally exempted from legal responsibility. The mentally ill were classified as "wrathful, mad, fools, insane, fatuous"; but the laws of Justinian established no legal difference between them. The meaning of the words crazy,* wrathful, and fool was based on legal usage. Later, other expressions such as lunatic and "possessed by the devil" were used, and later still, the word "innocent" came into use, as the mentally ill were considered irresponsible and in need of care and special protection.

Roman doctors were more interested in the classification of their patients than in their treatment, and the most they did was call in a "healer" to take care of them. From the therapeutic point of view, thermal baths were the most significant innovation. The Roman baths at Alange, a small village in the province of Badajoz, have survived and are still visited by patients with nervous complaints and mental disorders. This thermal resort is now quite run down; a depressive patient, reporting his visit there, said to me: "I was so concerned with taking care not to fall, as it was so difficult to reach the baths, that I

---

* Loco (crazy), a Spanish and Portuguese word, comes from *Laucu*: of doubtful origins; perhaps from the Arab lanqa, lauq, feminine and plural of the adjective "alwaq:" stupid, crazy.

was made free of my anxieties." In addition to the famous thermal baths of Alange in Badajoz, the Romans installed other spas to whose waters were attributed various medical virtues, as those located in Lora del Rio and other villages, one of them now submerged by the reservoir of Buendia.

In Seville, the mentally ill were cared for by devout Christians, some of whom were later proclaimed saints, like the famous St. Cosmas, and St. Damian. Following the orders of Diocletian and Maximilian, they were tortured and beheaded in the year 303, but devotion to these saints persisted and centuries later encouraged the spirit of Christian charity which dictated that the innocent and the mentally ill should have care and protection. In Spain, this attitude gave rise to the Brotherhoods of St. Cosmas and St. Damian, founded exclusively by doctors with deep religious feelings and especially dedicated to the care of the sick.

The Roman Empire in Spain fell under the pressure of the invaders from the north of Europe: the Visigoths, the Vandals and the Alans. Of these, the Visigoths established themselves and stayed for several centuries. Great invasions, and occupation of vast territories, can never take place unless the invaded country is well on the way to decline and disintegration. One of the best examples of this is the last 30 years of Visigoth rule in Spain. When Rodrigo, the last Monarch of the Goths, succeeded Witiza, the Arabs had already conquered the north and center of Morocco; but instead of heading south they decided to cross the Channel and penetrate into the Iberian Peninsula; it was not hard to decide between the Sahara Desert and the lands of the Peninsula! Muza ben Nusayr and Tari ben Ziyat, with the collaboration of the so-called Count Julian, a Byzantine exarch from Ceuta, organized the expedition. The conquest of the Peninsula, except for the northerly isles, was easy.

The path of Arab influence started from the Syrian cultural centers and proceeded towards the east, where Nisius and Edejsa occupied the main positions and where the Syrians were introduced to Nestorianism along with the *Corpus Hippocraticum*. In 489, Nestorian immigrants under the protection of the Sassanides founded a medical school of Gudishapur, called the Hippocratic Academy, and provided the Islamic Baghdad and its caliphs with physicians. Mahomet taught the quest for *Salam*—integration. Persia, Syria, Palestine, Egypt, and Alexandria were conquered. The Arabs entered Spain between 711 and 732, when Carlos Martel checked them in Poitiers.

The Arabs distinguished themselves by their capacity to make contact with the people they invaded and defeated. Aristotelian arabism,

Jewish monotheism, and scholasticism successfully achieved what was more a mutual influence than a co-existence. When the Arabs extended their empire, they were interested in scientific as well as in military problems. Around the year 1000, Al-Bermin said that all the knowledge and science from all over the world had been translated into Arabic, so that the new heart, given impetus by so many life forces, would start beating and be able to maintain the great new body that had been created. The Greco-Roman inheritance spread not only through the Christian West, but also toward China, India, Byzantium, Africa, and all the area which constituted Islam itself. The Arab culture took its place between the Greek culture and the new Christian West; thus its influence was greater than the Arab conquests. It has left its traces in Sicily, the Iberian peninsula, and in the Far East.

The difference between the Greco-Roman and the Arab culture is better summarized in the following commentary by Watt and Cachia rather than by lengthy discussion:

> There is a difference between the Parthenon and the Alhambra. When we admire the Parthenon, we do so from without, while the Alhambra can only be looked at from within. . . . It has been suggested that the lithe pillars of the Alhambra, with their elaborate and massive super-structure, express the coming to the world from the heavenly kingdom of something of an eternal value and significance, while the other structures express man's aim to get to heaven.

The Arab physician was a *hakim*: a philosopher-physician. Because of its language, no culture has been able to assimilate a traditional learning better than the Arab culture. Avicena proposed to create an oriental philosophy of Aristotelian foundations. Up to the 17th century the *Isagoge des Johannitius,* by Hunain Ibn Shad, a Syrian physician of the 9th century, was studied in Paris, Padua, Salamanca, and other universities.

During the first part of the Middle Ages, psychology and psychiatry in Spain were much influenced by the convergence of the Arab and Jewish cultures with the inheritance of the classic world. In the *Koran* the soul is considered more from a theological point of view than from a psychiatric one. While there are few mentions of mental disorder in the *Koran,* it does mention that Mahomet forbade the application of leeches on the nape of the neck, because this produced loss of memory, which was believed to be located in the rear part of the brain.

In the Moslem villages, from around the 7th century, there were places of confinement for the insane, similar to those of Baghdad and

Fez. Between the years 711 and 1200—about when the first Spanish university was founded in Valencia—all scientific knowledge lay in the hands of the Arabs. They were especially attracted by the climate of southern Spain, which is why the Emir Al Ha Kem sent philosophers to Cordova to translate the medical works of Hippocrates and Galen. But the classical tradition passed to the Arabs mainly through Toledo's "School of Translators," which contributed to the preservation of a great part of the ancient culture. Thanks to this school many psychiatric practices of the Classic Period were recorded; they are significant because they resulted from the efforts of Philo Judaeus who, in the 1st century A.D. endeavored to affect a union between Greek philosophy and Jewish thought.

The separation of Christians and Muslims was the first schism which later led to Descartes enunciating his theory of duality of body and soul. Earlier psychiatry, as practiced in medieval convents, regarded man as a whole and medicine as part of a wider program of learning.

Spanish historians have recently speculated whether Spanish Islamism has made any contribution to Western culture in general. Americo Castro relates how the Christian Army, when entering Seville in 1248, was awed before such art treasures. The fusion or cultural symbiosis between Islamism and Christianity allowed Greek philosophy to reach Christian Europe. At the end of the 12th century, Toledo was in the hands of the Christians and Cordova was Islamic, but there was free exchange of ideas between the two cities, and Aristotelian philosophy reached Christian Europe through Spain.

When Baghdad declined as the sole capital of the caliphate, other centers appeared from which new forms of knowledge burst forth. This hispano-arabic period lasted as long as the Caliphate of Cordova. The end of the Arabic rule was accomplished in 1492, after the Catholic sovereigns, Isabel of Castille and Ferdinand of Aragon, captured Granada.

The real unity of Spain began in that period and coincided with Columbus' discovery of America. It took a long time for Spain to emerge with her own language. According to Americo Castro, Spain was non-existent until it acquired its own language, which is like saying that a child is not a human being until it learns to talk. As important as the early differences in language was the presence of three religions which co-existed in Spain during the Middle Ages, a fact of exceptional historical importance: these were Christianity, Judaism, and Mohammedanism. From them the Spanish people drew their characteristics.

3

EARLY CONTRIBUTORS

Among the philosopher-physicians who influenced medical practice in Spain during this early period was Avicena (978-1036).* He was inspired by the writings of Aristotle which he adapted in his own doctrine. His *Canon* maintained its validity throughout the Middle Ages. In his treatise *De Anima,* he wrote about the relationship of body and soul in man and discussed the causes of melancholy. Avicena agreed with al-Farabi (870?-950 A.D.), the Arab philosopher, although he differed with him by not considering matter as an emanating product. Like Aristotle, Avicena accepted matter as something not created and forever lasting. Avicena, and the Arabs in general, believed that the functions of the brain originated from the innermost part of the ventricles. According to him psychic changes depended upon the proportions of the compositions of the brain. He devised a classification which recognized disorders of imagination and memory; in another group he included melancholia, mania, imbecility, and dementiae. Anomalies in the forebrain produce perception disorders; those of the medium-brain imbecility, and those of the fourth ventricle, as I have already said, have to do with memory. Avicena had the sharpest mind of his time.

The poet and philosopher Avicebron, or Ibn-Gabirol (c. 1021-c.1071), systematized the Aristotelian notions about the soul; according to him, the vegetative soul produces the necessary movements for reproduction and development; the vital soul, those of sensation and movement; the rational soul takes care of thought. Even though 9th century Arab and Jewish philosophers were more concerned with theological than medical problems, they evidently contributed to a psychology which partly served as a basis for the development of subsequent psychiatric notions.

The Arabian physician Avenzohar (1072-1163) was born in Peñaflor (Seville); he had a more practical approach to illness than Avicena and based his teachings on experience.

Abulcasis (1106) was inclined towards surgery: "When melancholia is produced by corrupt dampness and thick phlegm, it must be cauterized." He also propounded various cauterizations of the head.

Avempace (Ibn-Bejah, who died in 1163) occupies a special place among his contemporaries, who were also inclined towards a neo-

---

* Ibn-Sinah, Ibn Ali Abdulla Ibn Sinai, his real name, was probably not Spanish by birth.

platonic tradition, understanding the development of the soul by
means of the emanation of the "Nous," while he followed the Aristotelian tradition. He thought that, just as animals possess instincts, so
must man, and that intellectual power must be something like an
emanation from God. In this sense, Avempace followed the Aristotelian
point of view more than the Platonic.

Averrhoes (11-26-1198), a philosopher and physician, was completely
influenced by the Aristotelian philosophy and favored it even when
it contradicted the writings of Galen. Yet he could not conceive the
"Nous" of Aristotle and, influenced by the thoughts of Alexander of
Aphrodisios, he affirmed that the potential "Nous" was individual, but
not eternal, disappearing after death. What is more, while Averrhoes
searched for a compromise between Alexander of Aphrodisios and
Temistos, he maintained that the potential "Nous" is not only a
capacity whose necessity is demonstrated by its activity, but could be,
at the same time, active and in possession of its own potentiality—
yet this "Nous" was not individual, but tied to the "active Nous," and
shared by all. Each man has only the power of taking a few active
particles of this "existential Nous," in the same way that all men
possess the capacity to see the light. After death, the "Nous" goes on
existing, not individually but as something common to every man, and
this is the "Nous" which, as an emanation of God, human beings
possess. That is to say, in every individual soul there exists a particle
of the immortal spirit as it originates there. However, there are differences between individuals, depending on their greater or lesser
participation.

The Jewish philosopher Moses Maimonides (1113-1205), lived in
Cordova and studied under Arab scholars. From the psychological and
psychopathological point of view, his treatise *Guide of the Perplexed*
is even now of great interest, not only on account of its historic importance, but also for its contents. According to Fidel Fernandez, his
knowledge of psychiatry was considerable for the time: "One should
not consider as mentally ill those who run wild in the streets, throw
stones, or wreck household goods, but those whose mind is clouded by a
fixed idea, although they are normal in that which is not related to it."
In this way he formalized the idea of monomania.

An important work of this period was that of the philosopher
Suhar. According to Suhar, God made himself manifest in word and
act since he was the creator of Adam Kadmos (Cadmus, according to
Greek mythology). This original man is made up of ten forces, from
which psychological or animalistic faculties derive on one side, and
virtues on the other. The spiritual and immortal soul of man (Nne-

schama) is part of the spiritual world. The soul which maintains life (Ruach) pertains to the psychic world, and respiration (Nphesch) belongs to the third materialistic world. Suhar was under the influence of Plotinus and Plato.

In the writings of Solomon ben Dubuda ben Gabirol (1020-1070) we find that all that which does not come from God has matter and form; the soul is explained in this way, which combines the Aristotelian and neo-platonic doctrine with the Jewish philosophy.

4

EARLY SPANISH MENTAL HOSPITALS

There have been many detailed controversies as to whether the first psychiatric hospital in the world was in Valencia. In many hospitals, the mentally ill were admitted to small, isolated rooms, and insane patients were crowded together with others who were not so afflicted. In 1326, the Georges Hospital of Elbing, belonging to the order of Teutonic Knights, built a few cells, called *Doll-haus,* for the mentally ill. Similar cells are mentioned in the documents of the Municipal Hospital of Hamburg in 1375. They could also be found in the great hospital of Erfurt, rebuilt in 1385.

In England, in France, and in Germany some general hospitals accepted a few mental patients, but the hospital in Valencia was the first in Europe dedicated to them exclusively. It is difficult to pinpoint when psychiatric hospitals as such originated. In his *History of Insanity,* Foucault points out that those institutions that in France were known as "asylums" were not for the mentally ill, nor were they hospitals in the modern sense of the term, but rather places for the commitment of those regarded as anti-social: vagabonds, prostitutes, delinquents, and so on.

There are some references to mental hospitals established by the Arabs in the 12th century. The 18th century Spanish traveler Benjamin De Tudela wrote in his *Travels* that in Baghdad there was a great palace called *Dar-el-Morestán,* where the insane were committed in the summer; they were tied with great iron chains until they recovered their reason, and, if they did, were then freed.

Valencia

One of the most important events in the history of Spanish psychiatry is the foundation of the first lunatic asylum in Valencia, in

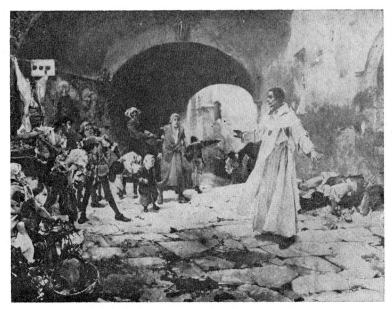

PLATE XIII. Painting by Sorolla showing Father Jofré protecting a madman.

1409. The story of its foundation is both curious and moving. On the 24th of February of that year, Fray Juan Galiberto Jofré, a monk of the Order of Our Lady of Mercy, was going to preach in the Cathedral of Valencia on the feast-day of our Lady of the Helpless when he beheld a group of boys insulting and stoning a poor madman. He was so moved that he abbreviated the sermon he had planned and instead delivered a plea for the founding of a hospital for the mentally ill. Sorolla—the great contemporary painter—has immortalized the scene (Plate XIII). Descending from the pulpit of the Cathedral, he was accosted by various citizens who had been present during his sermon; led by Lorenzo Salom, they decided there and then to supply the means needed for the founding of the hospital, which was named Our Lady of the Innocents. King Martin I of Aragón granted permission for the project and, in 1410, Pope Benedict XIII issued a Papal Bull to the same end.

Father Jofré's initiative arose not from abstract theories, but from the direct experience of seeing an insane person being pursued and persecuted by the healthy near the Cathedral of Valencia (Plate XIV). His action was not motivated by a wish to protect anti-social or psychopathic individuals, but by a wish to protect mentally ill patients from the thoughtless assaults of the healthy. His end was to assist them

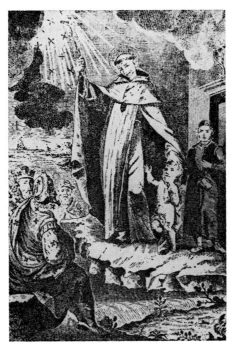

PLATE XIV. An old engraving showing Father
Jofré with all his attributes: the halo of sanctity, the miraculous shower of crosses, ships
for the redemption of captives, a foundling,
and, behind him, the mental hospital he
founded and a mental patient in characteristic garb of two colors, the left and right
side of the tunic contrasting.

and try to cure them. Hence, the foundation of the insane asylum of
Valencia holds great interest. It has also been said that Father Jofré,
as a Mercedarian, dedicated to the rescue of prisoners in Arab hands,
was acquainted with the existence of mental hospitals in the Moslem
Empire, but after careful study of these establishments, it seems that
they were similar in function to the general asylums in France and in
other parts of Europe not dedicated exclusively to the care of the
mentally ill.

Saragossa

In 1425 King Alfonso V founded a hospital in Saragossa dedicated
to Our Lady of Mercy; on the front of the building was placed the

inscription *Urbis et Orbe* (for the city and for the world), as anybody could be admitted, without regard to religion or nationality. A part of the hospital was set aside for mentally ill patients; this section was later destroyed by fire, but was re-erected in 1829. Saragossa Hospital was noted for introducing what was later called "moral treatment" for the mentally ill. In 1549 it housed nearly 100 mental patients. The following statement comes from Inverti:

> Fresh water baths are employed for refreshing, although this kind of treatment is generally without results. This treatment is difficult to carry out under outbursts of madness; most of all it is hard to bleed them as the patients may tear out their bandages; but continuous experience has demonstrated in this hospital that the most efficient treatment is providing the patients with an occupation or work.

The greater part of the patients were employed in workshops and were made to clean the house, with the exception of the wards; they carried water, coal, and firewood. They were also employed in the pharmacy and on the hospital farm: in threshing, harvesting grapes, and olives. They fulfilled the function of stretcher-bearers, under the supervision of one of the custodians whom they called "father." In 1859 Desmaissons wrote a description of this hospital and of the one in Toledo, which he regarded as perfect for that time.

Seville

In 1436 Marco Sancho or Sanchez founded in Seville Spain's third mental hospital. Little is known of Sanchez, but tradition has it that he was wont to collect the insane who wandered through the streets and bring them to the hospital. He was put in charge of the institution and left to struggle with its problems. Many of the insane from neighboring villages took refuge there, and some—according to the data of the provincial records of Seville—were sent for treatment to the thermal baths at Alange, which were the nearest. In 1481 Henry IV took the hospital under his protection and his example was later followed by Isabella and Ferdinand. According to the records, the hospital building was found to be inadequate and it was improved in 1686. Another hospital was built in Palma de Majorca in 1456.

Granada

In Granada during the Moslem rule (probably from 1356) a center existed for the confinement of anti-social individuals. As we can see by the information collected by Delgado Roig, the building of a hospital in Granada was begun in 1356, during the reign of Mohammed V, and was completed in 1367. It was erected in the suburbs, in a locality known as the Pleasure Place (Haxasir), and it was always called "the house of the insane and the innocents."

Lamperez, the architect, describes it for us and says that it covered a rectangular area, was two stories high, had one small courtyard, porticos on its four sides, and a number of galleries. At the back there were a patio, four stairways, and a room in each of the four corners. The porticos and the galleries were the walking areas for convalescent patients, while the infirmaries were probably on the corridors. Piped water spurted from the mouths of two stone lions, which today are placed in front of the Ladies' Tower in the Alhambra. Lamperez called attention to a series of ridges in one of the rooms which divide it into small areas, like little cells, similar to those of the Dar-el-Morestán of Baghdad in the 13th century.

The plans of this institution show that this was not the insane asylum which was founded later by King Ferdinand and his wife Isabella in the year 1492, at the corner of the Plaza del Triunfo.

Others

One of the best known psychiatric hospitals in Spain was the Hospital of the Innocents in Toledo, founded in 1483 by the Papal nuncio Francisco Ortiz, who placed it under the protection of the local Council. In 1700 it was enlarged by annexing to it a large building called the House of the Nuncio. An engraved inscription on the door of the hospital read *Mentis integrae, Sanitari procurando Aedes, Concilio, Sapientes constitutae, Ano Domini MD CC XX II.* The rules of the hospital were formulated in detail.

In 1489, Don Sancho Velazquez de Cuellar, auditor for the Chancellery of the State, founded the hospital in Valladolid.

The hospital in Barcelona was called the Hospital of the Holy Cross. It admitted all classes of patients, irrespective of nationality or disorder. Hence, it was not exclusively a psychiatric hospital. It was rebuilt in 1680. It seems that in 1412 clerics and emotionally ill people were also taken in. In 1836 the Academy of Medicine produced a report proposing the building of a new insane asylum and psychiatric hospital; a modern hospital was erected, following the advice of Pi y Molist, a famous psychiatrist from Barcelona.

5

THE 16TH AND 17TH CENTURIES

It is usually assumed that the Middle Ages came to an end in 1490. After a period of darkness it seemed that the new light of the Renaissance would spread through Europe. Later, between 1590 and 1630, the change from the somber medieval night to the sunny Renaissance midday was to take place. And history tells us that in the time of Bacon, Montaigne, Descartes, and many others, the gatherings of witches so increased that in Hendaye, in the south of France, near the present frontier between Spain and France, about 12,000 witches gathered in "covens." Witches abounded in Catholic territory as well as in Protestant areas. It was only in the Age of Enlightenment that all this superstition began to subside. A careful study of this contradiction, comparable to the anti-semitism which arose in Central Europe in our time, leaves us no alternative but to admit, as Trevor-Roper does, that the change in social structures is different from that produced by intellectuals and what we call superstition in one era might be rationalism in another.

Admissions to Spanish insane asylums built at the time were enforced only when absolutely necessary; moreover, as soon as they were better, the patients enjoyed a certain freedom, as demonstrated by Don Miguel de Cervantes in his book *Don Quixote,* in which he describes a sick man who thought himself cured, but was recaptured by an envoy of the Archbishop.

Those called today feeble-minded or imbeciles were often found employed in palaces, as shown by paintings by Velazquez, who could imbue with humanity and nobility the figures of those wretched people, as he did the portraits of kings. Anyone who is acquainted with Velazquez' paintings can confirm this statement.

The Inquisition

The period we shall now refer to, from its beginning up to the 18th century, is the age of sorcery and witchcraft. It is useful to comment briefly on the Spanish Inquisition, in the light of recent studies devoted to it and in the perspective allowed by time.

The Inquisition already existed in many European countries before it was introduced into Spain. The heresy of the Catharists, a dissenting sect, and the spreading of witchcraft moved Pope Innocent III towards its institution. In Spain, the problem which worried Ferdinand and

Isabella was how to produce a modern state from people of many races and religions which were spread throughout the peninsula. Once the paternal archaism of the Middle Ages was overcome by the European monarchs, a new problem arose on how to restructure the country so that its unity would be maintained.

The criminal laws in the Europe of the 15th century regarded heresy as the worst crime. The Catholic sovereigns asked the Pope to extend to Spain the power of the Inquisition, which had already been established in many countries since the 13th century. Isabella and Ferdinand were convinced, on a visit to Seville in 1478, that the pseudoconverts who remained loyal to Judaism would cause trouble in the Christian community. "The true grounds for that conviction by and large escape us," states the historian Suarez. It was not until November 1, 1478, that Pope Sixtus IV granted the bull establishing the Inquisition in Spain. On September 27, 1480, Miguel de Morcillo and Fray Juan de San Martin were named inquisitors with the mandate to cleanse Seville. It has been calculated that about 500 people were burned in three years. Fray Thomas de Torquemada was inquisitor for Aragon; he was said to be very tough, in accordance with his personality, but he was not in his sovereigns' good graces. Catalonia, Valencia, and especially Aragon put up a hard fight. The Inquisition met with much resistance, but it persisted because of that same feeling of danger— justified or not—that motivated Isabella and Ferdinand, who wanted to achieve the Christian unity of the country at all costs.

The synagogues were obliged to move to other places, and the Jews—those who were not converted—were made to leave Spain. The decree ordering non-Christians to leave claimed to be based on religious criteria. Some of the Jews were converted and changed their names, as, for example, the chief rabbi of the synagogues, Abraham Senor, godchild of the King, who took the name of Ferdinand Numez del Corral. The estimated number of Jewish homes in Castille in 1492 was 15,000—with around 80,000 people. The number of Jews was not so great in Aragon. The way in which the economy of the country was influenced by the banishment has been much debated, and continues to provoke controversy. Yet the Moslems banished from Portugal in 1497 were welcomed in Castille, although soon after the desire for unity was to cause the expulsion of the Moors, after they organized a few serious revolts. By 1503 no "infidels" were left in Spain, except for the Mudejars of Aragon and Valencia.

The Catholic Church was confronted by these errors, which makes it strange that ordinary people should be so involved in polemics about them. "Madness" was usually considered to be a "preternatural error."

Both the Church and the Inquisition distinguished between those possessed by the devil and the insane. This confusion was very common in the Middle Ages and in part of the Modern Age, but Trevor-Roper has recently stated that Spain burned or punished the least number of witches, because they simply considered them to be sick. This opinion is shared by Kamen, in more modern times. The Inquisitor Alonso de Frias put an end to the persecutions of witches.

Philosophers and Physicians

The most outstanding physicians of this period, and others who, although not physicians, had a decisive influence on the medicine and psychiatry of the time, are best grouped together, because they give a clear image of the evolution of ideas in this long period of time. They are Pedro Hispano, Raimundo Lulio, Arnaldo de Villanova, Luis Vives, Juan Huarte de San Juan, and Dona Oliva Sabuco de Nantes.

Pedro Hispano (1226-1277), was a Galenic physician. As a philosopher he followed the wake of Aristotle, and was very interested in astrology. His main book, discovered by Grabman in 1927 in Codex 3314 of the National Library, was entitled *Treatise of the Soul.* He was Portuguese, and he should be in the last part of this chapter, but he so much influenced the whole Peninsula that it is justifiable to include him here.

Arnaldo de Villanova (1250-1303) had an extraordinary personality (much has been said of him by the great medical historian Diepgen in a number of publications). Although born in France, Villanova is considered by Diepgen to be Spanish, because most of his life was spent in Spain and because there are doubts about his birthplace.

His many interests and the span of his knowledge, exceptional for his time, were similar to Paracelsus, physician to a number of Kings of Aragon. In addition to his medical activities, he was also an alchemist. In his *Medical Practice,* he discusses mania and melancholia; according to him, the former is caused by a defect in the anterior ventricle of the brain which at the same time prevents imagination; he attributes melancholia to the animal spirit which produces fear, sadness, and dumbness. Among the nourishments which produce melancholia is wine, because it burns humors and produces black bile. Black bile may also be produced by other causes, such as wrath, anxiety following excessive study, a retention of the menstrual flow, or corrupted sperm.

Raimundo Lulio (born in Majorca in 1232, died in 1272) was a Franciscan monk and a man of exceptional worth for that time. A philosopher and alchemist, rather than a physician, he always yearned for the fusion of faith and reason, and the solution of all problems by basic knowledge. Giordano Bruno called him "divine" and Trithemius, Cornelius Agrippa, Father Kirchner, and many others were inspired by him. Carrera y Artau has made a detailed investigation of Lulio's views of the structure and functions of the rational soul. According to Lulio, the different activities of the soul may lead to normal personality or to psychopathology. Typically of his race, he was a man of great imagination and of extraordinary activity. It is astounding to look at all he wrote. His *Tree of Science* shows what a large field his studies covered. He was of the opinion that the normal activity of the soul demands or supposes the normal activities of the main faculties: memory, understanding, and will-power; but in abnormal functions, the soul suffers a change of its activities (for example, a faulty memory, an ignorant intelligence, and a will-power directed more towards hate than towards love). He left us his work on *Liber de instrumento intellectus in medicina*.

Juan Luis Vives (1492-1540) was among the famous humanists of his time, but his writings on psychology give him the right to be included here. Of interest are his views on the association of ideas, which have been pointed out by Foster Watson as well as by others. In his *Treatise on the Soul* he bases his views not only on the external continuity of time and space, but also on the internal continuity. He believes that the study of the human soul was indispensable for educators, priests, and politicians, and that the doctor moves between body and soul; he continuously refers to the soma in order to reach the psyche. The mind should be healthy, and a man with a sick mind should be taken to the hospital for treatment. Perturbation of the imagination might produce perturbation of the mind. His detailed analysis of the passions has been discussed by Zilboorg, who has not hesitated to compare him with Freud.

Some authors believe that Vives and Fox Morcillo were only collaborators of the anti-scholastic movement represented in the Renaissance by other Italian and French dissenters. Such a statement is inexact as well as emotional. Vives did not attack Aristotle or Plato, but placed the principle of reason before that of authority. He ardently affirmed the urgency of the progress of science: *"Milla ars simel est et enventer et absolute."* As Bacon had done, he also underlined the need to experiment: *"experiments et usum rerum."*

Although not properly pertaining to psychiatry but to psychology, one of the most outstanding writers of his time was Juan Huarte de San Juan (c. 1530-1592). His book, *Probe of the Mind,* written in

1575, has been translated since into other languages because of the fame it acquired. Following Plato and Aristotle, Huarte believed that man's different dispositions depend on three qualities: heat, humidity, and dryness. He distinguishes a vegetative, a sensitive, and a rational soul, each with innate intelligence which determines the temperament of each. The brain's temperament depends on the intelligence of the sensitive soul; the task of the rational soul is to hear, imagine, and exercise the memory. When man is born, he is incapable of such activities related to the rational soul, and can exercise only those controlled by the sensitive and the vegetative soul.

If man is stricken by illness, like mania, melancholia, or frenzy, it is because the temperament of his brain has changed, and the reverse happens when he is cured. Huarte gives some clinical examples, among which is the case of a frenetic woman who described to anybody who visited her all his virtues and, worst still, his vices, because "the heat is near the east of the spirit." Climate and cultural environment exercise influence on the spirit. The more the cultural advances, the more numerous the mental diseases. The climate influences passions, "influences feelings," as Huarte says.

He also wrote on the education of children, on physiognomy and on the motley collection of racial influences which makes up the Spanish temperament.

In 1570 Huarte observed a mentally ill patient, called Luis López, whose sickness derived from a malignant fever, and who, like Don Quixote, regained soundness of mind in the last years of his life; another person, however, who had received the same treatment for the same infirmity, died insane. He cited other clinical examples which are both interesting and picturesque; from them we may perceive the intellectual climate in which he moved. He carefully studied the influence of the "ecological factors" in the formation of the personality and of its morbid deviation, although he asserted that atmospheric influences can not cause mental illness. His work also discussed "cultural influences" as causative agents of sickness and of psychopathies.

A brief mention must be made of Dona Oliva Sabuco De Nantes, although many believe that the real author of the book attributed to her was her father. Others think that some worthy Arab or Jewish physician who had escaped from Alcaraz may have initiated Dona Oliva in her studies of philosophy and medicine. She wrote a colloquium on *The Nature of Man* and *A Dialogue on True Medicine* (1587). Her psychological understanding could be considered well above psychiatric knowledge proper, as she studied the various emotions and feelings with great appreciation of the heart and of human behavior.

The brain, according to her, receives all the sensations of the damages and noxas of the body, although not of itself, because it is the beginning and the cause of all feelings. Elsewhere she affirms that the Spaniards, against all reason and motives, persist in the common practice of using black garments, despite the fact that black causes sadness, influencing moods like light and darkness do. Some of her thinking has the same characteristics as that of Heraclitus as for instance when she says that maturity and perfection are the origins of imperfection and putrefaction, or that health causes illness and life begets death. Life is a prolonged death, forever diminishing and destroying life. The principal general remedy of "true medicine" is to reconcile the soul with the body and remove all discord and the best remedy is speech, which, in adults, produces joy and hope for the better. She thus developed what was a genuine treatise of psychotherapy.

Having mentioned this group of thinkers, whether physicians or not, but who so much reflected the thoughts of medicine in those days, let us now review briefly the physicians of that Age.

Luis Mercado (1520-1606) was royal doctor to Philip II and Philip III. His work appeared in Frankfurt and Venice and was published in three parts (1605-1620). In the second, he discussed a series of disorders such as epilepsy, phrenitis, lethargy, hypochondric melancholia, etc. In the third part, he is concerned with melancholia, repeating the ideas of the Greeks. Along with Vallés he was one of the outstanding doctors of his time. The passions of the soul are divided into five parts, of which the fifth is melancholia, which he considered from the classic Greek point of view. In volume two, he offers some unusual clinical examples, including that of an epileptic girl, another on a phrenitis which degenerated into lipemania and lethargy, and still others of a hypochondric melancholia nature, etc.

Andres Velazquez published a book on melancholy in 1585; it followed the theories of Galen. In the fifth chapter, he explains the meanings of the term melancholy and points out the mechanisms of its etiology. Following Galen's footsteps, he refers to the four humors. Melancholy is the alienation of the understanding or reason, but without fever. Doctors distinguish two kinds: melancholy in its proper sense, and mania. Melancholic moods place those affected in a sorry state of discouragement; he completes the picture by explaining how, apart from this symptomatology, some patients are besieged by scruples, others by prodigality; some believe they are a rooster and try to crow and beat their arms, while others believe they are bricks and are afraid to drink, lest they are dissolved, etc.

Andres Laguna was called the Spanish Galen. He was born in Segovia in 1499, and died in 1560, after having been the doctor of the Emperor Charles I. His best known work deals with the various opinions concerning the soul, taking the ancient Greek theories as his base and accepting Plato's distinction of the rational soul and the sensuous soul to which he adds the natural or vegetative soul. With regard to sleep, he leans towards the theories of Heraclitus and the Stoics, although he also refers to Acmeon's opinion when he asserts that sleep occurs when the veins are drained of blood. Laguna is a good example of the influence exerted on the physicians of that time by ancient Greek medicine.

Francisco Vallés or De Covarrubias (born in 1524) raises the question in his book, *De Sacra Philosophia,* whether demoniacal illness existed and whether it required the same therapy as the illness which was not related with demoniacal possession. He concludes by stating that demoniacal illnesses do not exist, and that melancholy and epilepsy are produced by natural causes. His exposition is somewhat obscure, but he is often right in his interpretation of "lycanthropy" as well as in that of the phenomena of somnambulism and similar disorders.

It is very important for Vallés that exorcism, predictions and Biblic prophecies be separated from the auguries and magic of Romans and Arabs; in other words, he wanted to keep the theological and philosophical from what was properly medical. According to him, mental illness could be divided into amentia, dementia, mania, insane fury, melancholy and other disorders, which are not to be considered as such, but are vices, including lust, irascibility and greed. Melancholy could not be produced without the presence of the humor or melancholic juice, which would involve the brain itself if the influence was direct, or some other part if it were by "consensum."

An important author during the revival of Greek medicine in Spain was Don Christophoros De Vega. He was physician to Don Carlos, Philip II's son, and was Professor of Medicine at the University of Alcalá in the middle of the sixteenth century. It is known that he died in 1573. In his works he deals with mania, which he considered as synonymous with insanity and furor; he defines it as follows:

> Insanity is a delirium which has no fever of the hot humour which affects the brain's membranes. It is preceded by certain symptoms which may be considered as antecedents, such as pain and throbbing of the head, terrible insomnia, untimely laughter,

rage with no cause and nightly pollutions. After that comes a more violent period, with loquacity, strange fantasies and verbal and bodily aggressions. The sick person sometimes throws himself out of the window, tears his clothes, etc. This disease frequently attacks young people.

De Vega's interpretations are in general still based on the Greek theory of the four humors; irritants and purgatives were employed in treatment and most of all was used what was called "anti-inflammation derivation" which consisted in bleeding near the brain or in its periphery, etc. He also dedicates an extensive chapter to melancholy, referring its etiology to a plethora of blood and black bile, as well as to sorrows, sadness and griefs. He dwells on "flatulent melancholy," which is followed by whole chapters on "lycanthropy" and "erotho-mania." In order to deal with this last, he mixes medical measures with psychological advice, recommending distractions, games, reunions, tours through pleasant places, etc. In any case, the fundamental symptoms of melancholy were those the Greeks pointed out: fear and sadness, with no fever.

It is strange that this Hellenic tradition on the origins of melancholy survived side by side with the Moslem tradition, as may be seen for example in *On the government of health and the sterility of men and women,* written by Luys Lovera of Avila (1540), Royal Doctor to Charles V. He is completely in agreement with Avicena and asserts that when the lochia of women who have just given birth are suppressed, they fall in a state of melancholy; he also describes the suppression of menstruation as the origin of this illness.

Gomez Pereira opposed Galen's theories in his famous *Antoniana Margarita* (Valladolid, 1605), which owes its title to the fact that his father was called Antonio and his mother Margarita. He wrote that "Animals do not possess a sensory life, otherwise their organs would be influenced by objects or ghosts." He denied that animals have sensitive souls. He did not know if this denial was spontaneous or if he was guided by a religious feeling. "He wanted to elevate man to heaven as an image of God, and pull down to earth the animal."

Alfonso Ponce De Santa Cruz, physician to Philip II, wrote a book on melancholy (Plate XV); published in 1622, it is one of the most interesting books in all the history of Spanish psychiatry. It is divided in various dialogues on the nature and origins of melancholy, on its symptoms, its treatment, etc. Melancholic humor is a product of the bile which attacks the brain. When this humor attacks memory in particular, it produces sadness, fear and anxiety. If its attack is focused on the womb, then nymphomania is produced, and if the humor attacks the hypochondriacs and is accompanied by obstructions, then it produces hypochondria. In his collection of case histories we find strange cases, like the one of the patient who believed that he had been transformed into a glass vase and was covered with straw for a time until he was cured; once his delirium was over he stated that there

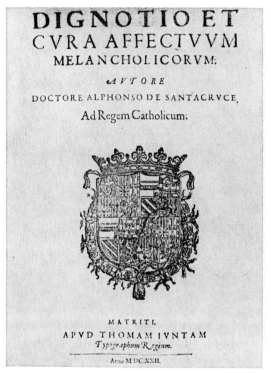

PLATE XV. Title page of book on melancholy by Alfonso Ponce De Santa Cruz.

was no such monomania, but that he really was a wretched man (see Cervantes' book on the *Glass Bachelor*). Another example was that of the thirty-year-old patient who first fell into a melancholy, then developed a monomania which made him believe that he was transformed into a wolf (lycanthropy); he fled from men and sought refuge in the mountains, where he spent the nights howling, visiting the graveyard and invoking the dead. He was treated by bleeding, purgatives, general baths and good food.

Alfonso Ponce De Santa Cruz should not be confused with Antonio

Ponce De Santa Cruz, Jr., doctor to Philip IV, who died in 1650. In his book he criticized Avicena. He followed Aristotle's theories, insisting on the four main humors which have always characterized Hellenic medicine. He worked at a more natural-scientific level than other authors of the time, especially the great metaphysicist Francisco Suarez. His book starts with a collection of case histories.

Other interesting authors include Esteban Pujasol, who wrote an *Anatomy of Intelligence* (1637). Before him, authors divided the skull into three areas. In the first and foremost, they placed common sense, fancy and imaginative powers; in the second or middle area, mental faculties and reason, and in the third, they placed memory or the faculty to remember. From the physiognomic point of view, he said, for example, that a big head denotes kindness and intelligence, courage and strength in inner feelings, and that those with large heads are prudent and wise. He established similar comparisons, relating the size and the shape of the head with the personality traits of the patient. The third part of the book is more a treatise on astrology, as he discusses the influence of the stars over the temperament.

Francisco Nuñez De Oria, in his *Regimen of Health and Good Advice* (Madrid, 1562 and 1572), deals with the influence nourishment has on good habits. A sanguine nature is apt to have a quick understanding and sound judgment. The melancholic personality is wise, clever and meek. The phlegmatic is cold and bound to routine, and the choleric is bold, rash and direct.

Tomas Murillo Velarde y Jurado, born in Belalcazar, was physician to two Kings, Philip IV and Charles II. His work is entitled *An appraisal of intelligence and the cure for hypochondriacs* (Saragossa, 1672); it is full of strange observations and remedies. This book is not very original, apart from maintaining that witches and demons may be the cause of melancholy, and explaining that the devil resides in the spleen and in the black bile. He considers hypochondric melancholy to be produced throughout the body, although there is a type which is especially linked with the brain.

6

RECENT HISTORY

Eighteenth and Nineteenth Centuries

Andrés Piquer (1711-1772) became one of Spain's greatest medical celebrities, being physician to both King Ferdinand VI and Charles III.

In his treatise he described convulsions, tremblings, epilepsy, vertigo, phrenitis, insomnia, lethargy, catalepsy, coma, apoplexy and paralysis, melancholic and hypochondriac afflictions. This last is especially developed in another manuscript by the same author.

Some authors, like the well-known medical historian Chinchilla, say that this last essay includes a description of Ferdinand VI's illness. This manuscript is reproduced in the fourth volume of the *Historic Annals of General Medicine in Spain,* published by Chinchilla. Piquer insists that mania and melancholia are one and the same illness, to be distinguished only by the degree of the morbid activity of the spirit. "His Majesty," says he, "had since five months a fixed idea about death which was accompanied by such anxiety, that he had no other subject of conversation."

Gaspar Casal established himself in Oviedo as a doctor after having practiced in Madrid. He wrote a work on the *Natural and Medical History of the Principality of Asturias* (Madrid, 1762), published by Juan José Carica Sevillano after his death. He studied the endemic illnesses of that province—before it was a Principality—and described as endemic the mania or insane fury in the village of Piñola. In another chapter he calls attention to the frequency with which epilepsy and melancholy appear together, but his main merit arises from having described the psychic symptoms of what was then called "the rose's evil" which was no other than the "pellagra."

To the nineteenth century belongs Don Ignacio Maria Ruiz de Luzmiaga (1763-1822), who wrote a dissertation on mania, and another on the treatment of dementia, basing these dissertations on experience he had acquired in England.

In 1810 Ramón Lopez Matias wrote a book on the *demonmaniacs or the possessed,* half seriously, half in jest. In another publication of 1810 he discussed the problems of mental perturbations caused by external influences, insisting on the power of melancholy, especially the religious kind, and that of persistent mania, regarding the problem from the forensic or medico-legal point of view. His main concern was to determine how much freedom of action man has in these cases and what was the relation between crime and the punishment. At the time, the influence of Pinel and Esquirol was quite extraordinary; their works were translated from the French as soon as they appeared. From a philosophic point of view, apart from Descartes, Kant, Fitsche, Schelling, etc., a second-rate German philosopher called Krause greatly influenced Lopez Matias.

In the nineteenth century started the enormous influence of French psychiatry in Spain; it was felt through the work of Pinel and Esquirol, without forgetting Cullen, who, in his lifetime, was already translated and read by Spanish doctors. However, the most outstanding Spanish workers of that period were Pi y Molist, Pedro Mata, Jose Maria Esquerdo, Jaime Vera, Juan Gine y Patagas, Arturo Garceran Granes, etc., but it was French psychiatry which influenced their ideas.

The nineteenth century in Spain is not noted for its brilliancy in sciences nor in psychiatric achievements. As Menéndez Pelayo said, mostly about the first half of that century, all possibility of a scientific creation withered between the declining royalists and the Frenchified leftists. In philosophy and psychology Spanish psychiatrists professed the empiricism of Condillac, Destull de Tracis and Cabanis.

German idealism, mostly that of Schelling through the books of Victor Consin, also had some influence. Among the Spaniards, only Balmes and Quadrado were successful amidst the passionate fights between carlists and liberals. In those times, civil wars absorbed all the available energy of the Spanish people. One could speak of the slow suicide of a people, referring to that period, and the words of Shakespeare could be applied to Queen Isabelle II: "Farewell, woman of York, queen of sad destinies." A great writer, Menéndez Pelayo, was able to say of that century "we are less inside Europe than we were at the end of the eighteenth century, a period which nobody can call enviable or victorious." Spain reached her lowest point in 1898, when Cuba was lost and she suffered her greatest defeat by the United States' powerful army.

The Twentieth Century

In the nineteenth century the scientific decline of Spain increased. In a work covering half a century of psychiatry, referring to the nineteenth century, Marañon cites Esquerdo, Jaime Vera, Perez Valdes, Achucarro and Sanchis Banus. They form two different groups which extend into the twentieth century. Some of them, like Esquerdo and Jaime Vera, were attracted more towards politics than towards science, in spite of their great talents and their ability as psychiatrists. Different reasons crippled the work of Perez Valdes, Valle Alda and Sanchis Banus. Achucarro was more inclined towards pathological anatomy. With the appearance of Cajal, Spain seemed to lose her inferiority complex. Marañon writes, with good reason, that this inferiority was felt only in the field of experimental science. The work and example of Cajal proved to be decisive in the creation of a new atmosphere for experimental sciences. Cajal, a professor of Histology, won the Nobel Prize while struggling against poverty; the prize impressed both the public and the Government, and later the Cajal Institute was created. Cajal was an histologist; hence his most important discovery was in the histology of the nervous system. Among the disciples who followed him more or less closely are Tello, Villaverde, Lafora, Prados, Such, Castro and Rio-Hortega. However, the interests of Cajal as an investigator did not touch psychiatry. It is of interest that he wrote:

> I must refer to Freud and criticize some of his most audacious assertions. Because in more than five hundred dreams I have analyzed (without counting those others done by people I know) it is impossible, except in rare cases, to prove the doctrines of the bold and slightly egotistic Viennese author, who has always appeared to me to be more anxious with the idea of establishing a sensational theory than having the desire to serve with austerity the cause of true science.

In other parts of Spain psychiatrists were further removed from this influence. During the century we are referring to and at the beginning of the present one, eminent psychiatrists could be found in Barcelona, but none of them produced creative work; among them were Pi y Molist, Gine and Pertegas, to name a few. From the end of the first quarter of the century, a new generation of psychiatrists made their appearance, many of whom were trained in Austria, Germany, England, United States, Switzerland and in other countries. This new generation has given a new orientation to Spanish psychiatry, as proved by the World Congress of Psychiatry which took place in Madrid in 1966.

From these beginnings, developed, slowly at first, but more rapidly later, a new Spanish renaissance. The account of these adventurous origins could be more extensive. What is important today is the building and organization of new hospitals, psychiatric dispensaries, centers for the care of various types of patients and private hospitals for treatment and research. The change in the last ten years has been extraordinary. Clinical psychology and psychiatry have been integrated with other disciplines in the curricula of the medical schools. Schools for post-graduate students have been created for those who choose these specialties. Spanish psychiatry has experienced a great change. What is more, after the World Congress of Psychiatry which took place in 1966, its progress in therapy as well as in its scientific aspects is very evident.

It would be falsifying the truth to offer a brilliant perspective of Spanish psychiatry in the years of the country's decline, but apart from the present renaissance, even in its most distressing periods, its humanitarian spirit towards the sick could always be distinguished. Look, for example, at the attention, respect and love for the patients which characterized the foundation of the insane asylum of Leganés in 1885; they were advocated, in 1859, by Pedro Maria Rubio, who proposed the building of a "Model Insane Asylum," which was erected, although the Spanish Parliament promulgated, in 1821, a general Regulation for charitable institutions. At the time about 1,626 mental patients were admitted there, of which 1,475 were sustained by "private charity" and the remaining 151 by their families. Another 5,651 mental patients were cared for in their own homes, by their own families.

7

PORTUGUESE PSYCHIATRY*

In 1539, in Portugal, mental patients started to be admitted together with syphilitics to the special infirmary of the "Hospital of All Saints" of Lisbon, where Fernandes Gonveia, a priest, treated them. Gonveia, curate of the Hospital and chaplain to King John III, was considered very experienced in the art of healing the mentally ill.

In the sixteenth century, another Portuguese, J. Cidade, later sanctified with the name of St. John of God (San Juan de Dios), dedicated himself to the care of the mentally ill. Yet organized psychiatry did not begin until the nineteenth century, starting in 1848 with the opening of the Hospital of Rilhafoles in Lisbon, today known as the Hospital of Miguel Bombada, which had 300 beds and where occupational therapy was already mentioned in the rules.

In 1889 was promulgated the first special law regulating assistance for the insane; it had been inspired by A. M. Sena, the director of another hospital for the mentally ill, which was opened in 1883 in Porto.

Two more hospitals for the mentally ill were established on the outskirts of Lisbon in 1893 and 1895 by initiative of the Order of San Juan de Dios. A new law was proclaimed in 1889 which made obligatory a medico-legal examination of all accused persons suspected of being mentally ill.

In 1911, the year after the proclamation of the new Republic, a new decree promoted the reform of psychiatric care following the proposals of Julio de Matos, who established the official teaching of psychiatry in the universities of the three main Portuguese cities, Lisbon, Porto

---

* I am in debt to Prof. Barahona Fernandes of Lisbon for most of these data.

and Coimbra. This new law foresaw the creation of clinics for the seriously ill, as well as out-patient departments, agricultural colonies, etc.; however, not everything that the law envisaged was put into practice.

In 1945, inspired by Professor A. Flores and on the basis of his experience in hospital work, Julio Mateos brought psychiatric care up to date, giving importance not only to treatment, but also to prophylaxis. The government undertook the basic orientation, and a new law defined the principles of psychiatric services, which included medical aid and child psychology. This law foresaw the division of hospitals into various types, as, for example, agricultural colonies for children and adolescents, places for the mentally handicapped, provisions for dangerous and anti-social patients, for invalids, etc.

Naturally, the legal conditions of psychiatric care were also defined, especially the admission and discharge of patients, having in mind the necessary guarantees demanded for individual freedom. In those hospitals similar to the one in Lisbon were established psychiatric clinics independent of the School of Medicine; at the same time, consulting services were established also for psychology and mental hygiene. Presently, there are about 20 psychiatric establishments which allow for a greater mobility of care.

The most important Portuguese psychiatrists were born in the nineteenth century, like Vizarro (1805-1860), Gómes (1806-1877), Abrandes (1812-1872), Pulido (1815-1876), and Antonia María de Sena (1845-1890)). Because of his scientific approach, Sena was the first to stand out among the Portuguese psychiatrists; he had studied in Germany and France and had published some work on delirium and acute illnesses, and on the state of the mentally ill in Portugal.

Rodrigues Bettencourt (1845-1923) studied under Charcot and Bull. In 1888 he founded the first Portuguese *Journal of Neurology and Psychiatry*. The first free courses on these specialties were organized by him in the Hospital of Rhilhafoles, where he taught an empiric and anti-metaphysic type of psychiatry. Better known was Miguel Bombarda (1851-1910), director of the Rhilhafoles Hospital, which was later called "Bombarda Hospital." A man of strong and spirited personality, of an ideological materialistic background, he paid special attention to the organization of psychiatric services in his country; he also published a number of psychiatric papers in the journal *Contemporary Medicine*.

The successor of Bombarda was Julio de Matos, who inspired many psychiatric reforms in the first quarter of this century. Professor of Psychiatry at the Medical School of Lisbon, he published various psychiatric works, which include a study on paranoia and three volumes on the mentally ill appearing before the courts. While he was still young, he founded a journal. Magalhaes Lemos (1855-1931) was a disciple of Charcot, Magnan and Legrand de Saulle in Paris. In Portugal he was director of the Hospital Conde Ferreira and University Professor of Neurology and Psychiatry. Although materialistically oriented he published over 40 works, among which excels his work on unilateral hallucination due to damage of the temporal lobe and a study on the localization of the aphasias.

Sobral Cid (1877-1941) was Professor of the School of Medicine of Coimbra, and later of Lisbon; he distinguished himself by his polished investigations into psychopathology, which are reflected in his book entitled *The Psychic Life of the Schizophrenic,* published in 1925.

A. Costa Ferreira (1879-1922) initiated the study of child psychiatry in Portugal; he taught anatomy in the School of Medicine of Lisbon and was particularly dedicated to anthropologic investigations. A number of his papers have been published, including his lessons on psychiatry and pedagogy, and on occupational therapy for the mentally retarded.

A very distinguished worker, relatively recent, was Egas Moniz, world-wide famous Nobel Prize winner for his discoveries on cerebral angiography and pre-frontal leucotomy. His books and papers have been translated into many languages. There is a large bibliography on frontal leucotomy, and also an excellent German translation of his work on cerebral angiography. He was honored with many titles, decorations, etc., and he headed the Portuguese delegation to the Peace Conference held in Paris in 1918.

Today's psychiatry has reached a high level of development, thanks to the efforts, amongst others, of the Professors Barahona Fernandes, Seabra Dinis, Pedro Polonio, and of the neurosurgeon Almeida Lima, who closely collaborated with Egas Moniz in the development of leucotomy and arteriography, etc.

The ideas of contemporary Portuguese psychiatrists are not characterized by materialistic limitations, which were so fashionable with their predecessors. Barahona Fernandes is the originator of the "point of view embracing materialistic biologic, psychic and spiirtualistic phenomena in the personality as a whole." He has a good knowledge of foreign literature and of psychiatric services in various European countries; his works have received the widespread acclaim they merited. He has described the psychological action of leucotomy "as a regressive conduct accompanied by the syntonizing of the environments." He has not abandoned his work and is now Professor of

Psychiatry in the University of Lisbon. Fernando Fonseca, today a Professor in Porto, was trained in England. Diego Furtado, a military neuropsychiatrist who died a few years ago, excelled in neurology and in the investigation of certain states of avitaminosis.

For many years child psychiatry has been, and still is, fostered by Victor Fontes, who, with a number of collaborators, has directed an Institute for the observation and mental hygiene of children. In Lisbon, the "Egas Moniz" center promotes investigations in neurology and psychiatry, as well as practicing psychology in close collaboration with psychiatric clinics. There is also a small group of psychoanalysts.

The Portuguese Society of Neurology and Psychiatry was founded in 1949 in Lisbon, and in 1951 the Portuguese League for Mental Hygiene was established. During the last 20 years, Portuguese and Spanish psychiatrists have published the *Actas Luso Españolas de Neurologia y Psiquiatria y Ciencias Afines*.

REFERENCES

1. DELGADO ROIG, J. (1948): *Fundaciones Psiquiátricas en Sevilla y Nuevo Mundo*. Madrid: Paz Montalvo.
2. FOUCAULT, M. (1967): *Madness and Civilization*. Translated by Howard, R. London: Tavistock Publications.
3. SUAREZ HERNANDEZ, L. (1970): *Historia de España*. Edad Media. Gredos.
4. ULLERSPERGER, J. B.: *History of Psychology and Psychiatry in Spain*. Spanish translation by Peset.
5. WATT, W. M. & CACHIA, P. (1965): *History of Islamic Spain*. Edinburgh: Edinburgh University Press.
6. ZILBOORG, G. (1947): *A History of Medical Psychology*. New York: Norton.

4

FRANCE

YVES PELICIER, M.D.

Professor of Psychiatry, Paris, France

1

INTRODUCTION

French psychiatry is not a separate branch of European medicine. Throughout its evolution, the relations with England, Germany, Italy, and Spain were close. However, to circumscribe the field, this chapter will discuss the development of psychiatry within French territory.

2

THE MIDDLE AGES

Till the 13th century, Western medicine was entirely supported by Greek and Latin tradition, mainly through the works of Galen. Mental illness was described in many works, like the great theological *Summa* of Thomas Aquinas, or of Albert the Great. Cassian, abbot of Saint Victor, near Marseille, described "acedia," a kind of moroseness with spiritual apathy common in monks. Medical works of this period had no originality: in teaching and in practice, mental illnesses were not distinguished from physical disorders. The foundation of Montpellier University (1220) originated a famous medical center. Students and teachers came to it from all parts of Christian Europe. The Catalan physician Arnauld de Villeneuve (1250-1313), taught an eclectic medicine: he pointed out the role of inflammation of the brain ventricles (cellulae), of alimentary excess, and of passions in the production of mania. Villeneuve did not contest the humoral theory and advocated blood-letting, purges, and cauterization. Popular medicine was more original: there was a kind of specialization of the cult of saints and relics. Saint Mathurin de Larchant in Beauce, Saint Leu d'Esserant near Paris, and Saint Dymphne at Geel in Belgium, became places of pilgrimage for the insane and the epileptics.

Irrational phenomena were common and demonstrated the "contagion" of madness: they were exemplified by the children's crusades (1212), and in the many sects of mystics and prophets, such as Pierre de Bruys in Languedoc, Eon de Loudeac in Brittany, Pierre Valdo in Lyon, and so on. The adamites in Austria, the flagellants, the Saint Vitus dancers, and many others were the signs and proofs of a collective anxiety, aggravated by wars, starvation, and epidemics. People tended to confuse religion with superstition. At the end of the Middle Ages, and mainly since the 15th century, witchcraft and magic monopolized minds and appeared as an actual heresy, a new paganism. Modern psychiatry can find here the changing masks of hysteria and demonopathies.

3

THE RENAISSANCE

The psychological medicine of the Renaissance did not produce an influx of new ideas as we find in other disciplines, such as surgery and anatomy. Nevertheless, it did ask basic questions. What is madness? How does one become insane? The humanists answered that insanity is the key to wisdom, whereas the claim of understanding everything is a sign of the incurable madness of the so-called wise men—the theme of Sebastian Brandt (*Das Narrenschyff*, 1492), of Erasmus (*Encomium Moriae*, 1511), of Thomas More (*Utopia*, 1516), of Rabelais, of Montaigne, and others. But this represented merely a literary or philosophical attitude. In reality the law penalized insanity which was confused with magical practices and witchcraft. The court physician of the Duke of Cleves, Johan Weyer (1515-1588), wrote a famous book, *Histoires, disputes et discours des illusions et impostures* (1566); he claimed that almost all the so-called witches were old hags, completely out of their minds. King James I of England and the French jurist Jean Bodin (1580), supported by the judges Nicolas Remy, Henri

Boguet, and Pierre de Lancre, fanatically refuted Weyer's thesis. Some famous physicians, such as Fernel, Platter, Ambroise Pare, and Paracelsus, agreed with the witchcraft myth. On the other hand, those physicians who examined the so-called witches, by request of the Church, were skeptical and prudent; among them were Pigray, court physician of King Henry III, Michel Marescot, and Du Laurens.

Psychological medicine remained in the tradition of Galen. Hence Fernel's classification (1486-1557) included: 1. illness with fever (frenesia or parafrenesia); 2. illness without fever (simple melancholia); 3. mental debility (amentia, soporous states, catalepsy). Jacques Dubois advised the draining of humors—*humeurs peccantes*—in melancholy. Nicolas Lepois (1527-1587) asserted that every mental illness can produce acute and frenetic crises. Guillaume Baillou (1538-1616) and Du Laurens described erotic melancholy or melancholy *d'amour*.

4

THE 17TH CENTURY

In the 17th century, classical medicine was torn between two schools, the iatromechanical and the iatrochemical school. The first was represented in France by Claude Perrault, physician and architect of the Louvre, and by Hecquet. The second school, under the flag of Van Helmont and Thomas Willis, was represented by Deleboe (1614-1672), Lazare Rivière, and Nicolas Blegny. The influence of moralists and philosophers was important; they read Pascal, Cureau de la Chambre, Senault, and Descartes on the passions of the soul, not neglecting the works of the theologians (Bossuet). More often, essays on passions were support by an ingenious "neurophysiology" where animal spirits were believed to flow through nervous "fibers." The older the body, the harder and dryer the fibers, the more difficult the circulation of the spirits: passions were for young people!

Nevertheless, psychiatry was mostly in the hands of the moralists: the treatises on the passions were many, and usually copied one another. Physicians, in their *praxis medica,* repeated the classical teachings. For example Lazare Rivière (1589-1665), in his *Treatise* of 1662, included in the chapter devoted to the affections of the head: 1. cold humor of the brain; 2. soporous states (coma, lethargy, apoplexy); 3. watchfulness; 4. catalepsy (catochus); 5. palsies; 6. epilepsy; 7. convulsions; 8. children's epilepsy; 9. vertigo; 10. tremor; 11. frenesy;

12. brain abscess; 13. mania; 14. melancholy; 15. catarrh; and 16. headache.

In the chapter which concerns the spleen, Rivière wrote about hypochondria, whereas he relegated hysteria (furor, *passio hysterica*) to the section dealing with illnesses of women. However, Charles Lepois, like Thomas Willis, localized the source of hysteria in the brain. Lazare Rivière was an iatrochemist. Other physicians, like the famous Fagon, preferred an eclectic position, as Sydenham in England. The work of a physician from Toulouse, Jacques Ferrand, was devoted, once again, to erotic melancholy (1612).

Three important trials during the 17th century focused on the problem of the relationship between madness and witchcraft: the trial of the priest Gaufridy (Aix en Provence, 1611), the trial of Urbain Grandier (Loudun, 1632), and the trial of the Ursuline nuns (Louviers, 1633). They all had tragic results. In 1640, the Paris Parliament ceased to prosecute witches and the possessed. In 1670, there was a general prohibition of such trials, covering the whole kingdom.

There were some new trends in treatment of the insane. The Order of Charity, founded by a Portuguese friar, Joao Ciudad or Saint Jean de Dieu, had several hospitals in France: La Charité, in Paris (1601), Charenton (1642), Senlis, etc. Another famous priest, Saint Vincent de Paul (1581-1660), transformed an old leper-hospital, Saint Lazare, in Paris, into a lunatic asylum, where he advocated the humane management of patients. With the help of the Duchess of Aiguillon, he founded a general hospital for poor people. The royal edict of April 22, 1656 ordained the confinement (*le grand renfermement*) of beggars, tramps, vagabonds, free-thinkers, prostitutes, and the insane. The general hospital included five institutions in Paris: *La Pitié, La Salpêtrière, La Savonnerie, Bicêtre,* and *Scipion.* The promiscuity was awful and the treatment almost nonexistent. The confusion between vice and illness, sin and misfortune was complete. The general hospital of Colbert was mainly an instrument of social defense, used to protect Paris against marginal groups. For over a century, the charitable spirit of Saint Vincent de Paul was forgotten.

5

THE 18TH CENTURY AND THE ENLIGHTENMENT

The century of philosophers and reformers was a crucial moment for psychiatry. The basic principles were tolerance, respect of humanity, and philanthropical ideals. We find them in the works of moralists, of

men of letters, and of legal writers. Then again, the science of nature
and physics underwent an extraordinary development and gave medicine new patterns and methods. No doubt, the spirit of free inquiry did
not gain a complete triumph, as the medico-philosophical systems of
the past were always present, but the conceptions of experience and
observation prevailed over tradition and dogmatism.

Hence, Boerhaave corrected the theories of the hippocratic and of the
iatromechanic schools by insisting upon the solids (fibers) and not only
upon humors. He allowed the fiber to possess its own force. His disciple, Albert von Haller, from Switzerland, described a fundamental
property of fiber, irritability, different from Glissom's irritation. The
German physician, Friedrich Hoffman, imputed to fiber movement by
nervous fluid or "ether" the main power in the organism. Stahl (1660-
1734) refuted iatromechanic and iatrochemical theories; according to
him, the sensitive soul is the only motor of activity and dictates body
preservation. The "soul" governs all organic functions, growth, nutrition, circulation, and humor equilibrium. The message of the period
was that true medicine respects nature: that is the meaning of prudent
"expectation."

The Montpellier School modified the animism of Stahl into the
famous theory of vitalism. Boissier de Sauvages (1722-1776) and Barthez
(1734-1806) admitted a vital principle which mobilizes and keeps the
organism alive; it is the true "medicatrix" force. Indeed vitalism came
very near to discovering psychological forces.

Philosophical contributions were also considerable: the empiricism
of Locke, the theory of Berkeley, the phenomenism of Hume, and the
sensualism of Condillac supplied Pinel and the French "ideologues,"
Destutt de Tracy and Cabanis (*Rapports du Physique et du Moral*,
1802), with an actual pattern for the study of psychic life. In an
opposite direction, some of the encyclopaedists, Diderot, Helvetius,
d'Holbach, and La Mettrie (*L'homme—machine*, 1748), equated the
body to a machine and the mind to a natural function of the brain.

New classifications were produced by the physicians. The systems of
Linné, Vogel, Sagar, William Cullen, are well known. In France,
Boissier de Sauvages distinguished: 1. mental aberrations provoked by a
general cause; 2. delirium caused by brain fibers injury: mania, melancholy; 3. transitory delirium; and 4. dementia or feebleness of mind
(children, old people). We find the same classification in the *Medecine
pratique* by Lieutaud (1759). Melancholy was attracting much attention. The abbot Guyot Desfontaines (1685-1745) from Rouen used the
word *suicide* for the first time, in 1737. Bienville (1771) studied erotic
delirium. Tissot, from Genève, wrote about onanism. Pierre Pomme

(1763) was the author of a *Treatise upon vaporous affections*. He included hysteria, melancholy and spasmodic disorders in this group. The so-called *vapeurs* were attributed to the contraction and humidity of the fibers. English medicine, mainly through George Cheyne, Richard Whytt, and Richard Mead, had an important influence on French thought.

Psychiatric assistance in this period enlarged its scope, philanthropy succeeded charity. Chiarugi, in Italy, and William Tuke, in England, were the precursors of a movement which culminated with Pinel. Nevertheless, in spite of all these promises, the general conditions of the insane were very poor during the 18th century.

This panorama of pre-scientific psychiatry would be incomplete without taking into consideration more unorthodox factors. Witchcraft and trials were rare at the beginning of the century. There were the strange epidemics of Saint Medard cemetery, with the *convulsionnaires* around the tomb of Diacre Pâris, the Jansenist theologian. Later, interest in the mysterious became associated with interest for science, but quacks were often confused with scientists, as in the case of Cagliostro of Saint Germain and other adventurers. Sex problems were much in evidence with Casanova, the Marquis de Sade, Restif de la Bretonne, and others. There was a dark side to the century of enlightenment.

In Europe, and particularly in France, the success of Mesmer (1734-1815) with *animal magnetism* made it necessary to elaborate a scientific theory of psychic life, to counteract stage tricks. The need for explanations led also to the acceptance of Gall's phrenology and of Lavater's physiognomony. Through lack of truth, man accepts dreams.

6

THE 19TH CENTURY

In 19th-century France, intellectual life was dominated by two divergent currents. First, reliance on the exact sciences was complete, but the progress of knowledge was less bound to the absolute power of reason that it was in the preceding period: success and scientific results were considered the only valid facts. Accordingly, truth was believed to originate not only from the human mind, but from phenomena which man observes. On the quality of the method depended the quality of observation and of the doctrine. On this principle was based the French positivism of Auguste Comte and of all the scientific movements, from Littré to Renan. French medicine aimed at precision based on anatomy, clinical practice and the rules of experimental medicine. The *Introduction à la Médecine Expérimentale* by Claude Bernard appeared in 1865; the *Traité de l'auscultation médiate* by Laennec was published in 1819; and *Traité de la Diphtérie* by Bretonneau in 1826. They were the models for French alienists. In addition there were developments in biology, the introduction of Darwinism in France, and the important influence of associationism (Stuart Mill, Taine) on psychological research.

Diverging from that positivist and scientific current, we have to take into consideration the romantic stream, which was the field of emotions and temperament; man, according to the romantics, is moved by impulses that cannot be repressed. Turmoil is his law, sensibility and yearning his masters. Passions were no longer contrasted with reason; emotions were regarded as creative—even despair was thought of as a stimulus to create. *Moesta et errabunda,* as Baudelaire says, the romantic soul devotes its energies to insight and egotist contemplation. From this period until the rise of socialism, humanity is nothing more than a declamatory theme.

Over a period of several decades, French alienists have had to evolve a difficult method of studying and managing mental patients, taking into account all these philosophical currents.

Philippe Pinel and the Psychiatric Revolution

Pinel (1745-1826) (Plate XVI) was born in the southeast of France, near Albi, the son of a physician; he studied in Toulouse, then in Montpellier, where he attended the lectures of the vitalist school. Pinel knew the works of Locke and of Cullen and was specially interested in Condillac's methods and in the sensualist theory. During the most dramatic period of the French revolution, in 1793, he assumed the direction of the department for the insane, at Bicêtre, which was then a dungeon, a jail where excited patients were locked up in narrow cells. With the help of an experienced hospital attendant, Pussin, Pinel made history at Bicêtre by abolishing the use of chains for most of the patients. It was not merely a philosophical attitude; the release of the insane was medically important, and Pinel was perfectly conscious of it. Irons create agitation, hatred, and danger; conversely kindness allays excitement and allows contact, confidence, and cure. In 1795, Pinel was put in charge of the Salpêtrière hospital and here too he adopted the same generous attitude. He was not the first to advocate a more humane treatment of the insane; Tuke, in England, Chiarugi, in Italy, and Joseph Daquin (1733-1815), in Chambery, were also convinced of the value of such principles. But Pinel was more than a generous reformer; he was one of the most learned physicians of his generation. In 1798, he published his famous *Nosographie Philosophique;* in 1801, the *Traité médico-philosophique de l'aliénation men-*

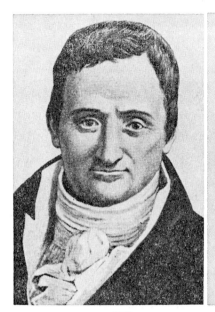

PLATE XVI.	PLATE XVII.
Phillipe Pinel (1745-1826).	Title page of Pinel's "Traité."

tale, one of the masterpieces of psychiatric literature (Plate XVII). At that time, Pinel was internationally known. He received many honors from Napoleon and the first Empire, but with the Restoration he lost his professorship at the University.

Pinel was a nosographer, but his own classification was inspired by Boissier de Sauvages and Cullen; he aspired to scientific precision, in the manner of botany; nevertheless, the resulting system is not original, for Pinel lacked an essential instrument of his analysis, a good hospital, where patients could be observed. The fourth class of Pinel's classification is that of *neurosis* which includes five orders: *Order 1*—neurosis of senses (sight, touch, etc.); *Order 2*—neurosis of cerebral functions: *suborder 1*—comata; *suborder 2*—vesania including mania, melancholy, hypochondria, etc.; *Order 3*—neurosis of locomotion and voice; *Order 4*—neurosis of generation (satyriasis, hysteria). As a therapist, Pinel advocated hygiene, good food, and a benevolent approach. He rejected systematic polypharmacy.

Esquirol and His Disciples

Pinel was a symbol, while Esquirol (1772-1840) was the leader of the French school of alienists. He was an observer who distrusted theory. Like Pinel, he was convinced of the importance of moral factors, but was also aware of organic factors. In fact, all his pupils became supporters of the organic approach in psychiatry.

Esquirol's classification of mental illness includes:

1. monomanias, i.e., partial delirium, which does not affect intelligence

   a) intellectual monomania (systematized delirium)
   b) affective monomania (perversions)
   c) instinctual monomania (homicide, pyromania, drunkenness, etc.)

2. general delirium, like mania
3. dementia
4. idiocy

This classification and the concept of monomania in particular were severely criticized. The main work of Esquirol was *Des Maladies Mentales considérées sous les rapports médical, hygiénique et médico-légal* (1838).

Among those who carried on the work of Pinel and Esquirol, J. P. Falret was one of the most important (1794-1870); he described alternate moods of mania and melancholy (*Folie circulaire,* 1854); Felix Voisin (1794-1872) devoted his efforts to mental retardation; Etienne Georget (1795-1828), who died prematurely, was the author of *De la folie,* illustrated by Gericault, in which he described stupidity as an acute dementia; Scipion Pinel (1795-1859) was a somatist, who believed that every mental illness is provoked by a peculiar brain vascular lesion, which he called *cérébrie*; Ulysse Trélat (1795-1879), a politician and physician, described "lucid insanity."

Francois Leuret (1797-1851) was the father of "moral treatment": delirium, he thought, is an error which can be refuted and corrected with persuasion and intimidation. It sounded like Celsius: *"fame, vinculis et plagis. . . ."* One of his followers, Louis Delasiauve (1804-1893) observed the primitive mental confusion.

One of the most original personalities of French psychiatry in this period was Moreau de Tours (1804-1884) (Plate XVIII), tried to consider madness within the whole patient. He recognized the links between dreams and delirium, analyzed the effect of hashish intoxication upon psychological functions, and he had an early concept of unconscious process, experimental psychosis, and so on. His main book was *Du haschich et de l'aliénation mentale* (Paris, 1845).

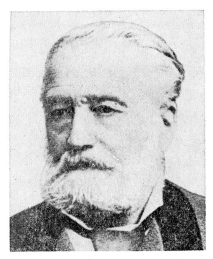

PLATE XVIII.
J. Moreau de Tours (1804-1884).

Jules Baillarger (1809-1890), a friend of Leuret, was the editor, with Cerise and Longet, of the *Annales Médico-Psychologiques* (1843), one of the oldest psychiatric reviews. He described "circular insanity" and psychic hallucinations, as opposed to the psychosensorial. Brierre de Boismont (1798-1881) made a special study of suicide, homicide, and hallucinations.

A very important event in psychiatry was the description by Antoine Bayle (1799-1858) of meninges inflammation in cerebral palsy (1822). This was the first time that an anatomical injury had been found responsible for insanity. In 1905, Alfred Fournier recognized the syphilitical origin of insanity. Unfortunately, the description of cerebral palsy will remain a lonely monument to organic psychiatry.

Legal Provisions

Two of the main disciples of Pinel, Esquirol and Ferrus (1784-1861), were the artisans of the famous law of 1838, one of the oldest regulations still in form in France. The basic principle of the law is the creation, in every *département,* of a lunatic asylum where poor or lonely people could be admitted. In order to avoid arbitrary confinement, admissions are strictly controlled by public authority. Voluntary admission (*placement volontaire*) is decided by the family, or by close relations, who can obtain the discharge of the patient at any time. The official admission (*placement d'office*) is decided by public authority, in case of emergency or danger, under the control of the *Préfet.* In any case, the mental health of the patient must be attested by several physicians and, if the patient protests against the confinement, a new investigation must be ordered by the administrative authority. During his stay in the hospital, the patient loses the right of conducting business and managing his property and an administrator is appointed to do this for him till his complete recovery. This law was an effective step forward; nevertheless, it was considered a menace to private freedom. However, misuses seem to have been very rare and the benefits important. The building of new hospitals was the only means to advance clinical psychiatry and to protect patients against the intolerant industrial society of the 19th century. All the modern criticism of the "fortress hospital" and segregation of the insane in this pre-therapeutic period of psychiatry is unjustified. Some psychiatrists, brought up with chemotherapy and psychoanalysis, should mitigate their comments and relate them to the historical development of psychiatry in the last century. Even if we admit the necessity of reforming the law of 1838, it appears to have been a good and an effective tool. Among the followers of Esquirol, Parchappe (1800-1866), called the *Napoleon des asiles,* was the most famous; he was against the segregation of curable from incurable patients and recommended the building of small hospitals.

Degeneration Theory: Morel and Magnan

Under the influence of evolutionism and of new discoveries about heredity, the French alienists since the middle of the 19th century had adopted a rigid conception of mental illness.

Benedict Morel (1809-1873), a friend of Claude Bernard, observed mentally retarded patients in the Maréville asylum, near Nancy. The cause of mental retardation was searched for in hereditary constitution or in infantile illness. Alcoholism, misery, and infections were often regarded as responsible for that kind of deviation from the norm which was called degeneration. Morel's theory was generally accepted, mainly in Germany by Krafft-Ebing. In France, Victor Magnan (1835-1912) was at first interested in alcoholism, but later adopted Morel's views. Magnan considered two kinds of madness: one among "normal" people, under the influence of violent and severe stress, who become delirious, melancholic, manic; the other among degenerates, where there is no link between stress and reaction and with physical stigma of degeneration (morphological asymmetry). The "superior degenerates" show disorders of character, impulsivity, obsessions, perversions, but no mental retardation as do the "inferior degenerates." The influence of the Morel-Magnan theory was important in Italy (Lombroso) and in England (Maudsley). In France, it was the origin of naturalist topics: atavism, alcoholic fatality (Zola), and heredity of delinquency.

Among the great French alienists of this period was Ernest Lasègue (1816-1883), who described the persecution delirium, the *folie à deux,* and the "dream-like" alcoholic delirium. Jules Falret (1824-1902), with Lasègue and Magnan, defined the systematized chronic delirium which develops in four acts, as a tragedy: 1. interpretation and anxiety period; 2. delirium organization period with hallucination; 3. megalomaniacal period; 4. ultimate dementia. This unitary conception of delirium did not stand up to the analytical orientation of future clinicians.

Neurological and Psychological Trends

During most of the 19th century, alienists were fascinated by positivist patterns: mental illness was described as a physical disorder. Almost no attention was given to the problems of personality. Etiology was limited to hereditary or accidental physical conditions. Psychological disturbances were the field of poets or novelists.

Nevertheless, the french psychological school was very active: Ribot (1839-1916), the founder of abnormal psychology, wrote his main works: *Maladies de la volonté* (1883), *Maladies de la Mémoire* (1881), and *Maladies de la personnalité* (1885).

During the same period, the cerebral localization theory prevailed: in 1861, Broca designated the third frontal circonvolution as the responsible area for aphemia. In 1863, Gustave Dax pointed out the left lateralization of the language area. Lordat, Baillarger, and Trousseau studied aphasia. After Wernicke, in Germany, Charcot, the "Master of La Salpétrière Hospital," separated many verbal images, corresponding to centers. The French philosopher Bergson was severely opposed to that mechanical conception. In 1906, Pierre Marie described motor aphasia (*anarthrie*). The neurological pattern, based on the study of language, became very powerful at the end of the 19th century.

Charcot (1825-1893), faced with the problem of hysteria, had no doubt about its neurological origin. Hence, he applied to it the effective criteria of his previous researches. For him, hysteria was comparable with convulsive or spasmodic illness, such as chorea, epilepsy, and shaking palsy. The hysterical crisis, according to him, comprises four stages: the epileptoid phase; the large movements phase ("clownism"); the passionate attitudes phase; and termination delirium and muscular resolution. Charcot emphasized the permanent stigma of hysteria (anesthesia, hysterogenic zones). With Richer and Gilles de la Tourette he considered hypnosis as a form of experimental hysteria. Nevertheless, his disciples were not convinced: Binet and Féré were in agreement with Charcot, but Babinski and Pierre Janet were hesitant to accept his theories.

In fact, hysteria was not a new problem in France. Mesmer had been expelled from Paris in 1784, but animal magnetism still had some defenders: the Marquis de Puysegur, Deleuze, the abbot of Faria and Azam and Broca, and the disciples of James Braid. Liébeault, a physician from Nancy, pointed out the importance of psychological factors in production of hysteria, especially concentration and imitation. Despite the fact that by 1866 psychological factors were recognized, when Charcot took over the Salpétrière psychiatric department, he ignored the psychological theory of Liébeault. In 1884, another physician from Nancy, Bernheim, believed that hysteria has no physical etiology, but all is mental, provoked by the observation itself. The main phenomenon of hysteria is suggestibility which is at its highest during hypnosis. Charcot was eventually obliged to agree with the mental theory of hysteria. Babinski (1901) proposed the name of "pithiatism" to designate a special condition, where suggestion is able to produce or suppress clinical symptoms. The mistake of Charcot was of historical importance for psychiatry: in 1885 Freud was a pupil of Charcot, in Paris, and, in 1889, he visited Bernheim in Nancy. But the works of Pierre Janet also sprang from the Charcot school.

7

THE EARLY 20TH CENTURY

During the development of psychoanalytical theory in Austria, Switzerland, Germany, and Hungary, French psychology proceeded in two main directions. On the one side, abnormal psychology, initiated by Ribot, was represented by Janet, by Georges Dumas, and by Binet, while experimental psychology, in the hands of Henri Pieron, took a leading place. On the other side, child psychology, with Henri Wallon and Jean Piaget, provided psychiatrists with helpful patterns of analysis.

Pierre Janet

Pierre Janet (1859-1947) observed a hierarchy of tendencies and functions in the complexity of human behavior: he placed at the bottom automatic life; at the top, rational, experienced, and finalized actions; and in the middle, immediate actions and beliefs. According to him, the different levels of action corresponded to special levels of psychological tension. When psychological tension is low, only an automatic life is possible, as in neurosis. Tension is regarded as an activator of psychic life, but "psychological force" is necessary to produce emotions, thought, and behavior. Neuroses are, more or less, exhaustion illnesses. The central concept of Janet pathology was asthenia. In his description of psychasthenia, Janet developed the picture of an hypotonic and asthenic personality economizing its poor forces by narrowing the field of action and limiting its penetration of reality. Equilibrium is the true problem and we can consider Janet's works as a dynamic psychology. Recently, Janet's conceptions have been utilized in efforts to analyze the effects of chemotherapy in mental illness.

The bibliography of Janet's works is considerable; among them are: *L'automatisme psychologique* (1889), *L'état mental des hystériques* (1893), *Les obsessions et la psychasthénie* (1903), *Les médications psychologiques* (1919), *De l'angoisse a l'extase* (1926), *L'amour et la haine* (1932).

Para-Kraepelinian Psychiatry

Within the first edition of his handbook of psychiatry in 1883 and the edition of 1896, Kraepelin enclosed European psychiatry in a terrifying system: every clinical picture had its place, every patient's destiny was predetermined. The psychiatric hospital was like the firmament of Kepler in which the positions and movements of stars and planets are determined.

French psychiatrists, like those in other countries, were impressed by the Kraepelin system, but they tried, progressively, to defend their traditional nosography. The great tragedy of the chronic systematized delirium (Magnan, Lasègue, Falret) was forsaken. Paul Serieux and Capgras (1902) described the "reasoning madness" which corresponded to systematized delirium without hallucination. Ernest Dupré evolved the notion of cenesthopathia (1907) and of imaginative delirium (1910). Gilbert Ballet and Logre defined the clinical picture of chronic hallucinatory psychosis (1911). Dide described the "passionate idealists" and the "delusions of grandeur," as a special chapter of paranoia.

At the same time, Bleuler (1857-1939) in Zurich was revising Kraepelin's concept of Dementia Praecox by proposing the notion of schizophrenia; a French psychiatrist, Chaslin, was doing the same. The work of Bleuler was published in 1911, the Chaslin book in 1912. To the Bleulerian concept of dissociation corresponded the Chaslinian concept of discordance. Later, in 1926, Claude described the group of "schizoses," with mild forms (schizo-neurosis), and severe forms (schizomania). The work of Claude gave rise to contemporary researches on borderline types which we call états-limits. In 1927, the French clinician Eugène Minkowski, a disciple of Bleuler and Bergson, made a prominent contribution to the study of schizophrenia: he pointed out the central concept of "vital contact with reality," lacking in schizophrenic patients; his thesis of "morbid rationalism" and "pathological geometrism" was noteworthy. In the last decades, Paul Guiraud, a clinician and histopathologist, refused the Bleulerian concept and used the old term of hebephrenia to designate a primitive failure of instinctual forces, explained by a neurobiological disturbance in the mesodiencephalic structures.

Clerambault and Mental Automatism

Gaetan de Clerambault (1872-1934) was a famous Parisian psychiatrist (Plate XIX). His approach was mainly organic; he distinguished an autonomic and automatic nucleus of ideation in pathological think-ink which provokes hallucinations of hearing, the impression of actions commentary, a feeling of predicting the thoughts of other people, a feeling of being spied upon, influenced, and so on. This syndrome of mental automatism depends, according to Clerambault, on brain irritation (toxic or infectious). Clerambault defined, too, a group of psychoses with a peculiar prominent and fixed idea (jealousy, prejudice). He described also erotomania, or the illusion of being loved.

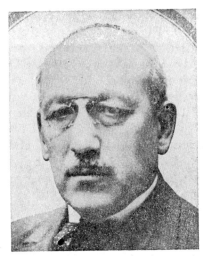

PLATE XIX.
Gaetan de Clerambault (1872-1934).

8

CONTEMPORARY TRENDS

Until the 1960's, the influence of psychoanalysis in France was limited. In spite of a brilliant school (Nacht, Hesnard, Lagache, Lacan), there was no great following in psychiatric circles. In the 1970's, the situation is changing: the new generation of psychiatrists is more interested in psychodynamic problems. This change was made easier by the development of chemotherapy and social therapy. Since 1952, with the use of chlorpromazine in mental illness by Delay and Deniker in the University Clinic of Paris, progress has been more evident and French psychiatrists have experimented with many of the most important psychotropic drugs, especially neuroleptics (phenothiazine derivates). More often, French clinicians rely on the biological treatment of psychosis.

French psychiatry is eclectic and tries to keep midway between the psychological and the chemotherapeutic techniques.

In the field of social therapy, since the famous report of Paul Serieux (1903), who severely criticized the French system of hospitalization, various attempts were made to transform the old psychiatric hospital. In 1922, Edouard Toulouse opened a "free service," based on the provisions of a law enacted in 1838, in Sainte Anne Hospital. Following Hermann Simon, in Germany, and Maxwell Jones, in England, Daumezon has propounded the notion of "institutional psychotherapy" and Paul Sivadon has insisted upon the necessity of a special type of architecture for mental hospitals; egotherapy and sociotherapy is being developed. A new form of assistance out of the hospital is proposed too, whereby the medical team—psychiatrists, psychologists, nurses and social workers—is responsible for a geographical "sector" of about 70,000 inhabitants. All the psychiatric work, from detection to after-care, is conducted by the same people, thus providing continuity of care. Hospitalization is as short as possible. This type of assistance is helpful to suppress "institutional illness" and chronicity. There are about 120,000 patients in the French psychiatric hospitals and it is hoped to reduce this number by increasing the rate of ambulatory discharged.

REFERENCES

1. BARIETY, M. & COURY, CH. (1963): *Histoire de la Médecine*. Paris: A. Fayard.
2. BARUK, H. (1967): *La psychiatrie francaise de Pinel à nos jours*. Paris: Presses Universitaires de France.
3. DELAY, J. (1953): *Etudes de Psychologie Médicale*. Paris Presses Universitaires de France.
4. EY, H. (1952): *Etudes Psychiatriques*, 1º série. Paris: Desclée de Brouwer.
5. HUNTER, R. & MACALPINE, I. (1963): *Three Hundred Years of Psychiatry*. London: Oxford University Press.
6. MUELLER, F. L. (1960): *Histoire de la Psychologie*. Paris: Payot.
7. PELICIER, Y. (1965): *Intégration de la sociologie à la psychiatrie clinique*. Paris: Masson.
8. PELICIER, Y. (1971): *Histoire de la Psychiatrie*. Paris: Presses Universitaires de France.
9. PELICIER, Y. (1972): *Psychiatrie compréhensible*. Paris: A. Fayard.
10. SEMELAIGNE, R. (1930): *Les pionniers de la psychiatrie francaise*. Paris: Baillère.
11. STAROBINSKI, J. (1960): *Histoire du traitement de la mélancolie*. Bâle: Documenta Geigy.
12. ZILBOORG, G. (1941): *A History of Medical Psychology*. New York: Norton & Co.

5

BELGIUM

R. PIERLOOT, M.D.

Professor of Psychiatry, University of Leuven, Belgium

1

INTRODUCTION

As an autonomous state, Belgium is less than 150 years old. During the preceding centuries, it was repeatedly occupied by other nations and was often the battlefield on which feuds between greater powers were resolved. Thus it is difficult to take a long backward look at the history of psychiatry in Belgium; one can only consider how the mentally ill were treated in those regions that later formed the territory of Belgium.

There are no records of any systematized attitude towards the mentally ill in the period prior to the Roman conquest; moreover, Greco-Roman medical principles, which may have found acceptance through the Roman occupation, were completely lost during the successive invasions of the Franks, the Germans, the Vikings, and various hordes from the East. The most ancient known forms of psychological medicine and provisions for the mentally ill date from the 8th to the 15th century and are manifestations of the culture of the Middle Ages, which reached a high level of development in the Low Countries. Traditional medical views were mixed with Christian religious elements, as they had been introduced for the major part from Italy and France by preachers and derived from monastic medicine. With the development of lay medicine and the foundation of the first university centers in the 13th century, the same general principles continued to be proclaimed for quite some time.

The influence of the Christian Church on psychiatric care persisted in the later expansion of psychiatry in Belgium, although in different forms. The importance of Christian charitable institutions in this country cannot be ignored and was, until recently, still paramount. They stimulated to a large extent the humanizing of psychiatric treatment, but probably they also contributed to a certain paternalistic rejection of the more modern concepts.

From the historical viewpoint, it is a remarkable phenomenon that at Geel, from an original medieval pilgrimage to the shrine of St. Dymphna, developed a form of foster family care for the insane, which preceded in practice the theoretical insights developed in more recent times.

2

THE MENTALLY ILL IN MEDIEVAL CULTURE

After extensive study of original lay and ecclesiastical documents, Beek (2) produced a global outline of the picture presented by the mentally ill and the concern they engendered in medieval times. In the following account, we shall rely greatly upon his study.

The differentiation of the mentally ill in various clinical pictures shows that, in this period, a certain descriptive nosological knowledge already existed. Manifestations of insanity with accompanying somatic symptoms and often fatal issue were described as *frenesis;* the *insania* were manifestations without somatic symptoms. They were divided into mania and melancholy, which were respectively characterized by unrestrained or inhibited behavior. Epilepsy, with sudden cramps and unconsciousness, was called the *falling-sickness,* or *lunatism,* because it was supposed to be influenced by the moon cycle. The symptoms of *rabies* following the bite of a mad dog were known, but under the more general term of *hydrophobia* were classified with other conditions characterized by refusal to eat or drink. *Hysteria,* ascribed to the displacement of the uterus in the body, was characterized by changes of consciousness. Moreover, it seems likely that all kinds of hysterical reaction and psychogenic psychotic manifestations were called *diabolic possession.*

Furthermore, mental derangements were classified according to three categories of the psychological doctrine of mental capacities. Hence, they were divided into functional disturbances of the imagination, of the intellect, or of the memory.

Medieval opinions about the origin of mental deviations show a remarkable compromise between the traditional humoral theories and demoniacal beliefs. A humor and its presence in a given organ, or the change of substance of an organ, were deemed the basis of behavior disorders, which, however, could also be ascribed to the presence of a demon in the body. In assessing the etiology and the course of a disease, supernatural, moral and cosmic forces, as well as human and material influences, were taken into consideration (17).

This multi-factorial view of the causality and genesis of the mental derangement unavoidably led to a wide variety of mutually complementary forms of treatment. Through surgical interventions, among which was trepanation, the removal of the diseasing agent was contrived. But the same goal was also aimed at with symbolic and magical formulae, which culminated in the exorcism ritual. At the same time therapeutic changes of the humors and the substance of the organs were expected from the intake of medicinal herbs or the following of a diet. Not only the physician and the priest, who were often the same person, but also the man in the street was involved in the administering of these forms of treatment.

Relatives and friends took care of the mentally ill, who were often allowed to wander about freely and thus, because of their wandering through forests and their unusual behavior, were called *wood men* or *fools* (jesters). The intellectually deficient or insane *wood man,* with his aggressive or sexual unbridledness, sought solitude, while the *fool* or *jester* was the prototype of careless folly, who, as an object of laughter, was imitated in the role of court jester or theater fool.

Gradually the city authorities concerned themselves with the care of the mentally ill and they were cared for in hospitals. At the beginning they were taken to the city hospitals, together with other types of patients. Later, the madhouses developed, often conglomerates of separate small madhouses, where the mentally ill were housed with vagrants and paupers.

The oldest known institution of this type in Belgium is the St. John's home at Ghent, founded in 1191 (5). Around 1400 a similar institution was functioning at Bruges (8), followed by others at Mons and Antwerp, in the 15th century. The modalities of admission, residence and dismissal and the legal status were officially laid down. In some cases, the relatives paid, but financial support from the city was foreseen.

An important aspect of the concern for mental patients was the pilgrimages to shrines of saints, to whom a special curative power was ascribed. At these places, medical interventions as well as exorcism

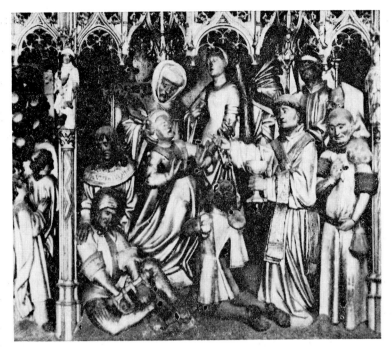

PLATE XX. Church of St. Dymphna, Geel. One of the 21 altar carvings executed by Jan Wave in 1515 showing the demoniacs, lunatics, and other sufferers succored by Dymphna.

rituals took place. The pilgrimage to St. Hermes Church in Ronse (1) and the cult of St. Dymphna at Geel became particularly important; the latter led to a system of foster family care in that city.

According to the description by Petrus Cameracensis in 1247 based upon a popular legend, Dymphna was the daughter of an Irish king, who ran away from her father when he wanted to marry her, after the death of his wife. She went to Antwerp and thence to Geel, where she was discovered by her father and, because of her continued refusal, was murdered. There are no precise dates, but one may assume that the facts of the legend should be placed in the 7th or 8th century. From the 11th to 12th century, Geel and the shrine of St. Dymphna (Plate XX) were known for miraculous cures of many affections, but were not yet limited to mental diseases. By the end of the 13th century, a hospital was built at Geel in addition to the already existing two chapels of St. Dymphna, where several priests took care of the pilgrims.

From the second half of the 14th century, Geel gradually became a place of pilgrimage specifically for mental patients. Since the church could not provide food and shelter for all the patients, the custom originated to lodge them in the houses of the local population, for the period of one to nine days during which they honored the holy relics. Only around the end of the 15th century was a sick room built next to the church. The miraculous cures made Geel famous as an ever-increasing number of pilgrims poured in, so that, in 1532, a college of ten curates was set up in the church dedicated to St. Dymphna and they were entrusted with the treatment of the sick. In 1562, the college was transformed into a chapter of ten canons (12, 13).

3

REPRESSIVE PRACTICES VERSUS NATURAL SCIENCES AND HUMANISTIC THEORY

At the end of the 15th century the general attitude towards the mentally ill became more rejective and repressive; this attitude left its mark until the 18th century. In the same period, however, a number of works on the natural sciences and on humanistic principles were published; they too provided important basic material for the subsequent development of medicine and psychiatry.

In 1486 the Emperor Maximilian officially approved in Brussels the book by the German Dominican fathers Sprenger and Kraemer, which under the title of *Malleus Maleficarum,* was to be drafted between 1487 and 1489 at Cologne University (18). Herein some psychopathological manifestations were reduced to various forms of witchcraft and diabolical possession. Sexuality, in its most varied utterances and outspoken role, was regarded as the link between witchcraft and mental illness. The work went through ten editions in the following 150 years, which points to its widespread influence and distribution. With its practical hints on how to recognize and treat witches, it provided the foundations for those repressive practices which victimized mental patients during the inquisition.

However, this did not prevent a certain Christian charity being shown towards those who were willing to entrust themselves to the bosom of the Church and to submit to the necessary rituals. Hence, in this period, the cult of St. Dymphna at Geel reached its climax. The canons had worked out a complex ceremonial of offerings, processions, penances and prayers, extended over nine days. In 1687, the sick room was rebuilt in the vicinity of the relics, against the southern side of the church tower (Plate XXI), so that two big and three small rooms were available for the nursing of the patients by specially appointed female nurses. This provision, however, proved insufficient and the patients had to be housed with the inhabitants of the city. As a result of this, after completing their nine days of devotions, some patients remained at Geel with the intention of performing the rituals once more at a later date or to see whether their recovery was constant. After having been accepted into their new community and having reached a certain adjustment to it, the stay of some of the patients became of an undetermined duration. It may be readily assumed that

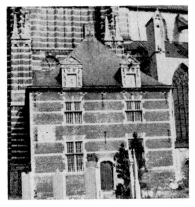

PLATE XXI. Sick room at Geel, built in 1687 against the southern side of the church tower.

ever since the 17th century quite a number of mentally ill have found shelter with the families of Geel. In the hospitals, madhouses, and places of pilgrimage, the use of rods and chains to restrain mental patients had become a general rule. At Geel, where the patients were lodged with private families, this created some problems. Thus we find reports of imprudent lack of restraint of dangerous madmen, or of arbitrary and superfluous interventions. In other places also, such as Stiphout, Herent, and Lebbeke, sick rooms connected with a shrine had been erected (20). St. Hubert's shrine was known as a miraculous site for people bitten by a rabid dog.

It is remarkable that at the beginning of this period the practical approach to mental patients developed independently of any medico-scientific institution. Yet at the same time it was characterized by a revival of scientific and humanistic interest. Cities such as Bruges,

Ghent, Brussels, and Leuven (where a university was founded in 1426) had developed into well known cultural and scientific centers. The work realized there contributed to a large extent to the development, later, of scientific medical psychology. It was at Leuven that Vesalius began the research that led to the publication of his volume on anatomy in 1553, one of the pillars of modern medicine. It was at Brussels that Erasmus stayed repeatedly and made public his humanistic ideas in select intellectual circles. At Leuven and at Bruges, Vives spent the 20 most productive years of his life; he died in 1540, at Bruges, aged 48.

Vives, called by Zilboorg (24) the first true precursor of Freud, disavowed his Spanish upbringing and his Paris scholastic education and went to Flanders and England to develop his personal creative theories. In his work *De anima et vita* (22), he describes in an empirical fashion the functioning of the mind. He was the first to recognize the importance of psychological associations, their influence upon emotional factors and the relation with forgetting and recollecting. His analysis of feelings and emotions as active and passive love, shame, ambivalence, and jealousy, has been accepted and further elaborated in modern psychodynamic theories. By recommending that, in the first place, the patient's perturbed mental functions should be observed and the causes of the perturbation sought, and that the patient should be treated humanely he emerged far above the prevailing views of his time. His concern for social justice, the paramount importance he gave to education, and his belief in the equality of women raise him to the level of one of the most universal humanists.

His views, however, found no repercussion in the contemporary approach to mental patients. Moreover, religious feuds, wars, and successive occupations for a long time produced a climate unfavorable to intellectual scientific development. The efforts of research workers from neighboring countries, such as the work of Paracelsus, Weyjer Ferrand, and Stahl, and the medical discoveries of the 18th century did not reach Belgium until later.

Although the ecclesiastical repressive attitude had abated in the 18th century, the fate of the insane was no better. In certain cities, they were confined to jail, without medical examination or juridicial sentence. Well-to-do people were left to their sorry plight in neglected lunatic's departments in hospitals. In the institutions, they were chained, ridiculed, mistreated, and even exposed as curiosities to a paying public. The civil authorities provided no regulations and interested individuals could make arbitrary decisions, whereby many abuses occurred (4).

At Geel, where in the meantime a few hundred patients continued to be lodged with the citizens, the local authorities issued, between 1676 and 1754, three regulations with the purpose of maintaining peace and order and regulating the relations between civil and ecclesiastical authorities in respect to the patients (21).

4

THE DEVELOPMENT OF INSTITUTIONAL PSYCHIATRY

At the end of the 18th century, under the influence of physicians like Pinel, Tuke, Reil, Chiarugi, and Franck, a movement started with the aim of providing humane and understanding treatment for the mentally ill. This new approach was termed "moral treatment." Throughout the French Revolution, the mental patient was gradually wrested away from the Church; in 1797, the church of St. Dymphna (Geel) with its sick room was closed.

The new regime made some attempts to bring some order in the care of mental patients, but some abuses still remained. Around the middle of the 19th century, a systematic structure for psychiatric care emerged. This was the result of important efforts from different sources. The government adjusted the legislation, while in the medical field a scientific systematization of therapy gradually developed. The contribution of the Catholic Church consisted of the erection of quite a number of new psychiatric institutions, administered by newly founded religious orders; in these institutions mental patients were given a more charitable and humane treatment.

The decrees, issued in France after the Revolution, became laws in 1797 and applied also to the annexed territories. They gave a more legal character to the incarceration in jail of mental patients, but brought no practical change to their plight.

The Civil Code of Law (1803) established a procedure whereby mental patients were placed in custody. When the tribunal decided this upon demand by a relative, the family council was allowed to decide whether to have the patient treated at home or in an institution. Thus cases of arbitrary confinement should no longer happen. In practice the application of the law was very poor. Some boards of civil hospitals tried to adhere to the legal regulations, but the enormous costs of a cumbersome procedure made it almost impossible. Thus, in numerous institutions, including that at Geel, a number of patients was illegally confined. The police officer at Geel, for instance, reported in 1809 that 200 insane patients were illegally in residence there. Because of the difficulties in redacting a local regulation, the higher authorities went so far as to threaten to forbid the residing of mental patients with the citizens (21).

In 1815, after the overthrow of Napoleon, William I simplified the judicial procedure, so that it became possible upon the simple demand of a relative or of a civil attorney to place an individual suspected of being insane for one year in an institution. In 1818, William I issued another decree ordering the closure of inadequate institutions and the construction of new institutions. The direction and the financial management of those establishments were also outlined. In practice little was accomplished, and the decree of 1815 was abolished with the Belgian independence in 1830.

In 1832 Ducpétiaux, who was appointed inspector general of prisons and charitable institutions, published a report (6) denouncing the miserable conditions of the insane and pointing out the need for a medical assessment. Through his intervention, a commission was appointed in 1841 which inspected the existing institutions and drew up a report (15). Of the 37 establishments then existing, only three were found where somehow satisfactory medical care was deemed possible. Poor material conditions, arbitrary confinement and other abuses were widespread.

Yet this situation lasted until 1850, when legislation dictated that medical advice was required before committing an individual to a mental hospital; the co-operation between medical, judicial and administrative authorities was also regulated. The legal position of the patient and the necessary material and medical requirements of psychiatric hospitals were also designated by law. To safeguard the implementation of these regulations a system of control and inspection was devised at the same time. This, then, was the basis, completed in 1872, on which was built a system that provided psychiatric care with a definitive legal structure (23).

From the medical side, the most important contribution was made by Guislain, who was professor at Ghent University from 1835 until his death in 1860 (19). In 1826 he denounced the abuses perpetuated in psychiatric institutions in his work, *Traité sur l'Aliénation Mentale et sur les Hospices des Aliénés* (*Treatise on Mental Alienation and Asylums for Lunatics*) (9). He was also one of the principal collaborators of Ducpétiaux in the struggle for decent medical and material conditions for these homes. Furthermore, Guislain was a typical representative of the scientists of that period. In 1833, in his *Traité sur les Phrénopathies* (10), he presented his views on the causes, forms, and nature of mental afflictions. According to him, mental illness was to be considered as a dynamic change of the brain, an alteration of the vital forces. The most important etiological factors are moral, although the physical ones should not be excluded. Hereditary, abnormally strong character features and a large group of emotions called *agents moraux* ought to be taken into consideration. The evil influences of the modern Occidental civilization were also strongly stressed and denounced by him. Heredity, however, is also given a major role.

Guislain considered mental illness to be a reaction to affective trauma, an *impression douloureuse*. He distinguished six main categories of reactions: melancholy, mania, ecstasy, phobia, delirium and dementia.

Later, in his *Leçons orales sur les phrénopathies* (11), he emphasized the importance of the various methods of treatment; good upbringing, education, and work must be offered to those patients who live in collective groups. He himself drew up the plans of a new psychiatric asylum to be built in a healthy environment, with gardens, fields, and workshops. In 1857, it was operational at Ghent, where it still exists as the Guislain Institute.

The contributions of as eminent a scholar as Guislain were a stimulus to the development of psychiatry as a science. Psychiatrists needed a common organ of communication, which was provided by the *Annales médico-légales*, first published in 1855; the *Société Phréniatrique Belge* was founded later, in 1869.

As already mentioned, one of the main problems facing the development of psychiatry was the poor medical and material conditions of most institutions for the mentally ill. With the laicization of the care of mental patients at the end of the 18th century, a series of homes, sometimes mere lodging for ten or twenty patients, were started by private individuals, who often exploited the plight of the mentally ill. A report prepared in 1841 states, "The managers of most asylums are nothing else but contractors, speculators who ply their trades in the most convenient and lucrative way for themselves. An honorable exception existed in certain religious congregations which aimed at offering relief to the suffering of the unfortunate people entrusted to their care" (15).

The initiative taken by ecclesiastical bodies with charitable aims was the basis of momentous improvements in the living conditions in psychiatric institutions. In the first half of the 18th century, various new religious orders were founded, which dedicated themselves entirely, or partly, to the nursing of mental patients. Pioneer work was accomplished in this field by Canon Triest, who in 1808 succeeded in persuading the authorities to entrust to his Sisters of Charity the nursing of female mental patients in the asylum of the city of Ghent. Afterwards, he contrived to obtain the same arrangement in other homes. This example was followed by various other founders of religious orders. Between 1830 and 1850, 18 new psychiatric hospitals operated by religious orders were founded. In the second half of the 19th century, about three-quarters of the nursing of the insane was undertaken by religious orders (3).

The lodging of patients with families at Geel had also progressively increased in the first half of the 19th century. From 284 in 1804, the number rose to 1,000 in 1847. Nevertheless, this was a period of transition which entailed many difficulties. There was an inevitable shift from the cult of St. Dymphna to proper psychiatric care in the foster family context. Although there was medical interest for this kind of nursing, as it appears from a visit to Esquirol in 1821, it was a long time before medical intervention became integrated at Geel. As late as 1855 it was possible to install a still rather primitive infirmary. Administrative supervision also brought some problems. Until 1851 a few cities which sent patients to Geel had a director on the spot, who could more or less act according to his own views. In 1851 the legislative body instituted a higher committee, dependent on the Ministry of Justice, which was responsible for the inspection and the protection of patients, but, because of local resistance, it could not function properly until some years later (21).

In 1851 a total of 3,841 patients were accommodated in the 60 existing institutions. Most of them, however, had fewer than 20 patients each. From then on reports from the permanent committee for inspection were regularly transmitted to the Ministry (16). This led to the closing down of several inadequate homes and to an obvious improvement in the medical and material standard of the remainder. In 1871, 5,909 patients were placed in asylums and the number increased during the following years. From 1860 the patients at Geel, too, were taken to a central infirmary and kept under observation before being placed in a family. Institutional psychiatry, by then, was in line with current practice and continued to prosper.

5

THE 20TH CENTURY

The first half of the 20th century is characterized by a further expansion and stabilization of psychiatric institutions, in which the total number of patients reached 25,000 in 1952 (14). This institutionalization of patients caused certain rigidity and a one-sided development of psychiatry. Hence the infiltration of new points of view and new forms of psychiatric theory and practice was slowed down.

The sole radical enlargement of the legislation, in 1930, was the providing of special measures and institutions for insane criminals. From the point of view of forensic psychiatry, this was a great step forward, but apart from this provision the legislation was left practically unchanged. Hence, the rigid juridical frame which originally was an excellent basis for the care of the mentally ill became an obstacle to new enterprises. Official interest in psychiatry, moreover, was scanty. Typical of this attitude is the fact that, with the establishing of an obligatory health insurance in 1945, insurance covering care in psychiatric institutions was excluded. The very few state mental hospitals seldom reached a high standard.

With a few exceptions, private institutions managed by religious bodies and organized in a spirit of Christian charity offered well organized psychiatric treatment, but a definite evolution towards a determined form of paternalistic establishment could not always be avoided.

Meanwhile, in the field of psychiatric theory, the principles of the French school of the 19th century were gradually being displaced by the Kraepelinian system. The views of Simon and other advocates of occupational therapy gained an easy audience in the psychiatric hospitals; in fact, they were very close to the earlier theories of Guislain.

Since it was practically impossible to practice psychiatry outside the institutions, clinical practice was limited to an organic approach to the more serious disorders. There was no place for a thorough exploration of neurotic problems and for the psychodynamic viewpoints. Freud's concepts reached Belgium with considerable delay, at least in the medical-psychiatric circles. This is strikingly illustrated by the fact that, in contrast to the surrounding countries, a psychoanalytic society was founded in Belgium only as late as 1947, and then by the initiative of non-medical individuals.

Social psychiatry also had a troublesome start. The foster family care at Geel, where the number of patients had passed the 2,000 mark, had been relieved by a similar attempt at Lierneux in 1884. But around 1950 an obvious drop in the number of patients was noticeable; moreover, often there was more interest in this form of treatment from abroad than from the country's own authorities and psychiatrists. Because of this, necessary innovations and adjustments could not take place (7).

In the last 20 years, however, the scope of psychiatric treatment has become wider; the possibilities created by psychopharmacology have largely contributed to this. Finally, the mental patient can now be considered as a sick person and his hospitalization entails treatment rather than custody. To this development psychotherapeutic methods have also largely contributed.

Ambulant treatment and shorter admissions in open clinic wards have gradually replaced institutional psychiatry. Programs of therapeutic community, rehabilitation, sector organization, and mental health care allow for hope that, in the future, there will be a differentiated psychiatric approach where the individual will be offered the maximum help in his psycho-social environment.

REFERENCES

1. BEEK, H. H. (1965): De hulp aan geestesgestoorden rond St. Hermes van Ronse. *Ann. Geschiedk. en Oudheidk. Kring Ronse,* 14, 163.
2. BEEK, H. H. (1969): *De geestesgestoorde in de Middeleeuwen.* Haarlem: De Toorts.
3. DEODATUS, BR. (1957): Onze verpleging in 't verleden en in 't heden. *Psychiatrie en Verpleging,* N⁰. 198, 2-40.
4. DEODATUS, BR. (1963): Historiek van de verpleging van geesteszieken. *Psychiatrie en Verpleging,* 5, 57-64, 84-96.
5. DE POTTER, F. (1921): *Gent van den oudsten tijd tot heden.* Gent: Annoot-Braeckman.
6. DUCPETIAUX, E. (1832): *De l'état des aliénés en Belgique.* Bruxelles: Laurent fréres.
7. EYNICKEL, H. (1971): *De uitbreiding en beoordeling van de gezinsverpleging van geesteszieken. Uitstraling van het Schotse en Geelse systeem, (1850-1970).* Unpublished study: Leuven.*
8. GILLIODTS VAN SEVEREN, L. (1871-1885): *Inventaire des archives de la ville de Bruges,* 9 vol. Bruges: Gaillard.
9. GUISLAIN, J. (1826): *Traité sur l'aliénation mentale et sur les hospices d'aliénés,* 2 vol. Amsterdam: Van der Hey et fils.
10. GUISLAIN, J. (1833): *Traité sur les Phrénopathies.* Bruxelles: Etablissement encyclographique.
11. GUISLAIN, J. (1852): *Leçons orales sur les Phrénopathies,* 3 vol. Gand: Hebbelynck.
12. KUYL, P. D. 1863): *Gheel vermaerd door den eerdienst der H. Dimphna.* Antwerpen: Buschmann.
13. MEEUS, F. (1921): *L'histoire de la colonie de Gheel.* Anvers: De Vlijt.
14. NIJSSEN, R. (1955): Psychiatrie en Belgique. *Encyclopédie Méd. Chir. Psychiatrie,* 3700, 9-11.
15. *Rapport de la commission chargée par Mr. le Ministre de la Justice de proposer un plan pour l'amélioration de la condition des aliénés en Belgique et la réforme des établissments qui leur sont consacrés.* (1842). Bruxelles: Haeyez.
16. *Rapports de la commission supérieure d'inspection des établissements des aliénés* (10 rapports). (1853-1872). Bruxelles: Gobbaerts.
17. ROSEN, G. (1968): *Madness in Society.* London: Routledge & Kegan Paul.
18. SPRENGER, J. & KRAMER, H. (1487-1489): *Malleus Maleficarum.* Cologne.

19. Van Acker, K. (1958): De roem van Prof. Dr. Guislain. *Psychiatrie en Verpleging*, No. 201, 29-32.
20. Van Craywinckel, J. L. (1658): *De triumpherende suyverheyt*. Mechelen: Joye.
21. Verachtert, K. (1967): *De krankzinnigenverpleging te Geel 1795-1860*. Unpublished study: Leuven.*
22. Vives, J. L. (1538:) *De anima et vita*. Fotacopia Faxsimile (1963). Torino: Bottega d'Erasmo.
23. Wouters, P. & Poll, M. (1938): *Du régime des malades mentaux en Belgique*. Bruxelles: Bruylant.
24. Zilboorg, G. & Henry, G. W. (1941): *A History of Medical Psychology*. New York: Norton.

* These studies are parts of a Research project on the foster family care in Geel, sponsored by the Universities of Columbia, New York, and Leuven, Belgium (General Director: Prof. L. Srole, Columbia University; Director of the historical section: Prof. H. Van der Wee, University of Leuven).

6

THE NETHERLANDS

F. C. STAM, M.D.

Professor of Psychiatry, Free University,
Amsterdam, The Netherlands

1

THE MEDIEVAL PERIOD AND THE RENAISSANCE

In the Middle Ages, disorders of behavior were hardly recognized as diseases. Medieval man tended to ascribe disasters, epidemics, and uncomprehended behavioral disorders to supernatural causes. It is not surprising, therefore, that mental disturbances were attributed to evil spirits and demons (demoniacal possession). Possessions were fought by expurgation, exorcism, or pilgrimages to sacred places; frequently these pilgrimages were embellished by ritual dancing as shown in a drawing from the school of Peter Breughel, depicting pilgrims near Brussels (Plate XXII). Other well known places of pilgrimage in the Low Countries were St. Hubertus in the Ardennes, and Ronse and Geel in Flanders. (See Chapter V, on Belgium.) The "dancing epidemics" were among the peculiar psychiatric aspects of medieval society. A large number of people took to the streets in a state of hysterical agitation, and many showed epileptiform fits. The agitation was further intensified by accompanying musicians. Such a mass psychosis occurred in Holland in 1373, and was called St. John's disease; on a smaller scale, similar psychiatric outbreaks occurred in monasteries and orphanages.

Witch Hunting

During the latter years of the Middle Ages and at the beginning of the Renaissance there was increasing acceptance of the view that not only did the devil take possession of innocent people, but many persons had forsworn their belief in God and the Virgin Mary and had voluntarily sold their soul to the devil. The devil was believed to have

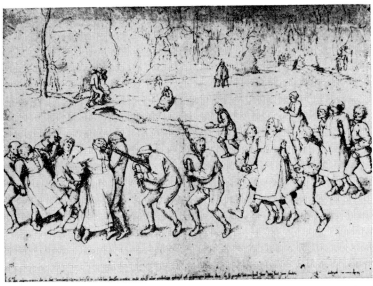

PLATE XXII. Pilgrimage on St. John's Day. Drawing from the school of Peter Breughel, 1569.

given these "witches" the power to cause illness and disaster, and even to transform human beings into animals.

Belief in the existence of witches was virtually universal among the clergy, even though some ecclesiastics thought more progressively. The monk Ofhuys (1456-1523) held that insanity could have either a natural or a supernatural cause; in the latter case there was divine intervention in order to convert the individual. He rejected demonism. But such voices were rare, and the widespread superstition of witchcraft almost automatically led to persecution of the witches. The belief in witches was born in the bosom of the Inquisition. The tribunals of the church based their trials on the *Malleus Maleficarum* (*The Witches' Hammer*), written in 1486 by Kramer and Sprenger. This nonsensical book had the approval of Pope Innocent VIII.

In The Netherlands, however, it soon became possible to call upon the civil authorities for assistance against self-styled witch hunters. And on many occasions the civil authorities did suppress witch hunts. It seems that no witchcraft trial has ever been held in the internationally oriented seaport of Antwerp. When an epidemic of witch hatred broke out in Bruges in 1542, the city fathers decreed that anyone who accused another person of witchcraft was to be imprisoned until the accusation had been proven. A less enlightened leader was the manor lord Bernard van Merode, who undertook a real witch hunt in Asten (Brabant) in 1595. Protests from the populace and the clergy prompted the Court of Brabant to call the high-handed lord to order. In Roermond (Limburg), by decrees of the Court of Gelderland, 64 witches were burned at the stake within six months in 1613. But, the Court of Gelderland came abruptly to its senses and the fires of hell in Roermond were extinguished. This brought the witch hunt craze in the southern provinces of The Netherlands to an end.

In the northern provinces of The Netherlands, Amsterdam played a leading role. In this city, two witchcraft trials were held in 1555, resulting in six executions. Nine years later, a woman stood accused of witchcraft on the basis of things she had said while delirious with fever. The patient died on the day after her conviction, and only her corpse remained for the executioner to burn. She was the last person to be tried for witchcraft in Amsterdam.

In 1566, mass hysteria occurred among the children in the Amsterdam orphanage. They shouted that they had been bewitched by a female street vendor, and demanded her death. However, the municipal authorities were sufficiently sober-minded to observe that those children allowed to visit relatives in the city did not suffer from this obsession. Consequently they boarded the affected children with foster families, and this brought their symptoms to an end. The woman accused of witchcraft remained unmolested. In the same year, a witch was brought before a court in Rotterdam; she confessed to almost every sin mentioned in the *Malleus Maleficarum*. The court's decision was to ban her from the city because of mendacity! The judges stated explicitly that their verdict was based on advice received from men of learning.

The darkest page in the history of witchcraft in The Netherlands concerns the trial held in Utrecht in 1595, which resulted in the death by fire of a number of peasant families. The last witch-burning in the northern Netherlands took place in Schoonhoven in 1597. The last trial for witchcraft in The Netherlands occurred in 1610 and concerned a woman from Goeree. At this trial the poet and statesman Jacob Cats

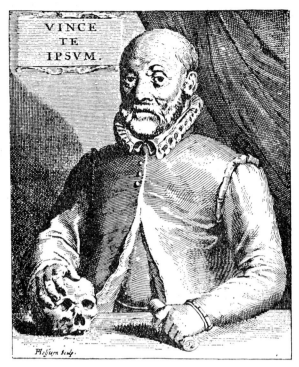

PLATE XXIII. John Wier. Illustration in *Opera Omnia*,
1660.

appeared for the defense. He described his experiences in a poem
ending thus:

> Behold Ye. After the court had passed sentence
> thus, all witchcraft from the nation seemed
> expelled at once.

> The woman, for a while by everyone despised,
> had quiet and blameless rest, by no one criticized.

In The Netherlands, the "witchcraft craze" never attained the same
extent as in Germany, France, and Scotland. This was due to a great
extent to the work of Jan Wiers, otherwise known as Johan Weyer
(1515-1588) (Plate XXIII). Weyer vehemently opposed the *Malleus
Maleficarum,* which he regarded as a nonsensical and godless book.
In his own book, *De Praestigiis Demonum* (1563), he refuted the
superstition that witches could cause disasters. He held that it was

only the devil that caused possession and disasters, deluding the witch into the belief that she was the cause. The soothsayers who indicated the witch as the cause of epidemics or disasters did so, in Weyer's view, at the instigation of the devil. Witches, he maintained, were sick people abused by the devil and therefore not punishable. But he regarded sorcerers as individuals who had voluntarily learned demoniacal tricks from books, and who were therefore punishable. Weyer maintained that the devil selected old, melancholic, or demented women, weakened sick people, and children as his victims. The same view was expressed by Levinus Leminius (1505-1568) of Zierikzee. Weyer's work reflects the spirit of Christian humanism as preached by Desiderius Erasmus (1469-1536), and it is therefore not surprising that his views were refuted by Catholics and Protestants alike. The French jurist Jean Bodin (1530-1569) fiercely opposed Weyer's work, and various Dutch Calvinist theologians were equally vehement antagonists.

In the period under discussion important political changes occurred in The Netherlands. Resistance to the Spanish Inquisition, which had many more victims than the *Malleus Maleficarum,* led the Netherlanders to rebellion. In 1581, the Seven Provinces rejected the king of Spain; this led to the separation of the northern Netherlands (under a reformed government) from the southern part, which was Catholic and remained under Spanish rule.

Unfortunately, it cannot be said that the Calvinists were able to change the then current views on demonism. An increasing controversy developed between medical men, philosophers, and jurists on the one hand, and theologians on the other. In 1594, three professors of medicine and two philosophers of the University of Leyden submitted a report to the Court of Holland in which they rejected the "water test" in witchcraft trials as nonsensical and illegal. The Leyden jurist Gerard Tuining (professor from 1599-1610) published a warning in verse, addressed to the witchcraft judges, in the book *Discovery of Witchcraft* by the Englishman Scot. This book was destroyed by order of King James I, a witch hunter who firmly believed in demons.

The Leyden theologian Danaeus (appointed professor in 1581) was a fierce advocate of capital punishment for the sorcerers who were believed to have made a contract with the devil. The theologians who adhered to the theory of demonism of James I of England had the ascendancy over the more tolerant theologians. In 1636 the Utrecht theologian Voetius delivered two lectures (Disputationes de Magia) in defense of demonism. Voetius was very firm in his rejection of the views of Weyer and Scot, but he also disapproved of the witchcraft trials which had caused so much misery elsewhere, and urged moderation. In the northern Netherlands of the 17th century, therefore, we encounter the remarkable situation that the belief in demonism was maintained as an article of faith, but its practical consequences, the trials and the death sentences, were abandoned.

Against this dark theological sky appeared, in 1691, the brilliant star of theologian Balthasar Bekker's book *De Betoverde Wereld* (*The Bewitched World*). But in 1693 the Voetian preacher Johan van der Wayen wrote a bulky volume against Bekker, holding that the latter had distorted God's word and was a heretic. On the other hand, Bekker's views were supported by the French philosopher Pierre Bayle, who lived in Rotterdam from 1681 to 1706.

Witches were believed to be weightless. A unique phenomenon in the history of the witch hunt in The Netherlands is the witches' weigh-house in Oudewater. Here, those accused of witchcraft were weighed and given an official certificate (Plate XXIV). Charles V is believed to have declared this certificate valid throughout the Holy Roman Empire of the German nation. Numerous foreigners accused of witchcraft were weighed in Oudewater during the period 1644-1773. Netherlanders were not officially weighed because prosecutions for witchcraft ceased in 1610. Nevertheless, Dutch women have occasionally been weighed at their own request, as, for instance, when they were accused of witchcraft by their neighbors. Without a certificate, after all, they could never prove that they were not witches. This fact demonstrates the strength of the belief in witchcraft that persisted in the population even after witchcraft trials were discontinued. Unfortunately, this belief was nourished by the theological followers of Voetius.

The Influence of Rationalism

The Voetians also met considerable resistance on the part of the followers of Descartes (1596-1650). At the age of 30, this French philosopher enrolled as a student at the University of Leyden. He lived in Holland from 1628 to 1639, and wrote his principal works during that period. Descartes paved the road towards scientific thinking.. He held that scholastic ideas would have to be replaced by methodical doubt, and that man must base his knowledge on rational thinking. In this way Descartes became the founder of rationalism. His significance for the development of psychology and psychiatry is mostly based on his thesis of the duality of body and soul.

Another important Dutch rationalist was Baruch de Spinoza (1632-1677), who also concerned himself with the problem of the relation

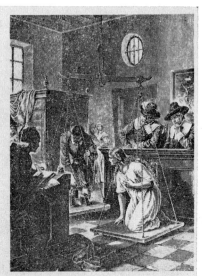

PLATE XXIV. The witches' weigh-house in Oudewater and an official certificate from 1729.

between body and mind. Unlike Descartes, Spinoza reached the conclusion that body and mind are two aspects of one entity. He advocated a parallelism between mental and physical processes. In his *Ethics,* Spinoza published treatises on theoretical psychology. He considered psychological phenomena to be as significant as material processes, and developed the most adequate theoretical system of personality of his time.

Despite resistance among the Voetians, the Cartesians gradually came to the fore in the Universities of Leyden and Utrecht. The Voetians reviled Spinoza's philosophy as much as they did Cartesian thought. But Spinoza made a deep impression on the famous Dutch physician Herman Boerhaave (1668-1738). In one of his famous lectures, Boerhaave stated that the natural causes of mental disorders had been insufficiently investigated. Too often, he maintained, physicians resort to spirits, demons, and similar notions to explain what they did not understand. This statement clearly shows that Boerhaave had rejected demonism. A good example of his sober-minded scientific attitude is his approach to a phenomenon of mass hysteria in the Haarlem orphanage, which, as the description indicates, showed the characteristics of hysterical pseudo-epilepsy. Therapies instituted by various physicians had failed to yield results. Boerhaave had a number of braziers placed in the rooms, in which iron hooks were brought to a glow. He announced that anyone who would have another attack was to be branded down to the bone with one of these irons. In this way he succeeded in bringing to an end the mass hysteria. This story throws a special light on the phenomena of mass hysteria which occurred in convents and orphanages during the Middle Ages. Probably the poor social conditions and oppressive house rules were the cause of these collective derangements. Abnormal behavior afforded a possibility of rebellion for which the patients could not be held responsible. After all, they had been bewitched by one of Satan's satellites!

Even though rationalism was gradually superseding demonism, there was as yet no trace of improvement in the fate of psychiatric patients. They were locked up in the dark little cubicles of city madhouses. If necessary, the "frenzied" were manacled. The first madhouse in the Netherlands was founded in Zutphen, by Engelbert Kreyninc, who was inspired by the eloquent testimony of Thomas à Kempis (1379-1471) and by the religious order of the Brethren and Sisters of Ordinary Life, which had been founded in Zutphen in 1425. In 1442, in den Bosch, Reinier van Arkel stipulated in his will that a fund be established for the foundation of an institution for mental patients. Willem Arntz of Utrecht did the same in 1461. In Amsterdam, Henrik Paulesz

Boelens made a gift of 3,000 guilders to the city council for the building of a madhouse (Plate XXV).

These madhouses were managed by a *"father"* and a *"mother,"* assisted by a number of male and female servants. The supervision was in the hands of a board of governors. There was as yet no question of psychiatric care. The care of the physically ill was entrusted to chirurgeons or doctors of medicine. At a small admission fee, the public could view the "fools." Not infrequently, this unhealthy interest

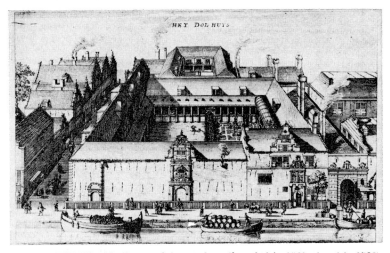

PLATE XXV. The Madhouse of Amsterdam (founded in 1561, closed in 1792).

degenerated to a baiting of the unfortunate inmates. This baiting of patients was one of the highlights of the so-called "madhouse fair" held annually in Utrecht until it was abolished in 1783. Viewing, however, continued until 1832!

Ambulant Treatment of Mental Patients During the Middle Ages and the Renaissance

Various methods of treating mental disorders were used in the Middle Ages; exorcism and pilgrimages have already been mentioned. In addition, experiments were made with the therapeutic effects of music on melancholic patients. Special therapeutic properties were attributed to the water of the river Senne, and in the 17th century convulsive patients were overpowered by their relatives and thrown into this minor Brabant river. The resulting shock often led to a "cure." The art of "stone cutting" became popular in the 16th century. This technique

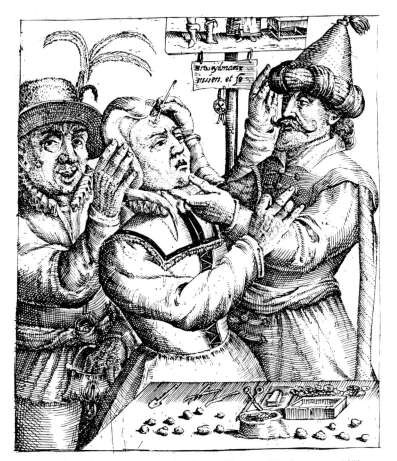

PLATE XXVI. "Stone Cutting." Print by Nicolaas Weydmans, ca. 1650.

was based on the superstition that madness was caused by a stone in the patient's head. Many charlatans made large profits from this superstition; they would make an incision in the skin of the forehead, whereupon an assistant saw to it that a stone did in fact emerge (Plate XXVI).

2

THE RISE OF MODERN PSYCHIATRY

A turning point was reached in Amsterdam in the early years of the 19th century. In 1820, Nieuwenhuys, a member of the provincial commission on medical investigation in Holland, published a survey of the medical situation in Amsterdam. In this survey he suggested that the city council should order improvements to be made in the local madhouse, which was to be divided into a department for chronic patients and one for curable patients. Niewenhuys maintained that the attending physician should administer not only medications, but also psychotherapy, which was to consist of rewards for good behavior and punishments for misbehavior. Moreover, he regarded work as a prerequisite to a cure, but believed on the other hand that chronic patients should be made as comfortable as possible. Niewenhuys censured his contemporary colleagues, calling them blind followers of Boerhaave and Van Swieten.

Nieuwenhuys' views found little sympathetic acceptance among the authorities until, in 1821, Schroeder van der Kolk (1797-1862) began to practice those principles in the Amsterdam "Outer Hospital" (Buitengasthuis). Soon after his appointment as professor of anatomy and physiology in Utrecht in 1827, he began to promote fundamental improvements in the treatment of the insane in the Utrecht lunatic asylum. His views were accepted there, and it can therefore be stated that the reform had its start in Utrecht. Schroeder van der Kolk's inspiring work increasingly persuaded Dutch authorities that the insane are patients, and that institutions to accommodate them are hospitals. Partly as a result of his efforts, the first Insanity Act was passed in 1841. He also wrote a textbook of psychiatry (1863). Schroeder van der Kolk (Plate XXVII) has the same historical significance in the Netherlands as Pinel and Esquirol have in France.

One of the first physicians outside the Utrecht circle to recognize the vitality of Schroeder van der Kolk's views was Johannes Ramaer (1817-1887). With great drive and vision he helped to make psychiatry an independent profession. He devised a classification of the psychoses, but it was never widely accepted. Of much more importance was his initiative to establish the Netherlands Association of Psychiatrists, in 1870. Ramaer should be honored for his achievement in uniting Dutch psychiatrists in a joint effort to persuade the government to concern itself more intensively with the care of the insane. As early as 1884, the young Association's efforts resulted in the promulgation of a law which regulated governmental inspection of the treatment of mental patients.

Van Deventer (1849-1916) became the pioneer of modern nursing care. In the Amsterdam Buitengasthuis he managed to gather a group of well-educated nurses, who were to form the nucleus of the nursing reform movement in The Netherlands. Tellegen (1848-1904) identified himself with the special training of mental nurses, while Cox (1861-

1933) took great pains to improve the primary and secondary working conditions for nurses.

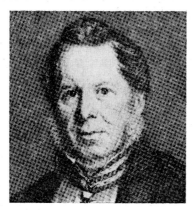

PLATE XXVII. Schroeder van der Kolk (1797-1862).

This brief outline has shown how, in the latter half of the 19th century, the "madhouse" developed into a mental hospital. Also how the insane came to be recognized and treated as patients. And one of the implications of these changes was that psychiatry had to be given a place in medical teaching.

The First Teachers of Psychiatry at the Universities

Halfway through the 19th century, there were as yet no teachers of psychiatry in the Dutch universities. In Utrecht, Schroeder van der Kolk filled this gap. In Amsterdam, psychiatry was taught by Schnee-voogt (1814-1871), professor of neuropathology.

In 1867 Van der Lith (1814-1903) was appointed honorary professor of psychiatry in Utrecht; but in 1878 he resigned because, when the higher education bill was passed, he was offered only a lectureship. In 1885 Winkler (1855-1941) accepted a lectureship which in 1896 was changed into a professorship. In 1896 he resigned because the government had made no efforts to found a university clinic. Soon after, Winkler joined the Amsterdam department of internal medicine with an assignment to teach neurology and psychiatry.

The establishment of a chair of neurology and psychiatry at Utrecht was strongly promoted by Donders (1818-1889), a professor of physiology. Unlike Ramaer, Donders believed that a combination of psychiatry and neurology was preferable to a separate chair of psychiatry. Donders had his way, and in accordance with this development the Netherlands Association of Psychiatrists, in 1895, became the Netherlands Society of Psychiatry and Neurology.

As already mentioned, the development of psychiatry remained linked to that of neurology. In Leyden, Jelgersma (1859-1942) was appointed professor in 1898. His successor, Carp, rightly described him as the grand master of early psychiatry in The Netherlands. Unlike his German colleagues, Jelgersma immediately understood the significance of Freud's psychoanalysis and it was partly through his efforts that Freud was made an honorary member of the Netherlands Society of Psychiatry and Neurology, in 1921. In 1907, Jelgersma acted as president of the First International Congress of Psychiatry and Neurology in Amsterdam. His textbook of psychiatry can be regarded as the first standard work of academic psychiatry in The Netherlands.

In 1903 the German Heilbronner (1871-1914) was appointed professor in Utrecht. Under his direction the University Clinic was built; it was completed in 1913. After Heilbronner's death, Winkler became professor and director of the Utrecht University Clinic. Winkler was above all a neurologist; he refuted psychoanalysis and believed that neurology was the only road to psychiatry. L. Bouman (1869-1936) was appointed professor of psychiatry at the Free University of Amsterdam in 1907. He built the Valerius Clinic and made it a center of neurological and psychiatric research. He succeeded Winkler in 1925; like him, he was no advocate of psychoanalysis. His pupil and successor Rümke (1893-1967) introduced Jaspers' phenomenological method into Dutch clinical psychiatry; his most important contribution was his study on symptomatology of schizophrenia.

In 1903, Wiersma became the first professor of psychiatry at the University of Groningen. He has occupied a special position in Dutch psychiatry because he was an advocate of psychic monism, taught by Heymans. Jointly with this famous psychologist he searched for similarities between psychological and physiological laws. According to Heymans, Wiersma also established the unity of psychological and psychopathological laws beyond any doubt.

Van der Horst, professor of psychiatry at the Free University of Amsterdam from 1936 to 1963, developed a very personal system of anthropological psychiatry based on existential philosophy. In 1915 K. H. Bouman (1874-1947) was appointed professor of psychiatry and neurology at the University of Amsterdam. He was one of the first to recognize the importance of social factors in mental disorders and became one of the founders of social psychiatry in The Netherlands. He was also among the pioneers of the young mental hygiene movement, founded in 1924 by Cox, Van der Scheer and Kat. Several societies for the promotion of mental hygiene were founded in the early 1920s; they were based on various philosophies. In 1934 these societies were brought together in the National Federation of Mental Hygiene.

This brief outline illustrates how, during the first decade of the 20th century, a wide diversity of views prevailed in University Psychiatric Clinics in The Netherlands.

During the past few decades, psychiatric teaching has been gradually detached from neurological teaching. Even before World War II, separate chairs of neurology were established in Amsterdam, Utrecht, and Leyden. After the war, the differentiation was made also in Groningen, at the Free University of Amsterdam, and at the Catholic University of Nijmegen. Nevertheless, the specialty of neuropsychiatry continued to exist until a differentiated training system (students majoring either in neurology or in psychiatry) was established in 1965. In 1972, the division into two separate specialties followed. In accordance with this development, the Netherlands Society of Psychiatry and Neurology was divided into two separate organizations of specialists in 1973.

3

THE 20TH CENTURY

The Dutch Mental Hospital

In the early years of the 20th century, bed nursing—in accordance with the German example—was the principle method of treatment. In 1926 Van der Scheer (1883-1957) became acquainted with the active therapy practiced by Simon in Gütersloh. He introduced this method in The Netherlands with such drive and authority that he achieved a complete change of approach in the treatment of mental patients. In this respect the importance of Van der Scheer's work can be compared with that of Schroeder van der Kolk in the 1840's. In 1950 Van der Scheer was appointed consultant to the Ministry of Public Health; his assignment was to promote active therapy in all Dutch mental hospitals.

Other factors which have substantially improved the therapeutic climate in mental hospitals in recent years have been the rise of psychopharmacology since 1952 and the establishment in some mental hospitals of therapeutic communities in imitation of those devised by Maxwell Jones and others. Day hospitals are now attached to several mental hospitals and mental hospitals work in close collaboration with the social psychiatric services.

Psychoanalysis and Psychotherapy

Although in the early phases of the development of academic psychiatry a few professors followed Freud's theories, the expansion of psychoanalysis has been promoted chiefly by investigators outside the universities. In 1917 the pioneers in this field established the Netherlands Society of Psychoanalysis, and four years later the work of A. Stärcke (1880-1954) was recognized with the award for medical psychoanalysis. Very important work was also done by Van der Hoop (1887-1950), who in 1929 was given a private lectureship in the theory of neuroses at the University of Amsterdam. But a split occurred in the Netherlands Society of Psychoanalysis in 1937 when Westerman Holstein, private lecturer in psychoanalysis at the University of Amsterdam, founded the more liberal Psychoanalytic Association. During World War II, Van der Waals, Lampl, Lampl de Groot, and Le Coultre laid the foundations for the establishment of a psychoanalytic institute, which was not publicized until after the war. During the past decade the influence of psychoanalysis in university teaching has greatly increased, because at four of the seven universities the chair of psychiatry is occupied by a psychoanalyst.

Psychotherapy, more or less limited to the privileged few until after World War II, has greatly expanded in recent years since health insurance companies began to cover this form of treatment. Moreover, psychotherapeutic assistance is now available on a much larger scale at government-subsidized institutes for medical psychology. During the past decade, psychologists have been teaching and applying psychotherapy at various universities; this applies in particular to behavior therapy.

The Development of Forensic Psychiatry

The Netherlands occupies a prominent position in the field of forensic psychiatry. The juridical climate in The Netherlands is characterized by a high degree of tolerance, rooted in the national character.

As early as 1823, the Netherlands Association for the Moral Improvement of Prisoners was founded; aiming at the rehabilitation of released prisoners, it provided a sound basis for the development of forensic psychiatry. Even before the end of the 19th century, many psychiatrists were reporting on the psychological features of delinquents.

In 1907 a discussion between jurists and psychiatrists led to the foundation of the "Psychiatric Juridical Association"—a study group of which Van Hamel, Winkler, Simon, and Heilbronner were the promotors.

In 1911 F. S. Meyers (1870-1953) received the first private lectureship in forensic psychiatry at the University of Amsterdam and, in 1928, he established a society for the protection of the social interests of mental patients. The care of psychopaths was organized throughout the Netherlands from this society. Meyers' work in forensic psychiatry had a strong focus on social psychiatry.

Other pioneers of forensic psychiatry were Mesdag in Groningen, Gerritsen in The Hague, and Overbeek and Tammenoms Bakker in Amsterdam. In Utrecht, Van der Hoeven (1880-1956) was the great stimulating influence. He paved the way towards psychotherapeutic treatment of delinquents, for which purpose the Van der Hoeven Clinic was founded in Utrecht in 1955. This clinic was the first experiment in forensic psychiatry in the world. Within its walls, jurists and psychiatrists collaborate in the treatment and resocialization of delinquents. The driving force behind this clinic was Baan, who in 1951 became the first Dutch professor of forensic psychiatry on the Law Faculty of the University of Utrecht. He rightly pointed out that forensic psychiatry is not a separate type of psychiatry, but merely psychiatry in court (*in foro*). The development of modern forensic psychiatry owes much to advances in the fields of psychotherapy and of social psychiatry.

Social Psychiatry and Mental Hygiene

In the early years of this century K. H. Bouman laid the foundations on which social psychiatry in The Netherlands was to be built. Van der Scheer pointed out the need for social structures to which the mentally handicapped could adapt themselves. Stärcke went so far as to regard insanity as a faulty relationship between individual and society. He emphasized the need to detect pathogenic factors in society, and considered the study of comparative sociology to be indispensable for workers in this field.

F. S. Meyers devoted his whole life to the practical realization of social psychiatric work. He was consultant to the municipality of Amsterdam from 1896 to 1933, and in this capacity he promoted several projects in social psychiatry, e.g., the foundation of workshops for the mentally handicapped, and the foundation of the first child guidance clinic.

Pameyer (1888-1956) founded, in 1926, the first pre- and after-care service in The Netherlands, in imitation of Kolb's work in Fürth-Erlangen. This service was organized from the mental hospital "Maasoord" in Poortugaal near Rotterdam. His initiative has had great significance for the development of social psychiatry in The Netherlands.

A. Querido, who succeeded Meyers as consultant to the municipality of Amsterdam, continued to build on the foundations already laid and achieved the establishment of a municipal social psychiatric service, which for many years attracted much attention in The Netherlands as well as abroad. Today, there are several social psychiatric services in The Netherlands, operated by municipal authorities, church groups, or provincial governmental agencies.

In the early phases of its development, social psychiatry attempted to reduce the increasing economic burden of the care of the insane by supervising hospitalization and the duration of clinical treatment (Barnhoorn 1955). This goal could be achieved only by the foundation of adequate services for pre- and after-care, and by engaging the services of social case workers.

In the course of the past two decades, social psychiatry has focused increasingly on mental hygiene and preventive psychiatry. This trend is reflected in the fact that, in 1969, Trimbos was appointed professor of social and preventive psychiatry; he maintains that pre- and after-care is not a purely sociopsychiatric field but one which also involves, in particular, mental hygiene. He greatly emphasizes mental health education and repatterning of pathogenic social structures. Thus social psychiatry and the mental hygiene movement, primarily organized as independent fields with separate objectives, are gradually coming together.

REFERENCES

1. BAAN, P. A. H. (1959): Forensische psychiatrie. Anniversary Volume. *Nat. Feder. v. geestel. Volksgezondheid.*
2. BARNHOORN, J. A. J. (1955): Sociale psychiatrie, geestelijke hygiene, geestelijke gezondheidszorg en geestelijke volksgezondheid. *Maandbl. geest. Volks-gezondh.*, 10, 449.
3. BASCHWITZ, K. (1964): *Heksen en heksenprocessen.* Amsterdam: Arbeiderspers.
4. BAUMANN, E. D. (1951): *Drie eeuwen Nederlandse Geneeskunde.* Amsterdam: H. Meulenhof.
5. BEEK, H. H. (1969): *De geestesgestoorde in de middeleeuwen.* Nijkerk: G. F. Callenbach.

6. BEKKERS, BALTHASAR, (1961): *De betoverde Weereld*. Amsterdam: Daniël van den Dalen.
7. BREUKINK, H. (1921, 1922): Overzicht van opvatting en behandeling van geesteszieken in oude tijden. I, II, III. *Ned T. Geneesk.*
8. COBBEN, J. J. (1960): *De opvattingen van Johannes Wier over bezetenheid, hekserij en magie*. Assen: van Gorcum & Comp.
9. DOOREN, L. (1940): *Doctor Johannes Wier, Leven en Werken*. Thesis. University of Utrecht.
10. ESCH, P. VAN DER, (1954): *Schroeder van der Kolk. Leven en Werken*. Thesis. Municipal University, Amsterdam.
11. HUT, L. J. POSLAVSKY, A., LOOIS, H. & VAN DER WAARD, B. (1961): *De Willem Arntsz Stichting 1461-1961*. Anniversary Volume. Utrecht: H. N. J. Oosthoek.
12. LINDEBOOM, G. A. (1958): Boerhave in het Weeshuis. *Ned T. Geneesk.*, 102, 1158.
13. SCHOUTEN, JOHAN (1972): *Heksenwaan en heksenwaag in oude prenten*. Alphen aan de Rijn: Repro-Holland.
14. SCOT, REGINALD (1886): *The Discovery of Witchcraft*. London: Brinsley Nicholson.
15. SPINOZA, BARUCH DE (1697): *Ethica*. Hamburg: Meiner.
16. STAM, F. C. (1971): *Honderd jaar psychiatrie*. Anniversary Volume on the occasion of the centenary of the Dutch Society of Psychiatry and Neurology. Velp: Meyer.
17. TRIMBOS, C. J. B. J. (1955): De ontwikkeling van de voor- en nazorgdiensten in het kader van de geestelijke volksgezondheid. *Maandbl. geest. Volksgezondh.*, 10, 1.
18. WAGENAAR, J. (1767): *Amsterdam zijne opkomst, aanwas, geschiedenis enz*. Part II. Amsterdam: Ynetma en Tieboel.
19. WAYEN, JOHANNES VAN DER (1693): *De betooverde weereld van Balthasar Bekker ondersogt en weederlegt*. Franeker, Leonardus Strik & Jakobus Horreus.
20. WIER, JOHANNES (1967): *De praestigiis demonus*. Amsterdam: E. J. Bonset (reedition).
21. ZWETSLOOT, H. (1954): *Friederich Spee und die Hexenprozesse*. Trier: Paulinus-Verlag.

7

GREAT BRITAIN

John G. Howells, M.D., F.R.C.Psych., D.P.M.,
DIRECTOR

AND

M. Livia Osborn, RESEARCH OFFICER

*The Institute of Family Psychiatry, The Ipswich Hospital,
Ipswich, England*

1

INTRODUCTION

Early management of psychiatric disorders in the British Isles is lost to us. Records are scanty until the Roman occupation—about 50 B.C.— although there were people in the islands from about 5,500 B.C. Of this history of 7,000 years, we have records relevant to psychiatry for only 2,000 years and written documents for only about 400 years. We must conclude that our history of psychiatry, with any certainty, can cover only a brief spell of the history of psychiatry in Britain.

We can reasonably assume that our ancestors had empirical knowledge garnered over five millennia in these islands and an inheritance of millennia from their ancestors elsewhere. There is a tendency for man, at any point in his development, to confuse contemporary knowledge with final knowledge. He also believes the latest knowledge to be superior to past knowledge. But early man had his own ways of contending with his handicaps—perhaps no worse and no better than our procedures today. Indeed, he was faced by the same essential situations. Furthermore, technological advances have hardly touched our understanding of matters of the mind.

We are impressed that these islands are but islands geographically; people in all countries have like circumstances and each influences the other. Thus our psychiatry has been enriched from many sources— the Iberian, Celtic, Roman, Nordic, and French invaders, the Christian proselytes, the Crusaders, Continental wars, the Renaissance, the influence of the continental universities, and the influence of a far flung Empire (64) all contributed in turn. Similarly, British psychiatry, through the founding of the Empire, Commonwealth links, Britain's position as a maritime nation, and intercourse with Europe, was to contribute to the psychiatry of other countries.

We have divided this chapter into three chronological phases. Naturally, each merges into the other with no absolute lines of demarcation. The first, the early period, covers the longest span of time, with the least certitude of knowledge. It begins in the mist of Celtic history, covers the early invasions of Britain, its emergence as a nation and its blossoming into a highly sophisticated world power. In psychiatry, these centuries were marked by primitive thinking, superstition, advancing or retarding influences from invading peoples, and, finally, a consolidation during which the theoretical teaching of classic authors remained unquestioned, based as it was on humoral theory and a rhetorical approach.

The second, the middle period, starts with the "scientific" approach to medicine inaugurated by Harvey. Although this period could be termed the "dark age" of psychiatry because of the drift away from psychopathology to organic pathology, at least it is a period when people became aware of neuropsychiatric problems, institutions exclusively for psychiatric patients were built in profusion, and the legislators vied with the architects in their efforts.

The third, the contemporary period, covers the present century. The advantage of living its history is counterbalanced by the difficulties in objectivity, the distortions of unrealized biases, the task of weighing the significance of events and of appreciating the broad sweep of change from one vantage point. Participation may blunt evaluation. The reader of the future must be the final judge.

Psychiatrist (*psyche-iatros*) literally means healer of the psyche. Thus a psychiatrist's main preoccupation is with psychonosis* (neurosis), pathology of the psyche. The first physician-psychiatrists saw

---

* The old terminology for reasons put forward elsewhere (30) is misleading and inaccurate; thus the term *neurosis* is replaced by the term *psychonosis,* and the term *psychosis* by *encephalonosis.*

this as their task although they sometimes confused organic, "mental" phenomena with psychic, emotional phenomena. Due to the swing to physiology in our second phase, the psychiatrist became a neuropsychiatrist with a prime interest in "mental" symptomatology arising from brain pathology—encephalonosis (psychosis). In our third phase we witness the slow movement back to psychonosis. Our history attempts to encompass both the history of psychonosis (neurosis) and of encephalonosis (psychosis).

We cannot claim exemption from the many errors of historians. To chronicle events is easy; to interpret them is difficult. We have learned to be critical of authorities (books are pale shadows of the events they portray), to suffer by relying on secondary sources, and to beware of giving undue weight to dramatic events. Our aim is to paint the picture of our knowledge of psychonosis and encephalonosis in its long history in the British Isles. We are also heedful of the warning of Polybius, a Greek historian writing before the recorded history of our islands, "That historians should give their own country a break, I grant you, but not so as to state things contrary to fact" (53).

2

THE EARLY PERIOD

The first phase in the history of psychiatry in the British Isles starts with early recorded history which comes at the end of a long period of occupation of the British Isles. It is an era of steady development enriched at its start by the Roman occupation and ending in a blaze of promise with the Elizabethan period, which was nourished by the English Renaissance. It extends over 1,600 years.

The Celts

Of those peoples that swept into the islands, at first over a land bridge until 5,500 B.C. and later by sea, by successive incursions, there are few records. Having passed through the Stone Age, Early and Late Bronze Ages, and the Iron Age, we find that the native people were largely Celts at the time of the Roman invasion. Caesar (50 B.C.) spoke of them—and commented on their unusual tribal life. It seems, he said, that they live in groups of ten or twelve men with their women and children, and that the men share all the women in the group (13).

Among these tribes were spiritual and intellectual leaders who were also teachers, versed in unnatural arts. These men, the Druids, were said by the elder Pliny (52) to have medical knowledge. Perhaps, too, they were the first psychiatrists. Britain became the purest center of Druidism in Europe and its last stronghold (41).

But of the Celtic management of emotional and mental illness we can only conjecture in the absence of a factual record. What is known is that primitive pagan people faced by similar hazards are dependent on almost identical acquired practices. Having pursued the same paths of trial and error, they tend to reach the same point of advancement and react in the same predictable ways. Unless their cause and effect are evident, phenomena are regarded as supernatural and the province of the priest-medicine man. The sick are assumed to be victims of demons, spirits, fiends, and devils (*the* Devil, in the Christian sense, comes later in history). These can be appeased by sacrifice, offerings, and prayers. Gods may counteract evil, and appeal to them is possible by incantation, ceremony, charms, and sacrifice. Sometimes the gods or fiends exist within the natural elements—stars, sun, moon, rain, wind, sea, rivers, pools, and mountains. They can reside in trees, plants, birds, and animals. So for the Celts we have, for example, Nodens, a god who dwelt in the Severn, and Coventina, a goddess who dwelt in the well of Carraw Burgh in Northumberland. The first Irish god of healing was Diancécht. Elaborate ritual can appease or bring support. These attitudes towards the ill—physical, mental and emotional—persist in some areas to the present day and we can surmise that they were there at the time of the Druids.

Later, the Celts were to be driven westward and northward to Wales, Scotland, and Cornwall by successive waves of Anglo-Saxon invaders. An outstanding Celt, a Welsh king, Hywel Dda (909-950 A.D.), codified the regulations of his people in The Laws of Hywel Dda (55). These laws reveal well defined attitudes towards the mentally ill. We quote three examples: 1) There were three persons who could not qualify to be a judge. One of these was a person with a defect and among those defective was an insane person—an individual whom it has been necessary to bind on account of his madness. 2) There were three releases from the obligation of a claim: by true swearing, by a guarantee, or because of madness. 3) The idiot was protected by law. Again, the physician's duties were carefully documented. The court physician had many privileges and at formal court sat next to the chief of the bodyguard. He was one of the three people with whom the king could have private conversation without his judge being present—the others were his wife and the priest. We may conjecture whether priest or physician, or both, were early psychotherapists. We cannot be sure that the humanity and understanding of these later Celts were to be found in the life of the early Celts, but humanity is not the monopoly of one era.

Roman Britain (43-410 A.D.)

Although Caesar's invasion of Britain took place in 54 B.C., after a brief exploratory incursion in 55 B.C., it was not until a century later in 43 A.D. under the Emperor Claudius that the Romans conquered Britain (64). The area covered by present day England and Wales experienced true Roman occupation, but it was only in the southeast that a process of temporary Latinization was effected. Elsewhere Celtic and Roman ways of life survived side by side, but the more sophisticated Roman civilization was able to check native development and impose its own values and customs. The protection of the traditional *Pax Romana* extended to Britain and was exemplified by a scattering of estates and country houses that needed no moats or fortifications.

The occupying legions had their own *medici;* they had no special training, but learned by experience and were expected to add to their usual military duties the task of looking after the wounded. It was only the high-ranking officers who took with them their own personal physician, often of Greek origin (58). Military hospitals were established in sheltered positions and were highly organized, but sick soldiers were sometimes left to recover in the care of a friendly local population. The agricultural estates that the Romans developed in Britain were worked by slaves and they too needed medical care. It is reasonable to suppose that an exchange of medical knowledge took place and that the practices of conquered and conquerors fused to a great extent, even if some of the theories brought in by the Romans were more sophisticated than those of the indigenous population (44).

In Rome, as in Britain, medicine was practiced at two levels. For the intellectual classes it was based on the knowledge of the philosopher-physicians, who attacked superstition and magic, unless it was the "scientific" magic of astrology and religion; for the masses medicine remained based on superstition, incantations, and amulets. Both levels, however, recognized psychonosis and encephalonosis among the illnesses that befell mankind whether they attributed the latter to imbalance of the humors or to possession by evil spirits; they agreed that the former resulted from "strong passions."

Since the 1st century A.D., physicians of high repute flourished in Rome: Celsus (25 B.C. - 50 A.D.), Dioscorides (c. 41-68), Soranus (c. 98-138), and Galen (c. 129-200). They understood the difference between insanity (encephalonosis) and illnesses due to emotional factors (psychonosis) and suggested remedies for both: purging, bleeding, diet, baths, massage, and rest were aimed to correct mental disorders with a physical aetiology; recreation, music, travel, and other psychological remedies were recommended for those disorders caused by grief, anxiety, anger, or excessive study. But their teaching reached only a small proportion of the population, and, in any case, their remedies were often expensive. The poorer classes retained their own folk remedies for physical, mental, and emotional ills: amulets to prevent disease, simple herbal concoctions, incantations, and visits to shrines. There were no public hospitals and the sick were cared for at home.

Temple sleep, or ritual incubation, whereby patients would spend the night at a temple and receive medical advice or an outright cure in their dreams, passed from Greece to Rome and from Rome to Britain. The ruins of a temple, probably taken over from the Celts, have been found on the banks of the river Severn at Lydney. They show a series of small cells, which suggest that patients slept there. No doubt offerings to the temple god were expected from the sick, but it still remained a form of treatment that could be afforded by most people. But Domitius Ulpion (c. 170-228) wrote: "those who chant, or those who expel evil spirits, should not be thought of as physicians."

From the 5th century B.C., the law of the Twelve Tables, an early Roman law code, made legal provisions for those who were mentally handicapped, assessed their state, appointed guardians and administered their property. The law distinguished between those who were irresponsible for their actions because of insanity or because of "strong passions," and those who were mentally deficient. These, however, were legal and not medical provisions; the jurist, and not the physician, was the authority, and he had no interest in ascertaining the cause of the disease, or its nature. The insane were ordered to be restrained and the responsibility for them rested with the family. Rich families delegated their care to a paid attendant; the poor left their sick to wander or kept them at home, often tied up or in stocks, in order to prevent them from harming themselves and others. These laws relating to psychiatric patients applied to Roman Britain. As can be seen, there is an indication of an early Roman classification of psychiatric states.

In general, the influence of Roman medicine in Britain seems to have been limited. Possibly the greatest contribution was in the field of surgery and hygiene. As a result of improving the standard of living, providing aqueducts, better diet and housing, the general health of the population may have improved and the incidence of infections and toxic states may have decreased, but it is unlikely that the incidence of emotional disorders was changed. Psychiatric diagnosis remained uncertain; aetiology, too, was no better understood: one evil spirit was perhaps replaced by another, some natural phenomena dependent on geographical features were discarded, and others accepted. The humoral theory of psychopathology was perhaps the biggest innovation, but reached only the educated few. Methods of treatment, again, may have varied but little; as the Romans brought with them some new herbs, the mistletoe of the Druids may have had to compete with the hellebore; warm baths took the place of less pleasant dips into cold springs; and Celtic incantations were replaced by Latin chants. The Romans were as superstitious as the Celts. The Roman attitude to mental disorders was more matter of fact, but then no stigma was attached to them in either culture even when insanity was considered divine punishment. Possibly this was so because there was no implication of an hereditary basis and thus the family of the sick did not feel contaminated.*

Even after over 300 years of Roman occupation, Latin culture had not made a permanent impact on Britain. The Celts were never Latinized, but from Rome they acquired Christianity, whose philosophy did indeed improve attitudes to mental disorders by introducing the care of the sick by dedicated people outside the family; but the perpetuation of the myth of devil possession and of the supernatural aetiology of insanity still retarded a rational approach for many centuries.

Anglo-Saxon Britain (410-1066)

Even while the Romans were in Britain, Saxon pirates raided the British coasts and, as the Roman power declined, invasion by the Nordic people (Angles, Saxons, and Jutes) increased, particularly in the 4th and 5th centuries. There are no chronicles of this conquest, but archeological research has led to a reconstruction of the general character of the invaders. They were mostly farmers, fishermen, and hunters, and they succeeded in permanently changing the nature of the peoples they conquered. The Romans had failed because they were too few to achieve racial assimilation, but the Nordic people came in great numbers, complete with women and children, and settled on the land, displacing or slaughtering the Romanized Britons in their unfortified villas and encampments. The newcomers were pagan, their civilization far inferior to that of the Romans, but they soon destroyed what the Romans had built and imposed their own language, customs, and institutions. The destruction was aided by the Celtic revival and was

---

* See also Chapter I, on psychiatry in ancient Greece and Rome.

stemmed only by the intensified efforts to convert England to Christianity, especially through the work of St. Augustine, a Benedictine monk sent by Pope Gregory to convert the Anglo-Saxons in Kent, in 597 (75).

Medical knowledge, like most other forms of learning, rested in the hands of the Church. The Church made use of it in propagating its beliefs: the devil was said to cause those illnesses whose aetiology was not immediately evident, and cures were attributed to the intercession of Christian Saints. This was a crude modification of previous beliefs (26).

Mental disease was regarded by the Anglo-Saxons as resulting from demoniacal possession and they seem to have equated it with epilepsy. The spirit responsible was *Wóden,* and the term *wód* meant "insane," hence the term "woodmen" (7). Miraculous wells, holy shrines, incantations, and exorcism as forms of treatment for the physically and mentally ill originated from this period, but unlike previous similar customs, they became connected with Christian beliefs. Bede (c. 673-735), for instance, reported that even the dust wetted by the water in which the saintly Oswald's bones had been washed "had the health-giving virtue of driving out demons from the bodies of the possessed" (6). Physical and mental diseases were often accepted as divine punishment for sin; hence the penances imposed on the sick were regarded as expiation for misdeeds committed.

The physician of this period was called "leech"; he was a lay practitioner of medicine, who lived and worked in the community, unlike the monastic physician, who was a member of a religious order based on a monastery. The *Leech Books* were the medical texts of the Anglo-Saxons, containing much material derived from Greek and Roman authorities, including Dioscorides and Pliny the Elder (23-79 A.D.). The most famous of the *Leech Books* was that of Bald (9th-10th century) (Plate XXVIII), which was written down by a scribe called Cild (78). In this manual the remedies for mental disorders were mostly based on herbal folklore; instructions were given about the correct way of gathering the herbs and the appropriate time, reminiscent of the elaborate ceremonies of the Druids. It all added to the mystique, contributing to the elements of supernatural, which fostered the belief in the curative properties of the plants. If the place where they grew was difficult to reach, unusual, or holy, this added to their placebo power.

The Anglo-Saxon herbal recommended dousing the head in vinegar "for the disease the Greeks call frenesis." "For lunacy" it said: "if a man lays the wort peony over the lunatic as he lies, soon he lifts him-

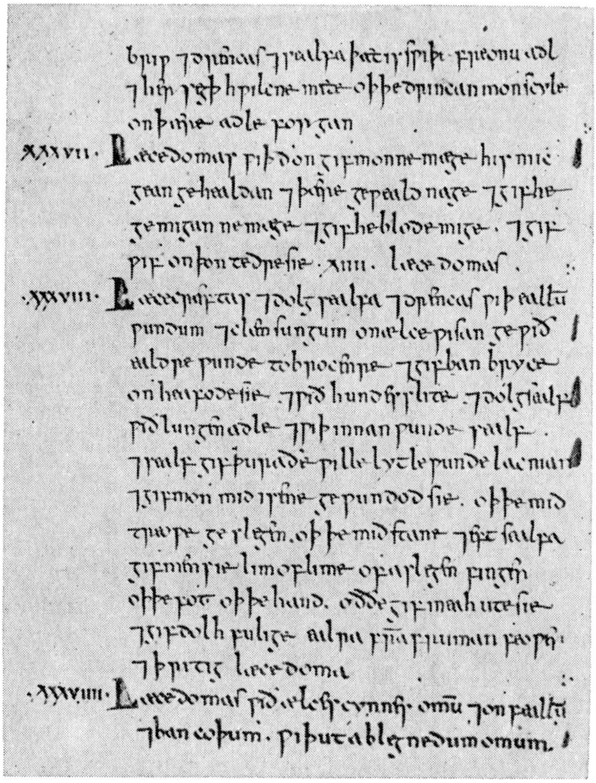

PLATE XXVIII. A page from Bald's Leechbook.

self up well: and if he has it with him, the disease never again approaches him." And again, "For a lunatic take cloverwort and wreathe it with a red thread about the man's neck, when the moon is on the wane." But common herbs, like sage or rosemary, were also included among those that "sootheth the brayne." Other mixtures were recommended as being more powerful if drunk out of a church bell. Some prescriptions were less practical and included such elements as the bark of a tree out of Paradise, or shavings from the horn of the mythical unicorn (51). Often revolting materials were pulverized and given to patients and one wonders on how many occasions St. Gildas' (c. 493-570) postscript to a prescription applied: "With God's help no harm will come to him."

  Charms and incantations were also in use and with them ceremonies of exorcism. These were extremely naïve and often resulted in a kind of dialogue between exorcist and demon-in-possession. St. Gregory (c.

540-604), for instance, recorded the case of a nun who became possessed when she neglected to cross herself before eating a lettuce; the demon resisted exorcism with the argument that it was not his fault, since he had been quietly sitting on a lettuce leaf when the nun had swallowed him! This example explains the use of purges, emetics, and sneezing powders, as their effect was presumed to be through the physical expulsion of the demon. Violence was used when exorcism and other remedies failed; again, the idea was to drive out the demon by beating his abode, the insane.

At a higher level the sophisticated teachings of Augustine of Hippo must have influenced the theory, if not the practice, of medicine. He had maintained that man is of one substance that includes the soul and the body; suicide was unremittingly condemned by him. Other influences may have come from Rome with the more learned monks who would have been aware, for instance, of the elegant works of Caelius Aurelianus (1st century A.D.); he wrote on mental disorders (*De re medica*) and offered a classification and methods of treatment, which included music therapy, travel, and reading, as well as the usual bleeding and emetics (51). But these and other learned works, although written in this period or earlier, became better known much later, when the printing press made them more readily available.

Religious orders in this period established the first hospitals attached to the monasteries, as the care of the poor and the sick was considered a part of Christian duty. It is difficult to establish whether they accepted those considered insane, but it is likely that they did care for all those ailing in body or mind, thus providing medical care outside the family circle. At St. Albans a hospital was in existence in 794 and St. Peter Hospital was founded in York, in 937, by King Athelstan (19). Their main purpose, however, was to shelter travelers, who often went on long pilgrimages which might take them as far as Rome. These hospitals sometimes required payment from their patients or looked forward to being included in their wills, so that a kind of private care was established. But it is likely that most patients were admitted for long stays, often until death, rather than for acute disorders, which were still catered for domestically.

The Middle Ages (1066-1485)

The Battle of Hastings (1066) marked the Norman conquest of England and the beginning of a period of national consolidation. The four centuries that followed saw the rise and decline of a social system based on feudalism, the struggle between the barons and the Crown, the establishment of national liberties (Magna Carta, 1215), and the conflict between civil and religious powers (64). Thus the Middle Ages were not a static era of dark barbarism, but rather an era of dynamic progress, of far-reaching changes; they were turbulent, anxious times. Medieval man was a pioneer, the father of the ages to come, more than the son of the centuries past.

Medicine, like other branches of science, was influenced by an import of new ideas from abroad brought about by the opportunities for traveling offered by the Crusades (1096-1272), the rise of trade and visits to foreign universities, and pilgrimages to holy places (72). Physicians went to continental universities to complete their training and thus brought back the teaching of the School of Salerno (first heard of in 848-859), of Avicenna (980-1036) (61), of Constantinus Africanus (1020-1087), etc. But it was still the humoral pathology of Galen (131-201 A.D.) that dominated diagnosis and treatment of sickness of body and of mind (36, 62). The writings of the "great teachers" depended on it and physicians were expected to accept on faith the established theories.

In England there were three languages: Latin, spoken by the clergy and used for the writing of learned works; French, the tongue of the gentry; and Anglo-Saxon, the speech of the peasants, which later became the English of Chaucer. Similarly, there were three approaches to medicine: that of the theologian-philosopher, who uncritically adhered to the traditional teaching; that of the scientist, who asserted the importance of experiment and learning; and that of the common people, who believed in folk remedies, in superstitious practices, and supernatural phenomena. This multiple approach applied also to the attitude to mental disorders, whose field was again a subject of controversy between physicians and clerics.

When the manifestations of insanity, or of emotional disorder, were regarded as sickness of the soul, it became impossible to disentangle the philosophical issues from the practical, as spirit and matter impinged on each other and neither released its secrets. But this dilemma was in fact the strength of medieval medicine, because it forced the concept of the "whole man" and made acceptable the principle that sickness was not always caused by physical, tangible agents. Thus the scientific approach of Roger Bacon (1215-1295) (3) was not in contradiction to the mystical philosophy of Duns Scotus (1265?-1308) even if Bacon advocated experience rather than deduction, whilst Duns Scotus defended his arguments on dialectical subtleties.

It was well understood that abnormal behavior could be due to emotional or to physical causes and that the treatment had to be appropriately directed to correct the damaged feelings or the disordered physical parts. This is demonstrated by the most popular treatise of the Middle Ages, *De proprietatibus rerum* (c. 1250), written by an English Franciscan monk, Bartholomeus Anglicus. He was not a physician, but a professor of theology, who collected what information was available at the time, and thus his work is a valuable witness of medieval attitudes. He dedicated part of his book to mental disorders and retained the classification of previous writers. Hence he recognized: "melancholie," which included what we would call "emotional disorders"; "madness," or mania; "gawrynge and forgetfulness," or stupor and dementia; "frensie," or delirium caused by a diseased brain and distinguished from febrile delirium, called "parafrenesi" (33). Confusion, however, arose in the use of the term "melancholie,'" as it covered the disease in the sense given above, and the black humor, which was the supposed cause of madness. Yet Bartholomeus makes it clear that some "madness" had its aetiology in anxiety and grief: "Madness cometh sometime of passions of the soul, as of business and of great thoughts, of sorrow and of too great study, and of dread." He then goes on to give physical causes, as bites of a mad dog, unsuitable foods, and too much strong wine, and advises restraint for the agitated likely to hurt themselves and others. Mental rest, music therapy, and occupation were his prescriptions for the depressed. Bartholomeus did not mention demoniacal possession, but it was regarded by some as a cause of insanity and exorcism was still practiced with varying degrees of success; true cases of insanity, of course, did not respond to it, but the ceremony with all its mystic implications must have been a powerful suggestive tool, which no doubt "cured" many emotional states.

Apart from the emotional prescriptions for emotional ills, it is irrelevant what kind of treatment was used. The important thing is that the disorders were "treated" and mental patients were not regarded as incurable. Herbal concoctions, bleeding, and beating continued to be used and it is possible that we underestimate their value as placebos.

The Hospital of St. Mary of Bethlehem (49) was founded in London in 1247; at first it was a place of rest for visiting clergy, and then it became a hospital, which, probably like most other hospitals, cared for a certain number of mental patients amongst others. Records show that in 1402, of its 14 patients, six were *mente capti,* or insane. St. Bartholomew's Hospital also gave shelter to patients suffering from a multitude of disabilities, including mental disorders. Another hospital may have existed in London for the care of the mentally ill, including members of the clergy, for in 1369, Robert Denton, a chaplain, applied and obtained a license to establish a hospital at All Hallows, Barking, for "priests and others, men and women who suddenly fell in a frenzy and lost their memories until such time as they recover"; but there is no proof that the projected hospital was actually founded. In 1414, the Rolls of Parliament refer to "hospitals . . . to maintain men and women who had lost their wits and memory." Salisbury was renowned for its hospital, Holy Trinity, which again did not segregate the mentally ill but cared for the physically sick as well as for "furiosi," or insane persons (15). It is likely that each small community was provided with some kind of hospital attached to the local monastery. As in previous centuries, the richer classes paid religious orders to look after their deranged members, either in monastic establishments or in special quarters set aside in castles belonging to the family.

In the Middle Ages, phenomena characterized by extremes of behaviour in large groups of people were common (46). The dancing mania, the hysterical behaviour of whole religious communities and the terrifying hallucinations reported by mystics may have been a product of stress, as for instance the unbearable anxiety caused by the Black Death (1349) (79), which reduced by perhaps more than a third the population of England, estimated then at about 4,000,000. On the other hand, some of these phenomena were due to toxic states, as for instance ergotism or alcoholic intoxication which was well recognized for producing insanity.

Towards the end of the 15th century, witchcraft gained a certain prominence in the thoughts of medical men, especially when they belonged to the ranks of the clergy. Again, it was an effort to explain baffling modes of behaviour that defied rationalization. Physical illness as well as mental pathology was sometimes attributed to witchcraft. The methods used in an effort to liberate the afflicted from the power of the devil may seem cruel and brutal to us, but the aim was to cure rather than to punish, and if the body could not be cured, there was still the soul to be saved. Astrology and occultism also found their followers and may have at times impinged on the field of mental illness with their pseudoscientific approach.

Legally, the mentally ill were reasonably well protected. As early as the reign of Henry I (1068-1135), the laws made the parents responsible for the insane, specifying that the care had to be benevolent (misericorditer): "insanos et ejusmondi maleficos debent parentes sui misericorditer custodire." Moreover, the principle of diminished responsibility was prominent and was taken into consideration in assessing guilt for criminal acts and in depriving the insane of certain civil rights or obligations (7). An example is the case of a man in Norwich who, in 1270, was tried for the murder of his wife and children. He was found to be insane; hence he was sent to a hospital rather than punished and his case was reviewed some years later, when the authorities decided that he had not recovered enough to return to the community. A statute of Edward II enacted in 1324 distinguished between lunatics and idiots and made provision for the protection of their estate. Henry VI (1422-1471), the pious, scholarly, but weak king, was less protected; he was deprived of his throne and much else when, after recurring periods of insanity, he was finally deposed and imprisoned in the Tower, where he died in mysterious circumstances.

The 16th Century

By the 16th century the population of England had increased to 5,000,000 people. After a long period of strife, Henry VII had reestablished law and order; Henry VIII, his successor, brought about drastic reforms (64). Two were of great import in medicine: firstly, he closed the monasteries, and secondly, he empowered the Church to issue licenses to physicians, reasoning that the Church reached everywhere, made no distinction between social groups, and was concerned with man from baptism to burial. The closing of the monasteries was no great disaster as they had fallen into disrepute, the conduct of the monks often caused scandal, and the public was eager for reform. Physicians, surgeons and apothecaries replaced the monks in the new Royal Hospitals, St. Thomas's, Christ's, Bethlem, Bridewell, and St. Bartholomew.

The practice of medicine continued to be influenced by the humoral theory of Galen (36, 62) and mental disorders were still regarded in the traditional way, which attributed them to imbalance of the humors, especially black bile and choler. Mental pathology occupied the thoughts of many physicians, but unfortunately much of the field still remained in the hands of theologians, philosophers, and lay people who prevented progress by their prohibitions, speculations, and superstition. An example of this non-medical attitude is found in the writings of Sir Thomas More (48), the Lord Chancellor of Henry VIII; he was of the opinion that many expressions of abnormal behaviour would be cured by a good thrashing (33). On the other hand, another layman, Sir Thomas Elyot, took it upon himself to write a manual of domestic medicine entitled *The Castel of Helth* (1539), in which he urged the depressed to seek the advice of a wise man in addition to the usual physical remedies (33).

Elyot's book was not the only work of this kind, as the impact of printing was by this time widely felt and books were being written for a readership that included the less educated, who could now afford to buy them; for instance, a bookshop in Oxford sold over 2,000 books in the year 1520. The vernacular replaced learned Latin, and in addition to works originally written in English, many were translated from the Latin, the French or other languages.

Andrew Boorde (1490-1549), a Carthusian monk and bishop of Chichester, who had studied medicine at Montpellier, wrote *The Breviary of Healthe* (54); in the section on mental disorders he discussed those due to possession by the devil, for which he predictably recommended exorcism; for toxic disorders due to the ingestion of henbane he prescribed goat milk with sugar and "merry company"; mania, a disorder he likened to the behavior of a wild beast, he attributed to corrupt blood in the head, to bile, or to a weak brain, and advised that the patient should be confined in a tranquil room, given a nutrient diet, kept cheerful and, if need be, punished and beaten if he tried to hurt himself or others. He also prescribed "dormitories" (hypnotics) for insomnia, while recommending bleeding and the washing of the head in rose-water and vinegar for the "phrenesic." Like many other books on herbs (57), Gerarde's herbal, published in 1597, also included many remedies for "melancholie" and its numerous symptoms. It was to become a very popular work, with many reprints in the years following.

But the most interesting 16th century work on mental disorders is *A Treatise of Melancholy* (8). It was written in 1586 by a physician who chose English, rather than Latin, for this learned book. The treatise was the first book of psychiatry to be written in English; its author, Timothy Bright (?1551-1615), also the inventor of a system of shorthand, set himself the task of explaining the causes and reasons of the strange effects that melancholy works in minds and bodies, and promised "physick cure, and spiritual consolation" for those in need of treatment. He made it clear that melancholy does not affect merely the body, but also the "soul," and thus he recognized two types of the disorder, one of organic aetiology, or imbalance of humors, to be treated by diet and other physical means, and another due to apprehension of the mind, producing anxiety, to be treated by psychological means. Thus his term "melancholy" includes much of what we would today call psychonosis (neurosis).

Apart from its clinical interest, Bright's work is also of note from a literary point of view, as it is thought that Shakespeare read it when it was being prepared for final printing; the description of melancholy in *Hamlet* is said to have been based on it (76). Be that as it may, Shakespeare provides in his works many examples of beliefs related to emotional illness, insanity, and mental retardation; the distinction between the latter and insanity is clearly stated in *Cymbeline*: "Fools are not mad folks." Emotional states and madness were likewise distinguished, as proved by the lines spoken by Constance in *King John*, in which she convincingly argues that her agitation is caused by grief, not madness:

> "I am not mad; this hair I tear is mine;
> My name is Constance; I was Geffrey's wife;
> Young Arthur is my son and he is lost.
> I am not mad—I would to heaven I were,
> For then 'tis like I should forget myself.
> O, if I could, what grief should I forget!
> Preach some philosophy to make me mad,
> And thou shalt be canonized, Cardinal.
> For, being not mad, but sensible of grief,
> My reasonable part produces reason
> How I may be delivered of these woes,
> And teaches me to kill or hang myself.
> If I were mad, I should forget my son,
> Or madly think a babe of clouts were he.
> I am not mad; too well, too well I feel
> The different plague of each calamity."

> (*King John*, III, iv, 45-60)

Linked with Shakespeare by his marriage to the poet's younger daughter, Susanna, John Hall (1575-1635), a Stratford-upon-Avon physician, also provides evidence of awareness of emotional disorder; his case histories give several examples of psychogenic disorders among his patients and of his sympathetic management of them (32).

The Elizabethan Poor Laws (43) provided some relief for the indigent mentally ill, even though they were not distinguished from the vagrants or the work-shy; the insane were simply regarded as a social problem when their behaviour caused a disturbance; they were the responsibility of the parish to which they belonged and, because their maintenance was expensive, they were often turned loose and encouraged to move on. Some parishes used the no longer needed leper houses as asylums for the sick of mind or body who could not work.

Despite obvious signs of progress and enlightenment, the 16th century is often regarded as a period during which the Inquisition took over the management of the mentally ill, cruelly persecuting them. This is a misconception. The intention was to protect the Church from heresies. The heretic had to be proved to be sane before he could be punished; punishment and repentance were aimed at saving the

all important soul from eternal damnation even at the cost of destroying the body, which was considered unimportant and in any case
temporal. Mass paranoia, which swept Europe, disregarded all principles of humanity and honour in the hunt for the heretic. He was the
target of the Inquisition, not the insane. It was the heretic, not the
insane, who was supposed to bear the marks of devil possession. The
mentally ill and the unbalanced were at times caught up in this net
of paranoia by accident, but when their plight was recognized, they
were treated humanely. As the onus of proving innocence rested on
the accused, it was not always easy to refute fanatical charges of witchcraft and pacts with the devil. Reginald Scot, a Justice of the Peace,
became convinced that the accused, and often the accusers, were sick
and asserted his belief in *The Discoverie of Witchcraft* (1584) (60).
James VI of Scotland and I of England (1566-1625), while refuting
Scot's dismissal of demoniac possessions in a book entitled *Daemonologie* (37), first published in 1597, could, on the other hand, personally
examine a young woman accused of witchcraft, and, finding her to be
emotionally sick, arrange for her treatment, rather than for her
punishment.

3

THE MIDDLE PERIOD

This period spans 300 years. Regarded as a time of much advancement, its evaluation may be biased due to its link with the contemporary views of our time. In years it covers a shorter period than the
Roman occupation of Britain. Materialism slowly but surely steered
medicine away from psychopathology and left the psychiatrist in
isolation, an alienist. In this context, these 300 years deserve to be
termed the dark age of psychiatry.

The 17th Century

The 17th century was rich in medical writings in the field of psychiatry, which, following the impetus of the previous century, became
more integrated into medicine, partly disentangling itself from theological speculations and philosophical discussions. The very first year
of the new century, 1600, provides an interesting document: the
licence to practice on the "melancholy and the mad" granted by the
Archbishop of Canterbury to one John Freman (33). This document
probably marks the official recognition in England of psychological

medicine as a specialty and also illustrates how melancholy (psychonosis) could at the time be differentiated from madness (encephalonosis). It was not long before the College of Physicians of London showed interest in those treating "mad people" by prosecuting a practitioner for incompetence, as recorded in the Annals of the College for 1614.

Nevertheless, the field of emotional disorders was slower to become a medical science and for some time the diseases of the soul, the passions of the mind and the troubled conscience continued to be of more interest and concern to the clergyman than to the physician. However, it was a physician, Edward Jorden, who in 1603 wrote the first English book on hysteria. It was entitled *A Brief Discourse of a Disease Called the Suffocation of the Mother*. He attempted to explain many symptoms of hysteria and of psychosomatic disorders by contending that their aetiology was of a sexual nature and the seat of the disorder was the uterus (the mother). Jorden was called to give evidence in a case of suspected witchcraft; he made history as the first psychiatrist to provide expert evidence in a court of law; "the mother," not the devil, in his opinion, was the cause of abnormal behaviour in the accused, Marie Glovers (68).

The most famous book on psychiatry of the 17th century is without doubt *The Anatomy of Melancholy* (12), first published in 1621. Its author, Robert Burton, a scholarly bachelor and a clergyman, who lived, on his own admission "a silent, sedentary, solitary, private life," poured into it all he knew, making the book into a kind of encyclopedia of general information rather than a medical work. Yet it mirrors not only the accepted views of mental disorders of his time, but also superstitions, misconceptions, and past influences, while offering a glimpse of future trends. The frontispiece of the book is a summary in itself (Plate XXIX) (the author, in fact, introduced his work with verses explaining what it represents). Democritus of Abderra, the 5th century B.C. Greek philosopher, appears at the top of the page surrounded by the animals he "anatomized" in search of black bile, the physical cause of melancholy; jealousy and solitude are represented as the emotional aspect of the disorder. At the sides firstly, a gloomy lover; secondly, a "hypocondriacus" and his many remedies; thirdly, a "superstitius" on his knees and fourthly, a "maniacus," show four types of melancholy. At the bottom of the page are engraved borage and hellebore "to purge the veins of melancholy and cheer the heart." The sign of Saturn, the planet of melancholy, occurs repeatedly. It all amounts to a statement of theory and practice of psychiatry in Burton's time. Much of what he wrote shows an understanding of emo-

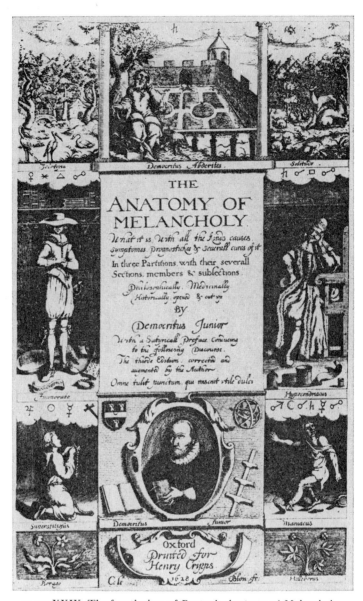

PLATE XXIX. The frontispiece of Burton's *Anatomy of Melancholy*.

tional disorders. According to Aubrey (23), Burton succumbed to melancholy and committed suicide by hanging himself in his chambers at Oxford.

A number of other writers were surprisingly attuned to various aspects of psychiatry which were subsequently lost and rediscovered much later; for instance, *folie à deux* was called by Sir Kenelm Digby "contagion of the imagination"; pseudocyesis was described by William Harvey; "Hypochondriacal complaints" were equated by Thomas Sydenham with female hysteria and included by him among psychological disorders (33).

Psychiatry would have advanced more rapidly if the learned men of this period had not become obsessed with a new approach based on measurement, classification, and localization. Theory had become all important. Thus, Francis Bacon was to influence psychology with his writings (56); a philosopher, he regarded the mind as his field, but suggested that more research should be done on the physical aspects of mental disorders by clinical and anatomical studies, more should be learned about the interaction of mind and body, and more attention should be paid to the influence of social factors. His organically-oriented doctrines were the most popular of his views.

Similarly, the publication of William Harvey's paper *De Motu Cordis* (1628) (27), claiming the discovery of the circulation of the blood, influenced the development of psychiatry by focusing attention on organic theories to the detriment of the understanding of psychological disorders. Bleeding, which for centuries had been used in the therapy of mental illness, became even more fashionable. Blood transfusion was attempted for the first time in England in 1667—the patient was a lunatic from Bethlem Hospital (73).

Meanwhile, neurology and neurophysiology were given new impetus (59), especially by the discoveries of Thomas Willis (1621-1675). He linked hysterical fits with disorders of the brain, classifying them with epilepsy; to a sick brain he also attributed madness with thought disorder and hallucinations; he described dementia praecox, and called "passions of the heart" those disorders like depression, which we would today call "emotional." His famous book on the anatomy and physiology of the nervous system, *Cerebri Anatome* (1664), was illustrated by plates drawn by Sir Christopher Wren, the builder of St. Paul's Cathedral (35).

But in general the new scientific language tended to dismiss psychological factors, or distort them until they fitted into the scheme of things; the emotions as aetiological factors were ignored and the causes of unusual behaviour, changes of mood, and psychosomatic

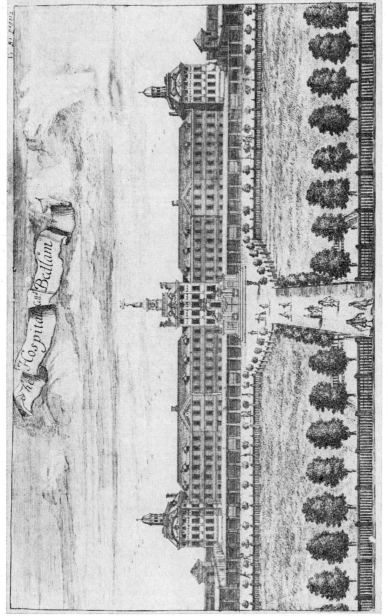

PLATE XXX. The new Bethlem Hospital at Moorfields.

disorders were explained in terms of biological changes due to physical agents. There were exceptions, as is testified by the following letter, written by James Howell, a much-traveled politician and historian, and quoted in Hunter and Macalpine's valuable text (33).

> Wer ther a Physitian that could cure the maladies of the mind, as well as those of the body, he needed not to wish the Lord Maior, or the Pope for his Uncle, for he should have patients without number: It is true, that ther be som distempers of the mind that proceed from those of the body and so are curable by drugs and diets; but ther are others that are quite abstracted from all corporeall impressions, and are meerly mentall; these kind of agonies are the more violent of the two, for as the one use to drive us into Feavers, the other precipitate us oft-times into Frensies.

Many sick people sought relief in the herbs and the charms of old and the healing power of people like Valentine Greatakes (33), the Cromwellian soldier who brought about strange cures by "stroking" the afflicted with his hands; or Nicholas Culpeper who combined herbal remedies with astrology.

London suffered the Great Plague in 1665, and the following year it was almost totally destroyed by the Great Fire (18). But from the ashes rose a better planned, more splendid city. The urge to rebuild spread to institutions for the mentally sick and a new Bethlem Hospital was built at Moorfields in 1676 (49) (Plate XXX). It was designed by a physician, Robert Hooke, a many-sided genius who, among other things, wrote on memory and on the properties of Indian hemp. The new Bethlem, then considered the finest public building in London, was spacious and, from the outside, resembled a French royal palace, the Tuilleries (which did not please Louis XIV of France), but despite some bleeding, purging, and administration of emetics, its function remained mostly custodial and the sounds, the sights, and the scents associated with the insane were soon to pervade its wards. Outside London, mental patients who could not be looked after at home were still admitted to public general hospitals, but no special provisions existed for them until, in 1696, St. Peter Hospital in Bristol provided special wards for the insane poor. Affluent lunatics were boarded out with clergymen or physicians, thus giving rise to the first private "madhouses."

The 18th Century

As the geographical and intellectual horizon of the Englishman expanded, the influx of new ideas from other countries increased and with it came a stimulus towards research, experimentation, and systematization. The English psychiatric literature of this period is enormous and can be divided into two groups. The first group was small and was exemplified by George Cheyne, who, in 1733, wrote on the "English malady" (14). By this term Cheyne referred to depression, which he attributed to the moist air of these islands, to our variable weather, to a too-rich diet, and to overpopulation. To it he added many other "distempers" of "nervous" origin, basing his findings on his own condition. According to him, "These nervous disorders" accounted for about a third of the complaints of the people in the upper classes. The second group, by far the largest, dealing with insanity, epilepsy and other organic disorders, is represented by the publication of William Battie's *Treatise on Madness* in 1758 (5). The author based his writings on his experience as physician to St. Luke Hospital for Lunaticks as well as on observation of paying patients in his own private establishment; his example was followed, among others, by Thomas Arnold with his *Observations on the Nature, Kinds, Causes and Prevention of Insanity* (33), and by William Prefect with his *Select Cases of Insanity*.

Classification of mental disorders continued to occupy many physicians. The classifications derived from the system employed in botany. Disorders were grouped by symptoms, rather than by aetiology, resulting in errors and perpetuation of old concepts. The most prominent classifier was William Cullen (1710-1790) (33); he rejected the psychological causation of some disorders and favored a cerebral aetiology; he coined the term neurosis, to indicate disorder of neurone. His views, based on little practical experience, influenced medical practice both in his country and abroad and contributed to a system of treatment built on coercion.

The economic changes brought about by the Industrial Revolution resulted in prosperity for the middle class and increased insecurity and discontent among manual workers, who were being replaced by machinery. The poor were living in appalling conditions of overcrowding and filth. Infant mortality was high; in London only one child in four survived. Antidotes to this kind of life were found in drink, violence, and gambling. Social contrasts were extreme (63). The plight of the sick poor, of abandoned children, and other distressed groups was partially alleviated by an upsurge of charitable institutions, both private and public. Lunatic asylums were not populated solely by adult and aged men and women; records show that between 1772 and 1787, of about 3,000 patients admitted in Bethlem Hospital, 132 were between the ages of 10 and 20 and one was under 10 years of age (33).

The oldest English mental hospital outside London was founded in

1713, in Norwich, with funds provided by Mrs. Mary Chapman, a clergyman's widow (4) (Plate XXXI). It is the oldest existing mental hospital building in Britain. In London, because of disquiet at bad conditions in Bethlem, although a special ward for lunatics was established at Guy's Hospital in 1728, St. Luke Hospital for Lunaticks (70) was founded in 1751, mostly by the efforts of William Battie, who became its first physician; he was the first psychiatrist in Britain to teach

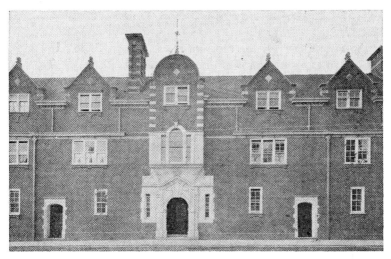

PLATE XXXI. Bethel Hospital, Norwich. The oldest standing mental hospital in Britain.

psychiatry to medical students. Psychiatry, based on organic pathology, survived in institutional form, although patients were hospitalized without a proper diagnosis and "dangerous lunatics," by the Act of 1714, could be locked up if two justices of the peace so directed. Though they were chained, they were not usually whipped, but the curious could still buy an admission ticket to visit the wards of Bedlam and be amused by the antics of the insane.

A new development was the multiplication of private madhouses (50) that accepted patients for payment and acted either as nursing homes, providing board and lodgings while leaving treatment to the patient's own physician, or offering a "cure," often on the basis of "no cure, no payment." Private madhouses, 15 of them in London alone, became a profitable trade; they often remained in the same family for generations and some were owned by reputable physicians, Battie among them. Their reputation, with a few exceptions, was so bad that public opinion eventually forced the government to intervene and appoint, in 1763, a Select Committee to inquire into their affairs and conditions. Daniel Defoe, the author of *Robinson Crusoe,* was among those active in the campaign for the control of private mental institutions. Another writer, Jonathan Swift, best remembered for his bitter satire *Gulliver's Travels,* was so interested in mental illness that in 1714 he became one of the Governors of Bethlem; on his death he left the bulk of his estate for the foundation of a "House for Fools and Mad"—St. Patrick's Hospital, in Dublin, Ireland, founded with his gift in 1746.

In the second part of the century, psychiatry in England was given impetus by the events surrounding the life and illness of George III (1738-1820) (9). This unhappy king was submitted to enormous stresses, political pressures, and personal anxieties in his family life. He was believed to be insane, but was possibly suffering from hereditary porphyria (45). He was ill on five distinct occasions, separated by periods of remission and concluded by a final breakdown and death. The official bulletins on the state of his health were a matter of national interest and familiarized lay people with insanity, its nature, its symptoms, and its management. The treatment of the royal patient was entrusted to a number of physicians until Dr. Francis Willis and his son, John Darling Willis, took charge of him. Nothing was spared: the suffering and indignities meted out to the King of England included bleeding, blistering, scarifying, purging, emetics, and solitary confinement away from his family. To him psychiatry owes much. Two attempts on his life and subsequent trials of the would-be assassins contributed to changes in the law of criminal responsibility, as the accused were found insane and sent to an asylum, rather than to prison (42). The emphasis on treatment was also evident in the Act of 1774, which stressed that the inmates of asylums were to be "cured"; they were no longer regarded as hopeless incurables to be incarcerated for the protection of society (38).

In Manchester, a Lunatic Asylum was founded in 1766, followed by the foundation of similar institutions in York in 1777, and in Liverpool in 1792 (70). Treatment was less harsh than in the past, but chains were still in use, although the regulations provided for periodical inspection of chained patients, to make sure that the circulation of the blood was not impeded. Blood-letting was the usual remedy for manic patients, who were also calmed by warm baths, tartar emetic, and purgatives; melancholic patients were given similar treatment, but they were immersed in cold water. Sores were artificially produced, as it was believed that they provided an outlet for "bad humors." General conditions in these asylums gradually deteriorated and they too were found lacking when officially inspected.

The century closed with an event that is considered a landmark in British psychiatry; *The Retreat* (67) at York was founded in 1796 by the Society of Friends (Quakers) at the instigation of one of their members, William Tuke. Here he instituted a new system of care based on minimal restraint and constructive treatment. The patients enjoyed an unusual degree of freedom and were treated like guests, often being invited to tea by the superintendent or the matron. For an extra fee and if they so wished, they could be looked after by their own servants.

The 19th Century

George III's illness had made mental disorder almost respectable; when he died his obituary spoke of the King's courage and honesty, linking his physical illness and his blindness to his insanity, which was referred to as "mental darkness." It could have been the beginning of a period of enlightenment, but, unfortunately, psychiatry too, like the old King, was enveloped in darkness.

As early as 1808, an Act was passed allowing, but not compelling, justices in every county in England and Wales to provide asylums for the lunatic poor, but by 1827, only 7 out of 52 counties had done so. Asylums were regarded with justified suspicion and distrust which culminated in a parliamentary inquiry into the conditions in mental hospitals. The situation had become a scandal following the discovery, in 1814, of William Norris, who was found in a dark and damp cell in Bethlem, where he had been kept in irons for ten years, despite his illness, tuberculosis, of which he died a year after being removed from Bethlem (42).

The first report of the committee of inquiry into private madhouses and public institutions was published in 1815. It brought to light a most unsatisfactory state of affairs, revealing overcrowding of patients, insufficient staff to look after them with consequent need for physical restraint, indiscriminate mixing of patients with various types of disorders, lack of treatment, unnecessarily harsh restraint, the poor confined in asylums and workhouses for lack of other accommodation, detention of people who were not insane, improper certification of certain patients, and superficial inspection of private madhouses. It was a dismal picture, which demonstrated the wide gap existing between practice and theory, the latter represented in the many textbooks of the period. Public opinion was outraged at these infringements of human rights and dignity and the findings of the committee of inquiry led to a number of Acts being passed with the aim of providing proper care and treatment, safeguarding against wrongful detention and establishing an efficient system of inspection and licensing of public and private institutions.

The Lunacy Act of 1845 marked the beginning of many reforms (38); it established the Commissioners in Lunacy with jurisdiction over the whole of England and Wales. In the same year another Act made compulsory the provision of asylums by counties and boroughs. Asylums were thus being built up and down the country; their solid walls closed around a small but permanent group of patients, the chronically insane. On the problems of the insane, real or misdiagnosed, were concentrated the efforts of most psychiatrists, who were now being called alienists, since their patients were considered to be "alienated" from society. The various Acts culminated in the Lunacy Act of 1890, which consolidated and brought together previous legislation and remained the most important Act until 1959.

The construction of purpose-built hospitals gave rise to studies and suggestions about their architectural structure together with the search for more efficient methods of management (11, 16). Some medical superintendents went to the Continent to see what was being achieved there and came back eager to apply what they had learned. An example of this was W. A. F. Browne (1805-1885) (10); his observations of continental practice, especially of the work of Esquirol in France, inspired his series of lectures on *"What asylums were, are, and ought to be"* (16). When these lectures were published, they came to the notice of a philanthropist, Mrs. Elizabeth Crichton, who was so impressed that she offered Browne the position of superintendent in the charitable institution for the insane (now Crichton Royal Hospital) which she was founding in Scotland. Thus he was able to put into practice progressive methods of treatment, based on kindness, understanding, a reasonable amount of freedom, and occupation. Browne was also a pioneer in the training of mental nurses, for whom he instituted a course of lectures. At the Lincoln Asylum the house surgeon, Robert Gardiner Hill, and the physician, Dr. Charlesworth, introduced a policy of no restraint (71). John Conolly (1794-1866), after spending some time in France, was influenced by the work of Pinel there and was able to put into practice the same enlightened methods at the Hanwell Asylum, when, in 1839, he became the resident physician. His book, *The Treatment of the Insane without the Use of Mechanical Restraints* (17), was influential in bringing about many reforms.

Treatment continued to be based on purging, emetics, and bleeding; however, these procedures were now carried out with more sophistication, while, inevitably, some "mechanical" methods were introduced, this being the age of the machine. Contraptions were devised to tranquilize manic patients. Some of these machines were no less restraining than the chains of old, but achieved immobilization by means of leather straps, canvas jackets, or shirts with ties for arms and legs. Other machines were constructed to spin the patient. Whirling chairs and spinning beds caused the unfortunate patient incontinence, vomiting and, often, loss of consciousness, yet they were not abolished until a number of fatal casualties proved how dangerous they were. Other devices employed included the douche, whereby water was made to fall from varying hights on to the head of the patient, and a padded hollow wheel, big enough to contain a person. To us these contraptions may look like instruments of torture and, no doubt, the rationale behind them had a thinly disguised element of punishment in their application; their crude construction makes them even more repelling to our eyes, used to the gleaming sophistication of an E.C.T. machine, but at the time they were regarded as progressive.

Much has been written about the cruelty, neglect, and gloom pervading the asylums of the 19th century; it is often forgotten that they instituted many beneficial innovations, only recently rediscovered. For instance, they were self-supporting; at times this led to exploitation of patient labour, but it provided agricultural, domestic, and light industrial work which today we would call occupational therapy and sheltered workshops. They encouraged diversions in the form of plays, dances, parties and fêtes, at which the asylum brass bands played with great pride, showing off the musicians' quasi-military uniforms and their well-polished instruments (Plate XXXII). Again, some asylums made good use of what talent they could find among the patients in writing, editing, and printing their own journals. The isolation of the asylums in remote parts of the country also had some advantages, as it provided spacious grounds where a certain freedom of movement was possible, away as they were from the censorious attitudes of the community.

The construction of these large institutions resulted in an apparent increase in the number of mental patients, but the true situation was that a need was now being met and those mentally sick individuals, who were previously denied institutional care, were now provided for. Nevertheless, some insane poor were still being sent to the workhouse; as they were transferred to asylums, the latter, already large, were forced to become larger still to accommodate them and to accept a number of poor who should, on the other hand, have been in the workhouse. Institutions varied in quality of care: some were bad, some were good, and all contained a number of patients who would have been better served by remaining in the community. In Scotland many patients were boarded out in the community. Towards the end of the century, in England, about 30 percent of all mental patients were still being cared for at home or in private institutions. Diagnosis was still uncertain and the wards were filled with mixed groups of

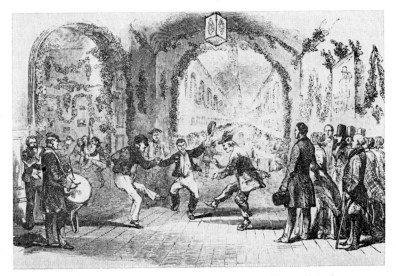

PLATE XXXII. Twelfth Night Entertainment at Hanwell Asylum.

patients that included epileptics, paralytics, patients suffering from the effects of past encephalitis, from toxic states, or from dementia. The physicians in charge of their care were medical officers, with little experience of psychiatry or neurology.

As already pointed out, the emphasis in psychiatry was on insanity. The treatises, the textbooks, the reports on its causes, course, treatment and nosology multiplied. Samuel Tuke (grandson of William Tuke, the founder of the Retreat at York) wrote a description of that institution (67); Henry Monro, the physician of St. Luke's Hospital for Lunatics, published his *Remarks on Insanity; Its Nature and Treatment* (47); John Conolly advocated his methods in *The Treatment of the Insane* (17), while others argued its genetic aetiology (Joseph Adams on hereditary disposition (1)), its prevention (G. Ness Hill,

Prevention and Cure of Insanity (28)) and its many aspects from the legal, social, and ethical points of view.

The psychiatric disorders of children were beginning to attract attention; Charles West, the founder and physician of the famous Hospital for Sick Children, in Great Ormond Street, London, included disorders of the mind in childhood in his series of lectures delivered in 1847 (74).

A professional organization for psychiatrists, the first in Great Britain and in the world, was founded in 1841. It was called the "Association of Medical Officers of Hospitals for the Insane," and in 1971 was to become the Royal College of Psychiatrists (31). In 1853 it published its own journal, the *Asylum Journal,* which later became the *Journal of Mental Science* and is now the *British Journal of Psychiatry.*

From the middle of the century, mental defectives, who had been kept at home, boarded out, put into prisons and workhouses, or mixed indiscriminately with the insane in asylums, were beginning to be regarded as a separate group, needing their own facilities. This trend was encouraged by the work of Seguin in France. The first institution dedicated to the care of the mentally subnormal was the Royal Earlswood Asylum in Surrey, founded in 1855 by the Rev. Andrew Reed. From 1870, the Metropolitan Asylum Board provided special institutions and training establishments for them, the most famous of which was the Darenth Training Colony (39). Interest in mental deficiency was further encouraged by the work of J. Langdon Down, the Medical Superintendent of the Royal Earlswood Asylum, who was the first to describe mongolism, or Down's Disease. William Ireland, better remembered for his psychiatric biographies in *The Blot upon the Brain,* also wrote on mental deficiency (34).

While works and trends concerning insanity and mental deficiency were following an evolutionary course, other ideas were making their influence felt in less well defined areas. It was obvious to some workers that not all disorders could be linked with heredity, or with defects and deterioration of the nervous system. A large number of patients still suffered with disorders that in earlier times had been recognized and accepted as "sickness of the soul," a sick psyche, emotional illness, psychonosis. These patients did not respond to physical means of treatment. Psychiatrists in many asylums were advocating "moral treatment," an ill-defined approach consisting of firm persuasion and re-education—almost, but not quite, psychotherapy (69). It could have been an early breakthrough, but it was damned by the 19th century obsession with "morality," which tended to attribute all kinds of disorders to a life which offered various pleasurable ways of destroying the physical and mental health of the rich, leaving alcoholism to the poor and self abuse to the poorest. Hence, "moral treatment" tended to remain just what it was called, aiming as it did at reforming the patient.

However, a new theory, first acclaimed, then ridiculed, was spreading to England from the Continent. It started towards the end of the previous century with the work of Mesmer in Austria and in France and led to the experiments of James Braid, a surgeon. After attending a public demonstration of mesmerism in Manchester, Braid embarked on a journey of discovery through experiments which convinced him of the existence of a psychic life of great importance in health and disease. In 1843, he wrote a book entitled *Neurypnology, or The Rationale of Nervous Sleep,* in which he suggested the word "hypnotism" for a therapeutic approach that would directly influence the patient through verbal suggestion. It was the middle link of a chain between mesmerism and psychoanalysis (24). At first mesmerism led to techniques that were in turn pathetic, ludicrous, or just plain deceitful. As always, the emotionally ill, in their need for support, counsel and, above all, hope, were easily taken in by charlatans who promised them a solution to their problems. Furthermore, the impossibility of exact measurements and assessment made emotional disorder, as today, a fruitful field for the unscrupulous and the untrained to infiltrate and do much harm.

The need for better psychiatric education and for more research was advocated by Henry Maudsley (1835-1918), whose efforts in that direction culminated in the foundation of an institution, the Maudsley Hospital, dedicated to intensive therapy and offering some facilities for research.

4

THE CONTEMPORARY PERIOD

We approach the last 73 years of our history. Tuke, the younger, introduced his *Dictionary of Psychological Medicine* (66) with an historical sketch of psychiatry. Writing at the end of the 19th century, he had this to say of his predecessors up to the 19th century: "One general observation is warranted. . . . That is the total absence of any original departure from the beaten track in which they had moved." He implies that things were different in his own 19th century. This we can question. What will be the judgment on the 20th century? Can we turn the tide of neuropsychiatry that flowed so strongly in the previous three centuries?

The 20th Century

The first half of this century brought an upheaval in British political life that indirectly proved to be of considerable potential benefit to psychiatry. The trappings of Empire were discarded, material prosperity increased, the country survived two World Wars and, most significantly, especially since World War II, a strong movement towards social reform began. As Adrian (2) has remarked, wars can have the compensation of being periods of creativity. Alas, the far-reaching health and social legislation of great benefit as a background to psychiatry is hampered by the country's economic situation and by the state of psychiatry itself.

The start of the 20th century saw British psychiatry in the grip of neuropsychiatry, a hold which has still not been released as we write today. That psychiatry should truly devote itself to the psyche and redress the imbalance in its practice is far from achieved, although here and there we find progress. The grip of neuropsychiatry is to be seen in the training programmes for psychiatrists, in teaching institutions, in mental hospital practice, and in legislation. The nosology of psychiatry is still chaotic and the lack of agreed criteria for the description of syndromes hampers research and clinical practice, e.g., schizophrenia is confused with severe states of emotional illness and findings relevant to the latter are ascribed to the former. In many areas, clinical practice tends to concentrate more on neuropsychiatry than psychiatry; the minor field of encephalonosis (psychosis) has prominent attention as against the major field of psychonosis (neurosis) with its crippling and life endangering conditions. Treatment is hampered by the extremes of drug therapy, or of psychoanalysis.

This century has seen the foundation of two new professional bodies. The first, the Society of Clinical Psychiatrists, was founded in 1959, mostly by senior clinicians. The Society's initiative led to changes in the Mental Health Act, 1959, which in effect abolished the Medical Superintendent whose preoccupation with administration hampered clinical developments. The Society then turned its attention to reshaping and strengthening the status of the professional body of British psychiatrists, the Royal Medico-Psychological Association, by campaigning for its metamorphosis into the Royal College of Psychiatrists; this was achieved in 1971 (31). The effort of the Society then went into establishing a number of study groups on topical issues and the publication of their progressive reports in readable form.

The formation of the second professional body, the Royal College of Psychiatrists, saw the most significant development in psychiatry in the United Kingdom in the last 200 years. Its importance was that psychiatry released itself from the control of the physicians of psychological medicine and thus dependence on the Royal College of Physicians. The formation of its own College meant that psychiatry could now frame its own practice, control its own training, manage its own examinations, and have a responsible voice in the affairs of medicine (31). In time it will influence medical training, redress the excessive slant towards the organic, and in turn improve recruitment into psychiatry.

Early in the century there was some progress in psychopathology. Shell-shock and acute emotional situations were so glaringly obvious that they aroused the interest of a number of clinicians. After the First World War, out of the imagination of J. R. Rees, Crichton Miller, and J. A. Hadfield, a British school of psychopathology was founded. From this emerged the Tavistock Clinic. However, into Britain came psychoanalysis and, in 1939, Freud himself. The analytical movement was never large, but it was distinguished. This extraordinary doctrine throttled the home product, and psychoanalysis or Jungian analysis became the vogue alongside some Adlerian analysis.

Despite psychoanalysis and neuropsychiatry, further progress in dynamic psychiatry (77) took place. General medical practitioners, pediatricians, physicians, and some psychiatrists displayed a great deal of interest in it and in psychosomatic medicine. The Institute of Family Psychiatry, Ipswich, sponsored family psychiatry, whereby the family rather than the individual became the patient; this led to experiential psychopathology and vector therapy. A mental health section within the Society of Medical Officers of Health reflected the interest of physicians in preventive medicine in social psychiatry. This latter concept was often vague and could amount to little more than nursing the mentally ill in the community rather than in hospital, and the after-care of patients following discharge. Enthusiasm and good intention are unfortunately inadequate substitutes for knowledge. The most promising element is the growing inclination of the family doctor to practice psychiatry in the community.

Until 1930 mental hospitals continued to admit patients mostly by certificate, i.e., by compulsion, but in that year came the Mental Treatment Act, which encouraged treatment while also allowing voluntary admissions. Psychiatric treatment was a new concept in law and a new concept for the psychiatrist. Hitherto the psychiatrist was essentially the medical officer in an establishment and physical care, but not psychiatric treatment, was his main function. Now came the era of metrazol, modified insulin therapy, deep insulin therapy, psychosurgery, and electroconvulsive therapy. Each form of treatment was adopted with the same lack of discrimination with which it was abandoned. But while discrimination was lacking, enthusiasm was not. Thus the very impetus of the therapeutic movement opened doors, threw down railings, and gave enormous help and encouragement to both staff and patients—but particularly to staff. The most therapeutic element in this therapeutic programme was enthusiasm harnessed to the belief in the possibility of change.

Then came legislation neither willed nor wished for by the psychiatrist, but bringing him and his patients considerable benefit. This was the foundation in 1948 of the National Health Service, from The National Health Service Act of 1946. This Act gave mental hospitals benefits equal to those of the general hospitals. Furthermore, it gave specialists in psychiatry the same grading, salaries, and opportunities as specialists in other fields. This was an unsought for but fortunate boost for the morale of psychiatrists. Inevitably, it helped recruitment into psychiatry. While still not quite respectable, the field now had the potentiality of respectability. Matters were enhanced by the Mental Health Act of 1959. Hitherto, the Medical Superintendent had been the first doctor in the mental hospital and his senior colleagues had often found themselves frustrated, as he controlled the clinical programme with the power of admission and discharge. This responsibility was now given to the Responsible Medical Officer—the clinician.

More recently, another significant change of attitude has taken place, whereby a Committee (20) advocated that psychiatry should geographically be placed at the district general hospital. Additional general guidance (21) was then given, whereby it was made clear that in future the mental and the general hospitals would be amalgamated into one hospital—the hospital. It may take 20 years fully to achieve this target, but the intention and legislation are there. So, as far as institutionalization is concerned, psychiatry has returned to the pattern it had left four centuries ago, i.e., a single hospital or hospice for all those in need of help. Unfortunately, modern thinking in organization has yet to match some of the old concepts. For instance, in the early hospitals of the Middle Ages, the long-term care was thought of in terms of a domestic layout; the contemporary general hospital's impressive mechanized accommodation is intended for short-term care, what could be termed hotel accommodation, but is most unsatisfactory for long-term care which requires home-like accommodation in an annex.

All the above changes were a background to a number of developments in patient care—the open door policy that led to the absence of locked doors and of the incessant jangling of keys, abolition of padded cells, progressive patient care to eradicate institutional neurosis, milieu therapy, group discussion, rehabilitation programmes, sheltered workshops, and community psychiatry. Some of these programmes were sad in their implications, for they were a consciously contrived humanization movement, when humane management should have been a natural component of hospital management. Nevertheless, the British mental hospital improved greatly and was emulated in other parts of the world (40).

The history of child psychiatry in Britain has been outlined elsewhere (29). Essentially, the impetus came at first from the paediatricians and from psychiatrists who had founded children's clinics, for instance the Tavistock Clinic and the Maudsley Hospital. Later came the child guidance movement, together with educational psychology. All these varied approaches led to a state of considerable confusion. As the government tended to regard the psychiatry of children as an educational matter, children were not given the services due to them within the Health Service. This, together with bad advice and the lack of impetus by the main training centres, delayed the development of child psychiatry. Only now, with the amalgamation of the hospital, general practice, and public health sectors of the Health Service, is the clear differentiation between clinical services for the emotional health of children and educational services for their educational improvement likely to develop. However, child psychiatry has one great strength— it employs the concepts of dynamic psychiatry.

In recent years the psychiatry of old age has been an expanding field within psychiatry because, as the number of beds in mental hospitals diminished, they were increasingly taken over for the admission of elderly patients, who should have been admitted elsewhere, had there been beds available. Thus, the psychiatrist was forced to become a psychogeriatrician and often a geriatrician. At first, there were no organized services for the elderly within the mental hospital. This is in the process of being put right, either by a comprehensive physical and mental service for the elderly, or by the psychiatrist operating his own psychogeriatric service (22, 25).

Psychiatric training remains mostly based on neuropsychiatry. The principal training centre, the Institute of Psychiatry, London, has practically held the monopoly of postgraduate teaching since World War II. The picture in psychiatric research is rather similar. In 1965, the Medical Research Council had only three research teams relevant to psychiatry. The large number of research workers at the Maudsley

Hospital, in London, again constitutes practically a monopoly of resources. Elsewhere, research goes on, but is less well endowed.

Monopolies hamper progress. The case for wider distribution of opportunities in research and teaching is undeniable. This is happening in psychiatric training which, in common with all postgraduate training in every branch of medicine, is moving to graduate teaching centres at district hospitals away from the university hospitals, which in future will concentrate on undergraduate teaching. Clinical research can be expected to follow the same path.

5

CONCLUSION

It is often argued that psychiatry is outside medicine proper. A glance over its history in Britain shows what a poorly justified viewpoint this is. Man found it necessary to train not only farmers to provide food, soldiers for protection, priests to study and guard ethics, but also healers to tend him in disease. Healing was required not only for physical wounds, but also for psychic hurt. The argument that psychiatry is not an healing art can be sustained only if it were possible to limit medicine to the art of healing for physical hurt alone. From the earliest times this has been shown to be impracticable. Disease (literally lack of ease) applies equally to psychic and physical trauma. And the two are indivisible.

We have seen the effort, from very early times, to find, not a pathology to explain psychic disorder and another for physical disorder, but a common pathology. From Hippocrates through Galen to Timothy Bright this was the quest. The materialism that followed the 16th century led to the quest for a common pathology being abandoned and to an overemphasis on organic pathology. Today we stumble, half discerning and beset with false prophets, to redress the balance.

Our knowledge and therapeutic efficiency has improved little over the centuries. All that we hold so dear is not new and can be found in the past—sleep therapy, electric treatment, neurosurgery, occupational therapy, rehabilitation, milieu therapy, psychiatry in a general hospital, drug therapy (in the form of herbs, gentle on the soma but powerful in their placebo effects), and psychotherapy (cautious and realistic). The words of Tuke in the last century are apposite:

> If the success of the treatment of insanity bore any considerable proportion to the number of the remedies which have been brought

forward, it would be my easy and agreeable duty to record the triumphs of medicine in the distressing malady which they are employed to combat. But this, unhappily, is not the case . . . (65).

One clear lesson emerges. Progress follows knowledge. For advances in the field of encephalonosis we need a sure understanding of its organic pathology; without this, the blind drug therapy of today is as indiscriminating as the blind purging of yesterday. For advances in the field of psychonosis we need a sure understanding of its psychopathology; without this, blind psychotherapy is as indiscriminating and damaging as the "blood letting" of yesterday.

And one day, an holistic approach will again prevail in medicine. We shall then be better able to understand and help the troubled man.

REFERENCES

1. ADAMS, J. (1814): *A Treatise on the Supposed Hereditary Properties . . . Particularly in Madness and Scrofula.* London: Callow.
2. ADRIAN, E. D. (1968): Introduction. In: Howells, J. G. (Ed.). *Modern Perspectives in World Psychiatry.* Edinburgh: Oliver and Boyd. New York: Brunner/Mazel.
3. BACON, F. (1605): *The Advancement of Learning.* Annotated by G. W. Kitchin, 1958. London: Dent.
4. BATEMAN, F. & RYE, W. (1906): *The History of the Bethel Hospital at Norwich.* Norwich.
5. BATTIE, W. (1758): *A Treatise on Madness.* Facsimile, 1969. New York: Brunner/Mazel.
6. BEDE. *Ecclesiastical History of the English People.* Colgrave, B. and Mynors, R. A. B. (Eds.), 1969. London: Oxford University Press.
7. BONSER, W. (1963): *The Medical Background of Anglo-Saxon England.* London: Wellcome Historical Medical Library.
8. BRIGHT, T. (1586): *A Treatise of Melancholy.* Facsimile, 1969. New York: Da Capo Press.
9. BROOKE, J. (1972): *King George III.* London: Constable.
10. BROWNE, W. A. F. (1837): *What Asylums Were, Are and Ought To Be.* Edinburgh: Black.
11. BURDETT, H. C. (1891): *Hospitals and Asylums of the World.* London: Churchill.
12. BURTON, R. (1628): *The Anatomy of Melancholy.* Jackson, H. (Ed). Everyman's Library, No. 886-8. London: Dent.
13. CAESAR. *De Bello Gallico.* Trans. by H. J. Edwards, 1917. London: Heinemann.
14. CHEYNE, G. (1733): *The English Maladie.* London: Strahan.
15. CLAY, R. M. (1909): *The Medieval Hospital of England.* London: Methuen.
16. CONOLLY, J. (1847): *The Construction and Government of Lunatic Asylums.* Facsimile, 1968. London: Dawson.
17. CONOLLY, J. (1856): *The Treatment of the Insane without Mechanical Restraint.* London: Smith, Elder.
18. COWIE, L. W. (1970): *Plague and Fire of London, 1665-6.* London: Wayland.
19. DAINTON, C. (1961): *The Story of England's Hospitals.* London: Museum Press.
20. Department of Health and Social Security (1969): *The Functions of the District General Hospital.* Report of the Committee. London: H. M. S. O.

21. Department of Health and Social Security (1971): *Hospital Services for the Mentally Ill*. London: H. M. S. O.

22. Department of Health and Social Security (1972): *Services for Mental Illness Related to Old Age*. London: H. M. S. O.

23. DICK, O. L. (Ed.). (1968): *Aubrey's Brief Lives*. London: Secker & Warburg.

24. ELLENBERGER, H. F. (1970): *The Discovery of the Unconscious*. London: Allen Lane The Penguin Press.

25. ENOCH, M.D. & HOWELLS, J. G. (1971): *The Organization of Psychogeriatrics*. Society of Clinical Psychiatrists.

26. GRATTAN, J. H. G. & SINGER, C. (1952): *Anglo-Saxon Magic and Medicine*. London: Oxford University Press.

27. HARVEY, WILLIAM (1628): *The Circulation of the Blood*. Franklin, K. J. (Ed.). Everyman's Library No. 262. London: Dent.

28. HILL, G. N. (1814): *An Essay on the Prevention and Cure of Insanity*. London: Longman.

29. HOWELLS, J. G. (1965): Organisation of child psychiatric services. In: Howells, J. G. (Ed.), *Modern Perspectives in Child Psychiatry*. Edinburgh: Oliver and Boyd. New York: Brunner/Mazel.

30. HOWELLS, J. G. (1971): Classification of Psychiatric Disorders. In: Howells, J. G. (Ed.), *Modern Perspectives in Adolescent Psychiatry*. Edinburgh: Oliver and Boyd. New York: Brunner/Mazel.

31. HOWELLS, J. G. (1971): *Royal College of Psychiatrists*. Society of Clinical Psychiatrists.

32. HOWELLS, J. G. & OSBORN, M. L. (1970): The incidence of emotional disorder in a seventeenth-century medical practice. *Med. Hist.*, 14, 192-198.

33. HUNTER, R. & MACALPINE, I. (1963): *Three Hundred Years of Psychiatry 1535-1860*. London: Oxford University Press.

34. IRELAND, W. W. (1877): *Idiocy and Imbecility*. London: Churchill.

35. ISLER, H. R. (1968): *Thomas Willis, 1612-1675. Doctor and Scientist*. New York: Hafner.

36. JACKSON, S. W. (1969): Galen—on mental disorders. *J. Hist. Behav. Sci.*, 5, 365-384.

37. JAMES, I . (1597): *Daemonologie*. Facsimile, 1969. New York: Da Capo Press.

38. JONES, K. (1955): *Lunacy, Law and Conscience 1744-1845: The Social History of the Care of the Insane*. London: Routledge & Kegan Paul.

39. JONES, K. (1960): *Mental Health and Social Policy*. London: Routledge & Kegan Paul.

40. JONES, K. (1972): *A History of the Mental Health Services*. London: Routledge & Kegan Paul.

41. KENDRICK, T. D. (1966): *The Druids*. London: Cass.

42. LEIGH, D. (1961): *The Historical Development of British Psychiatry*. Oxford: Pergamon Press.

43. LEONARD, E. M. (1900): *Early History of English Poor Relief*. Cambridge: Cambridge University Press.

44. LIVERSIDGE, J. (1968): *Britain in the Roman Empire*. London: Routledge & Kegan Paul.

45. MACALPINE, I. & HUNTER, R. (1969): *George III and the Mad-Business*. London: Allen Lane The Penguin Press.

46. MACKAY, C. (1841): *Extraordinary Popular Delusions and the Madness of Crowds*. Facsimile, 1932. New York: Page.

47. MONRO, H. (1851): *Remarks on Insanity: Its Nature and Treatment*. London: Churchill.

48. MORE, T. (1556): *Utopia*. Trans. by R. Robinson. Facsimile, 1970. Menston: Scolar Press.

49. O'DONOGHUE, E. G. (1914): *The Story of Bethlehem Hospital*. London: Unwin.

50. PARRY-JONES, W. LL. (1971): *The Trade in Lunacy. A Study of Private Madhouses in England in the 18th and 19th Centuries.* London: Routledge & Kegan Paul.

51. PAYNE, J. F. (1904): *English Medicine in the Anglo-Saxon Times.* Oxford: Clarendon Press.

52. PLINY, *Natural History.* XXIV. Trans. by W. H. S. Jones, 1956. London: Heinemann.

53. POLYBIUS, *The Histories.* Book XVI. Trans. by W. R. Paton, 1922-27. London: Heinemann.

54. POOLE, H. E. (Ed.) (1936): *The Wisdom of Andrew Boorde.* Leicester: Backus.

55. RICHARDS, M. (1954): *The Laws of Hywel Dda.* Liverpool: Liverpool University Press.

56. ROBERTSON, J. M. (Ed.) (1905): *Francis Bacon: Philosophical Works.* London: Routledge.

57. ROHDE, E. S. (1973): *The Old English Herbals.* London: Minerva Press.

58. SCARBOROUGH, J. (1969): *Roman Medicine.* London: Thomas & Hudson.

59. SCHERZ, G. (Ed.) (1968): *The Historical Aspects of Brain Research in the 17th Century.* Oxford: Pergamon Press.

60. SCOTT, R. (1584): *The Discoverie of Witchcraft.* Facsimile, 1971. New York: Da Capo Press.

61. SHAH, M. H. (1966): *The General Principles of Avicenna's Canon of Medicine.* Karachi: Naveed Clinic.

62. SIEGEL, R. E. (1968): *Galen's System of Physiology and Medicine.* Basel & New York: Karger.

63. TREVELYAN, G. M. (1944): *English Social History.* London: Longmans, Green.

64. TREVELYAN. G. M. (1959): *A Shortened History of England.* Harmondsworth: Penguin Books.

65. TUKE, D. H. (1882): *History of the Insane in the British Isles.* London: Kegan Paul, Trench.

66. TUKE, D. H. (1892): *A Dictionary of Psychological Medicine.* London: Churchill.

67. TUKE, S. (1813): *Description of the Retreat.* Facsimile, 1964. London: Dawson.

68. VEITH, I. (1965): *Hysteria: The History of a Disease.* Chap. VII: Hysteria in England. Chicago: University of Chicago Press.

69. WALK, A. (1954): Some aspects of the 'moral treatment' of the insane up to 1854. *J. Ment. Sci.*, 100, 807-837.

70. WALK, A. (1964): Mental hospitals. In: Poynter, F. N. L. (Ed.), *The Evolution of Hospitals in Britain.* London: Pitman Medical.

71. WALK, A. (1970): Lincoln and non-restraint. *Brit. J. Psychiat.*, 117, 481-496.

72. WALSH, J. J. (1920): *Medieval Medicine.* London: Black.

73. WARRINGTON, J. (Ed.) (1964): *The Diary of Samuel Pepys.* London: Dent.

74. WEST, C. (1854): *Lectures on the Diseases of Infancy and Childhood.* London: Longman.

75. WHITELOCK, D. (1952): *The Beginning of English Society.* Harmondsworth: Penguin Books.

76. WILSON, D. (1964): *What Happens in Hamlet.* Cambridge: Cambridge University Press.

77. WOLFF, H. H. (1970): *The Place of Dynamic Psychiatry in Medicine.* Society of Clinical Psychiatrists.

78. WRIGHT, C. E. (Ed.) (1955): *Bald's Leechbook.* Copenhagen: Rosenkilde & Bagger.

79. ZIEGLER, P. (1969): *The Black Death.* Glasgow: Collins.

8

SCANDINAVIA AND FINLAND

Nils Retterstol, M.D.

Professor of Psychiatry, University of Oslo, Oslo, Norway

1

INTRODUCTION

Scandinavia entered the history of civilization at a relatively late date. We know little about our history before the Viking age. Our sagas date from this period and constitute a valuable source of the oldest historical times in Scandinavia. Few places in the world can boast of such traditional and well-kept genealogical tales as the Scandinavian countries, thanks to the Icelandic traditions. The people of Iceland originally migrated from Western Norway in the Viking age. They have maintained their oral traditions up to the present day, probably because of the geographical isolation of an island realm situated between Europe and America. The principal older historical events in Scandinavia are recorded in the sagas which also provide our best source of information about the Norse traditions.

For the old Northerners, as for other primitive peoples, the concept of disease at the time of the sagas and, no doubt, also for centuries before, was linked to religious conceptions (10, 14). Mental diseases were supposed to be caused by demons and spirits, and the therapy was aimed at appeasing these forces by offerings allied to more powerful sorcerers. It was also a widespread belief that people with magic power could evoke diseases, including mental disorders, by associating themselves with the spirits and using magic formulas, like spells, witchcraft, and runes. The sorceresses were feared; they were believed to

207

have the power to inflict illnesses on their enemies by means of songs and conjurations. In the old Norse mythology (Åsatroen), the goddess Eir was the best doctor, but the most important—Odin—was the main god of medicine too, and he knew all the secrets of this art. Most of the practitioners of medicine in those days were lay women, who were much respected. Most of our information on Norse medicine in Norway and Iceland is due to the fertility of the Icelandic saga literature. The concept of that time is well illustrated by Egil's saga (Chapter 72). It tells of a young girl who has been ill for a long time and is suffering from complete asthenia. A young man who is in love with her tries to cure her by means of runes, but he carves the wrong runes and she sinks lower still. Egil undoes the wrong runes and carves others that bring about her recovery.

Mention of mental disorders is not infrequent in the sagas. They tell of anxiety and brooding, sometimes leading to suicide. They describe fits of rage in which the party concerned is so violent he has to be tied up. Some of the mental disorders are presented as familial diseases. To tie up the "possessed" appears to have been the standard method of treatment in the saga age. Thus, the mental disorders are termed "surveillance diseases" in the old Iceland laws. Thrashing was also applied as the patient was assumed to be possessed by an evil spirit (in Icelandic, Djöfulódr means devil's spirit), and this spirit had to be thrashed out.

Several warriors in our sagas are described as "running berserk" during combat. In Old Norse, this term means that they were clothed in bearskin, and men who were assailed by paroxysms during combat so that they did not feel pain were called berserks. In 1958, Howard Fabing (7) advanced the theory that such attacks were caused by fly agaric (Amanita muscaria), which contains the substance bufotenin, or N-L-dimethyl-serotonin, a hallucinogenic drug which, taken intravenously, may cause symptoms reminiscent of the berserker rage described in the sagas. The theory that the berserks may have taken plant poison is quite old (22). As early as 1784, the Swedish theologian Ödeman of Uppsala had suggested that they ingested fly agaric, a suggestion also put forward, in 1885, by the Norwegian physician and botanist F. G. Schübeler, who had no foreknowledge of Ödeman's work. However, according to others, there is little to support such theories.

Among all the Norse sagas, none is better known than the Snorre's king sagas, which are the sagas of the Norwegian kings. The work includes few descriptions of psychiatric disorders and even fewer explicit comments concerning the therapeutic measures available in such cases. From the tales about three of the kings mentioned in Snorre's sagas, it is evident that they must have passed through a mental disorder, if the saga is to be trusted (22). This applies to Harald Hårfagre who founded the kingdom of Norway in about 872. According to the saga, Harald Hårfagre went through a deep depression lasting for three years caused by the death of his concubine, the Samic girl Snefrid. The saga says that he mourned because she was dead, and that the people of the land mourned because he was insane. He later

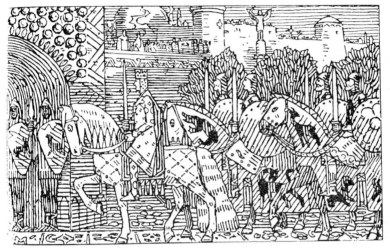

PLATE XXXIII. King Sigurd Jorsalfar and his men, riding into Constantinople (Istanbul).

recovered from this state. The symptoms of this king, as described in the saga, seems to fulfill the present day's criteria for a diagnosis of reactive psychosis.

Håkon Jarl, another Norwegian royal personage, developed a depressive disorder of stuporous character while in exile in Denmark in 962. His depression was not as deep or of as long duration as that described for Harald Hårfagre, as it lasted just through the winter. Also in Håkon Jarl's case, the depression appears to have been precipitated by psychogenic factors, as he was banished from Norway and brooded upon the problem of how to win his country back. He never had a relapse and he is most honorably mentioned in the saga in all other ways.

Sigurd Jorsalfar's mental disorder appears to have been of another type, characterized by anxiety, hallucinations and delusions, symptoms

which at times appeared suddenly and necessitated that his men hold
him back (Plate XXXIII). His men were in constant anxiety about
these sudden attacks, and the saga recounts how they speculate about
the king's instability. The nature of Sigurd Jorsalfar's mental disease
must remain an open question. The described visual hallucinations
with agitation might point to a delirious state, possibly due to alcohol.
There is, however, little to suggest that Sigurd Jorsalfar was inclined
to overindulgence. A more likely explanation might be a manic depressive psychosis with mood swings between depression and elation. However, King Sigurd is remembered as a good king and his brief psychotic
episodes have left no shadows upon his glorious name.

2

LEGISLATION AND PROVISION FOR THE MENTALLY ILL
UP TO THE 19TH CENTURY

Before and during the Middle Ages, there was no systematic mental
care in Scandinavia. The mentally ill were cared for by their families,
whereas what legal remedies might be called for were for the court
sessions—the *thing* (*tinget*)—to decide. The first legal measures for
improving the care of the mentally ill in Norway were laid down in
the Gulating Law, the Frostating Law, and the Common Country
Law of Magnus Lagaböter of 1274. The latter includes rules on the
compulsory boarding-out system, which applied to the poor, but more
particularly to the mentally ill. The decree was unpopular and was
frequently disobeyed. However, it is incontestable that, according to
Old Norse Law, the jurisdiction of the mentally ill was vested in
courts, although during the Middle Ages this function gradually passed
to the king's officials (20, 23).

The old Swedish county laws include rules for the protection of
society against the insane, who was called *afvita*, "*galin man*" or
vetvilling (8, 9). Thus the older Westgötha Law and the more recent
codex of the same law contain provisions that the galin man (madman)
should be imprisoned, and the same provisions are included in the
Upland Law. According to the Sudermanna Law, the relatives should
keep the *afvita* (insane) in *haptum* (safe custody), and they were
liable to fines if the insane escaped or did injury to himself. There
is an interesting report, dated 1698, from the governor of West
Norrland concerning a parson's daughter who had become "enraged."
A decree was issued to the effect that whenever she had a meal it should

consist of bread, boiled in good water or a weak brew, and devotions should be performed with reading of the Lord's Prayer and David's *Psalms*.

Danish legislation contained clear rules on the family's duties to the sick and to society (11). In Erik's Zealand Law, which was in force from the middle of the 13th century, it is set down (Chapter 36) that:

> Should it so happen that anybody has a brother or a close relative who loses his mind and is the owner of soil or property that he does not want him to dispose of, then he should take with him to the courts the best men of the district who know his relative, and they should give notification that he is not of sound mind and not responsible for his actions. When this has been done, he cannot sell his property, nor make good any contract of purchase whether this has been confirmed by handshake or by conveyance. And if he beats, cuts, or kills anybody then the person who got himself registered as his guardian shall pay for it just as if he himself had been guilty of the deed. Should he become so mad that he cannot cope with him without tying him up, he should give notification to the court and, with the court's men consent, restrain him. If he becomes so mad that he cannot bring him to the session without tying him up, then he shall tie him up in the legal manner and set out for the court and let this body appoint men to see his condition for themselves. If they likewise say that necessity forced him to tie him up, then he shall pay for it neither to the one he tied up nor to the King.

Thus, in the Middle Ages, the mentally ill were largely the responsibility of the family and the courts. Most of the mentally ill in Scandinavia, as in the rest of Europe, roamed the streets of the towns or wandered the country and were regarded as "originals" or "cranks." Later, the most afflicted were taken care of to the extent that they were lodged in outhouses, attic rooms, county jails, or in the town hall vaults. When "madness," "lunacy," and "insanity" first came to be accepted as diseases, it also had to be accepted that those suffering from such disorders should be treated as sick people. Since the hospitals were responsible for the care of the sick, it was natural that they should take over the treatment of the mentally ill.

Early Mental Hospitals

The oldest hospital in Norway is mentioned by the bishop Öystein in 1170 (15). It was attached to Trondheim Cathedral and became the Hospitale Infirmorum built in 1380 in the same place. In 1538 mention is made of Oslo Hospital, attached to a Franciscan convent. The first provisions for a more organized placement for the mentally ill were set down in the Royal Ordinance of July 14, 1736, which stated that the charitable institutions, or at any rate the main hospitals, "should furnish one or two rooms, where one could place and keep 'poor deteriorated persons' in such a manner that they could not escape easily" (4, 6).

The events leading to this ordinance were related to the killing of a child by a woman, and the finding of the theological faculty in Copenhagen, who came to the conclusion that she was suffering from "insanity." No appropriate place could be found for her in Christiania (Oslo) at that time, hence the ordinance, which caused cells for the insane to be established again in many of the country's hospitals. It was natural for the hospitals to regard the care of the mentally ill as a part of their activity, but it soon came to be accepted that the insane should be sheltered in separate buildings. These buildings with cells for the mental patients were slowly established, and were called *dollhus, dårekister,* or *dårehus* (madhouse, nut-house, loony-bin). From the beginning, conditions in this accommodation were very poor. On the whole, the mentally ill lived in wretched circumstances in the 17th and 18th centuries, and in several countries—among which was Norway—the Ministries of the Interior appointed committees to investigate the matter.

From the Middle Ages until well into the 18th century, the psychiatric hospitals in Sweden were badly underdeveloped (9, 12) (Plate XXXIV). Shelters for the sick and the poor existed during the 11th, 12th, and 13th centuries under the protection of the convents. During the Age of the Reformation, the convents were confiscated and some of them were converted into "Holy Ghost houses" for the poor and the sick. The Franciscan monasteries in Malmo and Ystad were opened in 1528 and 1531 respectively; the Holy Ghost house established by Gustav Vasa was opened in 1551 at Danviken, Stockholm, after confiscation of the Franciscan monastery in Stockholm (Plate XXXV). From Gustav Vasa's letters it appears that he gave particular thought to the care of the mentally ill. Danvik madhouse, which was an annex of Danviken hospital, was founded in the beginning of the 18th century. For many years, Danvik madhouse was the sole institution in Sweden which could accommodate a large number of mental patients. The number of hospitalized mental patients in Sweden can be gathered from the figures for Danvik hospital, where there were 19 lunatics in 1706, 24 in 1741, 50 in 1756 and 80 in 1779. The so-called Crown hospitals (*kronohospitaler*), originating from the convents, started as doss-houses but, by the Royal Ordinance of October 19, 1775, their sole mission was to admit lunatics and seriously ill people. During the

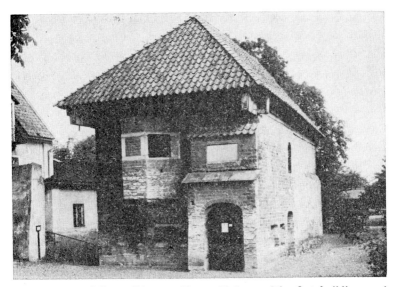

PLATE XXXIV. Mårten Skinnares House, Vadstena. The first building used as a hospital.

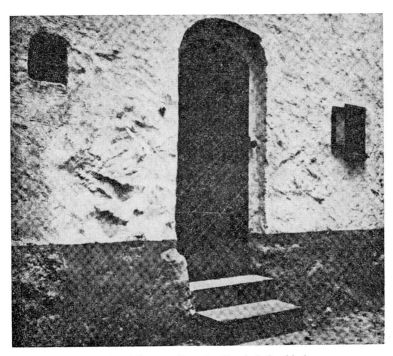

PLATE XXXV. The gate, Danviks Hospital, Stockholm.

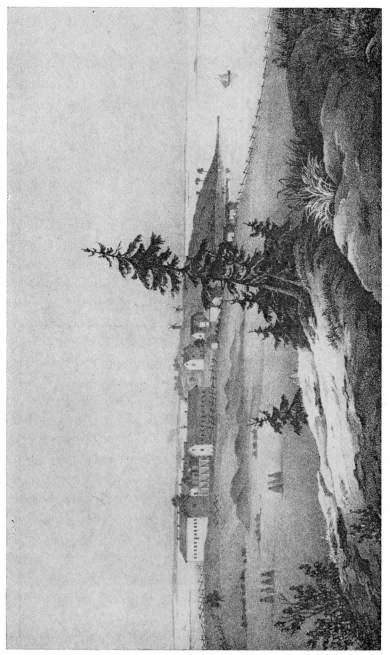

PLATE XXXVI. Seili Hospital.

period 1773 to 1876, the Order of the Seraphim had charge of all hospitals in Sweden. The number of mental patients increased during the 18th century. However, provision for the mentally ill were poor and reports of the time show that it was a kind of public entertainment to visit asylums, to watch compulsive measures being applied and unruly patients being locked up in houses, or even put in irons. According to the Order of the Seraphim, in 1822: "The hospitals do not fulfill their purpose which is to help the deranged to regain their reason by kind and appropriate treatment; on the contrary, the institutions are nothing but storerooms for these unfortunates." As late as the 1860's, Gadelius referred to the conditions for the mentally ill in Sweden as "scandalous."

Conditions in Denmark had much in common with those in Sweden and in Norway (11). As early as 1527 and 1528, there is mention of the establishment of a state asylum, which became the precursor of the present St. Hans Hospital, Roskilde. There are tales of utterly primitive conditions and a more or less animal existence for the "stark mad" in Denmark.

In Finland, too, there were, in the Middle Ages, houses of the Holy Ghost, which probably provided accommodation for the mentally ill (1, 2, 3). From the one in Åbo (Turku), mentioned in 1396, the patients were transferred to Seili hospital (Plate XXXVI), when this was founded in 1623, by the order of King Gustav Adolf II. It was a combined hospital for lepers and the mentally ill.

The worst repercussions of this limited ability to recognize mental disorders are the witch trials, which had their peak during 1480 and lasted into the 18th century. There can be no doubt that in this period many mentally ill in Scandinavia met their death on the torture bench or at the stake. However, the witch trials did not flourish to the same extent as they did in Middle Europe. Thus the first Norwegian witch trial, against Ragnhild Tregagas, conducted in 1325 by the bishop Andfinn, ended in acquittal, the accused being declared insane (*non mentis suis compotem*).

3

DEVELOPMENTS DURING THE 19TH CENTURY

Not until the 19th century did the circumstances of the mentally ill take a noticeable turn for the better. The humanitarian ideas of the Age of Enlightenment, the French Revolution, and the first Declaration of the Rights of Man played an important part in bettering the social position of the mentally ill. There is no doubt that the first impulse came from France, where the pioneers of the reform movement were Philippe Pinel, Jean Etienne Esquirol, and the principal of the Bicêtre, J. B. Pussin. These men introduced new methods in psychiatry and laid the foundation for a more appropriate and humane treatment of the mentally ill. The Declaration of the Rights of Man stipulates that it is the duty of the State to take care of the ill and the poor. The foundation was laid for the great reforms to come.

Norway

The first Norwegian to plunge into reform work was the physician Fredrik Holst (1791-1871), who later became professor of medicine at the University of Oslo (4, 6, 20, 23). He was the prime mover of a commission set up by the Norwegian Parliament in 1824 to investigate the circumstances of the mentally ill. This commission presented its recommendations in 1827: ". . . on the circumstances of the mentally ill in Norway, as they are today and as they might come to be." Their recommendations were to be of great importance for future developments. One of the main points was a proposal to establish four mental health institutions in Norway: one in Christiania (Oslo) with 100 beds, and one in each of the towns of Bergen, Trondheim, and Kristiansand, each with a capacity of 50 patients. However, decades were to pass before the Norwegian authorities granted the funds for building such institutions. Those who could afford to do so sent their afflicted relatives out of the country. There was a steadily growing aversion to the madhouses.

This was the situation when Herman Wedel Major (1814-1854) (Plate XXXVII) took over the work started by Holst. In the first place, Major regarded it as essential that there should be legislation about insanity in keeping with the times. On the request of the Parliament and without collaborators, he worked out a draft for Norway's first law on mental health, The Act for the Treatment and Care of the Mentally Ill, which was passed on August 17, 1848, based on Major's bill. With it, Norway had one of Europe's most adequate laws of mental health. When planning the building of hospitals, Major followed the ideas of two German psychiatrists, Damerow and Roller. According to them, the separation into curative institutions and nursing homes was "impossible from a scientific viewpoint and inadmissible from a practical and financial viewpoint." This style of building has been termed "the principle of the relatively associated nursing and curative institutions." The "curable" and the "non-curable" should be joined in one institu-

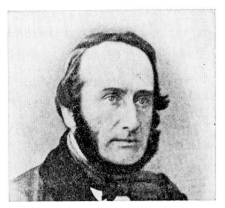

PLATE XXXVII. Herman Wedel Major.

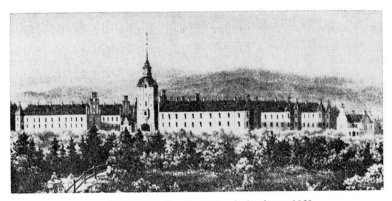

PLATE XXXVIII. Gaustad Hospital, about 1860.

tion, under the same roof, and with the same administrative and medical staff. Even so, the Pinel-Esquirol principle—advocating separation of the two categories—was followed soon after Norway's first psychiatric hospital, Gaustad Asylum (Plate XXXVIII) had been opened in 1855. After some years, the Damerow-Roller principle was applied in the Scandinavian countries, as in other Western European countries, up to World War II. Then Norway became one of the first countries to switch back to the Pinel-Esquirol system, with psychiatric nursing homes for long-term patients who had been submitted to modern therapeutic measures but were still unable to manage outside an institution.

The Act of 1848 made the development of the mental health system a national task. During the years 1855 to 1881, three psychiatric hospitals were built by the State: Gaustad, Rotvold, and Eeg. Neevengården Hospital, in Bergen, which was completed in 1891, was the first to be financed by the county. Gradually it became apparent that the State was not equal to providing the necessary psychiatric hospitals and private institutions were built, as, for instance, Möllendal asylum and later Dr. Martens' hospital in Bergen.

Although psychiatric hospitals were slowly established in most parts of the country, conditions within the mental health sector were far from satisfactory until after World War II. There was a good deal of unrest in psychiatric hospitals, which were closed institutions and which the public associated with something sinister, prisonlike, and shameful to have dealings with.

Denmark

The modern Danish mental health system originates from 1816, when a hospital intended for the treatment of the insane from the capital was established in the main building of Bistrup estate, Roskilde (St. Hans hospital (Plate XXXIX), whose first chief physician was J. H. Seidelin) (21). At this time, there were madhouses of low standard in the bigger provincial towns. The first State hospital in Denmark was opened in Slesvig in 1820 with P. W. Jessen as its head (11, 21). Jens Rasmussen Hübertz (1794-1855) and Harald Selmer (Plate XL) are looked upon as the pioneers of Danish psychiatry. Both had studied the mental health services organized in Germany and, on comparison, found that there was much room for improvement within Danish psychiatry. Selmer is known as the father of Danish psychiatry. He translated Prichard's book on psychiatry and was influenced by Pinel, Esquirol, and the Germans Jacobi and Roller. Selmer succeeded in effecting the important reform that the chief physician of the hospital should also be the administrative leader in all matters concerning the treatment of patients. In 1841, Selmer published *On the State of Psychiatry in Denmark*, and Hübertz's *On the Organization of Lunacy Measures in Denmark* followed in 1843. Both criticized the existing conditions in Denmark and included a reform scheme for the country's mental health systems. This led to the establishment of a number of new mental hospitals: Århus (1852), Oringe (1857), Kurhuset at St. Hans (1860), Viborg (1877), and Middelfart (1888). Selmer was the first head of the mental hospital in Århus, previously called Jydske asyl (Jutland Asylum) (10). The small cell department opened in 1863 in the Copenhagen Municipal Hospital was transformed into a department for nervous diseases, in 1875.

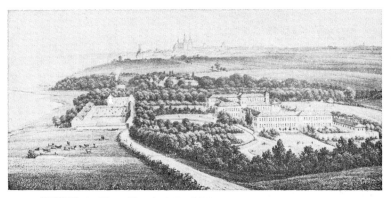

PLATE XXXIX. St. Hans Hospital, Roskilde, near Copenhagen, about 1860. In the background is the Cathedral of Roskilde, Denmark's most famous cathedral, where the Danish and Danish-Norwegian kings are buried.

In 1855 Hübertz founded a service for the care of the mentally deficient in Denmark, whereby the treatment of the mentally defective was separated from the mental hospitals (21).

Sweden

As already mentioned the Order of the Seraphim (with a board of six Knights of the Order) had charge of the hospital system in Sweden up to 1876. Not until 1877 did the hospitals come under the administration of the medical services. During the early part of the 19th century, the authorities occasionally lent support to the development of the hospitals, but it was not until 1851 that a recommendation was presented, largely based on reports by the head of Danviken hospital, Stockholm, C. U. Sondén (Plate XLI). It was pointed out that the treatment of the mentally ill was a medical problem and hence should be part of the medical services. It was suggested that patients with acute mental disorders and good chances of recovery, protractedly ill patients representing a danger to themselves and others, and persons requiring forensic psychiatric examination should be admitted to hospitals. According to the estimate, about 1,200 beds were needed (although the number of mentally ill in the country had been found to be 4,150 in 1841); the remainder could be treated at home or in institutions for the poor. Admission areas, each with its central hospital, were proposed; they were Uppsala, Vadstena, Växsjö, Gothenburg, and Härnösand. For comparison, it may be mentioned that in the middle of the 19th century it was estimated that accommodation

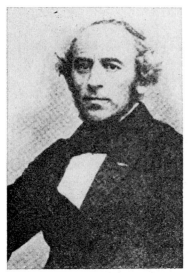

PLATE XL. Harald Selmer, the "father" of Danish psychiatry.

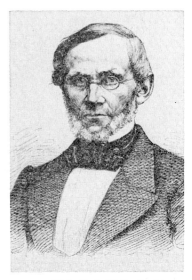

PLATE XLI. Carl Ulrik Sondén.

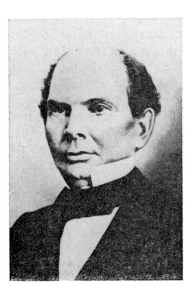

PLATE XLII. L. A. Fahlander.

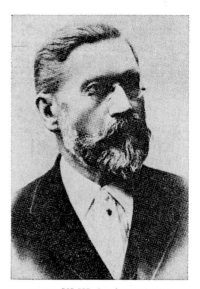

PLATE XLIII. Professor Saelan.

for 0.4 per 1,000 of the population would meet the requirement, whereas the corresponding estimate for 1965 was nearly ten times higher (13).

Finland

After having been part of the Kingdom of Sweden since the 13th century, Finland was connected with the Russian Empire as an autonomous Grand Duchy from 1809 to 1917. In 1835 the Senate appointed a committee to investigate the arrangement and organization of the care of the mentally ill in Finland. As a result of the work of this committee, the Lapinlahti hospital, the present psychiatric clinic of the University of Helsinki, was established; the first patients were admitted to it in 1841. The first medical director of the clinic was L. A. Fahlander, who held this post from 1841 to 1867 (1, 2, 3).

The Imperial Decree of 1840 was an important milestone in the history of the care of the mentally ill in Finland; the measures taken under it determined the course assumed by psychiatric care in the country for a long time. It included detailed stipulations concerning the care of "lunatics." For instance, the relatives, or the employer, of a mentally ill person were duty bound to notify the case to parish authority within eight days after the outbreak of the illness. The officer concerned would then visit the patient, in order to assess the situation, and notify the case in writing to the police or administrative authorities. The police or the servant of the Crown would take the patient to the provincial hospital. Prior to this, however, the governor of the province was to be notified and it was up to the governor to inform the persons concerned when a hospital bed became available. Hospital charges were fixed in detail. According to the 1840 decree, the State was exclusively responsible for the institutional care of the mentally ill, whereas under the 1889 decree the communes were also obliged to care for chronic mental patients of small means.

In 1853, the Emperor (Finland was at that time under the Russian Empire) requested the Directorate of the Care of Lunatics to assess the need for additional mental hospital beds and to find out how the hospital near Helsinki could be adapted to serve its purpose in the best way possible. The Directorate recommended that Dr. Leonard Fahlander (Plate XLII) be sent for a visit abroad to get acquainted with the result achieved in the field of the care of the mentally ill in Europe (2). On the basis of the knowledge thus gained, a long-range plan for the care of the mentally ill in Finland could then be drawn up. Fahlander visited Denmark, Germany, France, Britain, Austria, the

Netherlands, and Sweden. On returning home, he tried to introduce the no-restraint system in Finland. He also stressed how inappropriate it was to classify patients into curable and incurable and place them in two hospitals situated far away from each other, as was the case in Finland, where the Seili institution had been used for the incurables. In the annual report, submitted in 1858, he stated that the no-restraint system had been almost realized in the Lapinlahti Hospital (Plate XLIV) (1). However, later he had to reintroduce the use of physical restraint, apparently because of the opposition its abolition had met

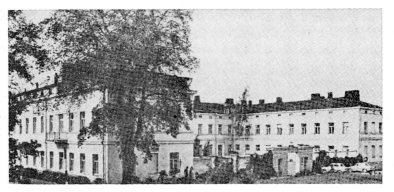

PLATE XLIV. Lapinlahti Hospital, Psychiatric Clinic.

from the hospital personnel, and these methods were not finally abandoned until 1904, when Professor Sibelius became medical director of the hospital.

Saelan (1867-1904) (Plate XLIII) was the second mental director of the Lapinlahti Hospital; he was followed by Christian Sibelius, the brother of the composer Jean.

In 1877, it was decided that a new mental hospital should be built near Kuopio, and in 1889 an asylum was founded in Käkisalmi, when the prison located there was converted into a mental hospital. The Pitkäniemi Hospital was opened in 1900, providing accommodation for 335 patients.

4

DEVELOPMENTS DURING THE 20TH CENTURY

During the years following World War I, the development of the psychiatric institutions within the Scandinavian countries expanded rapidly. A few psychiatric hospitals have been built. In Denmark, the large new mental hospital, Glostrup, has been constructed as a part of an important general hospital with many specialized departments. In the three countries a number of psychiatric departments attached to the central hospitals of the separate districts have been established. In these central hospitals, the psychiatric department is one of many specialized departments, usually with a staff of one doctor per ten patients. The first psychiatric department in Norway was established in 1917 as a part of the large somatic hospital Ullevål in Oslo. The second, the Psychiatric Department of the University of Oslo, was constructed as a detached institution in 1926. The clinical departments are intended particularly for short-term patients with psychoses, neuroses, etc., whose treatment should be completed in the course of three to four months. In Norway and in Denmark there are a few mental sanatoriums under private management which take in psychiatric patients needing more protracted treatment. In the Scandinavian countries, the psychiatric hospitals have undergone radical structural changes during the past decades. These have consisted in the adoption of the open-door system, the demolition of fences surrounding the hospitals, and the abolition of the hierarchic system, together with growing democratization and delegation of work. Milieu therapy has come to the fore. The therapeutic team is of interdisciplinary composition led by psychiatrists. The structure and the atmosphere of the mental hospitals have changed, though the developmental process has reached different stages, depending up on leadership and staff.

At first, the establishment of separate departments in general hospitals caused the asylums, which were designated as mental hospitals, to receive the more seriously ill mental patients, while the less severe cases were admitted to psychiatric clinics or departments. For a while it was "more distinguished" to be a patient or an employee in a department in a general hospital than in a mental hospital, a differentiation which is gradually disappearing.

It is also important to bridge the gap between the psychiatric hospital and society. In Scandinavia, the principal moves in this direction have been the establishment of after-care departments, with day-and-night hospitals whereby the patients spend only a part of the time in the institution, and the establishment of out-patient clinics with ambulatory personnel. The aim is a continuity of care, whereby the same institution provides a total and integrated psychiatric service from the onset of the disorder until recovery or transition into a more chronic or nursing home state. Also progressing is the division of the departments within the psychiatric hospitals according to geographical admission areas and not, as hitherto, according to sex.

Relatively few psychiatrists in the Scandinavian countries are private practitioners. The need for psychiatric services in the community is not fully met, but expansion of out-patient clinics, after-care departments and regional branches of such departments are in hand. The need for psychiatric hospital accommodation is decreasing, while there is an increasing need for out-patient facilities. The tendency is towards a shorter stay in the hospital and briefer treatment, but more frequent readmissions.

The rate of hospitalization of psychotic patients is well recorded in the Scandinavian countries (18). In Norway, we have had a central register for all hospitalized cases of psychosis for a number of years. The tendency during the last 40-year period, as reported by Odegard (19), is cited below:

> During the 30-year period between 1926 and 1955 the incidence of hospitalized psychoses in Norway remained at very much the same level, corresponding to a life-time risk of five per hundred. A relative stability of social conditions and a fairly adequate mental health care which developed gradually and undramatically explains this remarkably static pattern. The figure of five percent does turn up so consistently, however, in epidemiological studies from various countries and conducted by various methods, that it is tempting to regard it as an approximation towards true morbidity.
>
> Since 1955, an increase has taken place in the admission rates, which has brought the lifetime risk up to 8.2 per 1,000 for men and 7.7 for women. The greater part of this increase concerns senile and other organic psychoses; the admission rates from these conditions have been doubled in ten years' time, which is probably a result of increased hospitalization. The introduction around 1954 of modern drug therapy led to a shortening of hospital stay, whereby beds became available for an increasing number of 'non-therapeutic' organic cases.
>
> The non-organic or functional psychoses have had an increase of merely 33 percent, which is probably a result of an interaction of two opposite trends. The greatly improved environment in the mental hospitals, as well as the establishment of psychiatric departments in a number of medical centres, has encouraged the hospitalization of less serious psychotic conditions such as reactive depressions. At the same time ambulatory drug treatment has made it possible to avoid hospitalization of certain types of psychotic patients, notably excitement and paranoid states.
>
> Within the group of functional psychoses the diagnostic distribution has changed radically. From 1926 to 1930, the two classical disease entities of schizophrenia and manic-depressive psy-

chosis accounted for 89 percent of the non-organic cases, while from 1956 to 1960 their share had dropped to 44 percent. This trend is international, but it has been more drastic in Norway than in most countries. The figures from 1961 to 1965 indicate, however, that the tide may have turned.

The capacity of Norwegian psychiatric hospitals is approximately 8,000 beds; of the Danish about 10,000; and of the Swedish about 23,000. Of the latter, 2,190 places are reserved for the mentally deficient (13). In all three countries there are psychiatric departments distributed throughout the country and the number of beds is about 1,200, 1,700, and 5,400 for Norway, Denmark, and Sweden, respectively.

Care of the Mentally Deficient

In the Scandinavian countries Denmark has pioneered in the care of the mentally deficient. In 1934, the Act of Provision for Mental Defectives was passed in Denmark. Now, the care of the mentally deficient is organized according to the Act of June 5, 1959 on the Provision for Mental Defectives and Other Particularly Feebleminded Individuals (25). This type of work was formerly in the hands of various State authorized private institutions; now all the institutions are under a private foundation, The State Provision for Mental Defectives (*Statens Åndssvakeforsorg*), under the management of the Minister of Social Affairs. For children, compulsory education and training start when the child would normally have started primary school according to the valid provisions on compulsory education of the Primary School Act, and usually continue until the age of 21.

In Sweden, rules and regulations for the care of mental deficients were included in the Lunacy Act of 1929. By 1857, Sonden, who was then chief medical officer, had proposed the establishment of special institutions for the mentally defective and, around 1900, the first institutions were opened (Carlslund outside Stockholm and Vilhelmshöjd outside Värnmo). From the 1930's, the building of institutions for the mentally deficient progressed more rapidly. Since 1955, the government is responsible for providing treatment for mental defectives requiring institutional therapy. In Sweden, there are now a number of remedial homes (91 in 1968), 21 boarding schools for handicapped children, and 80 day schools (13).

In Norway, the Care of the Mental Defectives Act was passed in 1949 (5), but a general plan for the care of the mentally deficient was not achieved until 1952. In this country, provision for the mental defectives is not under one central administration; the Ministry of

Social Affairs has the care of the more serious cases, whereas the less severely handicapped are the responsibility of the Ministry of Church and Education. The law on special schools stipulates that backward children from the ages of 7 to 16 have the right and duty to attend a special school for seven years, and that backward youths from 16 to 21 years of age have the right and duty to attend continuation and vocational schools for the feeble-minded for three years. Norway is now divided into eight mental deficiency areas, each with its chief physician. In Norway, about 6,500 persons (1968) are taken care of by special services, against about 20,000 in Denmark (same year).

Care of Alcoholics and Drug Addicts

The care of alcoholics and drug abusers is fairly advanced in the Scandinavin countries. There are special therapeutic institutions for alcoholics, both public (sanatoriums) and private (Blue Cross, the Home Mission, AA, etc.). Most alcoholics receive their first treatment in psychiatric departments or in hospitals. According to the Norwegian Temperance Act of February 26, 1932, originally covering alcoholics only, but from 1956 also including drug addicts, abusers who are a heavy burden to their home environment and in need of treatment can be committed to an institution (5, 17). In all municipalities and parishes of Norway, there are temperance boards, elected by the people, whose responsibility it is to further sobriety and take care of the alcoholics within the region. In decisions on commitment, the boards must be supplemented by a lawyer.

An independent institution for drug addicts was established in Norway in 1961 (Statens klinikk for narkomane, Hov i Land). However, in Norway as in the other Northern countries, most of the drug abusers in need of institutional treatment are admitted to ordinary psychiatric departments or hospitals.

The problem of adolescent drug dependence has been felt in Scandinavia from the latter part of the 1960's. As yet, this has been much more of a problem in Sweden and Denmark than in Norway and Finland, occurring earlier and attracting a greater number of adolescents.

Child Psychiatry

For a long time, child psychiatry has been a neglected field in the Scandinavian countries. In Sweden, regulations for child and adolescent mental health services were stipulated by the King in 1945 and, on the whole, these are still in force (13). There are some child and adolescent psychiatric departments in each of the four countries, but we have still far to go before every central hospital will have its own child psychiatric department with a number of beds and adequate outpatient services. The number of remedial homes for children and adolescents is likewise limited.

Forensic Psychiatry

Forensic psychiatry has developed along much the same lines in all the Scandinavian countries. According to old Norse law, as previously mentioned, the jurisdiction of the mentally ill was vested in the *thing* (court sessions), but by and by an important part of these functions was transferred to the king's officials. However, some cases, especially those involving punishable offences, were still brought before the courts. The linked functions of administrative practice and judicial observation have continued up to the present. The old Norse legal proceedings did not include "experts" in the sense of the present criminal procedure. The tasks now imcumbent on the expert were disposed of by estimation and appraisal and by presentation of documentary evidence. During the 18th and 19th centuries, the duty of evaluation and appraisal rested with military officials and professors of medicine. Gradually this was extended to include State-employed doctors.

The first case involving forensic psychiatry in the Scandinavian countries occurred in 1735 in Sweden. Originally, the control of judicial cases requiring psychiatric assessment was in the hands of the medical board, but was later transferred to specially appointed commissions. In Norway, there has been a forensic commission from the year 1900, in Sweden, from 1913. If there is doubt as to the defendant's mental state, the prosecution or the court can demand a forensic psychiatric assessment. As a rule, two experts will then be appointed by the court. In Sweden, the subject of forensic psychiatry was singled out as a separate specialty in 1946 and at the same time the position of teacher in this subject (established in 1920) at Karolinska Institutet, Stockholm, was changed into a professorship (13, 24).

Whereas Norwegian and Swedish forensic psychiatry is founded on medicobiological concepts, a medicophilosophical orientation is adhered to in Denmark. Thus, in both Sweden and Norway proof of the presence of insanity or of other abnormal states is considered sufficient evidence of diminished responsibility. Danish criminal law, on the other hand, requires in addition an estimate of the degree of responsibility as a factor for consideration when presenting the verdict (16).

Care of Criminal Offenders

The care of criminal offenders has, traditionally, had little relation to psychiatry in the Scandinavian countries—Denmark has also been a pioneer in the field (16). In 1935, a psychopathic institution called Herstedvester was opened in Copenhagen. This institution is a detention and treatment establishment for criminal offenders unsuitable for imprisonment due to personality deviations, but who must be detained to protect the public. This type of detention is for an unspecified period. The court decides when the person concerned is to be discharged and submitted to less severe restrictions. The detention is designed to provide treatment consistent with the offender's personality; the therapy is of a markedly psychological and re-educative type aimed at motivating the detained to make the most of his possibilities for leading a socially acceptable life. After-care is well organized. The Scandinavian institutions most closely resembling Herstedvester, but not as well developed, are Ila detention home in Norway and Hall detention home in Sweden.

5

INSANITY LEGISLATION

The lunacy laws have developed along different lines in the Scandinavian countries. As mentioned, the Norewegian Lunacy Act drafted by Herman Wedel Major is the oldest, dating from 1848. This was in force until 1961, when it was replaced by the Mental Health Act. The Swedish Lunacy Act of 1929, first enacted in 1931, with amendments in 1949 and 1959, comprises the current rules for admission to and discharge from psychiatric institutions. The Danish law on hospitalization for insane persons dates from 1938 and was amended in 1954 (Christian V's Danish law from the 17th century was in force until 1938).

In principle, the admission procedure is similar in the three countries. It is a prerequisite that the patient, besides suffering from a serious mental disorder, should also be in need of treatment. Primarily, close relatives should act on the patient's behalf when he or she is incapacitated, and request admission. If the patient has no close family, the health authorities or the social agencies demand the admission; only exceptionally do the police authorities enter the picture.

6

IDEOLOGICAL TRENDS

Until World War II Scandinavian psychiatry was strongly influenced by German psychiatry. Griesinger, Kraepelin, Kretschmer, Rüdin, Kurt Schneider, Jaspers, and many others have left their mark on its development. During the last century and the beginning of the present, Scandinavians going abroad to study usually went to Munich, Berlin, Heidelberg, Göttingen, and Hamburg. The leading Scandinavian psychiatrists of the first part of this century, such as Wimmer and Helweg in Denmark, Kinberg, Sjöbring, and Wigert in Sweden, and Evensen and Vogt in Norway, cannot be said to have altogether adopted the views of the German classics. Helwig and Vogt in particular were greatly interested in dynamic approaches and warned against the exaggerated dependence on genetic or constitutional biology that pervaded German psychiatry. However, there seems to be no doubt that Scandinavian psychiatry up to the years after World War II was, and to some extent still is, greatly marked by Kraepelin's views. Freud's influence was late to arrive and did not really begin until after World War II, even though some leading psychiatrists, such as Vogt in Norway, had taken a positive attitude to his doctrines. Today, there is great interest in psychoanalysis, especially among younger psychiatrists, even if psychoanalysis as a method of treatment has never come to the front in the Scandinavian countries.

Few Scandinavian psychiatrists would call themselves Jungians or Adlerians, but both Jung and Adler have given important impulses to Scandinavian psychiatry and many Scandinavian psychiatrists have visited the Jungian and Adlerian centers in Middle Europe. Also the American neoanalysts, as Horney, Fromm, and Sullivan, have had considerable influence on Scandinavian psychiatry. The same applies to Wilhelm Reich, who lived in Norway in the 1930's before going to the United States. Adolf Meyer too has been of marked account for Scandinavian psychiatry. Generally speaking, Scandinavian psychiatry may be said to have been largely somatically and constitutionally oriented up to World War II, but has now become increasingly psychodynamically oriented. Most Scandinavian psychiatrists will probably profess themselves eclectics.

After World War II, Scandinavian psychiatry has become increasingly oriented towards English and, even more, American psychiatry. Thanks to the Rockefeller Foundation and to Fulbright scholarships, many young Scandinavian psychiatrists have spent considerable time in the United States and have returned home with new ideas of importance for the development of modern Scandinavian psychiatry. The contact between Scandinavian and German psychiatry is still close, and the same applies with regard to other Middle European countries (Switzerland, Austria, the Netherlands). The contact with Southern and Eastern European psychiatry has been less close.

During the past 10 or 20 years, social psychiatry has entered the picture. Psychiatrists have become increasingly interested in society outside the institutions. Preventive measures have come to play a more central role. There is no doubt that during the last 20 years Scandinavian psychiatry has become considerably more psychotherapeutically and psychodynamically orientated, on the one hand, and more socially orientated on the other.

The terminology in use in Scandinavia has much in common with that employed in Middle Europe. The concept of schizophrenia is less comprehensive than that currently used in the Anglo-American literature and is closer to the Kraepelinian concept of *dementia praecox*. The term manic-depressive psychosis is applied in the same sense as in the English literature. In Scandinavia, the concept of reactive psychoses is widely used, and goes back to Jaspers' psychogenic psychoses (1913). The Danish psychiatrist Wimmer's fundamental study on *Psychogenic Forms of Insanity* (1916) and Faergeman's *Psychogenic Psychoses* (1945, translated into English in 1963) have been important to Scandinavian psychiatry. A number of Scandinavian investigators have contributed to a better understanding of the reactive psychoses.

Schizophreniform psychoses likewise constitute a concept frequently employed in the Scandinavian countries (after Langfeldt, 1939). The Scandinavian concept of neurosis corresponds approximately to that employed in English literature. The concept of psychopathy was formerly used according to Kurt Schneider's criteria, but in most places this diagnosis is now applied in a much stricter sense, or even entirely replaced by the American concept of sociopathy. Dynamic views furnish the basis also when evaluating this concept.

The view of the psychiatric disorders as a multi-factorial phenomenon has penetrated to the Scandinavian countries.

7

THERAPEUTIC METHODS

On the whole, the historical development of methods of treatment in Scandinavia corresponds to that seen in the rest of Western Europe.

During the last century, treatment was very primitive (Plates XLV and XLVI) (1, 3, 4). Few hospitals existed. Coercive measures and isolation characterized the treatment. Many therapeutic procedures involved "expulsion" of the disease, as for instance treatment with mercurial ointments which were often applied several times a day for three to five consecutive days. The skin was irritated and ulceration was frequent.

From the middle of the last century opium preparations became a current therapeutic measure in melancholia. In mania, protracted baths represented the method of choice. The patient was placed in a tub with a lid, permitting only the head to emerge from the water; the water temperature was 33-35°C and the head was cooled by cold water; the bath lasted for up to eight hours. This method was in use until the 1930's. Various herbs, extracts, and oils were tried, like valerian, camphor, and ipecacuanha. Camphor was supposed to be beneficial for sexual excitation in man. Other drugs used in psychoses included tartar emetic and copper sulphate. Sodium phosphate was prescribed as an effective cathartic, and quinine was said to have a a soothing effect in hysteria. Iron and decoction of peruvian bark were mentioned as tonics, but the best tonics remained good food and Bavarian beer. Since about 1870, chloral was used as a sedative; the bromides came on the market about the same time. Blood-letting was employed in the middle of the last century, but gradually fell into disuse.

More active somatic methods were not introduced in psychiatric therapy until the present century; the first of these methods was Wagner von Jauregg's malaria therapy for paralytics, first used in 1922. Malaria therapy has been employed in Scandanavia since 1923. General paresis is now a rarity in these countries. From the 1930's, insulin shock therapy was used in schizophrenic disorders, but after the introduction of tranquilizing drugs, this therapy has been abandoned almost totally. The same applies to cardiazol shock therapy which was introduced at approximately the same time. Electroshock therapy was first used in the latter part of the 1930's and is still in use, although to considerably less an extent that it was ten years ago, when the anti-depressant drugs came on the market. Psychosurgery, especially lobotomy, was popular during the 1940's and 1950's. The first leucotomy in Scandinavia was probably performed by A. Torkildsen of Oslo, in 1942, and is said to be the first leucotomy undertaken in Europe after Moniz' preliminary trials in 1936. During the last part of the 1950's and 1960's,

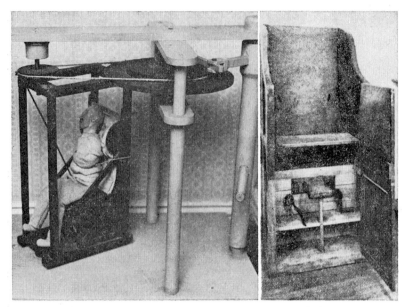

PLATE XLV. Model of an old swing-chair in Birgittas Hospital, Vadstena (Dr. Cox' svangstol). PLATE XLVI. Restraint chair in a cell from Birgittas Hospital.

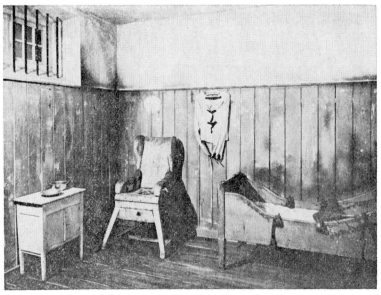

PLATE XLVII. A patient's cell, about 1830 in Denmark. Reconstruction from the exhibition "Københavns kommunes Sindssygevaesen."

lobotomy gradually fell into disuse together with modified procedures related to it. From the 1950's, the tranquilizers have represented the treatment of choice in the psychoses, and from the 1960's, the anti-depressants have also been widely employed. In the Scandinavian countries, there has been a cautious approach to use of the mild tranquilizers (benzodiazepines etc.), but they are nevertheless extensively used.

In Scandinavia, an attitude of reserve has always been maintained with reference to measures of restraint (Plate XLVII). In the middle of the last century, a conscious effort was made to combat coercive measures. The Norwegian Lunacy Act of 1848 includes, for instance, provisions on strict medical and administrative control of application of mechanical coercive measures. As an example, in the planning of Gaustad hospital, which was opened in 1855, the arrangements made for treatment aimed at non-restraint. Means of restraint were nevertheless employed, in the form of straitjackets, handcuffs, and belts. The statistics of a hospital, as for instance those of Gaustad Hospital, reveal that the use of restraint measures gradually disappeared. It is evident that the Scandinavian physicians had studied the non-restraint system in both England and Germany. Thus, in the records of Gaustad Hospital from 1874 onward it is reported that it was mainly a few particularly difficult patients who prevented the total abolition of coercive measures. The use of mechanical means of restraint came to an end as early as 1882 (Plate XLVIII) (4). However, occasional employment of restraint, especially in the form of belts, lasted up to the present days in Scandinavian psychiatric hospitals.

During the last century, epidemics were a frequent occurrence in psychiatric hospitals (typhus epidemics, the Spanish influenza of 1918-1919, diphtheria epidemics, and, not least, tuberculosis). Tuberculosis is no longer a public health problem in Scandinavia and is hence also disappearing from the psychiatric hospitals.

The focal infection theory had a certain following in Scandinavia, and during the first half of this century tonsillectomies and dental extractions were common operations in psychiatric hospitals.

At present, psychotherapy constitutes the principal method of treatment for the neuroses in Scandinavia; it also forms an important part of the therapeutic program for the psychoses and other psychiatric disorders. Freudian psychoanalysis as a form of treatment has never been adopted in the Scandinavian countries, even though Scandinavian psychiatrists have become increasingly interested in this method and psychoanalytic associations have been founded in the Scandinavian countries. Altogether, psychoanalysis had a far from flourishing start in Scandinavia, although a few leading psychiatrists, such as Bjerre in Sweden and Vogt in Norway, were favorably disposed towards it. Scandinavian psychiatrists did not become really interested in psychoanalysis until after World War II. It is now widely used as an educational measure for psychotherapists in self-therapy. In individual therapy, psychoanalytically oriented short-term therapy is steadily gaining ground.

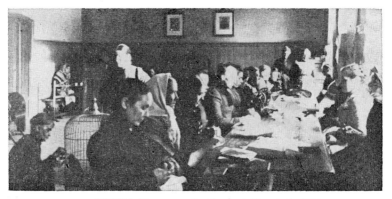

PLATE XLVIII. Day room in Gaustad Hospital, 1902.

From the end of the 1940's group therapy has come increasingly to the fore in the Scandinavian countries and is now practiced in all hospitals, especially for hospitalized patients. In a number of hospitals the entire hospital, or a department of it, is run according to the "therapeutic community" principle (in Norway, first introduced at Ullevål Hospital in the late 1950's).

Psychiatric treatment is becoming less and less "bed-minded." The requirement for beds in active therapeutic institutions is diminishing. Conversely, there is an increase in the number of institutions offering part-time treatment (day-and-night hospitals), consultative service (outpatient clinics), and ambulatory service to the homes (ambulatory personnel). Increasing emphasis is placed on ambulatory activities. The focus of the psychiatric services is shifting from the hospital to society.

8

UNIVERSITY EDUCATION

The first university in Scandinavia was established in Uppsala in 1477. There followed the Universities of Copenhagen (1479), of Åbo (1640), and of Lund 1666) (10). The University of Oslo (then Christiana) was not established until 1811. For a long time psychiatry was not included in the curriculum of medical education. The introduction of psychiatry as a separate subject for medical students seems to have occurred in the middle of the last century. Independent teaching in this subject was started in Sweden in 1856 (24); in the same year the director of Gaustad Hospital, Ole Römer Sandberg, started to give lectures on psychiatry at the University of Oslo (4). Not until this century did psychiatry become an examination subject. Slowly, the subject has taken its proper place in the curriculum and practical training in psychiatry has now become compulsory. The psychiatric training did not enter into the curriculum until the final period of study, but now it starts earlier. Whereas there are four to six professorships in psychiatry in Denmark, Finland, and Norway, respectively, Sweden has 14 such professorships.

Professorships in psychiatry are attached to all universities training medical students. Usually, the professorships in psychiatry are held by chief physicians in clinical departments.

9

RESEARCH

Research has old traditions in the Scandinavian countries. In some fields, psychiatric research has attained international heights. *Acta Psychiatrica Scandinavica*, originally called *Acta Psychiatrica et Neurologica Scandinavica*, has been the central organ for publication of Scandinavian research in the present century. Many important psychiatric works in Scandinavia have been reported in this journal, or published as supplements to it. Since 1946, *Nordisk Psykiatrisk Tidsskrift* has represented a forum for psychiatric debates in the Scandinavian languages, and to some extent for the publication of scientific articles. There have been psychiatric associations in each of the countries from the beginning of the 20th century.

Traditionally, Scandinavian research work has been mainly within certain spheres. Research on heredity and on the importance of the constitution has played a central part; during the later decades this has been partly superseded by epidemiologic studies and research on the course of psychiatric disorders. The Scandinavian countries have a small, reasonably stable, and easily accessible population. The registration system is advanced, not only with reference to domicile, and so on, but also from a medical point of view, with central registers of great reliability (central registers of statistics, psychoses, twins, cancer, etc.). Scandinavian psychiatry has been able to make valuable contributions also in more biologically oriented research (Gjessing, Fölling). No contemporary psychiatrist will be singled out here, as it is always difficult to estimate a living person's impact in historical perspective. No "school" of psychiatry of international standing can be traced back to the Scandinavian countries, but nevertheless Scandinavian research workers have greatly contributed to a better understanding of psychiatric disorders.

REFERENCES

1. ACHTÉ, K. (1971): The 130th anniversary of the Lapinlahti Hospital. *Psychiat. Fennica,* 9, 20.
2. ACHTÉ, K. (1972): Fahlander's second visit to European countries. *Psychiat. Fenn.* 10, 91-94.
3. ACHTÉ, K. (1972): On the history of Finnish psychiatry and the Lapinlahti Hospital. *Psychiat. Fenn.* 10, 65-84.
4. AUSTAD, A.-K. & ØDEGÅRD, Ø. (1956): *Gaustad sykehus gjennom hundre år.* Oslo:
5. EITINGER, L. & RETTERSTØL, N. (1971): *Rettspsykiatri.* Oslo: Universitetsforlaget.
6. EVENSEN, H. (1905): Grundtraekkene i det norske sindsygev aes ens undvikling i de sidste 100 aar. *T. norske La eg eforen,* 25, 21-28, 63-72.
7. FABING, H. D. (1958): On going berserk. A neuro-chemical inquiry. In: Reed, C. F., Alexander, I. E. and Tomkins, S. S. (Eds.), *Psychopathology, a Source Book.* Cambridge, Mass.: Harvard University Press.
8. GADELIUS, B. (1913): *Tro och öfverto i gångna tider.* Stockholm: Geber.
9. GADELIUS, B. (1913): *Sinnessjukdomar och deras behandling för och nu.* Stockholm: Geber.
10. GOTFREDSEN, E. (1964): *Medicinens historie.* 2 vols. Copenhagen: Nyt Nordisk Forlag Arnold Busck.
11. HELWEG, H. (1915): *Sindssygev aes enets udvikling i Danmark.* Copenhagen; Jacob Lund.
12. HJELT, O. E. A. (1891-1893): *Svenska och finska Medicinalverkets historia, 1663-1812.* Helsingfors:
13. HOLMBERG, G., LJUNGBERG, L. & ÅMARK, C. (1968): *Modern svensk psykiatri.* Stockholm: Almquist & Wiksell.
14. JONSSON, F. (1912): *Laegekunsten i den nordiske oldtid.* Copenhagen: Wilhelm Trydes forlag.
15. LAACHE, S. (1911): *Norsk Medicin i hundrede år.* Kristiania:
15a. LANGFELDT, G. (1939): *The Schizofreniform States. A Catamnestic Study Based on Individual Re-examinations.* Copenhagen: Munksgaard.
16. LANGFELDT, G. (1961): Scandinavia. In: Bellak, L. (Ed.), *Contemporary European Psychiatry.* New York: Grove Press.

17. LANGFELDT, G. (1964): *Laerebok i klinisk psykiatri.* Oslo: Aschehoug.
18. ØDEGÅRD, Ø. (1956): Den psykiatriske omsorg i Norge—organisasjon og opgaver. *Nord. psykiat. medl. bl.,* 10, 22-26.
19. ØDEGÅRD, Ø. (1971): Hospitalized psychoses in Norway: Time trends 1926 to 1965. *Soc. Psychiat. (Berlin),* 6, 53-58.
20. OSE, E. (1971): Forandringer i synet på, omsorgen for og behandlingen av de sinnslidende. *T. norske Laegeforen,* 91, 2165-2167.
21. RAVN, J. (1956): De danske psykiatriske institutioner. *Nord. psykiat. medl. bl.,* 10, 11-16.
22. RETTERSTOL, N. (1962): Psykiatriske synspunkter på persongalleriet i Snorres kongesagaer. *T. norske Laegeforen,* 82, 1219-1222.
23. RUD, F. (1966): *Betenkning vedrørende den psykiatriske service for Bergen fylke, dens nåvaerende status, den fremtidige utvikling og behovsdekning, med tillegg.* Bergen: Stensil.
24. RYLANDER, G. (1956): Rättspsykiatrin och dess stora chans. *Nord. psykiat. medl., bl.,* 10, 27-33.
25. STRØMGREN, E. (1969): *Psykiatri.* Copenhagen: Munksgaard.

9

SWITZERLAND

Oskar Diethelm, M.D.

Professor Emeritus of Psychiatry
Cornell University Medical College,
New York, New York, U.S.A.

1

INTRODUCTION

The essential features which have affected the development of psychiatry in Switzerland during the past centuries are still important today.

The present constitution of the country, based on the concept of confederacy of independent cantons of the Renaissance period, was written in the 19th century. Earlier efforts to develop a viable centralistic government through the Helvetic Republic (1797-1815) were not acceptable to the Swiss people. Many important liberal contributions that came out of this period were retained, but the power to deal with them was returned to the cantons. These included education, health, welfare, and fundamental economic decisions. Persistent efforts of the liberal party led to some further reforms, but they were increasingly rejected by the conservative party which dominated the seven Catholic cantons, resulting in a brief revolutionary conflict—Sonderbundkrieg, 1847. The religious factor was less important here than was an effort to protect the sovereignty of the small and sparsely populated cantons.

In 1847 a constitution was accepted which made the country a confederacy with a bicameral parliament. The rights and obligations of citizenship remained founded in the community, be it village or city. It was the community's responsibility to confer citizenship to outsiders and to take care of the needs of the inhabitants, including that of health. The communities expressed their will through the parliament of their canton. It became increasingly clear that more power had to be given to the federal government, but even at the beginning of the 20th century marked differences still existed in the civil and criminal laws of various cantons.

With the Helvetic Republic full political rights were given to all regions of Switzerland, and new cantons were formed in the French-speaking West, German-speaking North and East, and Italian-speaking South of the country.

In the 16th century, 13 independent cantons had formed a loose organization for mutual defense. With the Reformation their religious and cultural ties brought the country together, although the Catholic cantons formed a minority and disagreed on some political points.

In the medieval period and in the Renaissance, the cities of Basel, Bern, Zurich, and Geneva flourished through commerce and industry. Agricultural cultivation increased when laws against mercenaries in the 16th century prevented the struggling peasants from escaping into a life of adventure and gilded promises. The industrial development of the 17th and 18th centuries and the strong emphasis on agriculture in the middle of the 18th century increased prosperity where earlier, through the devastating epidemics of the 16th and 17th centuries, there had been great suffering and hardship.

Starting with the humanism of the late 15th century, the Swiss cities became a haven for persecuted emigrants from neighboring countries. This custom has continued throughout the centuries. Such emigrants from Italy and France helped stimulate the silk and wool industry in Basel, Geneva and Zurich. Other newcomers aided in building the country's political and cultural strength.

2

PSYCHIATRIC DEVELOPMENT IN THE 16TH AND 17TH CENTURIES

In the early 16th century humanism exerted a vast influence. Basel, Zurich, Geneva and Bern became educational and religious centers. Through Ulrich Zwingli (1484-1531) a religious reform was established in which a social-ethical radicalism attacked taxation by the Church, the sale of letters of indulgence, the adoration of saints, the celibacy of priests, dogmatic religious teaching, and the power of the Pope. An independent evangelical church was established in Zurich (1525) and its theological and cultural teaching was soon accepted in the cantons of the northern and western part of Switzerland, but the people of the mountainous central region retained their Catholicism (the religious separation in Catholic and Protestant cantons became less significant in the 19th century). In Lausanne and Geneva, independent influential reformers were preaching the theology of Calvin even before he came to live in Geneva, in 1536. Through the conciliatory attitude of the leaders of the Geneva and Zurich churches a formula was found (1541) which permitted the establishment of one evangelical church of Switzerland. However, efforts to find a solution for the theological differences between the Swiss and the Lutheran churches failed. For a historical understanding of the development of psychiatry in Switzerland, the spread of Calvinism into Holland, France, and Scotland is interesting because it offered cultural connections with these countries and their universities.

The aggressive leadership of Zwingli led to social reforms which became significant in his lifetime but more so in the succeeding years. Through his efforts the mercenary system of the 15th and early 16th centuries was abolished and political and military leaders were forbidden to accept pensions from foreign governments. He stressed the need for public education and founded a seminary for the education of preachers, which soon became an important school of higher education. Alcoholism, loose sexual morals, prostitution, and idleness were attacked. Pamphlets on marriage attempted to strengthen the life of the family. Support of the poor, i.e., those unable to work, became an obligation of the community. The great influence of Erasmus, whom Zwingli admired and had studied intensely, is readily evident. The son of a well-established family of a small village in Eastern Switzerland, Zwingli never lost contact with the farming population. He always stressed that a healthy society needs a healthy church.

Basel and Zurich were important medical centers. In Basel a university was founded in 1460. Its medical school began to flourish in the middle of the next century. Paracelsus, a native Swiss, taught there in 1527 but left after two years. Around this period he wrote his treatise on psychiatry (26), a stimulating presentation which, however, does not seem to have had much influence on medical theory and practice. An outstanding faculty at Basel, guided after 1562 by its dean Felix Platter (1536-1614) (7), attracted students from all the countries of Northern Europe. The publications of the professors and the printed dissertations of the students permit us to evaluate the

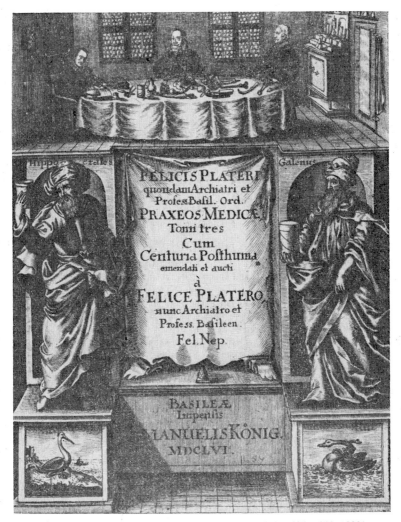

PLATE XLIX. *Praxeos Medicae*, 1656. (Editions 1602, 1625, 1656, 1666.)

psychiatric teaching and the significance of psychopathologic disorders which were described. Platter emphasized the need for careful clinical observations and students were invited to accompany him on his visits to patients in the hospitals. In his book *Observations* (1614) (29) Platter described concisely but vividly a wide variety of medical illnesses, including all known psychiatric diseases and their treatment. In his textbook *Praxeos Medicae* (Plate XLIX) (28), for the first time an attempt was made to classify psychiatric illnesses. He grouped them under mental weakness (caused by heredity, brain concussion, malformations of the brain, physical illnesses, imbalance of the humors, and excessive moisture or dryness of the brain), mental consternation (with symptoms of listlessness, stupor, paralysis, agitation, or catalepsy), deep sleep (the patient would be comatose or torpid and difficult to arouse, with or without delirium). In his chapter on mental alienation Platter emphasized that judgment, memory, or imagination might be affected and expressed in thoughts, words, or deeds, and hallucinations (including delusions) could be present. When the mental disturbance occurred without fever one was dealing with melancholia (caused by black bile); if accompanied by furor it was mania (yellow bile); if with fever, phrenitis. (Delirium was caused by inflammation of the brain, by toxins from disease in other parts of the body, or by the effects of alcohol or drugs.) This chapter was lengthy and additional space was given to hysteria and sexual excitement. As illustrated by his observations, melancholia included depressive and schizophrenic illnesses and mania embraced schizophrenic and manic excitements, while sexual furor was a disease of the uterus and therefore discussed under diseases of women. Epileptic psychoses were briefly mentioned.

We know little about Platter's personal contact with students but his textbook was widely read; it appeared in four editions between 1602 and 1670 and had its last printing in 1736. The English translation by Cole and Culpepper is dated 1662. His *Observations* (translated into English in 1669) contain illustrations of all known psychiatric disorders and frequently include enough details to understand the physical and environmental factors which were involved. The current treatment is always mentioned. The psychopathological descriptions stress the influence of various emotions, delusions, schizophrenic apathy, sexual unrest, and excitement. The intellectual disorders described under feeblemindedness include cretinism, at that time commonly found in the Swiss mountains. Accepting the current concepts of humoral pathology he advocated purgation by drugs and clysma, chemical treatment, diet, and bleeding. For sleep disorders he recommended opiates and alkaloids. Similar drugs, combined with a calm psychotherapeutic approach and at times restraint and isolation, were found to decrease excitement.

The printed dissertations on psychiatry in the period 1575 to 1629 (6) dealt with melancholia, including depression and schizophrenia (20 dissertations), mania (1), catalepsy (1), sexual excitement (1), delirious illnesses (12), hysterical reactions (7), memory disorders (1) and psychological discussions (6). The earlier dissertations reviewed the literature critically while after 1600 an increasing emphasis on psychopathology indicated the growing importance of the clinical experience of students who had observed patients. During this period 85 students from cities and villages of the whole of Switzerland graduated at Basel and later practiced in the regions from which they had come. Their psychiatric appreciation must have influenced their treatment of patients as well as the attitude of other physicians and the public.

The *Observations* of Fabricius Hildanus (1560-1634) (8, 9) were widely quoted by the physicians of the 17th century. He had received his surgical education in Jülich-Cleve, where he became a close friend of the son of Johannes Weyer. Later, he worked with the surgeon Griffon in Geneva before studying medicine at the University of Cologne. After a brief period of practice in his native town of Hilden, Germany, he went to Lausanne (1596) and later to Berne. He was a very religious man and devoted to his patients. Through his practice and his published works he attempted to improve the health conditions in the towns and villages of this large canton, warning against the danger of alcohol and offering advice on how to deal with disturbing emotions. An example of his interest in psychiatry is his study (9) of the catatonic Apollonia Schreier, which attracted wide attention. In his books he presents careful observations of all known psychiatric disorders, including somnambulism, hallucinations, dementia after brain damage, and the hitherto little-noticed relationship between mania and melancholia.

Medicine flourished in Zurich, but little was added to psychiatric knowledge. Zwingli's interest in the care of the poor brought an administrative reorganization of the medieval hospitals in Basel, Bern, and Zurich. In the Middle Ages, hospitals had been administered by monasteries or orders of knights. Hospices took care of pilgrims from German countries who, on the road to Rome or Compostella, visited the monastery of Einsiedeln. In the 13th century, the cities took the hospitals away from the monasteries. Hospitals were obligated to take care of those citizens who were poor, infirm, or sick, and acted in addition as hospices for travelers and pilgrims. It also became an established custom that a citizen, by paying a required amount of money, could spend the rest of his life as beneficiary in the hospital. Later, a home for foundlings was added to the hospital. The hospital was supervised by a public official and, under him, an administrator who exerted dictatorial powers over the patients. In 1513, the physician who was in charge of the services for maintaining health in the city was also requested to visit the hospital. When the care of the poor became the responsibility of the state (1520), it became necessary to find additional space and, in Zurich, a division for the sick was established in an old monastery (*Predigerkloster*). The physician now made regular rounds. Lay people were assigned to take care of the patients. Around the middle of the 16th century, the concept was accepted that the hospital should not merely take care of the sick, but the patient should also be treated and, if possible, cured.

Little is known about psychiatric patients in the Zurich hospital. We know from Platter (29) that some psychiatric patients were kept in cells in the basement of the Basel Hospital. Mentally ill people from a distant town or whose citizenship could not be established were expelled; many must have died on the roads from hunger, diseases, and exposure. In 1618, a special house was built in Basel to take care of violent patients. Later they were transferred to an annex of the hospital, called the *Almosen,* where idiots, drunkards, and the insane, together with chronically ill patients suffering from physical diseases, were kept in a large room. The quiet psychiatric patients were kept in a separate room. The most advanced development occurred in Bern (25) where, in 1328, the city took over the hospitals. The supervision of patients' care was undertaken by the city physician. In the early 16th century, the *Inselspital* became the hospital for curable physically and mentally ill, while chronic cases were admitted to another hospital. If chronic mental patients were not citizens of the city, they were sent to the poorhouses of their community which usually had a *Taubhäuslein* for unmanageable patients (these small buildings contained one to several locked cells). Whenever economically possible, patients were returned to the care of their families. In any case, whether in a hospital, poorhouse, *Taubhäuslein,* or family, the unmanageable patients were physically restrained by chains and often lived in filthy isolation. Rules for admission to and discharge from a *Taubhäuslein* were not established until the end of the 17th century.

Legally, mental illness was recognized in the early 16th century. A patient who committed suicide received a normal burial. Acts of violence, including homicide, in a recognizable psychotic state were considered a medical problem. On the other hand, among the members of religious sects that flourished in Switzerland and were cruelly punished, there must have been many who suffered from psychiatric disorders.

The persecution of witches occurred frequently and how many of them were mentally ill cannot be guessed. In the early 17th century, Platter still believed that exorcism was necessary for patients who were possessed. In isolated mountain districts belief in demonology existed well into the 18th century.

The number of psychiatric patients for whom help was requested increased greatly during the 16th and 17th centuries. In the Protestant cantons, monasteries became available for the care of these patients, but offered no medical treatment. Wealthy towns were also requested to take care of the poor insane from surrounding villages. The usually poor Catholic cantons could offer little help, except through family care or the *Taubhäuslein*.

From the beginning of the 16th century, efforts were made to change public attitudes towards psychiatric patients, but progress was slow. Yet it became possible to send chronic patients from the "hospital" to work on farms in the neighborhood.

Around the middle of the 17th century, the number of medical students in Basel decreased considerably. Many Swiss went to Dutch and German medical schools and to Montpellier, but Switzerland still produced significant works. Under the leadership of Wepfer, Schaffhausen became an influential medical center. In his *Observations* (40) Wepfer made valuable contributions to the clinical knowledge of psychopathology, including sexual disorders. The Basel dissertation on nostalgia by Hofer (1688) (16) attracted wide attention. His case illustrations emphasized psychodynamic factors. Further cases were published by Theodor Zwinger (45) and Johann Jakob Scheuchzer (32). In the 18th century, the topic of homesickness was discussed repeatedly in the Swiss medical literature (3, 15, 35, 42).

3

THE PERIOD OF ENLIGHTENMENT

During the 18th century, a striking feature in Swiss medicine was the increasing concern with the minor psychopathologic symptoms found so frequently in medical practice and with the ill effects of the culture of this period.

The outstanding physicians at this time were Simon André A. D. Tissot, Albrecht von Haller, and Johann Georg Zimmermann. Tissot (1728-1797), a graduate of Montpellier where he was greatly influenced by his teacher Boissier de Sauvages, was devoted to protecting and improving the health of the farmers and of the population of small towns in Western Switzerland. His many publications were soon translated into German and English and attracted wide attention. For two years he was professor in Pavia, but in 1783 he returned to Lausanne to become professor of medicine at the new Collège de Médecine. His dissertation (1749) (33) dealt with "mania, melancholia, and phrenitis." In 1758 (34) he published a small book on masturbation which in French and English translations was titled *Onanism*. It was the first medical discussion of this topic to offer broad information on male and female sexual functions, on the need for moderation in sexual activities, and on the pathological phenomenon of impotence and frigidity. The effect of this book is difficult to evaluate because of the emphasis on the dangers of excessive masturbation. His next book (1761) (35) offered practical advice on the preservation of physical and mental health, and in 1768 he stressed the need for physical and mental recreation (36). The three volumes, *Nerves and Their Illnesses* (1778) (37), offer a detailed presentation of the anatomy and physiology of the nervous system. The third volume includes a lengthy treatment on epilepsy, followed by a discussion of physical and mental (moral) factors that cause nervous illnesses. He devoted several pages to the problem of alcoholism. Under moral causes he presents in considerable detail the effect of strong emotions. To the list of causes which Cheyne blamed for the English malady Tissot added the effect of venereal diseases and the treatment by mercury. He emphasized that a physician, through questions and observations, should recognize if emotions play an important role. He also stressed that catalepsy (38) must be differentiated from religious ecstasy. His chapter on insanity included homesickness, and another chapter dealt with violent mania, hysteria, somnambulism, and hypochondriasis. Interestingly, in his therapeutic discussions he favored psychological explanations. In his neurological work Tissot leans on the teaching of his friend Haller who acquainted him with German medicine. The influence of Montpellier is seen in his acceptance of the relationship of emotions and physical functions. As a Protestant he had ties with Holland and England.

The influence of Zimmermann (1728-1795) was also widespread. Under Haller he presented in Göttingen an excellent dissertation and, on his teacher's recommendation, was appointed the physician of his native city of Brugg. During this period (1754-1768) he published a book, *The Experience in Medicine* (1764) (42), in which he discussed personality features desirable in a physician and emphasized the importance of critical observation and experience. His analysis of emotions and their effect on physiologic functions, especially those of the digestive tract, is interesting. He became recognized as an outstanding clinician and was appointed physician to the King of England (in Hanover). Despite his success he was often lonely and depressed. In 1784 he wrote *Solitude* (43), a medical-psychological study that gave him much public acclaim. In it he reviews the psychological aspects of solitude which may have desirable and undesirable effects. In a lengthy historical discussion he analyzes mysticism. In other volumes (41) he offers advice on how to deal with depressive moods and various psychological problems.

Through his political and social philosophy J. J. Rousseau made a lasting impression on Swiss life. At the same time, an unknown Swiss peasant, called Kleinjogg (5) (his correct name was Jacob Guyer, 1716-1785), who lived in a small village near Zurich, impressed his neighbors and citizens of the city with his marked success in cultivating the land. He achieved moral reforms by emphasizing the importance of the family unit and of being an active part of the community. Though publication of these ideas by the Zurich physician Hirzel, Kleinjogg became known and respected in Switzerland and in Germany. Both Kleinjogg and Rousseau influenced the thinking of Tissot and Zimmermann, and the educational theories of Heinrich Pestalozzi (1746-1827) (17). In his education of the poor, stimulated by Rousseau's *Emile* (31) and by visits to Kleinjogg, Pestalozzi taught not only a new method of elementary education, but also the dignity of any kind of work and thus the self-respect that even the poorest person deserved. In the novel *Lienhard and Gertrude* (27) he made people aware of the meaning of a strong family unit; in the novel, a courageous mother tries to support the alcoholic, weak husband, and keep the family unified. Alcoholism was a great problem in the countryside and physicians tried, largely unsuccessfully, to decrease this social disease.

The critical attitude of the leading physicians to Mesmer's animal magnetism was mostly hostile. One of them, Paul Usteri, had written a review of the literature in his Göttingen dissertation (1788) (39). His teacher, Haller, along with Tissot and Zimmermann, rejected Mesmer's theories and practice, while other Swiss physicians accepted the results of experiments with hypnosis obtained by critical German physicians, but were not willing to accept his theories. In Geneva Mesmer found considerable public, but little medical, support.

4

THE 19TH CENTURY

Medical and Public Interest in Mental Disorders

The French Revolution profoundly affected Switzerland, resulting in the new state, the Helvetic republic, and later the Swiss Confederacy. Both physicians and liberal political leaders supported reforms of hospitals and of education. Among the early 19th-century leaders was Ignaz P. V. Troxler (1780-1866), who graduated from Jena in 1803. In his younger years he was a follower of romantic medicine. While a successful practitioner, his psychologic-philosophic concepts matured and he presented in several books a dynamic concept of personality and its psycho-physical unity. After 1830 he became professor of philosophy.

In Geneva, physicians educated in Paris and Edinburgh presented the ideas of Pinel (1). J. A. Matthey, for instance, wrote a book on mental illnesses (1816) (24). Representing a continuation of the ideas of Tissot and Zimmermann J. P. I. Barras wrote on nervous diseases of the stomach (1827) (2).

In education the impact of Pestalozzi continued and was strengthened by his followers. The outstanding results were the establishment of general education, and the special attention paid to educating the poor, to advancing the technology of modern farming, and to training more teachers. The need for more universities with medical schools was recognized. The writer Jeremias Gotthelf (11) described the plight of the poor peasants, their hopeless attitude, and the marked alcoholism. The public and the physicians responded to his realistic stories with helpful social and political reforms, and his work promoted a lasting interest in the problem of alcoholism.

In medicine the principles of Pestalozzi were used by a Bernese physician, J. Guggenbühl (Plate L) (14), in the education of idiots and cretins. He taught them in a small institution, the Abendberg, located in the Bernese mountains. Instead of disdain he showed respect for the dignity of these patients. The result of his painstaking educational labor won him international recognition.

The Development of Psychiatric Hospitals

The ideas and therapeutic reorganization of Pinel and Esquirol found a ready response in Switzerland. They believed one must treat patients with respect, giving them as much freedom as caution permitted, offer them an acceptable if not attractive physical environment, and treat them according to the best available medical knowledge. They also believed the physician must have authority in the hospital. These ideas were welcomed, but did not become effective in all Swiss hospitals until some years after the middle of the century.

In Geneva, Abraham Joly (1), when he was in charge of the small psychiatric division of the hospital there (1787-1793), abolished restraint by chains, but it was not until 1838 that the patients were transferred to a psychiatric hospital at Vernets. At that time a law for commitment was established which preceded by a few months a similar law in France.

The monastery of Königsfelden (near Brugg), which had been used for some psychiatric and physically ill patients as well as for the poor, was reorganized and put under a medical director, but control of alcoholism and sexual activities in the hospital was difficult to main-

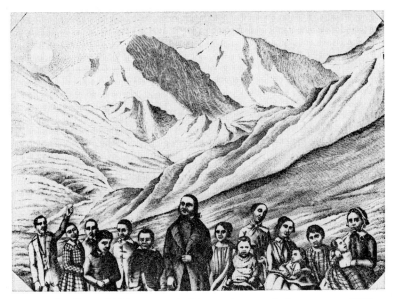

PLATE L. Guggenbühl, surrounded by patients and three nurses, 1853.

tain. On the other hand, by 1820, occupational therapy was used in a systematic way. A modern hospital was opened in 1872. In Basel, the *Almosen* (1842) was a psychiatric hospital reserved for treatable patients only. Chronic patients were cared for in a small separate institution. (The same separation was made in Bern in the 17th century.)

In the second half of the 19th century, psychiatric hospitals were recognized. Guislain's request for no-restraint was accepted in all Swiss hospitals as a basic principle, as was the recognition of the dignity of men. At a time when there were no Swiss psychiatrists, the guiding influence came from the psychiatric hospitals of the neighboring states where E. A. Zeller (22) at Illenau (Württemberg) and Ch. F. W. Roller (22) at Winnenthal (Baden) were the leaders.

August Zinn (1825-1897) (22) left Germany for political reasons in 1849. He was graduated in Zurich (1853) and became physician to the small psychiatric division which was attached to the department of medicine of the university hospital. Influenced by the teaching of Griesinger, who was the professor of medicine, and by a visit of several weeks to the progressive hospital of Roller, he felt ready to accept the directorship of St. Pirminsberg, formerly a small monastery, which, in 1847, had been converted into the psychiatric hospital of the St. Gallen canton. There he introduced non-restraint, and emphasized treatment, a well-planned daily routine, and occupational therapy. He made this hospital a model for all other hospitals in Switzerland. The most effective physician in the development of psychiatric hospitals was Ludwig Wille (1834-1912) (22), a Bavarian graduate of the University of Erlangen (1858), who became assistant in psychiatry under August von Solbrig (22), an excellent administrator and clinician. In 1864, Wille became director of the cantonal hospital in Münsterlingen (Thurgau), which in 1848 had been changed from a monastery into a psychiatric hospital. In 1867 he organized a hospital in the monastery of Rheinau (Zurich), and, in 1873, another in the monastery of St. Urban (Lucerne). In 1875 he was put in charge of the psychiatric division of the hospital in Basel and requested to plan the building and the organization of a psychiatric university clinic (*Friedmatt*). He was professor from 1886 to 1904 and proved to be a good clinician, devoted to the patients and to their relatives.

The small cantons in the mountainous part of Switzerland were neither populous nor wealthy enough to build large hospitals. Patients needing hospitalization were sent to public or private hospitals in other cantons. At that time, there were many private hospitals in Switzerland, usually very small and offering inadequate care. Government supervision was poorly carried out until the latter part of the 19th century. (Under the Swiss constitution of 1869 the patients are the financial responsibility of their community.)

While Zinn was in St. Priminsberg he founded a society that offered assistance to psychiatric patients. It proved to be valuable for finding work for them and offering help when it was needed. In addition the society acquainted the public with psychiatric needs and gained support for the hospitals. This society spread over Switzerland and smiilar societies were later developed in Germany. In 1850 a small society of psychiatrists were formed which, in 1864, became the Society of Medical Alienists and then changed into the Swiss Society of Psychiatrists (*Schweizer Gesellschaft für Psychiatrie*).

5

THE SCIENTIFIC PERIOD OF PSYCHIATRY

The psychiatric clinics of the Swiss universities offer treatment of both short and long duration. This development is related to the fact that each university is supported solely by the canton in which it is located. However, even if such a canton is large enough to need two psychiatric institutions (Berne and Zurich), the historically intimate connection between community and hospital makes the separation of hospitals for treatment and care unacceptable. In all hospitals the stress is on treatment. In recent years, all hospitals have modernized their therapeutic facilities and, whenever possible, the staff is active in suitable research. Cantons too small to need their own hospitals make suitable arrangements with other cantons.

In 1863 Zinn (44) submitted a long memorandum to the government of the canton of Zurich, presenting frankly and in detail the deplorable psychiatric treatment in the hospital. This published document gave much support to the plans of Wilhelm Griesinger (22), who was professor of medicine in Zurich (1860-1864), and had received a psychiatric education at Winnenthal. In 1845 he published his famous textbook (12), and in 1861 a second edition. In his ideas on treatment he was strongly influenced by Guislain and Zeller. Griesinger's ideal of a university clinic for curable patients also was not accepted and a large clinic (Burghölzli) for all types of psychiatric patients was built after he had left (4). Psychiatric education for the future Swiss physician began with his stimulating lectures (13).

The first professor of psychiatry (1869-1872), Bernard von Gudden (22), a Bavarian, was an outstanding brain anatomist who had received his clinical education under Roller and was greatly influenced by Griesinger. He established a well-functioning hospital but, dissatisfied by administrative difficulties, soon left. His first assistant, Gustav Huguenin, a good teacher from Zurich, succeeded him, but resigned after two years for the same reason. The most serious mistake in the organization was that independent authority had been given to the lay admiinstration, and this interfered with medical functions.

The new professor of psychiatry, Julius Eduard Hitzig (22) (1875-1878) was primarily interested in neurology and lacked a sound psychiatric education. His aggressive and uncompromising attitude made him disliked by lay staff and by many relatives of patients, but he succeeded in forcing the discharge of the administrator and achieved a sound reorganization. The responsibility for the entire hospital was transferred to the professor. Disappointed by the difficulties, Hitzig accepted the professorship in Halle. Being a native of Prussia he had little understanding of Swiss custom and people.

During the years from 1850 to 1870, the hospitals were directed by physicians who were poorly educated in psychiatry, but were devoted clinicians who learned much from their mutual exchange of ideas at meetings of the Society of Medical Alienists. Psychiatric education of medical students was strengthened in the universities of Basel, Bern, and Zurich and, a few years later, in Geneva and Lausanne. In 1887, the students were required to pass the examination in psychiatry to obtain their license as physicians.

The scientific period started with August Forel and Eugen Bleuler. Forel (1848-1931), born in the French-speaking Vaud canton, obtained his medical education in Zurich, and his scientific training in brain anatomy in von Gudden's laboratory (1873-1878). For about two years he was also put in charge of a ward of disturbed patients. Returning to Zurich, he became professor of psychiatry and director of the Burghölzli clinic (1879-1898). He devoted his first few years to establishing an outstanding clinical service, attracting promising young assistants and a reliable nursing staff. Although continuing his research in brain anatomy, he devoted his energy to patients, hospital organization, and teaching. The lay administration cooperated well. In 1883 Forel became actively interested in movements to combat the marked alcoholism of the country. He recognized the need for total abstinence for alcoholics and, with the help of physicians and many lay people, organized a widespread anti-alcohol movement, which he led for the greater part of his life. In the clinic he replaced von Gudden's fatalism with therapeutic activities, including occupational therapy. He recognized the need for psychiatry to play a strong role in forensic medicine. In 1887, he introduced the Nancy concept of hypnosis. A popular book on "the sexual question" (10) discussed sexual hygiene.

Eugen Bleuler (1857-1939) (23), a native of Zurich and graduate of its medical school, was director of the hospital in Rheinau (1886-1898), and a professor in Zurich from 1898 to 1927. He was a recognized leader in the study of clinical psychopathology, his work culminating in his concept of schizophrenia. In contrast to Forel, he accepted a great deal of Freud's psychoanalysis, but maintained a critical scientific attitude towards some of the theories. His clinic became the center of European dynamic psychiatry and of graduate education. His psychological interest in criminals led to legal improvements. He fought uncritical attitudes in medicine and urged his students to be open-minded and critical. From his clinic came a large number of clinical contributions.

Among his outstanding co-workers was Carl Gustav Jung (1875-1961) (23), who contributed greatly to the understanding of schizophrenia, to psychopathology, and to psychotherapy. He presented a new approach to the study and theory of the unconscious and its dynamics (19, 20). His *Analytical Psychology* (21) offered new psychotherapeutic approaches.

Psychoanalysis exerted a stimulating influence on the theory and practice of psychotherapy, on education and theology (O. Pfister) and on a new anthropology (Ludwig Binswanger). Psychoanalytic principles were applied to child psychiatry. In experimental psychopathologic investigations valuable results were obtained by association studies (C. G. Jung) (18) and interpretation of ink blots (Hermann Rorschach) (30).

Neurology and psychiatry have remained separate but mutually stimulating disciplines. In Bern, the neurologist Paul Dubois (1848-1918) (23), an autodidact in psychiatry, developed a psychotherapeutic method called persuasion, which became widely used, and he also clarified the concept of psychoneurosis. In Zurich, the neuropathologist Konstantin von Monakow (1853-1930) (23) made a strong contribution to a biological theory of psychiatry. Largely due to his influence neurologists and psychiatrists combined to publish the *Schweizer Archiv für Neurologie und Psychiatrie.*

6

CONCLUSION

In the 20th century, psychiatry in Switzerland has seen many new developments. University and cantonal hospitals have tried pharmacological treatment through prolonged sleep. Improvements in occupational therapy, early discharge of schizophrenics, and family placement of chronic patients have put these institutions in the forefront of psychiatric treatment. Out-patient departments have been established, various modifications of psychotherapy employed, community resources utilized to help ambulant patients and socially maladjusted individuals, including alcoholics, prostitutes, and unmarried mothers. Interest in these developments existed in all parts of Switzerland, fulfilling needs which had been recognized for centuries. An important aid to the rapid growth of Swiss psychiatry has been the close relationship of the staff of the university clinics and cantonal hospitals, of psychiatrists and neurologists, and of the medical practitioners and their communities.

REFERENCES

1. ACKERKNECHT, E. H. (1964): *La médecine à Genève surtout dans la première moîtiè du XIX siècle.* XIX Congrès International d'Histoire de la Médicine.
2. BARRAS, J. P. I. (1827): *Traité sur les gastralgies et les entéralgies ou maladies nerveuses de l'estomac et de l'intestin.* Paris: Béchet.
3. BILGUER, J. U. (1767): *Nachrichten in Absicht der Hypochondrie.* Kopenhagen.
4. BLEULER, M. (1951): *Geschichte des Burghölzlis und der psychiatrischen Universitätsklinik.* Vol. 2. Zürich: Züricher Spitalgeschichte.
5. BLEULER, M. (1962): Early Swiss sources of Adolf Meyer's concepts. *Amer. J. Psychiat.,* 119.
6. DIETHELM, O. (1971): *Medical Dissertations of Psychiatric Interest Printed before 1750.* Basel: S. Karger.
7. DIETHELM, O. & HEFFERNAN, TH. F. (1965): Felix Platter. *J. Hist. Behav. Sci.,* 1, 10-23.
8. FABRICIUS, HILDANUS, G. (1682): *Opera omnia, Observationum centuria, tertia et quarta.* Frankfurt a.M.: Chr. Wurstius.
9. FABRICIUS HILDANUS, G. (1682): *Opera omnia, Observationum centuria quarta, obs. IV. Frankfurt a. M.:* Chr. Wurstius.
10. FOREL, A. (1905): *Die sexuelle Frage.* München: E. Reinhardt.
11. GOTTHELF, J. (1887): *Uli der Knecht.* Leipzig: Univ. Bibl.
12. GRIESINGER, W. (1845): *Die Pathologie und Therapie der psychischen Krankheiten.* Stuttgart: A. Krabbe.
13. GRIESINGER, W. (1872): *Gesammelte Abhandlungen.* Berlin: A. Hirschwald.
14. GUGGENBÜHL, J. (1853): *Die Cretinen-Heilanstalt auf dem Abend-Berg.* Bern: Huber.
15. HALLER, A. (1732): *Versuch Schweizerischer Gedichte.* Bern: N. E. Haller.
16. HOFER, J. (1688): *De nostalgia oder Heimwehe.* Basel: J. Bertschi.
17. HÜRLIMANN, M. (1938): *Grosse Schweizer.* Zürich: Atlantis.
18. JUNG, C. G. (1906): *Diagnostische Assoziationsstudien.* Leipzig: J. A. Barth.
19. JUNG, C. G. (1912): *Neue Bahnen der Psychologie.* Zurich: Rascher.
20. JUNG, C. G. (1917): *Psychologie der unbewussten Prozesse.* Zurich: Rascher.
21. JUNG, C. G. (1953): *Two Essays on Analytical Psychology.* New York: Pantheon Books.
22. KIRCHHOFF, TH. (Ed.) (1921/24): *Deutsche Irrenärzte.* Vols. 1 and 2. (Biography of Roller, Zeller, Solbrig, Griesinger, Gudden, Zinn, Hitzig, Wille.) Berlin: J. Springer.
23. KOLLE, K. (Ed.) (1956/63): *Grosse Nervenärzte.* Vols. 1, 2 and 3. (Biography of Bleuler, Jung, Dubois, Monakow.) Stuttgart: G. Thieme.
24. MATTHEY, J. A. (1816): *Nouvelles recherches sur les maladies de l'esprit.* Paris and Geneva.
25. MORGENTHALER, W. (1915): *Bernisches Irrenwesen.* Bern: G. Grunau.
26. PARACELSUS, A.TH. (1568): *Von den Krankheiten so die Vernunft berauben.* Basel: A. von Bodenstein.
27. PESTALOZZI, H. (1781): *Lienhard and Gertrude.* Zurich: Gessner.
28. PLATTER, F. (1602): *Praxeos medicae opus.* Basel: Schroeter. (Eng. trans. Cole, A., and Culpepper, N. (1662), *A Golden Practice of Physic.* London.)
29. PLATTER, F. (1614): *Observationum . . . Libri tres. Basel.* (Eng. trans. Cole, A., and Culpepper, N., 1664. *Histories and Observations upon Most Diseases.* London.)
30. RORSCHACH, H. (1921): *Psychodiagnostik.* Bern: E. Bircher.

31. ROUSSEAU, J. J. (1762): *Emile, or Education*. Amsterdam (Eng. trans. Foxley, B. 1968. London: Dent)
32. SCHEUCHZER, J. J. (1705): *Von dem Heimwehe*. Zurich: Naturgeschichte des Schweizerlandes.
33. TISSOT, S. A. A. D. (1749): *De mania, melancholia et phrenitide*. Montpellier.
34. TISSOT, S. A. A. D. (1758): *Tentamen de morbis ex manustrupatione*. Lausanne.
35. TISSOT, S. A. A. D. (1761): *Avis au peuple sur sa santè*. Lausanne.
36. TISSOT, S. A. A. D. (1768): *De la santé des gens de lettres*. Lausanne: Grasset.
37. TISSOT, S. A. A. D. (1778/80): *Traité des nerfs et de leurs maladies*. Geneva: Grasset.
38. TISSOT, S. A. A. D. (1780): *Traité de la Katalepsie, de l'exstase, de la migraine et des maladies du cerveau*. Lausanne: Grasset.
39. USTERI, P. (1788): *Specimen Bibliothecae criticae magnetismi sic dicti animalis*. Göttingen: J. C. Dieterich.
40. WEPFER, J. (1727): *Observationes medicae-practicae*. Schaffhausen: J. A. Ziegler.
41. ZIMMERMANN, J. G. (1758): *Von dem Nationalstolze*. Zurich: Heidegger Co.
42. ZIMMERMANN, J. G. (1764): *Die Erfahrung in der Arzneykunst*. Zurich: Heidegger Co.
43. ZIMMERMANN, J. G. (1784): *Ueber die Einsamkeit*. Leipzig.
44. ZINN, A. (1863): *Ueber das öffentliche Irrenwesen im Kanton Zürich*. Zurich.
45. ZWINGER, T. (1710): *Fasciculus dissertationum medicarum selectiorum*. Basel: J. L. König.

10

GERMANY AND AUSTRIA

Esther Fischer-Homberger, M.D.

Privatdozent of Medical History,
Institute of History of Medicine,
University of Zurich, Switzerland

1

INTRODUCTION

Psychiatry is a medical specialty. Like other medical specialties it culti-
vates a certain domain intensively. Like social medicine, legal medicine,
or hygiene, it has close relations with non-medical disciplines. For the
psychiatrist it is less obvious than for other specialists how his contribution is separated from the contributions of other disciplines. Often
it is questionable whether he can fulfill his task if he approaches it
solely as a medical man—he may also have to function as a pedagogue,
a psychologist, a sociologist, an historian, a philosopher, a theologian.
Even as to the *methods* medicine furnishes to psychiatry, clarity does
not always prevail. Expectations of success often change from one approach to the other. Such difficulties and oscillations characterize the
history of psychiatry. While they have not been more prevalent in the
regions of present-day Germany and Austria than elsewhere, in these
places, perhaps more than elsewhere, they have challenged and pre-
occupied the profession.

---

* Translated by Professor E. H. Ackerknecht.

2

THE MIDDLE AGES AND THE RENAISSANCE

The recorded and continuous history of psychiatry in Germany and Austria starts in the Middle Ages, when we encounter simultaneously two great psychiatric traditions: ancient humoral psychiatry and demonological-theological psychiatry. They often fused.

Hildegard of Bingen

Hildegard of Bingen (1098-1179) (Plate LI) often used both approaches. This abbess was well known throughout Europe for her abilities and her prophetic gift. Her many books, typical of the period, include a medical book, *Causae et curae* (37). This work is permeated by ancient humoralistic theories; the human organism consists of four humors, among which, according to her, phlegm plays a particularly important role. However, she does not disregard the traditional black bile as an important cause of illness. On the other hand, the treatise is full of theological ideas. The fusion of medical and religious notions of disease is noteworthy; disease as disturbance of the humoral balance, and disease as punishment for sin, are not mutually exclusive. Diseases came into this world through the fall of the first man. "If man had remained in paradise, phlegm, which produces so much disease, would not be in his body, but his flesh would be healthy and free of phlegm." Through the eating of the forbidden fruit—with Hildegard it is an apple—black bile was formed in man, and he became simultaneously accessible to suggestions by the devil. Thus dietary mistakes and taboo violation are for Hildegard an inseparable pathogenic unit of great importance.

On this theoretical basis in *Causae et curae* rests an extensive psychosomatic system. In addition, there are passages which clearly deal with psychiatric material. Idiocy (*amentia*), insanity, despair, and other character disorders are rooted in humoral inbalance. This is also true for obsession, where, however, additional spirits are attracted by the humoral weakness, endangering the salvation of the patient's soul through production of heretic ideas. In idiocy and in nightmares the devils can exert evil influences only within certain limits.

In the Renaissance, the mixture of ideas typical of Hildegard's representative medieval work tended to be replaced through a separation of theological and scientific thought derived from the Greco-Roman tradition. Priest and doctor, sinner and patient, theology and medicine, became separate entities.

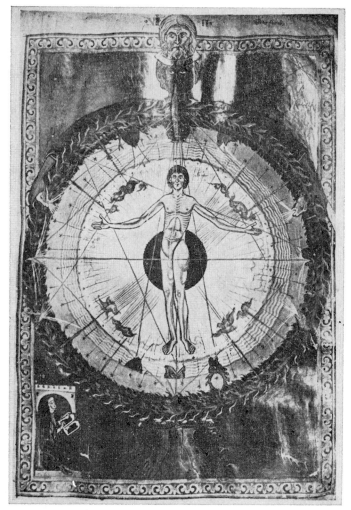

PLATE LI. Hildegard of Bingen seeing the Creator, Microcosm and
Macrocosm.

Paracelsus

Bombastus von Hohenheim, called Paracelsus (1493-1541), the Swiss-
born son of a German nobleman and doctor, has left two psychiatric
books which reflect the above situation. The first volume of his *Philosophia* contains magico-theological psychiatry. After a thorough discussion of the activities of devils and witches (up to and including rid-

ing on forks and distaffs), Paracelsus discusses the possessed. The state of possession is compared to the state of a wormeaten hazelnut (Satan has entered the healthy fruit—but, like the worm who can only enter the damaged shell of a nut, Satan can only enter humans who have been damaged by his previous attacks). Paracelsus also believed that the disease of the *lunatici* was caused by the separation of the spiritual soul from God (on account of this the corporeal soul can become diseased through the influence of the stars). Fools suffer from a malformation of their natural spirit—their corporeal soul—and therefore cannot be held personally responsible for their disease. It is the fault of Adam's and Eve's disobedience. Fools are even closer to God than we are, because their animal nature is not damaged; they should therefore be respected.

Thus Paracelsus, like Hildegard, discusses the connection between disease, especially psychiatric disease, and sin. He clearly associates psychic health with salvation through Christ, disease with sin and fall. But disease does not necessarily become punishable in the framework of these concepts, as is evidenced by his attitude towards fools.

In his earlier *Seventh Book of Medicine: Of the Diseases Which Deprive of Reason,* Paracelsus proceeds very differently. He pleads here quite definitely for a somatic-scientific approach to psychiatric diseases. He deals first with epilepsy. This "sacred disease" appears as early as in the Hippocratic book on epilepsy as a paradigm of a somatogenic disease, which affects the psyche and is therefore often erroneously derived from supernatural influences. Paracelsus deals with it in the same way. He then discusses mania, in whose pathogenesis processes of distillation and sublimation play a great role. The theological interpretations of the so-called Saint Vitus' dance are called by Paracelsus "useless chatter." Intestinal worms and retained feces play a prominent role in *suffocatio intellectus.* A fifth group of psychiatric patients, the "true senseless people," he characterizes specifically by the fact that possession by the devil cannot occur in them. The therapeutics of these psychiatric diseases are consequently somatically oriented. They consist primarily of drugs and the removal of corrupted humors (69).

Paracelsus hardly ever deals with the question of which of the two interpretations is to be applied to which psychiatric patients; that is, where one should assume a somatic etiology and where one should point to sin. His conversion-like concentration on religious problems and values, which characterizes his later life and works, perhaps made this question irrelevant to him.

Johannes Schenck

Other physicians of the Renaissance have dealt more intensively with this problem. Thus, for instance, Johannes Schenck von Grafenberg (1530-1598) tried to look at theological and medical theories of his time from a unified medical point of view. In the first book of his *Observations* (78), in which, according to the old scheme "from head to foot," he treats first the head, the discusses mental diseases among other disorders. According to him, epilepsy and other spasms, melancholy, mania, and hypochondria are pathological states which offer no difficulties, as their somatic causes are obvious. Corrupted humors, toxic vapors—especially the unavoidable black bile—are responsible. Lycanthropy, in which people believe themselves to be wolves, and incubus, are "natural" diseases.

On the advice of doctors, a manic patient was not treated by exorcism but by medicaments. Since he believed himself to be possessed, these were applied under the pretext of exorcising manipulations. The patient was cured, though he believed that not bodily medicine but exorcism had restored him.

Johannes Schenck does not dismiss possession; after the description of mania follows the description of the possessed, but even here he remains faithful to his point of departure. He underlines that there is a bodily predisposition to possession and reports that through blood-letting, purging, and sweating, he was able to increase the resistance of a woman menaced by possession against the demons so that she could be regarded as cured. The Renaissance physician mentions that the ancients too treated their possessed with drugs before and after exorcism.

The psychiatric theory of Schenck has very practical implications. During the Counter-Reformation it was dangerous to fall into the diagnostic and therapeutic machinery of the Catholic Church. Exorcism, the treatment of the possessed, could assume the form of torture (13); the purifying treatment of witches had this character to begin with. The chances of falling into this machinery were numerous. It is well known that the persecution of witches reached its peak in the 16th and 17th centuries. As physicians were often called for an opinion— whether in a given case possession, witchcraft, or natural disease was to be diagnosed (13)—the situation must have stimulated the production of medical writings concerning the subject. Here somatically oriented medical thought offered an alternative to theological and demonological thought, and in a given case could bring about the application of a purgative, where a rather disagreeable spiritual purgation was in the offing. Practical impulses and goals might thus have dictated some of Schenck's psychiatric observations.

Johan Wier (Weyer)

Similar thoughts are clearly formulated in the famous book of Johan Wier (1515-1588) who, though born in Belgium, spent most of his life in Germany and should therefore be mentioned here. In Wier's *De praestigiis demonum* (1563) (94), we find, together with somatic arguments in the style of Schenck, the theological argument that not the accused but the accusers could be under the influence of the devil.

3

THE 17TH AND 18TH CENTURIES

Iatrophysics and Iatrochemistry

During the 17th century the scientific interpretation of pathological phenomena was much extended. This development took place in the field of psychiatric phenomena as well.

During this period the two dominant trends in medical science were the physical and the chemical. Iatrophysics, stimulated by Harvey's discovery of the circulation of the blood and by the works of Descartes, analyzed physiological and pathological phenomena from the physical —especially the mechanical—point of view. Iatrochemistry, which derived from the ideas of Paracelsus, chose the chemical approach. Basically iatrochemistry and iatrophysics are different aspects of the same movement, so the limits within them are often unclear. Central Europe participated only partly in this evolution. The 30 Years War (1618-1648), and the devastation which it left behind, absorbed much of Central Europe's strength. Nevertheless, iatrochemistry in Germany had a prominent representative in the person of Michael Ettmueller (1644-1683) and iatrophysics were carried far into the 18th century by Frederic Hoffmann (1660-1742) of Halle.

An attempt was made to understand psychiatric diseases chemically or physically. Thus Ettmueller reinterpreted the old humoral theories of pathology. The chemistry of the kitchen, as cultivated by the ancients, was replaced by him by the chemistry of the alchemist's laboratory. The black bile of the ancients, the cause of melancholy, mania, and hypochondria, was for him essentially an acrid and acid humor, which could boil, ferment, and evaporate, and thus produce disease (14).

Frederic Hoffmann was inclined to use mechanical models in interpreting the cause and pathogenesis of mental diseases. According to him, spasms, atony, and difficulties of circulation played an important role in the evolution of hypochondria, of both manic and melancholic deliria and of phrenitis, the mental disturbance accompanied by fever (38).

The Classifiers and the Describers

Yet in Germany the movement, which arose as a reaction to and a compensation for these attempts at a scientific foundation of medical activity, became more important than iatrochemical and iatrophysical medicine and psychiatry. Suddenly it was realized that neither chemistry nor physics was able to give such foundations. Actually these basic sciences were far too undeveloped to be able to grasp medical phenomena without the use of speculation. Time and patience, necessary to promote the evolution of these sciences or at least to wait, were lacking. The pressure exerted by patients on their physicians and the physicians' own need for causal explanations were probably responsible for this situation. Consequently during the 18th century a tendency developed not to continue the search for scientific causes. Were there perhaps other methods that could be used to come to grips with medical experience and to orient oneself in physiology, pathology, and therapeutics? The Englishman Thomas Sydenham (88) had suggested that diseases should be classified as botanists classified their plants, or that they should be described according to their external signs, as painters depict people in their portraits (or as they did in Sydenham's times, at least).

In the 18th century, following these suggestions, very painstaking descriptions of diseases were made on the one hand, while on the other hand nosological systems were constructed, in which diseases were organized according to the model of the systematic botany of Linné. The most prominent German nosologist was Rudolph August Vogel (1724-1774), who subdivided diseases into 11 classes or 560 species. Psychiatric diseases are mostly found in his 5th and 9th classes. This was the one alternative to the search for the causes of disease "in nature's abyss of cause," as Sydenham termed it, which had been found unrewarding (18).

Animism and Vitalism

The other possibility for grasping all physiological and pathological facts without using scientific causal deductions seemed to be provided by the assumption of a hypothetical general causality, by which the gaps of knowledge could be filled. Such a causality was offered by the notion of the "soul," a notion sanctified by tradition. This entity was derived from magico-theological thought, but had been again and again regarded as the *primum movens* of vital and pathological processes. Adam started his physical existence only after God had "breathed into his nostrils the breath of life and man became a living soul." In the framework of chemiatric thought, Paracelsus had known a soul-like principle: the *archeus,* the alchemist working in the laboratory of the organism.

The iatrophysicists too had not always been able to operate without such a primary principle: Descartes, the father of the "homme machine," had attributed to this machine a soul-like manipulator. Yet, for these iatrochemists and iatrophysicists, such principles had remained in the background. They were primarily interested in phenomena which they believed to be chemically or physically explainable. Now, as confidence in chemical and physical explanations had been badly shaken, these principles came again to the foreground. Psychical causes again became convincing.

It was the pious sectarian George Ernest Stahl (Plate LII) (1660-1734) who found the cause of all vital and pathological phenomena in the soul. Stahl was a professor at the University of Halle, which had been founded in 1694. Frederic Hoffmann had been instrumental in having him called to Halle. Stahl, like Hoffmann, defended in principle a mechanistic point of view. Tension and laxness of fibers, circulation and stagnation of humors were for him central notions too. Chemical thought was equally familiar to the author of the phlogiston theory. But Stahl found it nonsensical exclusively to interpret the functioning of the organism by natural laws. Our body is inclined to move according to mechanical laws, but there is no physical, mechanical necessity to move. And even if it would move this way, the body would not be able to move rationally (82). With this theory Stahl became an opponent of Hoffmann, who acknowledged the existence of psychological causes of physiological and pathological phenomena but did not derive any all-embracing principle from this statement. Stahl demanded a very far-reaching recognition of his psychic principle, the anima, as the cause of biological phenomena. His anima was the cause of all movement. In pathology, monsters, death, jaundice, meningitis, but also sudden cure of fevers and paralysis, were the consequence of emotions (83).

The "animism" of Stahl was accepted in Montpellier and spread from there as "vitalism." It was not so much a religiously conceived soul, as a secularized form of it, a natural vital force, which was to the vitalists the primary moving force of all life. The French vitalists in their turn influenced German physicians, who recognized the "vital force" as the specific principle of living matter. One of the most prominent of them was Johann Christian Reil (1759-1813), who worked

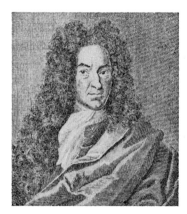

PLATE LII. George Ernest Stahl
(1660-1734)

most of the time in Halle and was known primarily as an internist. In 1795 he wrote a classic treatise on the vital force (71). Today Reil is remembered mainly for his contribution to psychiatry. It was he who first called the psychic method of treatment a part of the medical and surgical methods, and isolated its specific value in the treatment of mental diseases. Massage, flagellation, opium, and the seton were to him "psychic methods of treatment" like talking, rest, music, education, and occupational therapy, because he called "psychic" curative methods simply those therapeutic methods which "first of all influence the soul." This concept of Reil is connected with his vitalism insofar as he regarded mental diseases as diseases of the brain.

The brain, an organ presiding over the whole nervous system, is of central importance in the functioning of the vital force (72). In recommending his psychic methods of cure for mental diseases, Reil made a significant contribution towards the establishing of psychiatry as a medical specialty. Therewith an evolution, which had started with Stahl, came to an end. Stahl had by no means intended it; he had meant his animism to be the new foundation of all medicine, but the situation out of which he had created his doctrine had changed. There was no longer distrust of physics, chemistry, and anatomy. It became possible to attribute more and more diseases to somatic causes. Pathological anatomy, which was one of the most fertile methods in this respect, experienced a tremendous upsurge. Consequently the need for an etiological soul principle in medicine diminished. Wherever diseased organs could be found, it seemed possible to work without this principle. Only psychiatry remained untouched by this progress, as no clear-cut pathological lesions for mental disease could be found. Hence psychiatry began to separate from somatic medicine, and to become a discipline in itself (18). The work of Reil completed this evolution. Stahl became thus one of the most important founders of psychosomatics and Reil one of the most important founders of psychiatry as a medical specialty. Reil is also regarded as the founder of rational psychotherapy (48). He published in 1805 the first psychiatric periodical and the word "psychiatry" was coined by him (49).

Philosophical Psychiatry

During the 18th century, psychiatry was often in the hands of non-medical men. This is probably connected with the predominance of Stahlian thought in this discipline. Though, for instance, Reil had pleaded strongly for the inclusion of psychiatry in medicine, physicians could not monopolize the soul. Reil himself must have seen this difficulty. As long as psychiatric problems were those of the "soul," philanthropic clergymen (like Johann Friedrich Oberlin, made famous by George Büchner's novel *Lenz*), poets, and philosophers could be professionally concerned with such problems. The philosophical psychiatry of Immanuel Kant (1724-1804) (44) became widespread and influential. This philosopher felt that in dealing with psychiatric questions he was not only equal to, but more competent than, a medical man. He deemed it impossible that psychology could become an exact science (95). He demanded that a court in doubt as to whether a criminal had been insane when committing his deed, should submit this criminal for examination not to the medical, but to the philosophical, faculty, as this was a psychological question, and medicine was not yet sufficiently familiar with the human machine.

Johann Friedrich Herbart (1776-1841), Kant's successor in Königsberg, furthered another concept, which was to influence German-language psychiatry even more profoundly, if possible, than that of Kant. Herbart tried, in spite of Kant's opinions, to apply mathematics to psychology. He criticized the psychology of faculties which Kant had adhered to. This psychology operated with inexact notions like the faculty of representation, the faculty of feeling, the faculty of desiring, and was thus unable to become a science. Herbart therefore created a "hypothesis of representations as forces," which allowed to develop a "mathematical psychology" (36). "The lawful regularities in the human mind resemble completely those of the stars in the sky." Herbart regarded representations as forces which mutually support or inhibit each other. The association of representations was presupposed as a consequence of the unity of the soul. From these premises he derived notions like that of the darkened inhibited representation, of the threshold of conscience, and of the unconscious representation, which can influence conscience through desires. New representations provoke a movement in the total mass of the existing representations, and are in turn influenced through these. Herbart delineates here the idea of the mass of apperceptions forming experience. The dynamic relations of representations produce in the individual the phenomenon of different emotional states. This psychology spread in the German-speaking countries, together with Herbart's pedagogical doctrines, through books and the so-called "Herbart Societies" which were founded everywhere (87). Their influence is recognizable in the writings of many important contributors to psychiatry: Griesinger refers to Herbart (27); Wundt in his *Physiological Psychology* (94) calls him a great pioneer; the internist and neurologist Adolf Struempell grew up venerating Herbart (87); and as far as Freud is concerned, Maria Dorer has shown what enormous influence Herbart's theories exerted on him (11).

Simultaneously with the developments sketched out above, new approaches towards a medical-scientific psychiatry appeared during the 18th century.

Sensibility and Irritability

One of these approaches derives from Albrecht von Haller's (1708-1777) *De partibus corporis humani sensibilibus et irritabilibus*, published in 1752 (30). Haller, who by birth and allegiance was Swiss, but whose scientific life was spent mainly in Göttingen, wrote this book at the acme of his fame. Regarded as one of his most important contributions, it claims that sensibility and irritability are vital properties of certain tissues, that is, of nerves and muscles.

Those properties had nothing to do with each other. Haller tried thus to redefine these old animistic and vitalistic notions in an exact physiological fashion, and this makes his work so important for physiology (Temkin) (89). In our context it is significant that through his book the notions "sensibility" and "irritability" came into general use. The great researcher had made sensibility and irritability specific properties of all vital substances. It was not a very farfetched idea to use these entities as a key for a somatic interpretation of psychic phenomena, but Haller's definitions were rarely strictly observed.

Brownianism

One special speculative modification of neurophysiology which became particularly famous was Brownianism (Brunonianism). Its creator, John Brown, was a disciple of William Cullen, next to Haller one of the great Boerhaave-disciples, and the one who coined the expression "neurosis." To Cullen all diseases, but especially psychic diseases, were "neuroses," i.e., disturbances of the nervous function (9). In a similar fashion Brown claimed that all diseases were caused either by too much or too little irritation, irritability, and stimulus. All diseases could be treated by a corresponding stimulating diet which consisted primarily of large or small doses of alcohol or opium. It is well known that addiction-producing remedies have repeatedly been "successfully" used in therapy, including psychiatric therapy. Brownianism flourished in Vienna under Johann Peter Frank (1745-1821) and his son Joseph (59). In Germany Friedrich Wilhelm Josef Schelling (1775-1854) integrated Brownianism into his system of natural philosophy, which was to influence psychiatry profoundly. Thus many elements of the later German-language psychiatry are derived from a Haller-Cullen-Brown-neurophysiology, including the ever recurring dichotomy of psychiatric states of exaltation and depression (6).

Magnetism

The notions of sensibility and irritability were not the only means by which a scientific analysis of the "nervous force" was tried. The concept of "magnetism," as developed by Franz Anton Mesmer (1734-1815), can be regarded as another attempt to make psychic-nervous processes accessible to scientific thought. Galvanism was to play the same role later. Mesmer assumed the existence of a physical fluid which filled the whole universe. He conceived of this fluid on the model of electricity, but, after some hesitation, called it magnetic. This magnetic fluid also circulated in the human body, and irregular dis-

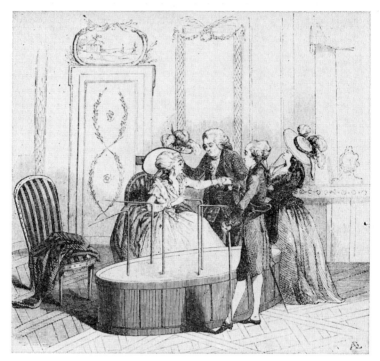

PLATE LIII. The "baquet" of Mesmer.

tribution in the body produced disease (62). On the basis of this concept Mesmer developed his therapy, which aimed to re-establish the magnetic equilibrium of the body. In the typical Mesmerian technique the patients sat around the famous *baquet* (Plate LIII) which, after the model of the Leyden jar, was regarded as the recipient of magnetic force, and let this force exert its influence on them. As a sign of cure, the patients experienced convulsion-like "crises," hence the room of treatment was called the crisis room (12). Mesmer connected his doctrine with the doctrine of irritability: the aim of his treatment was to adjust the disturbed "irritability" of the body, which was the cause of every disease. Mesmer, born and brought up in Germany, studied medicine in Vienna, where he developed his concepts. But he acquired his great reputation in the German-speaking countries only after leaving Vienna and his wife, and transferring to Paris (1777). Between 1790 and 1820 many prominent Germans defended magnetism. In the Universities of Berlin and Bonn special chairs were created (4). Magnetism was less criticized in Germany than in France.

This seems to be linked with the development of Romanticism in Germany, which will be discussed later.

Brain and Spine Localization

Meanwhile another conqueror of the realm of the psyche appeared in Vienna. Franz Josef Gall (1758-1828), who also completed his medical studies in Vienna, conceived his "organology" of the brain during the last decade of the 18th century (1). Neurophysiology and Mesmerism—insofar as they can be separated—like the animism of Stahl, were originally intended to be the foundation of the whole of medicine and became important for psychiatry *per exclusionem* only. But the organology of Gall was from the beginning conceived as a foundation for scientific psychiatry. Basically it was a doctrine of psychiatric localizations. Gall differentiated 27 "organs" in the brain. Each of these organs embodied a certain psychic function. Love of progeniture and libido were located in the occiput; the center of homicidal tendencies was parieto-occipital; the organ of theosophy occupied a central position in the apex (26); the organ of language was found bilaterally behind the orbit. The better these organs functioned, the larger they were. The skull was a "faithful cast" of these anatomical structures of the brain. This made possible the cranioscopic psycho-diagnostics which made Gall popular. The old faculties of the soul, character, the focus of mental diseases, could now be palpated. Lesky calls Gall a true son of the Viennese variety of Enlightenment medicine. The same desire to make the lesion of organs accessible to diagnostics, which had stimulated Auenbrugger's invention of percussion, was at the basis of Gall's "psychopalpation," as one might call it (59).

Gall, like Mesmer, left Vienna (1805). The Emperor had forbidden the continuation of his much frequented private courses, because his materialism was believed to be undermining religion and morals. Gall, again like Mesmer, settled in Paris, after having gained the recognition of many leading thinkers during a triumphal journey through Germany. The historical importance of Gall lies in two directions: first, in establishing a motor center of language, though in a different location from that found later by Broca; second, his "phrenology" (this term was never used by himself) drew the attention of science and of the general public to the brain as an organ of the soul (1). An old tradition of the localization of the soul thus reappeared and became for a long time an undisputed and dominant doctrine.

Before the brain gained dominance, the spinal marrow played a role as the seat of essential psychic functions. Johann Peter Frank, who later promoted Brownianism in Vienna, and helped Gall to obtain psychiatric patients from the "Narrenturm," and who for similar reasons left Vienna one year before Gall, is prominent in this respect (59). He developed the doctrine which later became well known as the skull-vertebral theory of the poet Johann Wolfgang Goethe. Frank pointed out the analogy between the skull and the vertebrae and between the brain and the segments of the spinal marrow. He replaced the old notion of the spinal marrow as a purely conductive organ by a theory of the spinal marrow as a chain of more or less autonomous organs (67). Gall too had regarded the spinal marrow as a chain of ganglia (1), and not simply as a conductor. If the segments of the spinal marrow were "small brains," they could be viewed as the seat of independent psychic functions. This idea obtained much support by Bell's and Magendie's neurophysiological explanation of the reflex, which was propagated in Germany by Johannes Mueller (1801-1858). The reflex of the spinal marrow seemed now an expression of the autonomous psychic activity of a spinal segment (19). Through a strange fusion with the notion of irritability, which Frank had introduced into the physiology of the spinal marrow, now the doctrine of "spinal irritation" arose. This supposedly very widespread disease of the spinal marrow was regarded as the root of the many symptoms which in the 18th century had been attributed to black bile or hypochondria. Palpitations, diarrheas, constipations, hysterical symptoms like headaches, convulsions, paleness, weakness, capriciousness, depressions, and other psychical symptoms as well as pain in the back were now no longer related to the upper abdomen but to the spinal marrow. The doctrine of spinal irritation has been promoted in the German language area primarily by Benedict Stilling (1810-1879), a friend of Magendie (17). Its great popularity in the German language area is undoubtedly also due to the Romantic movement.

4

THE 19TH CENTURY

Romanticism

German Romanticism, which started in the early 19th century, had a profound influence on psychiatry. To begin with, the Romantic aversion to science in medicine and psychiatry brought about an aversion to knowledge rationally acquired and a devaluation of "intelligence" as compared to "feeling" or "emotion." This alternative was thought by the Romantics to correspond to reality. Simultaneously, the notion of soul experienced a new flowering as is evidenced by *Psyche* (1846), this "precious sum of Romantic psychology" by Carl Gustav Carus (1789-1869) (8). Romanticism also implied a concentration on national history, especially the legacy of the Middle Ages. This brought about a revival of medieval thought, and a new German preoccupation with the personality and the work of Paracelsus became unavoidable.

As Romantic medicine was dominated by the natural philosophy of Schelling, the notions of polarity and evolution became central to it. Psychiatry, which even today is inclined to participate with a special intensity and sometimes lack of criticism in philosophical oscillations, was particularly stimulated by Romantic thought. Since Goethe, the Germans felt that they carried "alas, two souls" in their heart. The evolutionary model of natural philosophy seemed to be particularly fitted to psychic events. Certain ideas from the private lectures of Schelling on the soul (1810) became basic for the whole epoch (6). The Romantic-natural philosophy fusion of facts and their apperception and interpretation facilitated a "science of the soul." It made possible a tautological confirmation of psychiatric theses, by which any kind of psychiatric ideas could be made to look scientific. Good and bad, conscious and unconscious, unfree and free became the polarities around which Romantic psychology was arranged.

Johann Christian Heinroth (1773-1843) considered the principle of evil as essential in the aetiology of "disturbances of the soul." According to him, psychic disease is synonymous with absence of free will (32). Psychic health, virtue, and freedom are closely related in the traditions of the Enlightenment. In the therapeutic and legal field, in which the Romantics were particularly interested, such ideas had a humanizing influence insofar as punishment was replaced by treatment. On the other hand, therapeutics and punishment often overlapped (58). An example is provided by Ernst Horn (1774-1848), basically a very humane individual, who became notorious as the inventor of a bag, named for him, in which excited patients were enclosed as a form of therapy. His psychiatric career at the Berlin Charité ended in 1818, after he had been accused of first degree murder when a patient died in the bag (10).

Romantic psychiatry in the German speaking countries was fascinated by the alternatives: psychogenic or somatogenic (24). Heinroth believed in the primacy of the soul: "The body is submitted to the soul." He was considered a "psychicist," like Johann Gottfried Langermann (1768-1832) and Karl Wilhelm Ideler (1795-1860), who established the fame of Stahl and Langermann as the founders of psychiatry. The opposite to the "psychicists" were the "somaticists" like Maximilian Jacobi (1775-1858) and Johann Baptist Friedreich (1796-1862). For them, psychiatric disease was primarily somatic disease. In spite of this Romantic polarization of opinions, both parties agreed on basic issues, as Ernst Freiherr von Feuchtersleben (1806-1849) rightly stated (16). Both parties assumed an independent soul principle. Both had a very simplistic notion of causality. The somaticists were, in a certain sense, even more "psychic" than the "psychicists," since they supported their theory by the argument that the soul as such was unable to become primarily diseased (3).

German Romanticism also profoundly influenced Mesmerism, Brownianism, and the doctrines of spinal marrow and spinal irritation. Mesmerism was transformed under its influence from a psychophysical to a psychological speculative doctrine. This is obvious in the writings of the mesmerist Justinus Kerner (1786-1862). This poet-physician used magnetic methods in his clinical practice in Weinsberg in Swabia. One of his cases, Friederike Hauffe, born Wanner, the so-called seeress of Prevorst, has become famous. This patient was an incarnation of the Romantic problems of day and night, conscious and unconscious, the problems of double personality, the shadow, the demon-ego. In 1827-1829 Friederike lived as the object of intensive study and magnetic therapeutics with Kerner and his long-suffering wife. In 1829, Kerner published a work of 500 pages on Friederike, which carries the subtitle: *Revelations concerning the inner life of man and the interference of the world of ghosts with our own* (46). The "seeress of Prevorst," during sleep-like states, was able to speak a long forgotten language and could communicate with spirits. This case illustrates the close relation between medicine, especially psychiatry, and old demonological, theological ideas, which is typical of the Romanticism. However, the experiences and opinions of Kerner and other mesmerists and magnetisers became an important point of departure of later developments in the field of psychotherapy and psychoanalysis (12).

The Romantics popularized among doctors and the general public neurophysiological principles, especially those contained in Brownianism, in the form of the natural philosophy of Schelling (6).

The doctrine of the spinal marrow and its diseases was also modified in the Romantic period. The doctrine of "spinal irritation" can be regarded as a product of Romantic thought. This doctrine became popular because the spinal marrow tended to be regarded as the substratum of unconscious psychological processes, while the brain governed conscience; it was supported by the discovery of the relative autonomy of the segments of the spinal marrow. This theory was clearly expressed in the work of the physiologist Eduard Pflueger (1829-1910), who in his youth studied the spinal marrow. Pflueger, on the basis of his experiments, defended, with Romantic-religious zeal, the divisibility of the soul by operations (70). His doctrine became famous as the doctrine of the "spinal marrow soul." This "spinal marrow soul" is an early anatomical-physiological form of the "unconscious" (19).

Psychiatric Institutions in Germany

In the field of psychiatric institutions, decisive events took place during the first half of the 19th century in Germany (40). Romantic psychiatry undoubtedly retarded the theory of psychiatry, unless one thinks an exact science incapable of achieving progress in this field. But in the practice of psychiatry during this period, a thorough humanization of the treatment of the insane can be observed. These developments were stimulated on the one hand by the Romantic reintroduction of medieval ideals, the individualizing examination of experience, and the emancipation of psychiatry, its transformation into an independent, status-conscious specialty with its own journals and associations. On the other hand, these developments were a fruit of the revolutionary declaration of the rights of man by the Enlightenment and of its zeal to organize. In Germany, like in other countries, this transformation began with the spectacular act of the "liberation of the insane" (from their chains). In Germany this accomplishment is attributed to the "psychicist" Langermann (Bayreuth, 1805). On the other hand, Reil, whom we have mentioned previously, had indicated the directions in which the care of the insane had to be reformed. Reil counted the mental institution among the psychotherapeutic instruments. As he demanded psychic methods of cure for psychic diseases, Reil demanded special institutions for psychiatric patients. Above all, these institutions were to be therapeutically oriented. Therefore, the incurable and the curable insane should be housed separately. These institutions should receive mild names, like "pension for nervous diseases," they should not be too large, they should be located in agreeable surroundings, and offer security, stimulation, and comfort to the patients (72). During the first half of the 19th century, the construction and administration of institutions were seen for the first time in their full therapeutic importance. Steinebrunner goes so far as to call the institution "the main psychiatric therapeutic instrument of the 19th century" (84).

The contribution of Reil towards the organization of institutions had been purely theoretical; practical developments followed. Famous men of this period brought about these practical innovations; this is probably because they were closely connected with the current theories of the era. Maximilian Jacobi was one of the first who succeeded in obtaining an exclusively medical administration of an institution in his Siegburg (Plate LIV) (1825). Albert Ernst Zeller (1804-1877) be-

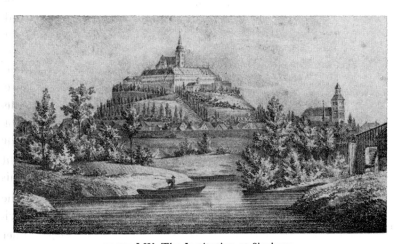

PLATE LIV. The Institution at Siegburg.

came famous through his exemplary administration of Winnenthal (Swabia), opened in 1834. Zeller had prepared himself for these activities by studying Jacobi's institution and by traveling in England and France. Christian Friedrich Wilhelm Roller (1802-1878) created, in the duchy of Baden, the Illenau (1842), in a new building which became the prototype for German institutions for the insane for the next 50 years (84). Roller became well known also through his books on practical management of the insane. In his book, *The Mental Institution in All its Aspects* (1831) (74), nothing is omitted which seemed of practical importance to the author: recommendations for the structure of case histories or recommendations on how to build floors and walls, considerations of dress for patients, or the management of convalescence, or the arguments against lying to the patient, or against observation holes in doors.

Another influential psychiatric institution was Nietleben near Halle, a product of the theoretical and practical endeavors of the psychiatrist Heinrich Damerow (1798-1866). It was opened in 1844 (68).

It is interesting that during the first half of the 19th century the non-restraint system of Conolly found little acclaim in Germany in spite of the fact that the reforms of this period had received strong stimuli from England. It was admitted that non-restraint might be good for English patients, but for German institutions a psychotherapy based on some constraint seemed preferable (39). The change occurred only in the 1860's, after the translation into German of Conolly's *The Treatment of the Insane without Mechanical Restraint* (1860), and after the influential Wilhelm Griesinger (1817-1868), in the second edition of his text (1861) (28), stressed his agreement with the non-restraint system.

Psychiatric Institutions in Austria

The situation in the practical care of the insane differed in Austria from the one in Germany. Not only the non-restraint system but the whole reform of the care of the insane did not take place until the second half of the 19th century. The so-called Narrenturm, erected in 1784 by the Emperor Joseph II, was a massive circular structure with a prison-like appearance, which proved to be an impediment for such reforms. Bruno Goergen (1777-1842), stimulated by the French and the Germans, had created, in 1819, an institution for the insane which corresponded to contemporary standards, but this was a private institution and flourished in the second half of the century. Narrenturm did not lose its function until 1853, when the imperial and royal institution for the cure and care of the insane (*k.k. Heil- und Pflege-Anstalt*) was opened. Here, Carl Spurzheim (1809-1872), the nephew of the collaborator of Gall, introduced the non-restraint system (59).

Brain Psychiatry and Psychophysics

The great advance of German and Austrian neuropsychiatry, "brain psychiatry," started with Wilhelm Griesinger (1817-1868). The psychiatry of Griesinger illustrates very well the relations of this new psychiatric trend with Romantic psychiatry. Griesinger was not primarily a psychiatrist but an internist. Together with his lifelong friends, the surgeon Roser and the internist Wunderlich, under the influence of Johannes Mueller and the French physiologists, he became the leader of a new, physiologically oriented, anti-Romantic medicine in Germany (2). In psychiatry too Griesinger's orientation was physiological.

In his confidence in physiology he felt related to the iatrophysicists of the 17th century, who had put similar confidence into the mechanic sciences (6). Following Gall and the somaticist Friedreich, he regarded the life of the psyche primarily as a function of the brain. Although Griesinger was an anti-Romanticist in psychiatry, it cannot be denied that his psychiatry, in the type of questions it asked and the type of answers it gave, exhibits many Romantic traits (6). Ackerknecht says that Griesinger put Romantic psychology "on its feet," like Marx claimed to have "put on its feet" Hegelian philosophy (3).

Griesinger, as a young physician, worked for two years with A. E. Zeller in Winnenthal. This was—except for the last three years of his life—the only period which he spent in full-time psychiatric practice. From this period derives his interest in psychiatry. Under the influence of his time and of Johannes Mueller, Griesinger inclined in the beginning towards a reflexological psychiatry. As early as 1843, he published an article entitled *"On psychic reflexes: With an excursion into the essence of psychic diseases."* Here he compared brain function and function of the spinal marrow, psychic activity and spinal reflexes. In 1844, in another article, he expressed the hope that this comparison could become as fertile for a correct analysis of psychic phenomena as the skull-vertebral theory had become for an understanding of the structure of the skull (29). In the first edition of his authoritative *Pathology and Therapeutics of Psychic Diseases,* he stated that psychic life is a function of the brain, psychic diseases are always "diseases of the brain." As the disease notion of Griesinger was physiological, a strict anatomical localization was not intended by him (27). These ideas of his combined without difficulty with Zeller's doctrine of the unitarian psychosis (96), according to which all psychiatric diseases followed a similar pattern, and different disease pictures were only stages of one and the same disease. This prevented Griesinger from seeing the importance of the discovery of general paresis by the Frenchman Antoine Laurent Bayle, in 1822. Bayle had found, for the first time in the history of psychiatry, a true nosological unit (66). Griesinger had created his theory of psychiatry to overcome the difficulties of differentiating clinical entities, and, to a certain extent, he succeeded. But his theory simultaneously preserved this difficulty; thus he regarded the paralysis of the syphilitic patients, just as the convulsions of epileptics, as mere "complications of insanity" (27).

Griesinger devised a psychology which was closely related to his brain physiology. His point of departure was the psychology of Herbart, It seemed to him that a psychological analysis of psychiatric phenomena was justified, because disturbances of the will and of representations were symptoms of brain lesions. Thus he regarded psychological descriptions as the adequate method of describing psychiatric disease. Griesinger developed certain ideas of Herbart into psychological concepts which seem very modern today. Numerous notions which were later appropriated by psychoanalysis can be found in his work (11). But Griesinger became famous not through his psychological contribution but for his somatic foundations of psychiatry. This is because he stands at the turning point from a "psychiatry of institutions" to a "psychiatry of university departments." The latter necessarily followed contemporary scientific thought.

Thus the second half of the 19th century became a period of intensive research into the somatic phenomena of mental disease (weight, temperature, pulse, composition of blood, electric reactions). It was the dictum of Griesinger that psychic diseases are "always diseases of the brain" (27); this formulation corresponded to the dominating pathologic localizing thought of his time. In Austria, especially in Vienna, the soil was well prepared through a tradition which already supported Gall's localizing doctrine. In 1860 Maximilian Leidesdorf (1818-1889) published his *Pathology and Therapy of Psychic Diseases* (58), which imitates the great example of Griesinger in more than just the title (59).

Theodor Meynert (1833-1892), a disciple of the eminent Viennese pathologist Karl Rokitansky, devised a detailed modification of Griesinger's doctrine of localization. Meynert had started his psychiatric career in 1865 by collaborating in the chapter on brain anatomy in the second edition of Leidesdorf's textbook (58). In his *Psychiatry. A Clinic of the Diseases of the Forebrain* (1884) (63), Meynert developed his views into an all-embracing system. In 1890 he believed that psychiatry had definitely entered a stage in which the explanation of phenomena could replace their description (64). Meynert's interpretations center above all on the contrast between the cortex as the seat of representations, and the brain stem as the seat of apperception and movement. The most important pathogenic mechanisms are, according to Meynert, of a hemodynamic nature.

The work of Meynert had in many respects a stimulating effect on the psychiatric research of his time (59). Carl Wernicke (1848-1905), the later chair-holder in Breslau, had worked in his laboratory. Wernicke's work reached a new stage in localization psychiatry. Wernicke continued the tradition of Gall in adding to the motor center of language, meanwhile discovered by Broca, a sensory center of language (92). Wernicke continued the tradition of Gall also in claiming that research in brain localization would be the true and certain road for psychiatric research. For him aphasia was the paradigm of psychiatric disease. With his "aphasia pattern," he believed he had found the model of all mental diseases, which to him were diseases of the "organ of association" (93).

Another attempt to find a scientific foundation for psychiatry came from the physiological laboratory. While for the brain anatomists aphasia was the model, for this scientific trend, sensory physiology was the model of psychophysiological function. This is obvious in the basic work of Gustav Theodor Fechner (1801-1887), *Elements of Psychophysics* (1860) (15). Fechner modified the law of Ernst Heinrich Weber (1795-1878) concerning the relation between the intensity of stimuli and the sensory reaction which follows. He called this a fundamental law, and Weber the "father" of psychophysiology. Hermann Helmholtz (1821-1894), through his *Doctrine of the Acoustic Sensations* (1862) (35), nourished the hope that psychology would be based on exact scientific notions. Wilhelm Wundt (1832-1920) eventually came to his "physiologic psychology" via sensory physiology. Sensory physiology is therefore in the foreground in his authoritative treatise (95). Wundt published in 1889 a second edition of the psychophysics of Fechner.

Towards the end of the century, anatomical and physiological aetiologies no longer satisfied the physicians' needs for causality. The rise of bacteriology in the 1870's and 1880's had provoked intensive discussion on aetiology in general. Pathological anatomists had prepared this evolution, and bacteriologists, who now believed they had discovered the true causes of disease, had started the controversy. This concern with aetiology spread also to psychiatry, where it was more intense, because aetiological knowledge, even knowledge of pathologic anatomical lesions, was mostly absent (20). Mental diseases of syphilitic origin were the much appreciated exception.

Theoretical psychiatry reacted to this situation in different ways. It partly exchanged somato-scientific research methods for other methods. Even within scientific thought, aetiological alternatives appeared. A certain eminence was achieved by toxicology, by the doctrine of heredity (which fused with Darwinian evolutionism, the degeneration doctrine imported from France, constitution doctrine, and later theories of memory (77)), and, eventually, hypotheses on the traumatic origin of mental disease. Alcoholism served as a paradigm for an exogenous toxic aetiology of psychic disease (55). It was predestined for this role not only on account of its great frequency, but also because an adequate therapy, abstinence, resulted from aetiological insight. Thyroid dysfunctions and autointoxications from the intestine served as paradigms of endogenous intoxication producing psychiatric disease (89). Evolutionary thought reinforced theories concerning stages of psychic function, and stimulated discussions which led to the emergence of child psychiatry (47).

Heredity and degeneration are regarded as the predominant aetiological factors in the works of Heinrich Schuele (1840-1916) (79) and his friend Richard von Krafft-Ebing (1840-1902) (57). Krafft-Ebing had been drawn into psychiatry by the example of Griesinger and became the successor of Leidesdorf and, later, of Meynert in Vienna. He is best known for his work in the fields of legal psychiatry and sexual pathology. His *Psychopathia Sexualis* (1886)—also a "forensic" study, by the way—was an enormous success and the signal for a wave of intensive research in sexual problems (12). Towards the end of the century, not only were sexual disorders much discussed but also the sexual aetiology of psychic disorders. Sexual aetiology, insofar as sexuality is somatically interpreted, can be regarded as an aetiological alternative in the framework of somatic-scientific thought.

Psychology and Sociology Toward the End of the 19th Century

In the 17th century chemistry and physics had not provided medicine with answers to its questions, and towards the end of the 19th century psychiatry remained dissatisfied by the answers provided by the somatic-scientific approach. Too many of the claims of psychophysiology and of "brain psychiatry" seemed to be speculative and unproven. Nissl spoke in this context of "brain mythology," Emil Kraepelin of "speculative anatomy" (3). Again, but this time only in the field of psychiatry, the opinion spread that scientific aetiological research was inadequate. Again two alternatives appeared: empiricism and the "soul." Both differed from their analogues in the 18th century insofar as they were only methodic alternatives, and, in the beginning, did not antagonize the results of other research methods. Stahl introduced his "anima" as an entity which science had overlooked. Freud and Moebius introduced the "psyche" as an element of a method of thought neglected by science: psychology. The "anima" of Stahl was the more or less scientific cause of all life and disease processes. The "psyche" of the late 19th century was, in the beginning, only the psychological aspect of something which was not yet accessible to natural science in psychiatry. Paul Julius Moebius (1853-1907) deliberately placed psychology as a method outside the natural sciences (65). In this he followed a suggestion of Adolf Struempell (1853-1925) who, through his father who was a professor of philosophy, was an admirer of Herbart and was psychologically oriented (87). Meynert's pupil, Sigmund Freud (1856-1939), spoke of his psychology as "psychological provisoriums" and never abandoned the opinion that "the building of psychoanalysis must at a given time be put on its organic foundations" (22). However, he did not continue in his early attempts to create these foundations (compare his *Project for a Scientific Psychology*, 1895) (12).

The reconquest of psychiatry by psychology began in the field of neuroses, especially hysteria. While general paresis and aphasia had been the paradigms for the somatic-scientific oriented psychiatry, psychological psychiatry found its paradigm in hysteria. Hysteria was, even more than other neuroses, in the framework of somatic-scientific thought, a disease of unknown aetiology. Hysteria was, even more than other neuroses, predestined to be interpreted psychologically: it was the old disease of dissatisfied women—the lying disease, with crises which reminded one of exorcisms and of the curative crises of Mesmer. Thus the psychological legacy of magnetism, hypnotism, suggestion, and the philosophic psychology of Carus, Schopenhauer, Nietzsche, and many others entered the field of hysteria theory (12). Now, all of a sudden, hysteria seemed to be understandable. Phenomena of suggestion, unconscious representations and desires, and split personality seemed to explain the disease picture. The French (Charcot, Janet) were the first to interpret hysteria psychologically (61). Now, pathogenic representations dwelling in the unconscious were considered the cause of this disease. Stahl had already known "pathogenic ideas" (51). Moritz Benedikt (1835-1920) of Vienna regarded the "pathogenic secret," often with a sexual content, as the cause of most cases of hysteria (12). Consequently, a psychotherapy based on such theories—in the case of Benedikt it was liberation from the secret— was the rational therapy for this disease. Ellenberger connects the ideal of uncovering, which is behind this concept, with a general "unmasking trend," characteristic of the *belle époque* (12). The idea of the psychological test might also be partially rooted in this trend. Not only Benedikt, but also Struempell, Moebius, Joseph Breuer (1842-1925), and Sigmund Freud (7) first developed their psychological ways of analysis in connection with hysteria. Departing from this doctrine of hysteria, the above-mentioned generalization of psychological analysis followed and led to the application of psychological interpretations to neurasthenia, to the whole field of neuroses, and to psychiatry in general.

The new psychological approach crystallized around forensic problems. It seems that again and again forensic problems provoked new approaches in psychiatry. The practical forensic application of ruling medical and psychiatric theories invites critical reexaminations of these theories. Such a mutual influence is observable as early as the psychiatric theories of the Renaissance. Gall and Griesinger were very much concerned with the implications of their ideas in legal practice. The intense preoccupation of the Romantic psychiatrists with forensic problems also suggests a stimulus exerted by practical forensic experiences on Romantic psychiatry.

"Traumatic neurosis" played an important role in the rise of a psychological view of neuroses (21). Whether traumatic neuroses should be recognized as true diseases, or whether they should be treated as a product of simulation, was a practical problem. In this sense Moebius classified traumatic neurosis as hysteria, and introduced its psychological interpretation in order to protect the traumatic neurotic against the aggressive diagnosis of simulation. According to Moebius, most cases of so-called simulation were misdiagnosed hysterias, misdiagnosed on account of the lack of psychological understanding and of psychiatric abilities on the part of physicians.

The early publications of Freud show a tendency to apply the traumatic aetiology of traumatic neuroses to the whole field of hysteria, i.e., of psychogenic neuroses (7). Later, trauma was replaced by sexuality as the universal aetiology of neurosis. Both had still in common a very material element—the "concussion" or Freud's "sexual toxin." As sexuality was more suited to psychological interpretation, trauma receded into the background of psychoanalytic theory and the sex theory was developed into the libido theory (22). The notions of the "traumatic moment" and of the "psychic trauma" still remind us of Freud's early endeavors.

5

THE 20TH CENTURY

The period from 1890 to World War I is characterized by a relatively peaceful pluralism in psychiatric thought. Somatic-scientific and psychological approaches appeared as different aspects of the same thing.

War Neurosis and Social Conditions

World War I brought about a profound change in this situation (21). Under the pressure of events, a polarization took place which

made science and psychology mutually exclusive. The immediate
reason was a special form of traumatic neurosis, war hysteria, which
from 1914 to 1918 was so widespread as to constitute a danger for the
nation. It was an act of national self-protection to refuse to regard
war neurotics and war hysterics as sick people. This was done by
applying psychological arguments. As hysteria was psychogenic, it was
not a disease. Thus the psychological interpretation, at least in the

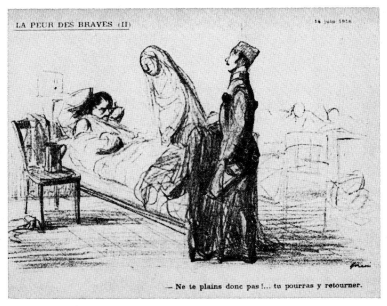

PLATE LV. The situation of the soldier in World War I.

field of neuroses, became dominant during World War I (Plate LV),
while the somatic medical approach was regarded as irrelevant,
if not erroneous. Psychoanalysis profited from this wave, in spite of
the fact that Freud did not participate in the discrimination of the
war hysterics and the devaluation of psychological aetiology. After
the two wars psychoanalysis and its byproducts were to monopolize the psychological market in medicine.

Again, during World War I, people realized that mental disease
could be regarded from a sociological point of view. We have reported
above that a sociological alternative in psychiatric aetiology developed
in the 18th century, and again in the 19th century, when there was

widespread disappointment with a somato-scientific foundation of psychiatry. During the 18th century, the sociological approach became particularly obvious in the analysis of hypochondria. Responsible for this disease were not only the "hypochondriac organs" (liver and spleen, the old sources of disease-producing bile, and stomach), or the "soul," but also social phenomena (17). Insofar as hypochondria was a disease of civilization, it was quite obvious that it had to be sociogenic.

Sociological aetiology receded in psychiatry, when, during the 19th century, the conviction spread that the causes of the earlier "hypochondria" could be found in the nervous system. Thus, these symptoms were described as "spinal irritation," "nervous disease," or "neurosis." The sociological interpretation reappeared when the supposed changes of the nervous system could not be identified. The same recurrence had taken place in the case of psychological causality. The discussion around traumatic neurosis served as the point of departure for this approach (21). This disease was the first to be explained by many physicians as caused exclusively by social situations, in this case by the existence of insurance policies. Thus, during the last two decades of the 19th century, a sociogenic doctrine of neurosis developed, helped by the myth of neurosis as a disease of civilization and by the political currents of the time.

Stimulated by the bourgeois historian Karl Lamprecht, Willy Hellpach (1877-1955) suggested a social pathology of hysteria in a bourgeois mood (34), while, under the influence of Karl Marx, Alfred Adler (1870-1937) studied the social roots and causes of diseases (81), starting in 1898 with his *Health Guide for Tailors*. The approach used in occupational hygiene became an integrated element of his later *Individual Psychology,* a study of social conditions and causes of disease.

During and after World War I, sociological thought entered psychiatry on a larger scale. Therewith Adler's ideas have become generally adopted in psychological medicine. It is a remarkable phenomenon that now his name is only rarely mentioned, although his terminology is still used (12, 81).

Forms of therapy which correspond to a sociological interpretation of psychiatric disease flourished after 1918. In the 1920's, the "active treatment" inaugurated by Hermann Simon (1867-1947) of Gütersloh (80) marked the beginning of modern occupational therapy. Political social therapy which does not aim at the patient, but at his environment, be it through racial hygiene or revolution, is another fruit of sociological thought in psychiatry.

Clinical Psychiatry and Research

Psychiatry found methodical alternatives for the unsatisfactory "brain psychiatry" of the 19th century not just in non-medical disciplines. Medicine itself had an alternative to offer: this was again the descriptive and classifying method, the so-called empirical method. Emil Kraepelin's (1856-1926) attitude towards a system of psychiatry in the style of Meynert was critical. His method was the method of systematic collection and description of facts (53). The eight editions of his little *Compendium* (52), later the multivolume "Textbook" of psychiatry (54), issued between 1883 and 1914, witness how faithfully Kraepelin followed this method. The work was not only continuously increased in size, it was changed again and again. In the course of these changes, the so-called "clinical" method of Kraepelin developed, which incorporates all experience and insight in the field of psychiatry based on science, insofar as such insight is relevant for clinical activities. Kraepelin differs from the empirics and systematics of the 18th century through a more highly developed consciousness of his methods. He did not want to give a "system of psychiatry" but rather a "system" which made possible an unencumbered survey of the total psychiatric knowledge of his time.

The clinical psychiatry which Kraepelin taught was, like contemporary speculative psychology, conscious of the farreaching ignorance of the causes of mental disease. It tried to bridge this gap by clinical delineation of disease entities. In studying the total picture, the evolution of the disease in individuals and statistics, a natural division of mental diseases was to be obtained in spite of the still lacking aetiological knowledge. In this sense Kraepelin established, for instance, the clinical entity *dementia praecox,* the predecessor of the "schizophrenias" of E. Bleuler. Important for this clinical psychiatry was the differentiation in principle between disease processes and psychopathological states. Kraepelin derived this differentiation from Karl Ludwig Kahlbaum (1828-1899) (55). Kahlbaum had differentiated in this sense between states or habitual forms and disease forms (43). He became famous for this accomplishment only with and after Kraepelin (45). The Kraepelin-Kahlbaum notion of the psychopathological state (*Zustandsbild*) implies no aetiological judgment. This makes possible an even more unprejudiced approach to psychiatric phenomena than that given by the Zeller-Griesinger concept of the unitarian psychosis. This approach also made possible the integration of general paresis into psychiatric theory, which had not been possible with the Zeller-Griesinger concept.

Besides his empirical clinical work, Kraepelin promoted basic sciences (50). This corresponded to his fundamental attitude as well as his education. As a young man he had worked in Leipzig with the neurologist Wilhelm Heinrich Erb (1840-1921) and with Wundt. In Leipzig, Fechner's adopted city, Wundt founded the first institute for experimental psychology (1879). Kraepelin furthered neuropathological talents like Alois Alzheimer (1864-1915) and Franz Nissl (1860-1919) (31) as early as in the 1890's, when he was a professor in Heidel-

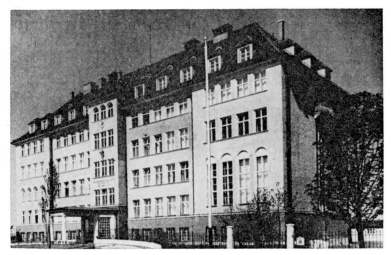

PLATE LVI. Kraepelin's Institute at about 1918.

berg. The name of Alzheimer is still remembered on account of the eponym "Alzheimer's disease," which Kraepelin introduced. The name of Nissl survives among other things in Nissl's "granules." Kraepelin brought Nissl to the Research Institute which he founded in 1917 in Munich. This Institute comprised, besides a brain pathology division, a clinical, a serological, and a genealogical division, and was a cradle of great names.

The Institute of Kraepelin was exemplary (Plate LVI), but it had predecessors. The Vienna Neurological Institute of Heinrich Obersteiner (1847-1922) (60) deserves a special mention in this context. Obersteiner had, like Freud, worked as a student in the famous physiological Institute of Ernst Wilhelm Bruecke (1819-1892). He then became *Dozent* for neuroanatomy and neuropathology and, in 1882, founded the institute which was the first brain research institute in the world.

The Obersteiner Institute stimulated numerous similar foundations which have produced important work and stimulated further research (60). Research in basic neuropsychiatry has also been cultivated outside the walls of such institutes. Hans Berger (1873-1941), the discoverer of the EEG (1924, published 1929), made his studies in a hidden room on the grounds of the psychiatric clinic of the University of Jena, which he directed (31).

The amount of somato-medical research in psychiatry is enormous, but therapeutic fruits are still sparse. The discovery of malaria treatment for general paresis by Julius Wagner von Jauregg (1857-1940), the introduction of the insulin shock therapy of psychosis by Manfred Sakel (1900-1957) (76), and of similar therapies which have been used in German-speaking countries, did not follow exact somato-medical deductions. Like the introduction of bromine and luminal, and like later discoveries in psychopharmacology, including the discovery of lithium, they are products of accident. The effect of fevers, and among them malaria, on mental disease had been known for a long time through accidental observations. The great scientific merit of Wagner is to have examined scientifically this phenomenon and applied it. He was not able to find how it works (91). Nevertheless, in 1927, he received the Nobel prize for his malaria treatment, so far the only psychiatrist to receive this prize, for the simple reason that this treatment was successful.

To this day, somato-medical research in psychiatry has produced few results in the field of therapy. If this were not the case, the question of what is the best research method in this discipline would not be so much discussed. But, under the circumstances, the old problems of psychiatry continue to be relevant in Germany and Austria as well as elsewhere.

REFERENCES

1. ACKERKNECHT, E. H. & VALLOIS, H. V. (1956): *Franz Joseph Gall, Inventor of Phrenology and his Collection*. Madison, Wisconsin: Department of History of Medicine, University of Wisconsin Medical School.
2. ACKERKNECHT, E. H. (1967): *Kurze Geschichte der Medizin*. Revised edition. Stuttgart: F. Enke.
3. ACKERKNECHT, E. H. (1967): *Kurze Geschichte der Psychiatrie*. 2nd edition. Stuttgart: F. Enke.
4. ARTELT, W. (1965): *Der Mesmerismus in Berlin*. Mainz: Akademie der Wissenschaften und der Literatur.

5. BENZ, E. (1971): *Theologie der Elektrizität. Zur Begegnung und Auseinandersetzung von Theologie und Naturwissenschaft in 17. und 18. Jahrhundert.* Mainz: Akademie der Wissenschaften.

6. BODAMER, J. (1949): *Zur Ideengeschichte der Psychiatrie. Wilhelm Griesinger. Das Leben und das Werk.* Heidelberg: Scherer.

7. BREUER, J. & FREUD, S. (1893): Ueber den psychischen Mechanismus hysterischer Phänomene. (Vorläufige Mitteilung). *Neurol. Zentbl.,* 12, 4, 43.

8. CARUS, C. G. *Psyche. Zur Entwicklungsgeschichte der Seele.* Nachwort by R. MARX. Leipsic: A Kröner.

9. CULLEN, W. (1786): *Kurzer Inbegriff der medicinischen Nosologie: oder systematische Eintheilung der Krankheiten von Cullen, Linné, Sauvages, Vogel und Sagar.* After the 3rd edition. Leipsic: C. Fritsch.

10. DOERNER, K. (1969): *Bürger und Irre. Zur Sozialgeschichte und Wissenschaftssoziologie der Psychiatrie.* Frankfort-on-the-Main: Europäische Verlagsanstalt.

11. DORER, M. (1932): *Historische Grundlagen der Psychoanalyse.* Leipsic: F. Meiner.

12. ELLENBERGER, H. F. (1970): *The Discovery of the Unconscious. The History and Evolution of Dynamic Psychiatry.* New York: Basic Books Inc.

13. ERNST, C. (1972): *Teufelaustreibungen. Die Praxis der katholischen Kirche im 16. und 17. Jahrhundert.* Berne: H. Huber.

14. ETTMUELLER, M. (1688): *Opera omnia.* Frankfort-on-the-Main: J. D. Zunner.

15. FECHNER, G. T. (1860): *Elemente der Psychophysik.* 2 volumes. Leipsic: Breitkopf und Härtel.

16. FEUCHTERSLEBEN, E. (1845): *Lehrbuch der ärztlichen Seelenkunde.* Vienna: C. Gerold.

17. FISCHER-HOMBERGER, E. (1970): *Hypochondrie. Melancholie bis Neurose, Krankheiten und Zustandsbilder.* Berne: H. Huber.

18. FISCHER-HOMBERGER, E. (1970): Eighteenth-Century Nosology and its Survivors. *Med. Hist.,* 14, 397.

19. FISCHER-HOMBERGER, E. (1970): Railway Spine und traumatische Neurose—Seele und Rückenmark. *Gesnerus,* 27, 96.

20. FISCHER-HOMBERGER, E. (1971): Charcot und die Aetiologie der Neurosen. *Gesnerus,* 28, 35.

21. FISCHER-HOMBERGER, E.: *Ursachen der traumatischen Neurose von der "Railway Spine" bis nach dem Ersten Weltkrieg.* Unpublished.

22. FREUD, S. (1940-1950): *Gesammelte Werke, chronologisch geordnet.* 17 volumes. London: Imago Publishing.

23. FRIEDREICH, J. B. (1830): *Versuch einer Literärgeschichte der Pathologie und Therapie der psychischen Krankheiten. Von den ältesten Zeiten bis zum neunzehnten Jahrhundert.* Reprint of the Würzburg edition, Amsterdam, 1965: E. J. Bonset.

24. FRIEDREICH, J. B. (1836): *Historisch-kritische Darstellung der Theorien über das Wesen und den Sitz der psychischen Krankheiten.* Reprint of the Leipsic edition. Amsterdam, 1964: E. J. Bonset.

25. FRIEDREICH, J. B. (1839): *Handbuch der allgemeinen Pathologie der psychischen Krankheiten.* Erlangen: J. J. Palm und E. Enke.

26. (GALL, F. J.) (1807): *Dr. F. J. Galls neue Entdeckungen in der Gehirn-, Schedel- und Organenlehre.* Karlsruhe: C. F. Müller.

27. GRIESINGER, W. (1845): *Die Pathologie und Therapie der psychischen Krankheiten.* Stuttgart: A. Krabbe.

28. GRIESINGER, W. (1861): *Die Pathologie und Therapie der psychischen Krankheiten.* 2nd edition. Stuttgart: A. Krabbe.

29. GRIESINGER, W. (1872): *Gesammelte Abhandlungen,* volume I: *Psychiatrische und nervenpathologische Abhandlungen.* Berlin: A. Hirschwald.

30. HALLER, A. (1755): *A Dissertation on the Sensible and Irritable Parts of Animals.*

Reprint of the London edition. Introduction by O. Temkin, (1936). *Bull. Inst. Hist. Med. Johns Hopkins Univ.*, 4, 651.

31. HAYMAKER, W. & SCHILLER, F. (Eds.) (1970): *The Founders of Neurology*. 2nd edition. Springfield, Illinois: Charles C Thomas.

32. HEINROTH, J. CH. A. (1818): *Lehrbuch der Störungen des Seelenlebens oder der Seelenstörungen und ihrer Behandlung*. 2 parts. Leipsic: F. C. W. Vogel.

33. HEINROTH, J. CH. A. (1825): *Anweisung für angehende Irrenärzte zu richtiger Behandlung ihrer Kranken. Als Anhang zu seinem Lehrbuch der Seelenstörungen*. Leipsic: F. C. W. Vogel.

34. HELLPACH, W. (1904): *Grundlinien einer Psychologie der Hysterie*. Leipsic: W. Engelmann.

35. HELMHOLTZ, H. (1870): *Die Lehre von den Tonempfindungen, als physiologische Grundlage für die Theorie der Musik*. 3rd edition. Brunswick: F. Vieweg & Sohn.

36. HERBART, J. F. (1816): *Lehrbuch der Psychologie*. Königsberg and Leipsic: A. W. Unzer.

37. HILDEGARDIS. *Causae et curae*, ed. by P. Kaiser (1903). Leipsic: B. G. Teubner.

38. HOFFMANN, F. (1748): *Opera omnia physico-medica*. 6 volumes. Geneva: De Tournes fratres.

39. JACKI, C. *Rezeption des Non Restraint in Deutschland*. Unpublished.

40. JETTER, D. (1971): *Zur Typologie des Irrenhauses in Frankreich und Deutschland (1780-1840)*. Wiesbaden: F. Steiner.

41. IDELER, K. W. (1835): *Grundriss der Seelenheilkunde*. Berlin: T.Ch.F. Enslin.

42. KAHLBAUM, K. (1863): *Die Gruppirung der psychischen Krankheiten und die Eintheilung der Seelenstörungen*. Dantzic: A. W. Kaufmann.

43. KAHLBAUM, K. (1878): *Die klinisch-diagnostischen Gesichtspunkte der Psychopathologie*. Leipsic: Breitkopf und Härtel.

44. KANT, I. (1833): *Anthropologie in pragmatischer Hinsicht*. 4th edition, with an introduction by J. F. Herbart. Leipsic: I. Müller.

45. KATZENSTEIN, R. (1963): *Karl Ludwig Kahlbaum und sein Beitrag zur Entwicklung der Psychiatrie*. Dissertation. Zürich: Juris.

46. KERNER, J. (1829): *Die Seherin von Prevorst. Eröffnungen über das innere Leben des Menschen und über das Hereinragen einer Geisterwelt in die unsere*. 2 parts. Stuttgart and Tübingen: J. G. Cotta.

47. KINDT, H. (1971): *Vorstufen der Entwicklung zur Kinderpsychiatrie im 19. Jahrhundert*. Dissertation. Freiburg: H. F. Schulz.

48. KIRCHHOFF, TH. (1921-1924): *Deutsche Irrenärzte*. 2 volumes. Berlin: J. Springer.

49. KOELBING, H. M. *Skizzen zur Geschichte der Psychiatrie*. Unpublished.

50. KOLLE, K. (1956-1963): *Grosse Nervenärzte*. 3 volumes. Stuttgart: G. Thieme.

51. KORNFELD, S. (1905): Geschichte der Psychiatrie. In: Neuburger, M., and Pagel, J. (Ed.), *Handbuch der Geschichte der Medizin*, vol. 3. Jena: G. Fischer.

52. KRAEPELIN, E. (1883): *Compendium der Psychiatrie*. Leipsic: A. Abel.

53. KRAEPELIN, E. (1887): *Die Richtungen der psychiatrischen Forschung*. Leipsic: F. C. W. Vogel.

54. KRAEPELIN, E. (1909-1915): *Psychiatrie. Ein Lehrbuch*. 8th edition. 4 volumes. Leipsic: J. A. Barth.

55. KRAEPELIN, E. (1918): *Ziele und Wege der psychiatrischen Forschung*. Berlin: J. Springer.

56. KRAEPELIN, E. (1918): Hundert Jahre Psychiatrie. *Z. ges. Neurol. Psychiat.*, Orig. 38, 161.

57. KRAFFT-EBING, R. (1888): *Lehrbuch der Psychiatrie auf klinischer Grundlage*. 3rd edition. Stuttgart: F. Enke.

58. LEIDESDORF, M. (1865): *Lehrbuch der psychischen Krankheiten*. 2nd. edition. Erlangen: F. Enke.

59. LESKY, E. (1965): *Die Wiener medizinische Schule im 19. Jahrhundert.* Graz-Cologne: H. Böhlaus.

60. LESKY, E. (1971): Hirnforschung in Oesterreich. *Oest. Aerzteztg.,* 26, 417.

61. LEVIN, K. *The Status of Somatic Models in Freud's Early Psychology.* Unpublished.

62. MESMER, F. A. (1812): *Allgemeine Erläuterungen über den Magnetismus und den Somnambulismus.* Halle and Berlin: Buchhandlung des Hallischen Waisenhauses.

63. MEYNERT, TH. (1884): *Psychiatrie. Klinik der Erkrankungen des Vorderhirnes.* 1st part. Vienna: W. Braumüller.

64. MEYNERT, TH. (1890): *Klinische Vorlesungen über Psychiatrie auf wissenschaftlichen Grundlagen.* Vienna: W. Braumüller.

65. MOEBIUS, P. J. (1894:) *Neurologische Beiträge,* 1st part: Ueber den Begriff der Hysterie und andere Vorwürfe vorwiegend psychologischer Art. Leipsic: A. Abel.

66. MUELLER, ST. (1965): *Antoine-Laurent Bayle. Sein grundlegender Beitrag zur Erforschung der progressiven Paralyse.* Dissertation. Zurich: Juris.

67. NEUBURGER, M. (1909): Johann Peter Frank als Begründer der Rückenmarkspathologie. *Wien. klin. Wschr.,* 22, 1341.

68. PANSE, F. (1964): *Das psychiatrische Krankenhauswesen.* Stuttgart: G. Thieme.

69. PARACELSUS: *Sämtliche Werke,* Ed. by K. Sudhoff, (1922-1960). 1st section: Medizinische, naturwissenschaftliche und philosophische Schriften. 14 volumes. Munich and Berlin: R. Oldenburg; Munich: O. W. Barth.

70. PFLUEGER, E. (1853): *Die sensorischen Funktionen des Rückenmarks der Wirbelthiere.* Berlin: A. Hirschwald.

71. REIL, J. CH. (1795): *Von der Lebenskraft.* Reprint ed. by K. Sudhoff, Leipsic 1910: J. A. Barth.

72. REIL, J. CH. (1803): *Rhapsodieen über die Anwendung der psychischen Curmethode auf Geisteszerrüttungen.* Halle: Curtsche Buchhandlung.

73. ROBACK, A. A. (1961): *History of Psychology and Psychiatry.* New York: Philosophical Library.

74. ROLLER, C. F. W. (1831): *Die Irrenanstalt nach ihren Beziehungen.* Karlsruhe: Ch. F. Müller.

75. ROTHSCHUH, K. E. (1958): Vom Spiritus animalis zum Nervenaktionsstrom. *Ciba-Zeitschrift,* 8, 2949.

76. SAKEL, M. (1935): *Neue Behandlungsmethode der Schizophrenie.* Vienna and Leipsic: M. Perles.

77. SCHATZMANN, J. (1968): *Richard Semon (1859-1918) und seine Mnemetheorie.* Dissertation. Zürich: Juris.

78. SCHENCK VON GRAFENBERG, J. (1665): *Observationum medicorum rariorum.* 7 volumes. Frankfort-on-the-Main: J. Beyer.

79. SCHUELE, H. (1878): Handbuch der Geisteskrankheiten. In: Ziemssen, H.v. (Ed.), *Handbuch der Speciellen Pathologie und Therapie.* Leipsic: F. C. W. Vogel.

80. SIMON, H. (1929): *Aktivere Krankenbehandlung in der Irrenanstalt.* Berlin and Leipsic: W. de Gruyter.

81. SPERBER, M. (1970): *Alfred Adler oder das Elend der Psychologie.* Vienna, Munich and Zurich: F. Molden.

82. STAHL, G. E. (1728): *Collegium practicum.* Leipsic: C. J. Eyssel.

83. STAHL, G. E. (1695): Ueber den mannigfaltigen Einfluss von Gemütsbewegungen auf den menschlichen Körper; . . . (1714): Ueber den Unterschied zwischen Organismus und Mechanismus; . . . In: Gottlieb, B. J. (Ed.), *Georg Ernst Stahl.* Leipsic 1961: J. A. Barth.

84. STEINEBRUNNER, W. F. (1971): *Zwei Zürcher Krankenhausplanungen des 19.*

Jahrhunderts. Ihre ärztlichen Experten, ihre Vorbilder. Dissertation. Zürich: Berichthaus.

85. STILLING, B. (1840): *Physiologische, pathologische und medicinisch-practische Untersuchungen über die Spinal-Irritation.* Leipsic: O. Wigand.

86. STRUEMPELL, A. (1892): *Ueber die Entstehung und die Heilung von Krankheiten durch Vorstellungen.* Erlangen: Fr. Junge.

87. STRUEMPELL, A. (1925): *Aus dem Leben eines deutschen Klinikers.* 2nd edition. Leipsic: F. C. W. Vogel.

88. SYDENHAM, TH. *The Works,* Ed. by R. G. Latham, (1848-1850). 2 volumes. London: Sydenham Society.

89. TEMKIN, O. (1971): *The Falling Sickness. A History of Epilepsy from the Greeks to the Beginnings of Modern Neurology.* 2nd edition. Baltimore: Johns Hopkins University Press.

90. WAGNER VON JAUREGG, J. (1902): Ueber Psychosen durch Autointoxication vom Darme aus. *Jb. Psychiat. Neurol.,* 22, 177.

91. WAGNER VON JAUREGG, J. (1936): *Fieber- und Infektionstherapie. Ausgewählte Beiträge 1887-1935.* Vienna-Leipsic-Berne: Verlag für Medizin, Weidmann.

92. WERNICKE, C. (1874): *Der aphasische Symptomencomplex. Eine psychologische Studie auf anatomischer Basis.* Breslau: M. Cohn und Weigert.

93. WERNICKE, C. (1900): *Grundriss der Psychiatrie.* Leipsic: G. Thieme.

94. WIER, J. (1578): *De praestigiis demonum.* Reprint of the German edition, Amsterdam 1967: E. J. Bonset.

95. WUNDT, W. (1880): *Grundzüge der physiologischen Psychologie.* 2nd edition. 2 volumes. Leipsic: W. Engelmann.

96. ZELLER, E. A. (1837): Bericht über die Wirksamkeit der Heilanstalt Winnenthal von ihrer Eröffnung den 1. März 1834 bis zum 28. Februar 1837. Beilage zu: *Medsches CorrBl. würt. ärztl. Ver.,* 7, 321.

11

HUNGARY

NÁNDOR HORÁNSZKY, M.D.

*Emeritus Chief Physician, Outpatient Department for
Mental Care of the Buda Area, Budapest, Hungary*

1

INTRODUCTION

Psychiatry, as a systematic branch of medicine, became established in Hungary in the middle of the 19th century. Because of the geographical position of the country and the political situation in Europe at that time, scientific developments reached Hungary through Austria only, and in particular through Vienna. Non-obligatory psychiatric courses for medical students were not introduced at the University of Vienna until 1843. More liberal attitudes towards the insane started by Pinel in France during the revolution were also late in reaching Vienna. Mihály Viszánik, the Hungarian-born chief physician of the Narrenturm ("Tower of insanes") in Vienna, had to remove a considerable number of chains still binding the patients there as late as in 1839.

At that time, Hungary had no mental institution, nor trained psychiatrists. Mental patients were kept together with other patients in the general hospitals, while others languished in prisons, or became tramps. Only a few hospitals had separate wards for the insane.

At the University of Budapest, the only Hungarian university at that time, no lectures in psychiatry were held, but a few physicians had taken an interest in mental diseases. For instance, Ferenc Bene, the elder, professor and later rector of the university, treated mental patients; he visited Western Europe several times and, in his travels, paid particular attention to mental institutions. He founded a travel scholarship, which enabled several Hungarian psychiatrists to study the problems of mental health abroad. His son, Ferenc Bene, Jr., also visited the mental hospitals of the western countries; in his diary, from 1826, he gives an account of the mental hospitals in Paris and of his meetings with Pinel and Esquirol.

At the beginning of the 19th century, psychiatric literature began to develop. For instance, several works by Mihály Lenhossék, the elder, university professor, later *protomedicus* of the country, deal with the importance of passions and changes of mood. Medical literature, however, became livelier from 1831 onward, following the foundation of the first Hungarian medical journal. At the beginning, the journal reported and reviewed foreign books only. Its concepts were organically oriented, as exemplified by an article by József Pólya (1802-1873) reporting his work on the cerebral localization of certain mental diseases. The self-taught and versatile Dr. Pólya arranged a few rooms for the observation of mental patients in the Municipal Hospital of Pest, later called the Rókus Hospital, and today the Semmelweis Hospital. This modest ward was the cradle of the first psychiatric clinic in Hungary. In 1841, Pólya opened a private sanatorium for mental patients, which closed down after a year. Pólya, despite his drive, failed to establish a school of psychiatric thought.

Later, the journal mentioned above published articles urging the establishment of a state mental hospital, which, in 1791, had already been approved in principle by a royal decree that had not been implemented. One of these articles suggested that the planning and control of the construction of the institution should be entrusted to the chief physician in Vienna, Mihály Viszánik (1792-1873) who, by his Hungarian birth, was best suited for this task. Unfortunately the construction of the state mental hospital was not completed until 1868. The planning, however, went ahead and some physicians optimistically applied for positions in it.

2

THE FIRST HUNGARIAN PSYCHIATRIC SCHOOL

The first physician to apply for a position in the future State Hospital was Ferenc Schwartzer (Plate LVII) (1818-1889). We owe to him the birth of Hungarian psychiatry. He was the son of poor parents; his

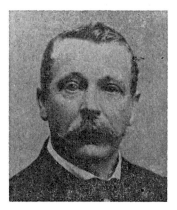

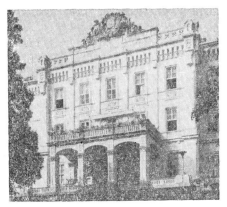

PLATE LVII. Ferenc Schwartzer (1818-1889).

PLATE LVIII. National Hospital for Nervous and Mental Diseases.

university studies, leading to degrees in medicine and surgery, were made possible by a rich relative in Vienna. He completed his psychiatric training at the Vienna Mental Hospital, where he had obtained a position. In his application, he stressed that his mother tongue was Hungarian, and asked for support for a study tour abroad. The latter was granted and, with his colleague, Konstantin Pomutz, the other resident of the Vienna Mental Hospital, he visited the best mental institutions of Germany, Belgium, England, and France, becoming personally acquainted with the best psychiatrists of the age—Ideler, Jacoby, Conolly, Foville, Guislein, Mitivié, etc. He wrote an extensive report about his experiences for the Hungarian government. In this report he made suggestions about the building of the planned institution and proposed Lipótmezö to be its site; this location was accepted, but the revolution of 1848-1849 postponed the venture for some time.

During the revolution, Ferenc Schwartzer worked as a field physician and then as a medical officer. After the revolution he settled in Vác. He continued to press for a mental hospital with the authorities, but without success. However, he was granted permission to treat mental patients in his own home. This was the first Hungarian mental hospital (1850). Because of the rapidly increasing number of patients, it was transferred to Buda in 1852, where it functioned for almost 100 years, providing accommodation for over 200 patients.

Hungarian psychiatry developed in this institution. In his growing and flourishing sanatorium Schwartzer engaged other physicians, who became the representatives of the first Hungarian psychiatric school.

Its members were as follows: Károly Bolyó (1833-1906), private docent, the first Hungarian psychiatrist to go to the United States on a study visit (he later became the director of the State Hospital); Gyula Niedermann (1839-1910), private docent at the faculty of law, later director of the State Hospital; Ottó Schwartzer (1853-1913), the son of Ferenc Schwartzer, private docent at the faculty of law, very active in the field of forensic psychiatry (he contributed to the establishment of medical legislation and founded the Forensic Medical Committee); Károly Laufenauer (1847-1901), the first professor of psychiatry at the University of Budapest; and Károly Lechner (1850-1922), the first professor of psychiatry at the University of Kolozsvár.

Ferenc Schwartzer wrote the first Hungarian textbook of psychiatry (1858), and in addition to lecturing at the University from 1847 to 1848, he taught psychiatry, as private docent, at the University of Budapest between 1860 and 1882.

3

INSTITUTIONS

Nagyszeben Hospital

Since 1849, Transsylvania was governed separately from Hungary and had separate *protomedicus* in charge of the health service. The separation of Transsylvania ceased in 1867, when its public health administration was transferred to the Hungarian Ministry of Internal Affairs. Due to this situation, Transsylvania, a richer country, was able to build a national mental institution of its own much earlier than Hungary. The choice of location fell on Nagyszeben, but while the building was in progress, a temporary asylum for the insane was established in Kolozsvár, with very few beds. The head of the asylum was Ferenc Bélteki (1827-1885). The institution of Nagyszeben was opened in 1853; its first director was Emil Schnirch (1822-1884), who had attended lectures in psychiatry in Vienna. As the chief physician of the Borsod county, he excelled himself in the segregation of mental patients in the hospital of Miskolc. In 1868, he was appointed director of the new State Hospital. He was followed at Nagyszeben by István Szabó (1813-1892), who introduced occupational therapy in the form of work in the fields and domestic work. His successor, Jeno Konrád (1854-1919), introduced the system of family care of mental patients, which was later further developed by Kálmán Pándy (1868-1945).

*National Hospital for Nervous and Mental Diseases**

The need for an institution had already been mentioned in a royal decree, in 1791. However, the devaluation of the currency caused by wars, the increasing threat of revolution, the war of independence in 1848-1849, and the 20 years of absolutism which followed did not favor its establishment. The plans were finally realized in 1860, but because the enterprisers went bankrupt several times, the hospital was not opened until the end of 1868 (Plate LVIII).

At the beginning the hospital could receive 300 patients; since then the number of patients has reached 1,600. As soon as it was opened, it was criticized for the number of cells built and for its prison-like appearance. Some of the equipment provided was inhumane and the medical board forbade its use. However, the location of the asylum had definite advantages, surrounded as it was by a large forest of 70 acres, in a very pleasant site in the hills of Buda.

The first director of the Hospital was Emil Schnirch from Nagyszeben; he was succeeded by Gyula Niedermann, whose great merit was the modernization of the building.

Gusztáv Oláh (1857-1944) was an ardent follower of the open-door system. In 1924 he joined the International League for Mental Hygiene and formed the Hungarian League for the Protection of the Mentally Ill; the aim of this organization was to prevent emotional disorders by establishing marriage councils; by fighting alcoholism and other addictions to control psychopaths and criminals, by promoting observation and treatment of abnormal children; and by following up discharged mental patients.

The next director was Rudolf Fabinyi (1879-1936), who believed in the same concepts and partially realized them. He succeeded in establishing the open-door system; he had a free ward built in the premises of the Hospital, called the Sanatorium of Hárshegy. Fabinyi also founded the Mental Care Service, which became one of the pillars of our present day psychiatry (see below).

During World War II, and immediately afterwards, the Hospital could not meet the demand for its services, but later, surmounting many difficulties, it developed at a rapid rate. It was reorganized, new departments were opened (for instance, for child psychiatry), and separate wards were built for tuberculous patients, for neurosurgery, and for infectious diseases. The number of beds in the open wards was increased. The Hospital was equipped with all the necessary labora-

---

*Previously National Insane Asylum of Buda, later Institution for Mental and Nervous Diseases at Lipótmező.

tories: EEG, x-ray, neurochemical, and psychological laboratories. More recently, an outpatient department for occupational therapy and a day sanatorium have also been added.

Since 1952, the Hospital has become a leading psychiatric center. All other mental hospitals in the country, except for the university hospitals, function under its supervision. It directs also the Institutions for Mental Care. The Ministry of Health has a supervisor of mental care, who coordinates the work of the various departments.

Valuable work has been carried out in the Institute. It was here that Kálmán Pándy (1868-1945) discovered the well-known test for CSF protein, named after him; István Hollós (1872-1957) carried out his psychoanalytic studies on psychotics; and it was here, too, that László Meduna (1896-1964) elaborated and practiced convulsive therapy, which has since become one of the most widely used therapeutic procedures in mental illness. The State Hospital is also in charge of the training of psychiatric nurses. The original study courses of a few weeks have been extended to three years. The lectures are delivered by the medical staff of the Hospital. The participants are qualified after passing an examination. Since the living standards of the nursing staff have been improved, the quality of applicants for these courses has also improved.

Mental Hospital of Angyalföld, Budapest

The State Hospital soon proved to be too small to meet the demands made upon it. The accumulation of chronic patients left no room for new cases. Therefore, in 1883, the Mental Hospital of Angyalföld was established to accommodate an additional 300 patients. The first director was Károly Lechner (1850-1922), who later was appointed to the chair of psychiatry at the University of Kolozsvár. He was succeeded in Angyalföld by Gusztáv Oláh, who later became the head of the State Hospital. In the Hospital of Angyalföld, approximately at the same time as in the State Hospital, an open ward was established similar to that of the Sanatorium of Hárshegy. One of the last directors of the Mental Hospital of Angyalföld was Gyula Nyiro (1895-1966), later professor of psychiatry at the University Medical School of Budapest.

The Hospital was changed to a general hospital, its character of a mental institution was eliminated, and only two mental departments were retained. This move made rehabilitation easier, as the certificate issued to discharged patients shows that they have been in a general hospital rather than in an asylum. Recently, a day sanatorium has been established in the Hospital.

State Mental Hospital at Nagykálló

The ever increasing demand could not be met even by the two institutions. Therefore, in 1896, an old public building was adapted to provide another mental institution with 300 to 400 beds.

János Kórház, Mental Care Department, Budapest

This institution was built as it now stands around World War I and, at that time, was one of the most up-to-date mental departments. During World War II, the patients from destroyed hospitals were accommodated here, causing much overcrowding, as originally it had been planned for 300 patients.

Annex Institutions

Pándy called annex institutions those mental departments which were established in general hospitals in various parts of the country, but most of them had no trained psychiatrists as chief physicians. These mental wards, considering their location, were mostly inadequate. Today the situation has changed, and trained psychiatrists lead every mental department.

Colony System of Care

Since the increase in the number of hospital beds did not solve all problems, and many patients became lethargic from complete inactivity, the possibility of introducing the colony system arose. In 1896, a number of expert workers went abroad to study the system. On the basis of their favorable reports, colonies were established in the districts of some county mental departments. The patients were kept occupied with agricultural work and were paid for their accomplishment. They were clinically supervised by the medical staff of the neighboring mental department.

World War II swept away these colonies, but soon after the war a few successful colonies were organized on abandoned estates and mansions. Near Budapest, a large estate was placed at the disposal of the Ministry of Health for the organization of a colony. This colony is also a center for the treatment of alcoholics, for whom after-care occupational therapy is also available. This institution is under the patronage of the State Mental Hospital.

Foster-Family Care

This system was started by Jeno Konrád and was under the control of the Mental Hospital of Nagyszeben; it was further developed by Rudolf Fabinyi, Kálmán Pándy and István Zsakó.

One or two suitable patients were placed with families who were willing to accept them as family members, allowing them to help with the easier household tasks. The patients were regularly visited by the physicians and the families were, of course, reimbursed for their keep.

Between the two world wars, family care developed around some larger institutions in the country, but after World War II, it was discontinued because it was felt that some patients were being exploited.

4

MENTAL HEALTH SERVICES

Outpatient Care

A system of after-care was organized in Hungary thanks to the endeavors of Oláh and Fabinyi. Fabinyi found, on the basis of German examples, that this system was extremely helpful. It helped reduce the overcrowding of the institutions and facilitated early patient discharge.

At the beginning, this form of care was restricted only to keeping under control the condition of discharged patients by way of district nurses; later, an outpatient department was opened in the State Mental Hospital, where help was offered not only to discharged patients and their relatives, but also to anybody else who felt in need of it. Later still, with the assistance of the capital, this outpatient department was moved to the center of the city. It screened patients who required hospital care and exerted a preventive function, insofar as it prevented the deterioration of prepsychotic patients. This outpatient department functioned so effectively that in 1942 it was taken over by the capital.

After clearing away the ruins of World War II, the outpatient department began to develop rapidly, new departments were opened, and today every one of the 22 districts of the capital has its own Outpatient Department for Mental Care. Accordingly, the number of psychiatrists increased to 30 and the number of nurses to 52. Each institution is headed by a director, while the overall control of mental care rests with the State Mental Hospital.

The activities of the mental care departments include care of patients discharged from hospitals, rehospitalization in case of threatening relapse, and assessment for hospitalization of mental patients. After-care consists of outpatient treatment in the consultation rooms, and study of the environment through home visits by the district nurses. If necessary, the physician too visits the home. Many individuals report voluntarily for consultation. The new law for mental patients emphasized the importance of the mental care departments.

Child Psychiatry

The study of child psychology started around the turn of the century. Pál Ranschburg (1870-1944) established a laboratory for the education of retarded children; this became an independent concern called the Psychological Laboratory for the Education of Retarded Children. Its main endeavor was in the field of research and theoretical work, which provided the basis for child psychology in Hungary. Ranschburg was a prolific writer; he left the laboratory in 1929, entrusting the leadership to one of his pupils, who turned it into the Outpatient Department for Educational Guidance, the first child psychiatric outpatient department in Hungary. Later the department was transformed into the Institute of Child Psychology and was suitably housed and staffed. After World War II, it merged with the Psychological Research Institute of the Hungarian Academy of Sciences. After many years, by general request, the former director of the Institute organized the Institution of Mental Care for Children in the capital, with a network of centers throughout the country.

It was an important step for child psychiatry when, in 1952, the first ward for mentally ill children was opened in the National Institution for Nervous and Mental Diseases, and a similar, though smaller, ward was organized at the Psychiatric Clinic of Szeged.

Since 1961, child psychiatry has been regarded as an independent discipline with a separate examination requiring previous service in pediatric and psychiatric wards.

Rehabilitation

Now that treatment of mental patients shows good results, rehabilitation has become a question of great importance. The open-door system and the new legislation simplifying the judiciary processes promote rehabilitation and eliminate some of the disadvantages.

A different type of rehabilitation technique is required for patients who are only partially incapacitated on account of their illness. In these cases special retraining is carried out in institutions which specialize in occupational therapy of patients with partial incapacity for work. These function under the supervision of certain cities or districts. Some of these institutions, in addition to training, supply the patients with work that can be done at home. Occupational therapy is one of the functions of the State Mental Hospital.

A plan is being devised to organize a workshop for partially incapacitated individuals; they would be supervised by foremen, a number of whom would be selected from ex-patients.

Forensic Psychiatry

Ferenc Schwartzer discussed certain aspects of forensic psychiatry in his textbook, published in 1858; he also wrote several papers on this subject and his son, Ottó Babarczi Schwartzer, became a pioneer in the field. Schwartzer was concerned with crimes committed during periods of disturbed consciousness and with the legal defense of the mentally ill. He was responsible for the Act which provided for the establishment of the Forensic Medical Committee. Its aim is to assess contradictory medical reports presented in the courts and to evaluate erroneous medical treatment.

The National Forensic Observational and Mental Institution was established in 1896. It is linked with the National Remand Prison and its task is not only the observation and assessment, but also the treatment of mental patients involved in crime. The first director of the Institution was Emil E. Moravcsik, a university professor. He and his successor were prolific writers.

Mental Health Legislation

The Law of 1876 concerning mental patients dealt with the judiciary control of hospitalization, admission, and discharge of patients; its main concern was with the patient's possible danger to himself and to others. This outdated law was replaced in 1966 by a law decree whose emphasis is on curability rather than security. It eliminates the complicated judiciary procedures of the old system and entrusts the control of the patient to a committee of experts. The patient can appeal to the court against the decision of the expert committee. The law also enables the hospitalization of the patient on his own wish. In the majority of cases the old practice of placing the mental patient in the temporary charge of a guardian has also been discontinued. The open-door system, promoted by the new legislation, contributes to facilitate rehabilitation.

5

THERAPEUTIC TRENDS

New techniques of active treatment started with fever therapy, first advocated by Gyula Donáth, who, in 1909, suggested sodium nucleinicum for this purpose. Fever therapy was introduced in Hungary shortly after it was first reported in the literature. In the 1920's, large-scale experiments were carried out with various methods and the published results of these trials have contributed to the final evaluation of fever therapy. Antibiotics for the treatment of psychiatric disorders due to syphilis were extremely difficult to obtain even after the war, but when their application became possible, this type of disorder has practically disappeared.

Insulin therapy for schizophrenia was introduced in Hungary shortly after the first attempts were reported in various foreign journals. The discovery and development of convulsion therapy in schizophrenia is linked to the name of the Hungarian László Meduna.

The introduction of neuroleptic and neuroanaleptic drugs and procedures in schizophrenia had been hindered considerably by the war. Immediately after the drugs became available, large-scale experimentation was begun, but it was not possible to use them widely. The supply has now improved and the Hungarian drug industry produces tranquilizers on a large scale. The outpatient treatment of restless patients and the extension of the open-door system were greatly assisted by these drugs.

Leucotomy and similar surgical procedures for the treatment of schizophrenia, after the first enthusiasm, have proved that the results are not commensurate with the inherent risks. Surgical procedures can now be carried out only on the recommendation of a special medical committee.

Conditioning techniques in the treatment of alcoholism were used between the two wars using Apomorphin. Antaethyl and Antabuse were introduced after the war. The official organ for the fight against alcoholism is the network of outpatient departments which, like the Institution of Mental Care, registers and treats alcoholics. The patients are followed up by district nurses, and, if necessary, hospitalized, but treatment is given in the outpatient units whenever possible. Drug addiction in Hungary is rare.

Psychotherapy—Psychoanalysis

Charcot's and Bernheim's experiments with hypnosis aroused interest among Hungarian physicians, many of whom had visited France. Among them were Gyula Donáth, who used hypnotherapy in preference to any other method of treatment, Károly Laufenauer, who wrote noteworthy studies on hysteria and hypnosis, and Erno Jendrassik and Sándor Korányi, later professors of medicine at the University of Budapest. Laufenauer's pupils, Schaffer and Moravcsik, wrote on the practice and effects of hypnosis. Today this mode of treatment is seldom applied, but simpler suggestion techniques are still used in certain cases. Group therapy procedures are also successfully employed.

The Hungarian psychoanalytical movement began in 1908, when Sigmund Freud met Sándor Ferenczi (1873-1933). Their friendship had a great bearing upon both of them, resulting in the exchange of more than a thousand letters. The idea of the obligatory analysis for psychoanalysts originated from Ferenczi. He was also the first to attempt the psychoanalysis of mental patients, followed by two more Hungarians, István Hollós and Endre Almásy.

The Society of Hungarian Psychoanalysts was founded in 1913. Its members were Sándor Ferenczi, István Hollós, Géza Szilágyi, Béla Felszeghy, and Lajos Lévy. During World War I, the Society could not function, but at the end of September, 1918, the International Congress of Psychoanalysts was held in Budapest and was attended by Sigmund Freud. The Congress nominated Ferenczi as president of the International Society.

The Hungarian Soviet Republic of 1919 appointed Ferenczi *private docent* and opened a clinic in a sanatorium for him. After the fall of the Soviet Republic, Ferenczi was deprived of his title and his clinic was closed. All university lectures of psychoanalysis ceased. However, in spite of these drawbacks, the psychoanalytical movement survived. Under the leadership of István Hollós (1872-1957) a new society was formed with a limited membership which included Mihály Bálint, Géza Roheim—the only ethnologist at the time who stood by Freud— and Endre Almásy. A result of this movement was the Psychoanalytical Polyclinic.

After 1945, psychoanalysis was rehabilitated. Wards, directed by psychoanalysts, were opened. At one time, the director of the National Institution was a psychoanalyst-physician, Mrs. Lili Hajdu-Gimes. Two psychoanalyst *private docents* were appointed at the University; at present, two departments of neurology and psychiatry function under the direction of psychoanalysts. In 1949 the Society was dissolved and university lectures discontinued, but the analysts have remained active.

6

TEACHING

For a long time, lectures in psychiatry were not obligatory for medical students; then they became optional and medical students could choose between psychiatry, pediatrics, and dermatology. But, beginning with the academic year of 1916-17, psychiatry was included in the curriculum with an obligatory examination. Since 1922, theoretical and practical examinations must be passed in this subject.

A psychiatric qualification requires the candidate to spend four years in a psychiatric ward, and to pass an oral and practical examination.

At the University of Budapest lectures in psychiatry were not held until 1847. (In Vienna non-obligatory lectures were started in 1843.) In the autumn of 1847, the medical faculty entrusted Konstantin Pomutz (1815-1883), resident physician of the psychiatric department of the General Hospital of Vienna, to deliver lectures in psychiatry, but attendance at these lectures was not made obligatory. Pomutz travelled with Ferenc Schwartzer during a study tour through Western Europe. He lectured for a few months only, as he did not return to Hungary. Until 1860, when Ferenc Schwartzer was appointed *private docent,* no lectures in psychiatry were held at the University of Budapest. Schwartzer continued these non-obligatory lectures until 1882.

The predecessor of the clinic was the small observation ward of the municipal Rókus Hospital. In 1865, Károly Bolyó became its director and his successor, Károly Laufenauer, became, in 1878, extraordinary and in 1891, ordinary university professor. The official lectures in psychiatry started with this appointment at the University of Budapest. At the beginning, the conditions were inadequate. Therefore, the clinic was transferred into an adapted building, which was not much better. Frigyes Korányi, professor of medicine, offered a room in his clinic to Laufenauer, where the latter could continue his observations of hysteria. Laufenauer, who was influenced by Griesinger and Meynert, under the influence of Westphal, had oriented himself to neurology; the difficult conditions under which he was forced to work limited his field to neurology and neuropathology. His interesting collection of neuropathological preparations attracted many visitors, even from abroad.

The second Hungarian psychiatric school, already recognized and appreciated abroad, developed around Károly Laufenauer. Among his prominent pupils were Emil E. Moravcsik, Károly Schaffer and Pál

Ranschburg. Pál Ranschburg (1870-1945) was the founder of Hungarian child psychology. His extensive scientific and research work was much appreciated at home and abroad. Of his numerous pupils, Lipót Szondi became the best known. Kálmán Pándy, the discoverer of the CSF reaction bearing his name, was one of the pioneers of the free treatment of mental patients and one of the leaders of the movement against alcoholism.

Gyula Donáth (1849-1945), though not actually one of his pupils, frequented his hospital. He was in contact with Charcot, DuBois Raymond, Helmholtz, and Westphal. In 1909, he suggested sodium nucleinicum for the fever treatment of paralysis. As the leader of the movement against alcoholism, he was involved in an extensive campaign of propaganda and was the first to point out the psychiatric aspect of social problems.

On his death, Laufenauer was succeeded by Ernö Moravcsik (1858-1924), who established clinical psychiatry. He was a sharp observer, who could evaluate things with great clarity; the interest of his patients was always his first consideration. As a recognition of his work he was given new, up-to-date buildings equipped with chemical, psychological, and neuropathological laboratories. His work, although essentially original, was influenced by Wundt and Kraepelin.

Of his numerous students, the most outstanding were Kamillo Reuter, professor of the University of Pécs, Ödön Németh, director of the Forensic Observation Institute and Károly Hudovernig, *private docent* and director of the Observational Department of Budapest.

Most of Moravcsik's pupils continued to work under his successor, Károly Schaffer (1864-1939), who gained a worldwide reputation for research in the histology of the normal and pathological conditions of the central nervous system. He recognized that the swelling of nerve cells in amaurotic family idiocy was due to lipoid accumulation. He also contributed to histopathological research of hereditary nervous disorders, primarily in the study of Tay-Sachs disease. To promote his work, in 1922 a neuropathological institute was established; he led this as extraordinary professor. In 1925 he became ordinary professor of neurology and psychiatry at the University of Budapest; he then incorporated his histopathological institute into the clinic as a research department. Among his pupils are Ernö Frey, who added to Alzheimer's disease; Hugo Richter, who clarified the pathogenesis of tabes; Kálmán Sántha, one of the founders of neurosurgery in Hungary; and others who occupy important posts in Hungarian psychiatry.

Schaffer was followed by László Benedek (1887-1945), previously professor in Debrecen, whose extensive work covered all branches of psychiatry as well as of neurology. He was particularly interested in the effect of insulin and the psychic disturbances it caused. He took over most of Schaffer's pupils and trained many psychiatrists who now occupy prominent positions in Hungary.

After 1945 the professors of the Medical Faculty were changed. Gyula Nyirö (1895-1966) became the professor of neurology and psychiatry at the Medical University of Budapest. He wrote a voluminous text-book of psychiatry comprising every up-to-date aspect of the discipline. Later the professorship was divided, and at present there are two chairs.

The University of Kolozsvár established a chair of psychiatry in 1889, before that of the University of Budapest. The first professor was Károly Lechner (1850-1922), an original man who, without knowledge of the relevant Russian literature, tried to attribute all normal and pathological functions of the nervous system to the reflexes. He built a large and impressive clinic for the University of Kolozsvár and lived long enough to see the transfer of the University to Szeged. After him, József Szabó (1886-1929), a neurologically oriented worker, became the head of the clinic. The temporary re-transfer of the University to Kolozsvár occurred under his successor.

At present, the Clinic of the University of Szeged limits its studies to psychoses and to biochemical research of nervous diseases. Károly Lechner's pupils are: Rudolf Fabinyi, István Zsakó, Gyula Nyirö, Sándor Stief, and László Benedek.

The first psychiatrist of the University of Debrecen was László Benedek, an active and versatile man, who later became professor in Budapest. He was followed by István Somogyi, one of the assistant lecturers of Schaffer. After his death, one of Schaffer's best pupils, Kálmán Sántha (1903-1956), was appointed professor; he was one of the first to establish neurosurgery in Hungary, after having visited the United States.

The first professor of the University of Pécs, Kamillo Reuter, was a pupil and follower of Moravcsik. His main interest was clinical psychiatry. He was succeeded by one of Schaffer's pupils, who introduced neuropathology and neurosurgery at the University.

7

CONCLUSION

In Hungarian psychiatry—from the first study tour to Western Europe of its founder—many influences have prevailed. Ferenc Schwartzer was inspired by Pinel and Esquirol, but was also influenced by important developments in German psychiatry. At times, foreign influences became stronger, as, for instance, the French influence emanating from Charcot and from Bernheim; the influence of German psychiatry and neuro-anatomy and the fruitful impact of the work of Griesinger, Kraepelin, Wundt, Meynert and Flechsig. The effect of scientific developments in English-speaking countries began between the two world wars, with the result that neurosurgery was established in Hungary. Since World War II, Soviet psychiatry and Pavlov's theory have gained a considerable influence.

From this brief summary it is evident that Hungarian psychiatry has always favored an eclectic approach and has been able to assimilate psychiatric trends from other parts of the world without prejudice.

REFERENCES

1. *Anniversary Volume of the János Hospital* (in Hungarian, 1970). p. 78. Budapest.
2. *Anniversary Volume of the Mental Institute of Angyalföld* (in Hungarian), 1933. Budapest.
3. CSORBA, J. (1858): *Commemoration Speech on Ferenc Bene* (in Hungarian). *Commemoration Speeches of the Academy.*
4. DONATH, GY. (1940): *Autobiography* (in Hungarian). Horizont.
5. EPSTEIN, L. (1897): *The Mental Care in Hungary* (in Hungarian). Gyógyászat.
6. GYŐRY, T. (1935): *The History of the Medical Faculty between 1770-1935* (in Hungarian). Budapest.
7. HORANSZKY, N. (1959): The Significance of F. Schwartzer and O. Schwartzer in the History of Hungarian Psychiatry (in Hungarian). *Communicationes ex Bibliotheca historiae medicae hungarica,* Tom. 15/16, 81.
8. HORANSZKY, N. (1826): The Travel Diary of F. Bene, Jr. in Paris. (in Hungarian). *Communicationes de historia artis medicinae,* Tom. 54, 205.
9. JONES, E. (1960-1962): *Das Leben und Werk von Sigmund Freud.* Vol. 3. (Translated by Katherine Jones). Bern-Stuttgart.
10. KÉTLY, K. (1902): Commemoration Speech on K. Laufenauer (in Hungarian). *Commemoration Speeches of the Academy.*
11. KOVACS-SEBESTYÉN, E. (1858): Commemoration Speech on F. Bene (in Hungarian). *Commemoration Speeches of the Academy.*
12. LECHNER, K. *Autobiography* (in Hungarain). Manuscript, in the possession of the family.
13. LENHOSSÉK, M. (1806): *Darstellung der menschlichen Leidenschaften.* Pest.
14. LESKY, ERNA (1965): *Die Wiener Medizinische Schule im XIX. Jahrhundert:* Graz und Köln.
15. MISKOLCZY, D. (1965): *Károly Schaffer* (in Hungarian). *Magyar Tudomány,* 7-8.
16. OLAH, G. (1903): *Treatment of the Mentally Ill* (in Hungarian). Budapest.
17. ORBAN, L. (1964-65): *Psychiatry in Transsylvania 50 years ago* (in Hungarian). *Hetilap—Horus,* 14.
18. ORBAN, L. (1959): The Insane Asylum of Kolozvár (in Hungarian). *Orvosi Ideggyógy.* Szle.
19. PANDY, K. (1905): *Care of Mental Patients* (in Hungarian). Gyula.
20. PANDY, K. (1914:) *Commemoration Volume on the 50th Anniversary of the State Mental Institute in Nagyszeben* (in Hungarian). Nagyszeben.

21. SCHAFFER, K. (1927): E. Emil Moravcsik (in Hungarian). *Commemoration Speeches of the Academy.*

22. SCHNELL, J. (1968): *Development, Scientific and Historical Antecedents of the Institute of Mental Care for Children in the Capital* (in Hungarian). Budapest.

23. SPIELMANN, J. (1956): K. Lechner, *Commemoration Volume* (in Hungarian). Bucharest.

24. *The 100 Years of the National Institute for Nervous and Mental Diseases* (in Hungarian), 1968. Budapest.

25. ZSAKÓ, I. (1935): Mihály Viszánik (in Hungarian). *Budapesti Orvosi Ujság.* p. 979.

12

UNION OF SOVIET
SOCIALIST REPUBLICS

Collated by the Editor from works by
JOSEPH WORTIS, M.D.* and A. G. GALACH'YAN**

1

EARLY RUSSIAN PSYCHIATRY

In medieval feudal Russia, before the great social reform initiated by Peter the Great, psychiatry fared as badly as in Western Europe, and probably worse. Superstitions of demoniacal possession, bewitchments, and visitation of godly punishments were the commonly accepted explanation of psychoses, though as early as the 11th century, some modest relief and protection was sometimes afforded to the unfortunate insane in the monasteries where they were more likely to be regarded as the involuntary victims of dark powers, whose devils might be exorcised by prayer. This charitable view was extended mainly to the wealthier and more pathetic psychotics. Psychotics without gross disturbances of consciousness were mostly left to their fate, and could be found wandering homeless and destitute through the land. The first governmental edict legalizing the monastic method of caring for the insane was promulgated in 1551 during the reign of Ivan the Terrible at the Higher Church Synod where provision was made for the care of the poor and sick, including "those possessed by the devil,

---

* Wortis, J. (1950): *Soviet Psychiatry*. Baltimore: Williams & Wilkins.
** Galach'yan, A. G. (1968). Soviet Union. In: Kiev, A. (Ed.), *Psychiatry in the Communist World*. New York: Science House.

308

and who had lost their minds." The edict provided for the segregation of these unfortunates in monasteries "that they should not serve
as an hindrance and source of alarm for the healthy," as well as for
religious and moral correction—the prevailing form of psychotherapy
of the time.

In one respect the Russian psychotic fared somewhat better than his
Western brother: he was not so liable to be called up before the ecclesiastical courts of the Inquisition, established in Western Europe by
Pope Innocent VIII, for the uprooting and destruction of heretics,
but often employed to destroy self-accusatory psychotics, and even to
extort confessions from healthy people. Instances of witch-burning in
Russia are, however, recorded in Russian history, and ukases were
published giving rules for the apprehension, inquisition, and burning
of witches and sorcerers. In 1677, just before Peter's reign, a law was
promulgated limiting the property rights of the deaf, blind, drunkards
and "fools." It was in this period that we encounter, as in Western
Europe, the first efforts to distinguish between bona fide mental disease
and possession by the devil, and by the eighteenth century, the question of mental disease was even sometimes raised in the defense of
criminals in the courts. In 1723 Peter the Great decreed the establishment of special hospitals for the insane, but the decree led to little
practical action. A similar decree was made in 1762 by Peter III
to build mental hospitals "as in foreign countries," and in 1765, during
the reign of Catherine the Great, fresh efforts were made to set up
mental institutions along Western lines.

2

THE 19TH CENTURY

In 1775 Russia was divided into states, each of which established its
own Department of Public Welfare, with appropriate insane asylums,
called "Yellow Homes." The first such home was opened in Novgorod
in 1776. In that same year a 26-bed psychiatric shelter was attached to
a Moscow hospital and in 1809 a special psychiatric hospital was finally
established in the outskirts of Moscow (Plate LIX). In successive years
similar shelters were established in St. Petersburg, Kharkov, and elsewhere. By 1810 there were 14 such shelters in all of Russia; by 1860
there were 43.

These bare figures tell us nothing of the sordid inhumanity of these
institutions. A contemporary account (1807) of one of these shelters

at Poltava reveals the following: There were facilities for the care of
20 patients, divided into "mean" and "quiet" ones. The annual budgetary allowance for each patient was 47 rubles, 57 kopeks. They slept
on straw spread over a brick floor; meat was given only to the "quiet"
ones, and even they got it only 60 days a year. The therapeutic arma-
mentarium consisted of a "dripping machine," which dripped cold
water on the patient's head, 17 cat-o'-nine-tails, and 11 lengths of
restraining chains. The staff of the institution consisted of one physi-

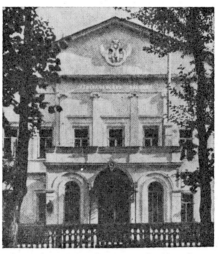

PLATE LIX. Moscow Preobrazhenskaya
Mental Hospital. Founded in 1809.

cian (salary 400 rubles per annum), two male "supervisors" (50 rubles
per year), two female "supervisors" (30 rubles), and a cook, two
laundresses, assisting soldiers from the invalids' brigade, or poorhouse
inmates, each of whom would receive 9 rubles a year. In other institutions, including the Moscow hospital, similar conditions prevailed. In
the latter institution, drastic reforms were introduced in 1828 by a new
director, Dr. Sabler. Its name was changed from Madhouse to Hospital.
Chains were abolished, occupational and recreational activity introduced, case histories utilized, and annual reports published. These
reforms were made possible, however, largely through the munificence
of private benefactors. One prosperous inmate, Koreishcha, who conducted a flourishing business while still at the hospital, became an
especially famous supporter of psychiatric reform.

Russian psychiatrists for the most part followed Western models in initiating reforms. Serbskii wrote a particularly glowing account of the new type of psychiatric agricultural work colony established in both France and Germany, employing the system—first introduced in Scotland—of the open door. Serbskii, who visited the colony at Alt-Scherbitz near Leipzig in 1885, made a moving appeal for the establishment of similar colonies in Russia. "It is hardly conceivable," he concluded, "that one would designate as an unnecessary luxury an institution that permits five hundred people to lead some sort of a tolerable existence, and that permits them some manner of pleasure."

At the close of the 19th century, a census of the mentally ill in the state of Moscow undertaken by Kashchenko reached the conclusion—on dubious statistical grounds—that the rate was 21.1 insane per

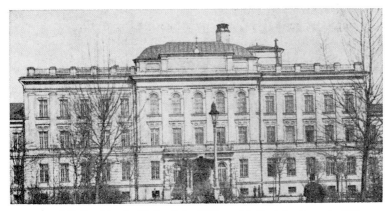

PLATE LX. Psychiatric Clinic of the Military-Medical Academy in 1891.

thousand for the entire population. An equally dubious investigation in the State of Petrograd in 1896 yielded a rate of 2.4 per thousand. A more careful study in the State of Orlov by Iakobii yielded a rate of 3 per thousand, which was close to rates found by similar methods at the time in Switzerland and Germany.

Meanwhile the rise of humanitarian feeling in the field of psychiatric treatment led to other efforts to relieve the oppressive conditions of asylum care. Korsakov, a famous figure in Russian psychiatry, was a public-spirited fighter for such reform and was responsible for the limited introduction of the family care system of psychiatric cases, again in imitation of the Western examples of the Belgian town of Gheel, the Scottish Connoway and the French Dun-sur-Auron.

Academic university psychiatry had its beginnings in the military medical academy of St. Petersburg (Plate LX) where the first professorship was held by the young physician Ivan Balinskii, a brilliant lecturer of wide knowledge and singular accomplishments, who had traveled extensively abroad, and who can be properly regarded as the founder of Russian scientific psychiatry. He was born in 1827 in Vilna, got his doctor's degree in St. Peterburg in 1846, and before entering psychiatry had lectured in pediatrics. He initiated his professorship with a thorough housecleaning of the military psychiatric hospital, organized a new clinic, and helped plan a wide system of new psychiatric hospitals in the main cities. Psychiatry for the first time became an obligatory part of the medical curriculum. Balinskii sponsored the use of psychiatric expert testimony in the courts, and organized the first Russian psychiatric society in St. Petersburg in 1862. He left no important literary or scientific memorials behind him, but fulfilled his main ambition to establish a setting in which his successor might find all the necessary material for study and scientific work.

He was succeeded in 1877 by his assistant Merzheievskii, who approached mental disease in a strictly biological spirit and who belongs to the line of materialists—though somewhat naive materialists—who formed so important a tradition in Russian psychiatry. Even his early dissertation, *"The Somatic Examination of the Violent,"* was entirely concerned with the physical changes in mental disease, such as changes in body weight, metabolism, temperature, and respiratory activity. With quite inadequate data he reached the mistaken conclusion that patients cannot satisfy their oxygen requirements in closed spaces, and led a vigorous fight against isolation rooms and in favor of open-air treatment, which served progressive ends in spite of his faulty reasoning. He traveled widely abroad and was especially influenced by Magnan in Paris and by Darwin. In a period of sixteen years he trained dozens of specialists, many of whom became teachers, and sponsored scores of scientific studies and publications.

In the succeeding years a number of new important centers of neuropsychiatric activity were established. Bekhterev (Plate LXI) was appointed professor of the University of Kazan in 1885 and soon rose to eminence. At this time the first Russian neuropsychiatric journal was founded in Kharkov by Kovalevskii, and many important foreign works were published. The renowned Kraepelin for five years held the chair of psychiatry in the old University of Dorpat (now Tartu, Estonia), before returning to Heidelberg in 1891. His predecessor was Emminghaus and his successor was Chizh, both distinguished names. In Moscow Kozhevnikov organized an active neurological school and established a modern 50-bed psychiatric hospital that was managed by the brilliant young Korsakov.

Contemporary Soviet psychiatrists take special pride in Korsakov (Plate LXII), a pupil of Meynert's, who exemplifies two prominent features of modern Soviet psychiatry: its close orientation to medicine, and its intimate concern for social factors in psychiatric disorder. It was Korsakov who first clearly defined a medical entity, polyneuritic psychosis, in psychiatry, and it was he who combined clinical activity with a wide interest in the organization of public mental health facilities. He recognized the importance of general

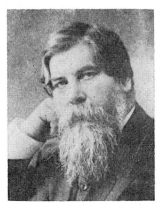 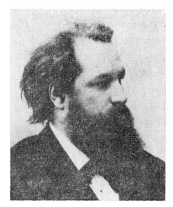

PLATE LXI. Prof. V. M. Bekhterev (St. Petersburg).

PLATE LXII. Prof. S. S. Korsakov
(Moscow)

hygienic conditions in psychiatry, and in sharp contrast to the trends prevailing in his time, advocated bed rest and quiet for certain types of mental disease. He played an important part in the no-restraint movement, and his name is intimately connected with basic reforms in Russian psychiatric institutions. He was a man of extraordinary clinical acumen, whose proposed system of classification of mental disease propounded over a half a century ago is almost completely in accord with prevailing concepts. In spite of his premature death in 1900 at the age of 46, he had attracted a wide circle of pupils and followers and left a deep impression on Russian psychiatry. In the succeeding decades Russian neuropsychiatry achieved world fame, and alone among the medical specialties in Russia—in spite of historical limitations—stepped forward boldly to advanced social tasks.

The first Russian medical congress devoted to psychiatry took place in 1887 in Moscow, attended by 440 physicians of whom 86 were psychiatric specialists. It is characteristic of the advanced social role that Russian psychiatry was assuming in those dark days of Czarist reaction that the proceedings stressed preventive medicine, and especially mental hygiene. The Congress (3) opened with an address by I. P. Merzheievskii, "On Conditions Favoring the Development of Mental and Nervous Diseases in Russia and on Measures Directed Toward their Control," which emphasized the importance of economic security as one of the factors in the prevention of mental disease. A paper was read against the use of restraints, and another on family care, both by Korsakov. The Congress ended with an address by I. A. Sikorskii on "The Task of Neuropsychic Hygiene and Prophylaxis," in which stress was laid on working conditions, particularly for women. These socially oriented strivings could never reach fruition under the conditions then prevailing, but they represented a significant trend for years to come. At one of the later meetings of Russian psychiatrists, in 1911, Serbskii, a former assistant of Korsakov's, made a famous speech attacking the government for its neglect of social services, and the Association of Russian Psychiatrists, formed at this Congress, became an advanced social organization which attracted the most progressive forces of psychiatry of the day.

During this period dozens of new institutions, some of them agricultural colonies, were developed, for the most part under capable and devoted psychiatrists, but desperate overcrowding prevailed and general psychiatric facilities were distressingly inadequate. In 1892 the *Zemstov,* or local government agencies, had 34 hospitals for mental cases, with 9,055 beds, staffed by 90 psychiatrists (15), out of a total of 12,433 physicians in all Russia at that time. A number of public-spirited psychiatrists of this period are recalled with pride in the contemporary literature. Virubov's study of the influence of social and economic factors on mental health was unique in pre-revolutionary Russian medical literature. Others, like Kashchenko, who created a central statistical bureau in Petersburg, found it easy to assume similar but larger responsibilities under the new regime. It was no accident that the Association of Russian Psychiatrists, under the leadership of Gannushkin, was among the first to offer its services to the new Soviet government at a time when suspicion and opposition were still widespread among the professional classes.

3

THE 20TH CENTURY

To the younger generation of Russian psychiatrists fell the task of developing a Soviet psychiatry after the October Socialist Revolution.

Soviet psychiatrists set about answering the urgent demands of Russian psychiatry, which were impossible to satisfy under the conditions of the Czarist regime but which now called for realization in the light of the new social attitudes in the nation. The prophylactic trend in Soviet psychiatry, as in all Soviet medicine, necessitated the prompt organization of a network of outpatient centers to bring psychiatric care to the populace. A regional psychiatric service was set up in Moscow in 1919 and similar services were later established in other large cities. The functions of these services included complete care of psychiatric patients who remained with their families, creation of the most favorable possible domestic and other living conditions for such patients, protection of their personal interests and rights, and, when necessary, provision of a fixed monthly allotment to their families. While carrying out medical observation of the mentally ill of the district and providing them with therapeutic aid, the regional psychiatrists sent all patients whose mental condition deteriorated to psychiatric hospitals for institutional care. With the organization in the same year of the Moscow regional network of neuropsychiatric sanitariums for patients with borderline conditions, the regional psychiatrists became responsible for those of the sanitarium patients who had been recommended for further observation and treatment upon their discharge. As the number of neurological sanitariums increased, their medical staffs were augmented by psychiatrist-physicians, so that the concepts of clinical psychiatry came to be applied to an ever greater extent to borderline cases. The increased workload of the regional psychiatrists and the need for dynamic observation of patients and establishment of dispensary services eventually resulted in the reorganization of the existing system into a network of neurological-psychiatric clinics with even broader prophylactic responsibilities.

Soviet psychiatrists devoted a great deal of effort to decentralizing psychiatric facilities and reorganizing the network of "major psychiatric" institutions. Since the large regional psychiatric hospitals which supposedly served vast areas were capable of caring only for the residents of the portion of the region nearest each hospital, it became necessary to open several smaller hospitals in the more remote areas. The building of psychiatric institutions in isolated regions of the national republics, which were largely neglected in this respect under the Czarist regime, became an especially pressing problem; an enormous amount of work was done in the construction of new institutions and in the reconstruction of the few pre-Revolutionary ones in these areas. In the early 1930's many psychiatric hospitals throughout the Soviet Union were converted to true therapeutic institutions by freeing the beds previously occupied by chronic patients, who required hospitalization in a different type of institution. Patients with acute psychotic conditions could be promptly and actively treated only with the facilities available at large, well-equipped psychiatric hospitals. To care for persons convalescing after an intensive course of therapy and for patients whose mental condition did not require confinement in restrictive therapeutic institutions, sanitarium branches were opened at psychiatric hospitals and neuropsychiatric clinics were established at neuropsychiatric hospitals and dispensaries. Psychiatric departments were organized at some large regional medical hospitals to handle cases of acute psychosis arising during the course of various infectious somatic diseases, after surgery, etc. The scope of this article does not permit us to consider this topic in greater detail, but we should point out one further achievement of Soviet psychiatry.

To bring psychiatric aid closer to the populace, Soviet psychiatrists (M. A. Dzhagarov, *et al.*) established a new form of semi-hospital, semi-clinical service, the *day ward*, which is set up as a special division of a psychiatric hospital. The patient spends the entire day, from early morning until evening, in this ward under a therapeutic regimen, receiving the necessary treatment, particularly psychotherapeutic aid, engaging in occupational therapy and cultural amusements, and being kept on a strict, full-valued diet; only in the evening is he permitted to return home to his family for the night.

In order to permit more thorough study of the problems associated with the operation of the network of prophylactic dispensaries, other outpatient facilities, and minor psychiatric clinics, the State Scientific Research Institute of Neuropsychiatric Prophylaxis was organized in 1925 on the basis of the State Neuropsychiatric Dispensary, which had already been in existence in Moscow for several years. L. M. Rozenshteyn, an enthusiastic advocate of the prophylactic-dispensary trend in psychiatry, was chosen to head the Institute, and Yu. V. Kannabikh, the scientific adviser and consultant to the large Moscow regional network of neuropsychiatric sanitariums, participated actively in its work.

The considerable scientific achievements of the Institute of Neuropsychiatric Prophylaxis in the clinical recognition and prophylaxis of latent forms of psychosis and borderline conditions were undoubtedly somewhat devalued by the methodological errors committed both in clinical psychopathological investigations and in psychoprophylactic and psychohygienic work. Sufficient attention was not always paid to the special features of the studies conducted by the Institute's dispensaries; no distinction was made among different groups of working data, which led to an incorrect application of psychopathological and diagnostic concepts taken from the field of "major" psychiatry to symptoms only remotely reminiscent of true psychiatric phenomena and mechanisms. All this naturally could not but have an unfavorable influence on psychohygienic and psychoprophylactic practice. As was the case at one time in child psychiatry, a deviation from strict clinical views and from a disciplined clinical way of thinking led to the un-

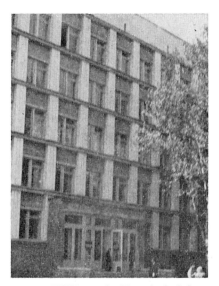

PLATE LXIII. Psycho-Neurological Out-Patient Clinic of the Viborgsky Region, Leningrad.

justified application of biological concepts and criteria to phenomena caused by factors of an essentially social nature.

Psychiatric-research institutes were opened also in other cities. Some of them served all of Russia, whereas others served only individual republics or regions; the former accordingly occupied themselves with solving the central problems of theoretical and clinical psychiatry, the latter were more concerned with theoretical, clinical, organizational, and practical problems at the local level. Psychoneurological institutes were established in Leningrad (Plate LXIII) (The V. M. Bekhterev Institute), as well as at Khar'kov, Kiev, Odessa, Baku, Tbilisi, Dnepropetrovsk, Tula, and other centers. Certain of these institutes were later closed as ineffective in line with the expansion of those in nearby cities. In 1920, even before the founding of the Institute of Neuro-psychiatric Prophylaxis, the V. P. Serbskiu Institute of Forensic Psychiatry was established in Moscow; the P. B. Gannushkin Municipal Psychiatric Research Institute was founded in 1933; and the Institute of Psychiatry of the Academy of Medical Sciences U.S.S.R. in 1944. Psychiatric departments were also organized at the Institutes for Evaluation of Working Capacity and Working Conditions of the Commissariats of Social Security in Moscow, Leningrad, and the Ukraine.

4

THE SCHOOL OF PAVLOV

At this point special mention must be made of Ivan Petrovitch Pavlov (Plate LXIV), who bridged the gap between 19th and 20th century Russian psychiatry (11, 12). For decades before his death in 1936 he was not only Russia's most distinguished physician, but her most renowned contemporary scientist as well. Born in 1849, the son of a poor priest, he also prepared himself for the priesthood, but decided at the age of 21 to leave the seminary for St. Petersburg University, where he became an assistant of the brilliant physiologist Elie Tsyon, and later a doctor of medicine. A fellowship award allowed him to spend the years 1884-86 with the two great German physiologists Ludwig in Leipzig and Heidenhain in Breslau. Upon his return to the Medical Academy in St. Petersburg he resumed teaching and re-

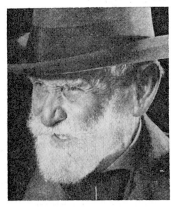

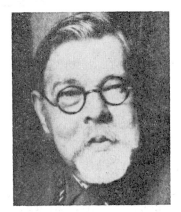

PLATE LXIV. Pavlov.   PLATE LXV. Prof. V. P. Osipov
                                 (Leningrad)

search and was appointed successively professor of pharmacology and physiology. In 1904 he won the Nobel Prize for his researches on the activity of the digestive glands—an interest which led him quite early to a consideration of the phenomenon of "psychic secretion" which laid the basis for his work on the higher nervous functions. After 1891 he was afforded laboratory facilities in the Institute of Experimental Medicine founded in that year by the Prince of Oldenburg, and later lavishly supported by the Soviet government. A vivid and picturesque character of enormous vitality, uncompromising honesty, and great courage, he lead a rich and productive scientific life which can fairly be said to have established a new branch of physiology and a new basis for psychology: the study of conditioned reflexes.

5

THEORY IN SOVIET PSYCHIATRY

The expansion of Societ psychiatry from the psychiatric hospitals into the broad field of borderline conditions, and the bringing of psychiatric help to new groups of patients, raised new theoretical and practical problems. Specifically required were the development of a clinical methodology for use in sanitariums, psychotherapeutic, psychohygienic, and psychoprophylactic techniques, and occupational therapy methods for institutions for borderline cases. The creation of a new, independent branch of clinical psychiatry, that dealing with children and adolescents, also posed a number of new problems for Soviet psychiatry; pre-Revolutionary Russian psychiatry had available only a few institutions for difficult and delinquent children and adolescents and a network of charitable orphanages and shelters for severely retarded and epileptic children.

Intensive work in the field of scientific psychiatry was undertaken after the October Revolution—despite the difficulties of the first years of revolution, civil war, and epidemics—at older university centers and at newly organized universities in outlying areas and the national republics. Investigative work continued to follow the traditional Russian psychiatric tendency toward solution of clinical problems, but also, in line with the requirements of the time, it became concerned with studying the scientific principles to be employed in reorganizing existing psychiatric institutions and planning new ones; the psychiatric consequences of the first World War and the civil war, of the epidemics of typhoid fever, of the prevalence of social diseases (tuberculosis, alcoholism, outbreaks of cocainism and other drug addictions during the civil war, etc.), and of other factors to be taken into account.

The theoretical basis common to all Soviet psychiatrists, the philosophy of dialectical materialism and, in biological science, I. P. Pavlov's physiological theory of higher nervous activity, united all research work and channeled it into a single methodological trend. It is thus understandable that Soviet psychiatrists had a not entirely consistent attitude toward the appearance in Soviet psychiatry of various types of idealistic, vulgarized, often inimical tendencies, which inevitably involved researchers in semantic tangles and fallacious constructs, ultimately creating a gap between theory and the pressing demands of public health. The physiological concepts traditional throughout the entire development of Russian clinical practice, which gave rise to I. M. Sechenov's physiological theory and then to I. P. Pavlov's theory of higher nervous activity, naturally entailed a tendency toward regarding the patient as a somatopsychic whole. This tendency was outstanding in all the theoretical pronouncements of Soviet clinicians and in everyday medical practice, and it was a natural outgrowth of the theoretical hypotheses of the leaders of Russian clinical practice during the first half of the nineteenth century. The clinical pronouncements of these luminaries are easily superimposed on the background of Sechenov-Pavlov physiological theory.

Pavlov's principles of protective inhibition, of the protective regimen followed at therapeutic institutions, and of the value of the physician's words as a therapeutic factor all provided a theoretical explanation of much that had long ago been deduced empirically in clinical practice. A new, "physiological" light was shed on the individual therapeutic approach to the patient, the psychotherapeutic "spirit," and the atmosphere of therapeutic institutions. A critical reexamination was then made of psychotherapeutic, psychohygienic and psychoprophylactic problems in order to eliminate everything foreign to the principles of Soviet psychiatry.

S. Freud's psychoanalytic method was unsuitable for the overwhelming majority of pre-Revolutionary Russian and Soviet psychiatrists. Individual adherents of Freudian psychoanalysis among Russian psychiatrists (N. A. Vyrubov, N. Ye. Osipov, O. B. Fel'tsman) attempted to popularize it in Russia during the period between 1910 and 1914; the journal *Psikhoterapiya* (Psychotherapy), which had a distinct psychoanalytic bias, was published in Moscow under the editorship of Vyrubov, with the close cooperation of a number of the most orthodox Viennese psychoanalysts. None of these attempts, however, had the desired success and, as before, Freudian psychoanalysis remained foreign to the majority of Russian psychiatrists. New attempts were made to popularize psychoanalysis in Soviet psychiatry after the October Revolution. During the 1920's, a whole series of volumes was published in the "Psychoanalytic Library" under the editorship of I. D. Yermakov, that were translations into Russian of the basic works of Freud and his closest followers. Attempts were made to relate Freudian psychoanalysis to Marxism (Yu. V. Kannabikh, V. A. Vnukov) as well as to understand communism from the Freudian standpoint (G. Yu. Malis). None of these attempts, however, met with any success and all went unnoticed by the majority of Soviet psychoanalysts. Modified, neo-Freudian forms were regarded by Soviet psychiatrists as blindly speculative, idealistic constructs having nothing in common with the philosophic methodology of dialectical materialism. In his very substantial monograph, *Current Trends in Foreign Psychiatry and Their Ideological Origins,* V. M. Morozov quite correctly points out that the adherents of all these idealistic trends "usually consider man only as a biological entity whose behavior and feelings are determined by a few innate instincts, subconscious impulses, or primitive mechanical reactions to the environment." Indistinctly seen in the origins and causative factors of morbid neuropsychiatric conditions is an obscure biological force hidden in the depths of the personality. In his classic monograph, *Psychopathological Symptomatology* (1933), P. B. Gannushkin, the head of the leading school of Soviet psychiatrists, and one who always maintained a very reserved attitude toward Freud's theories, felt it sufficient to relegate Freudian psychoanalysis to a footnote and pointed out that "the method by which Freud attempted to explain the genesis and symptomology of psychopathic conditions seems to us to be overly enigmatic, arbitrary, and indeterminate to be at all seriously applicable to such a vast and important problem."

The clinical-nosological trend and the tendency toward a pathophysiological view of mental disorders to a large extent protected Soviet psychiatry from fortuitous, methodologically foreign, and speculative elements. Discussions of theoretical problems in psychiatry and related biological disciplines, which took place over a period of years, uncovered the roots of the unwholesome, methodologically alien ideas and distortions that had crept into Soviet psychiatry and kept them from developing further. Thus, for example, the success of Soviet psychiatrists in the field of borderline conditions at the neuropsychiatric dispensaries and the sanitariums for neurological patients, and their direct guidance of extensive outpatient facilities for individual groups of workers, sponsored a tendency for individual physicians to accept extremely broad psychopathological criteria and to extrapolate uncritically the mechanisms of "major " psychiatric conditions to isolated neurotic and asthenic manifestations or to transient personality aberrations. Similar errors were committed in the psychiatry of early childhood.

This fact and the uncritical acceptance of Kretschmer's concept of the development of normal personality quirks into psychoses, a theory which erased the boundary between normal and pathological conditions, between normal personality traits and mental illness, led to an unjustified extension of the boundaries of such severe mental disorders as schizophrenia and to resultant severe consequences for persons thus classified as mentally ill. The necessary corrections were, however, made in all these overenthusiastic theories shortly after publication of a critical article by V. P. Osipov (Plate LXV), one of the most eminent Soviet psychiatrists, which caused a heated debate at the Second All-Union Congress of Neuropathologists and Psychiatrists in 1936. A nearly analogous situation arose in another case: Extremely intense interest in the problem of the localization of psychic functions led to complex psychopathological theories based on the functional integrity of the body and brain and positing localization in quite restricted areas of the central nervous system. Such simplified concepts could only promote an uncritical extension of operative intervention in schizophrenia (by prefrontal leucotomy)—a technique employed in the Western nations—to the Soviet Union. Soon after checking the results of such operations, the Soviet psychiatric community raised the question of discontinuing this practice as antiphysiological and undoubtedly harmful.

Pedagogical interest in the psychopathology of children and adolescents was also severely criticized. In addition to the usual clinical-psychopathological study of symptoms of mental retardation undertaken at psychiatric clinics for children and adolescents, the study of academic failure and of pedagogic and social neglect had been limited by the simplified investigative techniques used for children and adolescents, which were elementary in character and so universal as to be described in all psychology texts, and by the offhand treatment of mentally healthy but congenitally retarded children, or defectives, who were transferred to auxiliary classes for the retarded. On the theoretical level practices of this type entailed the establishment of a new, independent discipline, *defectology,* lying somewhere between the natural and medical sciences and the pedagogical sciences. The founding of a separate discipline was naturally not justified in actuality and pointed up the total erroneousness of attributing the diverse factors underlying academic failure or pedagogic and social neglect solely to biological defects. All the pedological pitfalls discussed above were finally brought into the open at the First All-Union Conference on Human Behavior held in Moscow in 1930. Also, a number of problems of heredity and constitution were critically reexamined in general discussions held by scientific societies for neurologists and psychiatrists in Moscow, Leningrad, and other cities.

These and subsequent discussions overcame theoretically inadmissible and speculative tendencies, which were causing Soviet psychiatry to stray from the clinical-nosological path. This was to the advantage of the discipline, and it subsequently progressed unhampered to indubitable achievements in both theoretical and clinical psychiatry.

The persistent interest of pre-Revolutionary Russian psychiatrists in the problem of infectious psychoses is to a considerable extent attributable to the not infrequent epidemics of acute infectious diseases in Czarist Russia. During the Soviet era the successful conduct of epidemiological measures sharply reduced the incidence of acute infectious diseases, some of which (such as malaria) were almost entirely eliminated, and the interest of Soviet psychiatrists in them naturally decreased. However, during the first few years after the October Revolution, a period of economic upheaval, the shortage of foodstuffs and the pandemics of typhoid diseases attracted a great deal of attention by psychiatrists. Their interest was concentrated on elucidating the differences rather than the similarities among the mental disorders observed in the various forms of typhoid. However the clinical observations of psychiatrists later (in some cases during World War I, 1914-1917) came to be centered in the infectious-disease wards of general hospitals or in special hospitals for such diseases. Only here could the entire spectrum of psychopathological manifestations be observed in ordinary infectious diseases not exacerbated by complications in the central nervous system. Kraepelin pointed out the extraordinary value to psychiatry of observations made in infectious-disease wards. Such observations by Soviet psychiatrists made possible detection of unusual psychopathological nuances in ordinary cases of infectious diseases and descriptions of them as characteristic of a given type of infection. In some clinically unclear cases of infectious disease, correct evaluation of these peculiarities in the patient's mental state is of material aid in making a differential diagnosis of the basic affliction. This is particularly true in typhoid infections, where such differences are most pronounced.

The attention of Soviet psychiatrists was drawn both to the infectious-disease wards and to other departments of general medical hospitals. P. B. Gannushkin was always interested in and tried to make observations in somatic hospitals and was, until his death, a constant consultant at the S. P. Botkin Clinical Somatic Hospital. He was a strong supporter of the idea of organizing a psychiatric service and psychiatric wards at general hospitals. After his death in 1933, Gannushkin's views were put into practice, first at the Botkin Hospital and then at other medical hospitals. The clinical data gathered at somatic hospitals are of great interest to psychiatrists: They are the most promising and accessible materials for studying problems of corticovisceral relationship and the clinical relationship of mental and somatic phenomena under clinical conditions. As was seen from the foregoing discussion, the attempts of Russian and Soviet physicians in this direction, which began during the first half of the nineteenth century, were based on strictly clinical principles and physiological concepts of neuropsychiatric manifestations. These attempts by Soviet doctors cannot, however, be confused with the current American theory of psychosomatic medicine, which is based wholly and completely on modernized neo-Freudian depth-psychodynamic concepts and is essentially idealistic. These artificial constructs of the American psychosomatic theoreticians, foreign to the truly materialistic clinical-physiological trend in Soviet psychiatry, could not but repel Soviet psychiatrists and reduce their interest in this problem. Substantial progress was made in determining the relationship of mental and somatic phenomena by Soviet physiologists of Pavlov's school who used experimental data and data of the symptomatology of internal illness to study corticovisceral and viscerovisceral relationships.

In connection with the great importance which Soviet society has always attached to the protection of workers and to industrial medicine, Soviet psychiatrists devoted a great deal of attention also to intoxication psychoses and to mental disorders associated with occupational hazards, particularly at chemical enterprises. Some of these investigations were carried out in close cooperation with the V. A. Obukh Institute of Occupational Diseases in Moscow. The problem of chronic alcoholism and the treatment of alcoholics also occupied Soviet psychiatrists. Much attention was devoted to studying the initial signs of chronic alcohol poisoning of the nervous system and the systems of hangovers, while methods and drugs were sought for treating chronic alcoholism, particularly in connection with the development of conditioned reflex vomiting associations with the drinking of alcoholic beverages. The traditional interest of Russian and Soviet psychiatrists in the Korsakov syndrome has persisted down to the present, and their many investigations, both purely clinical and clinical-physiological, have occupied a rather prominent place in their scientific publications.

Unfortunately, it has not been possible to establish anything conclusive about its physiological bases.

The problem of traumatic psychoses occupied Soviet psychiatrists throughout the entire period after the Otcober Revolution and even during World War I. From the very beginning, the concept of traumatic neurosis drew criticism as somehow paradoxical, although more from psychiatrists than from neuropathologists. The mass of data on traumatization of the central nervous system compiled during World War II naturally occupied a central position in research work, after problems of schizophrenia. Of special interest and value in this series of investigations are studies devoted to higher nervous activity in the presence of traumatic injuries to the brain and subsequent dynamic observations made on patients with traumatic mental disorders. Pathomorphological data on cerebral traumas terminating in death at various stages of morbidity are also important. In addition to a whole series of interesting individual scientific conclusions, data on trauma gathered by dynamic observation quite clearly showed that mental disorders following cerebral trauma are not residual phenomena but manifestations of a general cerebral morbidity with a characteristic dynamic course through its various stages, and that often (when the outcome is unfavorable) these should be regarded as traumatic disease. Besides establishing definite pathophysiological mechanisms, the numerous investigations of higher nervous activity in the presence of cerebral traumas brought about a number of new, physiologically grounded therapeutic measures.

Soviet psychiatry has made an especially large number of studies of schizophrenia. These have concentrated on clarifying its symptomatology and limits and on studying its pathogenetic mechanisms, the purpose being to confirm its nosological independence and to differentiate it from schizophrenia-like psychopathological conditions of differing nosological character. The expansion and concentration of research in this area and the search for the etiological and ophrenic conditions enabled the overwhelming majority of Soviet psychiatrists to take firm clinical positions and to recognize the nosological independence of schizophrenia as a processual disease. The extreme frequency with which diagnoses of "mild schizophrenia" were given played a positive role, since it properly attracted the attention of psychiatrists to the undoubted existence of cases of schizophrenia with a not very distinct processual symptomatology and a comparatively favorable course. This indubitable clinical fact, which was also noted in other branches of medicine, permitted a closer approach to the problem of the course and outcome of schizophrenia and the role played in this disease by the compensatory reserves of the nervous system; all these data also made possible reexamination of the validity of the almost universally accepted German hypothesis regarding the hereditary nature of schizophrenia.

A great deal of progress was also made as a result of the precise elaboration of the phenomenology of schizophrenia. In addition, Soviet psychiatrists devoted much attention to examining various aspects of disruptions of higher nervous activity in schizophrenia; there were numerous virological, immunobiological, and especially biochemical studies of the pathogenesis of the disease; and the problem of disruptions of cerebral electrical activity stimulated further interest. A broad range of purposeful, intensive, and successful research (both clinical-psychopathological and biological) studied the regularities in the course of syndrome sequence of the various stages of schizophrenia and its specific forms.

At the same time, intensive research was conducted at ordinary clinical institutions, psychiatric hospitals, dispensaries, and semiclinics. This work was directed primarily at clinical verification of old drugs and discovery of new, more effective ones for use in various types of psychoses; schizophrenia was naturally of primary interest.

Important investigations were conducted to elucidate the physiological bases of various types of hallucinatory phenomena and detrimental experiences (further developing I. P. Pavlov's theories on these problems) and compulsive phenomena. Soviet psychiatrists and physiologists also researched the physiological mechanisms underlying psychopathological manifestations in other nosological forms and clinically dominant syndromes.

Investigation in the field of "minor psychiatry" and borderline conditions was promoted by the fact that the most authoritative of the Soviet clinical psychiatrists, P. B. Gannushkin, a leading student of the classicists of Soviet psychiatry, S. S. Korsakov and V. P. Serbskiy, undertook his first clinical work in this area at the beginning of the century under the supervision of and in collaboration with his old colleague F. A. Sukhanov. The directions taken by their research subsequently diverged. While Sukhanov attempted to verify the possibility for pathological character traits to be psychopathologically intensified into corresponding forms of psychosis—a path taken considerably later in Germany by Kretschmer, which ultimately led him to his aforementioned theory unacceptable to Soviet psychiatrists—Gannushkin felt it impossible to stray from strictly clinical facts. This field of Soviet psychiatry is now wholly associated with Gannushkin. His classic, posthumously published monograph *Psychopathological Symp-*

tomatology (1933) reflects his thirty years of observation and theorizing in this area of clinical practice. His understanding of psychopathic conditions rested entirely on a sober evaluation of actual clinical data and lacked the often-encountered, simplified tendency to attribute all the diversity of specific data to the constitutional-hereditary roots of personality or to the action of fortuitous detrimental environmental factors. The former view completely ignores the significance of the external, primarily social environment in forming personality, whereas the latter overlooks the role of the biological bases of personality traits. As is well known, the majority of researchers, both Soviet and foreign, have adopted one of these two equally one-sided positions.

In taking into account the various aspects of the symptomatology of psychopathic conditions (static, dynamic, and phaselike), Gannushkin came very close to a physiological view of his clinical data and essentially paved the way for subsequent special physiological investigations in this area. He gave a clear account of the complications and difficulties which arise in any psychopathological investigation, and he emphasized that in his systematics of psychopathic conditions he proceeded solely from specific clinical data and did not permit himself to go farther than they warranted. At this stage of our knowledge we can consequently speak only of an empirical systematics of psychopathology, its statics and dynamics.

The entire force and significance of Gannushkin's theory of psychopathic conditions lies in his scientific strictness and thoroughness as a leading clinician and in his fear of premature, unverified, and speculative conclusions and generalizations. The majority of the work of other Soviet psychiatrists in this field is at the same level. Attempts to distinguish special types of psychopathic conditions based solely on social factors were unsuccessful both methodologically and clinically and have received no support in the literature. Unfortunately, no sufficiently convincing results have yet been yielded by attempts to construct a classification of psychopathic conditions on the basis of Pavlov's theory of nervous-system types. In recent years O. V. Kerbikov and his colleagues have tried to expand Gannushkin's theory of psychopathic dynamics by including transient psychopathoid conditions (which in some cases subsequently acquire a stable character), whose development is based solely on unfavorably complicated living conditions and unendurable situations, especially during the early stages of the formation of the conscious personality.

Specialists in mental illnesses of childhood and adolescence have introduced much of value into general Soviet psychiatry. In addition to working out the symptomatology of psychoses in these age groups, establishing precise differential-diagnostic criteria, and determining the symptomatological differences between childhood and adult illnesses, child psychiatrists furnished a great deal of support for the development of "adult psychiatry." They also contributed greatly to the clarification of the role of a number of other factors in the development of mental illnesses and abnormalities during the intra-uterine development of the fetus, delivery, and the postnatal period. Further, they increased our understanding of the functional development of the endocrine system and juvenile "brain infections" and other abnormalities to which children are subject but which are often overlooked in collecting anamnestic data at a later time and thus are not given sufficient consideration.

The scientific output of psychiatrists increased substantially during the Soviet era in comparison with that of the pre-Revolutionary years. This is attributable to the fact that the number of psychiatric workers rose considerably with the organization of special psychoneurological research institutes and medical schools with independent departments of psychiatry in many cities, while the instructors in these departments of psychiatry conducted a great deal of research in addition to their teaching, in keeping with the long-standing traditions of Russian universities. Research also attracted many physicians employed at psychiatric hospitals and dispensaries. The changes which took place in the publication of the results of scientific investigations are understandable if one takes into account the fact that the transactions of numerous scientific and scientific-practical conferences, meetings, and congresses had to be published. The situation gradually developed to the point that the majority of scientific papers appeared in collections, which were brought out as the scientific-research institutes and departments of psychiatry of medical institutes amassed material, as well as in special collections of scientific reports on the work of general and local psychiatric (sometimes in conjunction with neuropathological) congresses and meetings. At the same time, the number of journals of psychiatry and neuropathology was gradually reduced, so that there now remains only one, the oldest psychiatric periodical, first published in 1901, the S. S. Korsakov Journal of Neuropathology and Psychiatry. The advantage of this publication system for the majority of scientific papers lies, among other things, in the fact that it attracts local medical personnel to research and permits expansion and guidance of local investigative work. All this is of especially great importance for psychiatrists in the outlying republics, which were the most neglected in this respect in Czarist Russia.

The following facts also show the intensity of the research being conducted in the Soviet Union in comparison with that of the pre-Revolutionary period. During the entire era of the development of scientific psychiatry in Russia, i.e., from the second half of the 19th century until the Revolution in 1917, scientific and scientific-organizational problems and narrower problems of psychiatric practice were considered at four congresses of Russian psychiatrists and at the Congress of the Association of Russian Psychiatrists and Neuropathologists (in 1887, 1904, 1909, 1911), as well as at the Sections for Nervous and Mental Illnesses of five Congresses of Russian Physicians in Memory of N. I. Pirogov (between 1891 and 1904). After the February and October Revolutions of 1917, four All-Russian Conferences of Psychiatrists and Neuropathologists were held (in 1917, another in 1917, 1919, and 1923), as were four All-Union Congresses of Neuropathologists and Psychiatrists that involved a series of parallel sectional meetings on child psychiatry, forensic psychiatry, military psychiatry, and the function of the dissector in psychiatric clinics and hospitals (in 1917, 1936, 1948, and 1963). There were also many local psychiatric conferences, both in the central regions of the nation and in the various republics and territories. The majority of these local sectional meetings, especially those in the capitals of republics and the seats of territories, were well attended by participants from the entire Soviet Union. For example, the conference commemorating the 50th anniversary of the founding of the Psychiatric Clinic of Moscow University at Devichiy Polye attracted psychiatrists from almost all the regions and requblics, and the scientific conference held at the same psychiatric clinic by the First Moscow Medical Institute in 1951 to commemorate the 100th anniversary of the birth of S. S. Korsakov was no less well attended and saw many scientific papers presented. The same was true of the Combined Session of the Presidium of the U.S.S.R. Academy of Medical Sciences and the Executive Board of the All-Union Scientific Society of Neuropathologists and Psychiatrists in 1951, and of the psychoneurological congresses in the Ukraine, the Central Asiatic Republics (in Tashkent), the Baltic republics (in Riga), Armenia, Georgia, Azerbaydzhan, Moldavia, etc.

The Scientific Psychiatric Association of the Soviet Union comprises the All-Union Scientific Society of Neuropathologists and Psychiatrists and the corresponding scientific societies of neuropathologists and psychiatrists in the Union republics, which are affiliates of the All-Union Scientific Society. In turn the Psychiatric Association of the Russian Federation includes the All-Russian Scientific Society of Neuropathologists and Psychiatrists and its affiliates in the capitals of the autonomous republics and in the seats of the regions and territories. Each year, at an expanded plenary session, the Executive Board of the All-Union Society summarizes the work done during the year in the Report of the Chairman, which is followed by election of a new Executive Board. The plenary session of the Executive Board of the Society is usually coordinated with some scientific conference or meeting of interest to all psychiatrists in the Soviet Union.

Instruction in psychiatry is obligatory in all faculties of the medical institutes, but few hours are devoted to lectures and practical work in this area in the sanitation-hygiene faculty. Psychiatry, as the clinical discipline which culminates the development of a profoundly synthetic clinical way of thought in medical students, is taught in the last years of medical school, after the other clinical disciplines. The instructor in psychiatry thus has the very weighty task of using his clinical material to show the complex of causal factors producing the clinical pattern of illness in each patient and the importance of an integral view of the complicated individual psychosomatic organization of the patient. In former years, when the teaching load on medical faculties was not so heavy, psychiatry was taught in the last three semesters (of a five-year program). During the second semester of the 4th year, the students were familiarized with the history of psychiatry, the general principles of the organization of psychiatric aid, the place of psychiatry in medicine, etc., and they made a thorough study of the symptoms and psychopathological syndromes most frequently encountered in the clinic in mental illnesses. The final two semesters (the 5th year) were devoted to hospital work, to the study of the individual forms of psychosis and related problems of general clinical methodology, to acquisition of an integral view of the patient and a proper bedside manner, etc. As a result of the load on teaching programs in medical institutes, the number of hours now devoted to the teaching of psychiatry is greatly curtailed, not corresponding to the demands on or the value of psychiatry in general medical practice. The therapeutic faculties devote 36 hours of lectures and 50 hours of practical work to psychiatry, the sanitation-hygiene faculties 18 and 36 hours respectively. The specialized pediatric faculties devote a few hours as well.

The authors of Soviet textbooks on psychiatry have attempted to compensate for the lack of time devoted to teaching psychiatry, taking this circumstance into account and, as far as possible, improving both their manner of presentation and the character and sequence of their material. The most informative of these texts are the often-reissued *Textbook of Psychiatry* by V. A. Gilyarovskiy and M. O. Guervich and the *Handbook of Psychiatry* by O. F. Kerbikov, N. I. Ozeretskiy,

Ye. A. Popov, and A. V. Snezhnevskiy. The latter is based wholly on Pavlov's theory of the physiology of higher nervous activity. The psychiatric community also generally approves O. V. Kerbikov's *Clinical Lectures on Psychiatry*, A. S. Chistovich's *Manual of Psychiatry*, I. F. Sluchevskiy's *Psychiatry*, and G. Ye. Sukharev's *Lectures on Child Psychiatry*. The classical texts on general psychiatry are still those by S. S. Korsakov and V. P. Osipov; that on psychopathic conditions is P. B. Gannushkin's *Psychopathological Symptomatology*.

The large network of medical schools and scientific research psychiatric institutes in the Soviet Union necessitates serious attention to the problem of preparing scientific personnel and instructors in this field. The number of doctors employed at theraeputic institutions and simultaneously conducting fruitful research has increased considerably. The training of highly skilled specialists for hospitals and for the network of outpatient institutions is a major task. Because psychiatric aid is being provided for the populace by decentralization of clinics and expansion of the network of outpatient dispensaries and clinics, the network of psychiatric institutions requires more and more new medical personnel. After they have completed medical school, young physicians are given specialized training in psychiatry by institutes for residents at the psychiatric clinics of medical or scientific-research institutes and at the majority of municipal and regional psychiatric hospitals. The term of residence is two years. On completion of their residency the young specialists either remain at the local psychiatric institutions where they received specialized training or are sent by the Ministry of Public Health or the Region Public Health Services to therapeutic institutions in greater need of medical personnel; understandably these are for the most part in outlying areas. There is a system of graduate study for training scientific workers from among doctors who have completed their specialization in psychiatry. Graduate students in clinical psychiatry are selected from among young specialists with the greatest aptitude for research who have worked at least two years in therapeutic institutions of their specialty and have successfully passed entrance examinations in their basic specialty, in related disciplines, and in the principles of dialectic materialism. The maximum age for admission to graduate study is 35 years. The program for training of graduate students provides for completion of three years of study and successful defense of a dissertation at the academic level of Candidate of Medical Sciences. On completion of their studies the young research workers are assigned to permanent jobs, usually at one of the scientific-research institutes of psychiatry or at the departments of psychiatry of medical institutes.

The assignment is at the discretion of the All-Union or Republic Ministries of Public Health.

In addition to the extensive network of medical institutes, there are also Institutes for the Advanced Training of Physicians in a number of large cities and the capitals of the Union republics. Practicing physicians, including psychiatrists, are sent to these institutes in a definite sequence and at set intervals for advanced training in their specialty. Instruction is carried out in accordance with a strict program centered on problems of the symptomatology and diagnosis of mental illnesses and familiarization with modern methods for treating the mentally ill. In some cases, courses have been set up for requalification from one clinical specialty to another and for primary specialization in psychiatry. Individual short-term courses in the most pressing problems of psychiatry are organized sporadically.

BIBLIOGRAPHY

1. ANANIEV, B. G. (1947): *Ocherki istorii russkoi psikhologii XVIII i XIX vekov (Outlines of Russian psychology of the 18th and 19th centuries)*. Gospol.
2. BROZEK, J. & SLOBIN, D. I. (Eds.) (1972): *Psychology in the U. S. S. R.: An Historical Perspective*. New York: International Arts and Sciences Press.
3. EDELSHTEIN, A. O. (1944): *Puti otechestvenoi psikhiatrii* (Progress of Soviet psychiatry). *Sovetskaia Med.*, No. 3, 22, 24.
4. GALACH'YAN, A. G. (1968): Soviet Union. In: Kiev, A. (Ed.), *Psychiatry in the Communist World*. New York: Science House.
5. GILYAROVSKY, V. A. (1961): The Soviet Union. In: Bellak, L. (Ed.), *Contemporary European Psychiatry*. New York: Grove Press.
6. KANNABIKH, I. V. (1929): *Istoriia Psikhiatrii (History of Psychiatry)*. Moscow.
7. KIEV, A. (Ed.) (1968): *Psychiatry in the Communist World*. New York: Science House.
8. LONDON, I. D. (1949): The treatment of emotions in contemporary Soviet psychology. *J. Gen. Psychol.*, 41, 89.
9. LONDON, I. D. (1949): A historical survey of psychology in the Soviet Union. *Psych. Bulletin.*, 46, 241.
10. MONAKHOV, K. K. (1968): The Pavlovian Theory in Psychiatry: Some Recent Developments. In: Howells, J. G. (Ed.), *Modern Perspectives in World Psychiatry*. Edinburgh: Oliver & Boyd; New York: Brunner/Mazel.
11. PAVLOV, I. P.: *Lectures on Conditioned Reflexes*. Trans. by Gantt, W. H. Vol. I: *Twenty-five Years of Objective Study of the Higher Nervous Activity (Behaviour) of Animals*. 1928. Vol. II: *Conditioned Reflexes and Psychiatry*. 1941. New York: International Publishers.
12. PAVLOV, I. P. (1952): *Complete Collected Works*.
13. SUKHAREVA, G. E. (1955): *Clinical Lectures on the Psychiatry of Childhood*. Moscow: Medgyz.
14. TEPLOV, B. M. (1947): *Sovietiskaia psikhologischeskaia nauka za 30 let (30 Years of Soviet Psychology)*. Moscow: Pravda.
15. VALLON, C. & ARMAND, M. (1899): *Les Aliénés en Russie*. Montévrain.
16. WORTIS, J. (1950): *Soviet Psychiatry*. Baltimore: Williams & Wilkins.
17. YUDIN, T. I. (1951): *An Outline of the History of Russian Psychiatry*.

13

POLAND

T. Bilikiewicz, M.D., Ph.D.

Professor of Psychiatry,
Clinic for Mental Diseases,
Gdańsk Medical Academy, Debinki, Poland

AND

M. Lyskanowski, M.D.

Assistant Professor of History of Medicine
Institute of Social Medicine, Warsaw Medical Academy
Warsaw, Poland

1

LEGISLATION AND CARE OF THE MENTALLY ILL

Prior to the 16th Century

In prehistorical Poland mental diseases were associated with demonology and religion, as they were believed to be caused by evil spirits. The priests, as the mediators between spirits and men, were in charge of treatment.

When Christianity took the place of the old pagan religion, the ancient Polish beliefs and customs were tolerated, or even included in the new rites; thus sorcerers, fortune-tellers, and witch doctors were not persecuted. The clergy took over the care of the sick, but this activity was dictated more by custom than by a sense of duty. However, helping the poor and the sick was regarded as a most important Christian virtue and this promoted the building of hospitals, as they were considered charitable establishments (31, 36). Thus, for many centuries, hospitals were founded by the kings and run by religious orders (19). People unable to earn their living, invalids, old people, and those suffering from incurable diseases were cared for by the hospitals, until a time when they could again support themselves (18).

However, the government often acted independently from the resolutions of the ecclesiastical councils and also provided for the indigent ill and other people unable to work. The first bill dealing with provisions for beggars, paupers, indigent sick, and unemployables was passed, in 1496, by King Jan Olbracht. It recommended that municipalities in towns and rectors in villages should supervise beggars; those entitled to beg were issued with special badges, but those who were merely avoiding work were punished (27).

The first asylums for the mentally ill in Poland were founded in the 16th century—in Cracow, in 1534, and in Gdańsk, in 1542 (2). The asylum in Cracow was built by townsmen and the foundation act was passed by Bishop Tomicki. The establishment was called *Praepositura hospitalis foriosorum SS Fabiani et Sebastiani Martyrum*. The mentally ill from the Hospital of the Holy Ghost found shelter here. The other hospital, in Gdańsk, was founded by the town authorities and built on the site of the small-pox hospital (10).

The most important forensic act for the care of the mentally ill was the Lithuanian Charter, passed in 1529 by King Sigismondus the Old. Among other provisions it proclaimed that those insane accused of manslaughter were to be placed in the charge of their relatives as well as under the charge of the town or country authorities. The Lithuanian Charter was the first psychiatric bill in the history of Poland; in it the insane were treated as sick people, with justice and reason and without any trace of demonology (8).

The 17th Century

In the 17th century, the Order of Charity, or Bonifraters, appeared in Poland. In 1608 one of its members, Brother Gabriel (Count Ferrara, a physician in ordinary to the Emperor Ferdinand), was called to the bed of King Sigismund III who was seriously ill. The King recovered and the order became highly regarded for its medical skills. Hence, when Walerian Montelupi, a townsman of Cracow, founded a hospital in 1609, it was given to the Brothers of Charity. This order spread from Cracow all over Poland; the Bonifraters undertook the care of the male patients, while the Sisters of Charity of Saint Vincent a Paulo looked after the women. In 1728, the first bill was passed dealing with hospitals under the charge of the Bonifraters; the bill ordered the brothers to execute conscientiously the physicians' recommendations (32).

The question of witchcraft trials demands separate discussion. In Europe the trials for witchcraft took place earlier, in the 14th century, but in Poland the newly fashioned trials for witchcraft based on German legislation did not appear until the turn of the 17th century. Up to that time the legislation provided rules against witches, but witchcraft was not considered a crime to be punished by death. When, in 1261, the flagellants' movement came to Poland, regional princes, on the instigation of the Archbishop of Gniezno, punished the flagellants, but only by imprisonment and confiscation of property. Pope Innocent VIII's 1484 recommendation for the most severe punishments for witches was not heeded even by those members of the Dominican order who were already settled in Poland.

In 1447, a famous work by Johann Sprenger and Heinrich Kraemer appeared under the title *Malleus Maleficarum* (The Witches' Hammer); it became the textbook for the Inquisition and started a wave of mass destruction of "witches" throughout Europe. In Poland this procedure never flourished, and isolated instances are more often met in the 17th and 18th centuries than in the 16th century, as it was in those later centuries that Poland experienced an economic, social, and political decline and consequently a less enlightened attitude towards the mentally ill (21).

With the introduction of general education, new ideas spread in Poland in the period of enlightenment (17); wise reformers, newspapers, and progressive publications caused a decrease in the number of witch-trials; those that still occasionally took place were condemned by public opinion (37).

The 18th Century

In the 18th century a number of administrative regulations aiming at protecting the mentally ill were introduced in Poland. These regulations were issued when the highest administrative organ, the Permanent Council, faced with the danger of partition, worked out a new constitution and strengthened the administration. A bill, dated June 24, 1791, entrusted a newly founded Board with the protection of the national health, including mental health.

The Board took care of the mentally ill by the following procedures. Cases of psychosis were to be reported to the Board; special investigators were appointed, who interviewed persons seeking admission of patients and assessed their needs; a history relating to the patient was collected and passed to the physicians; medical examination and diagnosis were organized; the investigators made a report after reading the medical diagnosis; the insane were directed to the appropriate hospital and charges were fixed according to their means; the patient was again examined after treatment and a new assessment was made of his state of health; and cured patients were allowed to leave hospital. The *"Points for checking the reports of informants concerning mad minds"* are especially interesting. The informants were to tell how long they had known the patient, how he had behaved before, and how he behaved at that moment. They also had to tell where the patient lived, what he said, how he slept, how he was getting on with other people, and if his behavior, way of speaking, and manners seemed abnormal. They were also asked very exactly about the utterances and deeds of the patient which had caused the report to the Board. Archives make it clear that this procedure was not limited to privileged classes, i.e. the gentry and the aristocracy. The documents mention also a "charity fund," "the poor fund," and "charge of the government." These humanitarian measures for the protection of the insane were obviously developed from the enlightened promulgations contained in the Charter of 1529 (23).

The 19th Century

At the end of the 18th century, Poland lost her independence and was partitioned between Austria, Prussia, and Russia. Austria annexed 18 percent of the area of Poland and 32 percent of her population, Prussia 20 percent of the area and 23 percent of the population, Russia 62 percent of the area and 45 percent of the population. Each of these three countries introduced its own legislation and bureaucracy to the part it annexed (16). In spite of exceptionally difficult conditions the Polish people continued to care for their mentally ill.

In the Russian partition, in 1775, "The Polish and Lithuanian Committees of Hospitals were formed. The committees were to be central organs for management of hospital affairs, but ten years later they were abolished and the hospitals became the responsibility of the "Committees of Good Order," which were under the general direction of the authorities in charge of local administration in villages and towns (11).

In the Russian partition, since 1817, the General Supervising Board was in charge of all hospitals and Regional Supervising Boards acted in particular *voievodships,* or larger administrative units. After 1832, their functions passed to the so-called General Tutelary Board and the Regional Tutelary Boards, which survived, until 1870, as managing organs over all forms of welfare and treatment (39).

In 1839, "The General Regulations" for the Governing Body of Home Affairs of the Kingdom of Poland were devised; they included rules for sending mentally ill people to asylums destined for them. Police officers in towns and heads of villages were obliged to report cases of insanity to the medical supervisor, or the regional physician (26). In 1842, special forms were issued which were to be filled in before sending the sick to the hospital. The questions on the forms were about the state of health of the patient, his behavior, and his living conditions. In the same year, the Regional Tutelary Boards were replaced by County Tutelary Boards, which were in charge of all medical establishments within a smaller administrative unit (12). Hospitals became medical institutions in the full meaning of the word. Continuous medical care was provided by them and people were instructed to go to the hospital in case of illness.

In 1854, a collection of regulations appeared in Warsaw. It was called "Dispositions Concerning Charitable Establishments." These dispositions regulated the acceptance of the mentally ill into hospitals, and their management during treatment. One of the points stressed that the buildings should not be like prison (Plate LXVI). The more attractive the place the more effective the treatment and the more tolerable the stay for those who were destined never to leave the premises. This admonition was followed, in 1866, by other humanitarian rules about the transport of the mentally ill to hospital, their treatment during the journey, and less harsh forms of restraint (Plate LXVII).

The majority of psychiatric establishments in the Russian partition were in Warsaw. In 1891, one of the biggest psychiatric hospitals in Poland was opened at Tworki, near Warsaw. It was built by funds provided by the Polish people. It was a great achievement by a group of enthusiasts for modern help for the mentally ill, but it was little more than the proverbial "drop in the ocean of needs" for psychiatric facilities in Poland at that time (25). At the same time a discussion on modern methods of care for the mentally ill started in the columns of medical newspapers in Poland. Plans for building a new, large hospital for the mentally ill near Warsaw and criticism by outstanding Polish psychiatrists about the poor provisions for the mentally ill in Poland contributed to the discussion, but the vigorous and pointed remarks aimed at the authorities did little to improve the situation.

A greater contribution was that of those psychiatrists who, in spite of difficult conditions, did their best to secure medical care and humane treatment for the mentally ill (24).

In the Austrian partition, there was only one large hospital, the National Psychiatric Institute in Kulparków, near Lwów, founded in 1875. In addition there were two psychiatric wards, one in Cracow, founded in 1778, and one in Lwów, founded in 1789; two psychiatric

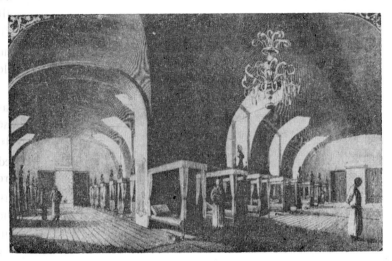

PLATE LXVI. Ward in The Warsaw Hospital of St. John of God.

wards in prison hospitals; and three private wards, including one for children. In 1912, the Neurologic-Psychiatric Clinic of Jagiellonian University came into being and it too gave a health service. The National Department of Governor-Generalship in Lwów, which was the capital of Galicja, was in charge of all the psychiatric provisions for this province.

In the German partition, there were, up to 1914, 26 different institutions for the care and treatment of the mentally ill. The total number of psychiatric beds in this area amounted to 9,000, or one psychiatric bed for 450 inhabitants (30).

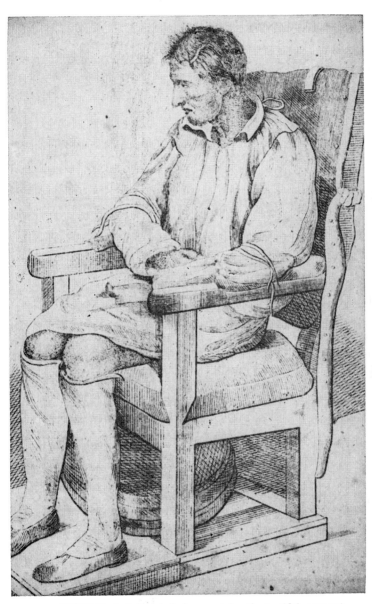

PLATE LXVII. Restraining chair for mental patients (19th century).

2

PSYCHIATRIC LITERATURE UP TO 1900

Despite partition and the loss of independence and the consequent exceptionally difficult conditions which impeded progress, scientific thought in Poland was not destroyed. Polish psychiatrists were in touch with scientific achievements of world psychiatry, and, as we can see from the compendium below, formed their own original concepts.

The first mentions of epilepsy, hydrophobia, headaches, and so on, are found scattered in 14th century herbals which, at that time, provided popular medical advice. The information included in them was not modern, nor was it influenced by medieval views; psychological matters were not at the high standard of Austria.

Jan of Glogów, the author of *Talks on the Action of the Human Limbs* published in 1501 and in 1515, and Andrzej Glaber of Kobylin, in 1535, dealt with problems of physiognomy and phrenology. Though they both imitated Aristotle, the approach to the problems they were concerned with is more empirical and their opinions could be checked by experience in everyday life. Andrzej of Kobylin can be called a predecessor of Lavater and Gall. His dissertation is illustrated with expressive sketches of human faces.

Sebastian Petrycy (1550-1626), professor of Cracow University, physician, historian, poet, and philosopher, translator of Aristotle, published *Aristotelian Principles* in 1605, with his own commentary. Among social suggestions included in the commentary, there are deliberations on sanity and responsibility for deeds committed while in a state of alcoholic inebriation. Petrycy suggested that ". . . frequent and intentional drunkenness should be punished, especially if someone commits an offense." This attitude is close to the modern forensic approach to psychiatric matters as expressed in the Polish penal code. Jan Jonston (1603-1675), called "Scoto-Polonus," a Polish physician of Scottish origin, was an encyclopedist, and the author of a work called *Idea Universae Medicinae Practicae,* published in 1674. In this work he discussed a number of problems concerned with neurosis and insanity. Ludwik Perzyna (1742-1812) challenged and corrected beliefs and superstitions relating to the mentally ill in his work *A Physician for Peasants,* published in 1793. His views were based on the preconception that the brain is the seat of mental diseases.

Jedrzej Sniadecki (1768-1838), professor of chemistry and later of medicine in the University of Vilno, became famous as an eminent physician, social worker, and author of distinguished works. His

Theory of Organic Beings brought him international fame. Among other topics, Sniadecki paid much attention to the neuropsychic functions of man, i.e. of psychophysiology. He considered all activities within the organism, and thus also mental processes, as symptoms of life. Life, in his opinion, is a process played out between the organism and the environment, and depending upon metabolism. Criticizing the thesis of the famous John Brown, Sniadecki emphasized the significance of the activity of each individual organism, but simultaneously believed that the activity of the organism may be apparent only thanks to the effect of the environment, especially to the effects of nutrition. Mental phenomena, he said, are life taking place in the nervous system. In particular, stimuli acting on the organism modify its metabolism and then "feeling" appears. Many eminent European scholars accepted with great respect the thesis that Sniadecki set out in his *Theory of Organic Beings,* which was translated into German and French. The originality of his views, which at some points were ahead of their time, prevented the work from being fully comprehended and appreciated (38).

Bartlomiej Frydrych (1800-1867), the author of the manual entitled *On Insanities,* published in 1845, in accordance with contemporary views, classified mental diseases into three groups. The first included mental diseases connected with the brain; the second those connected with the soul; and the third those related to both brain and soul. Frydrych seemed to be a believer in the first group; his hospital reports concerned with causes of mental diseases were based on scientific principles.

Andrzej Janikowski (1799-1864), who, in 1859, became professor of forensic medicine, criminology, and psychiatry in The Academy of Medicine and Surgery in Warsaw, was the author of *Principles of Medical Jurisprudence Investigations in Cases of Uncertain Health* (14), in which he discussed mental diseases in the chapter "On Doubtful Sanity." In *Pathology and Treatment of Mental Diseases* (15), Janikowski maintained that "mental diseases are illnesses of both mind and body, and any mental changes should be related with bodily changes and vice versa." He was a follower of the somatic school, because, as he maintained, "Psychiatry is not derived from theories but from truths observed in nature."

Romuald Plaskowski (1821-1896), who, in 1862, became the director of the Hospital of Jan Bozy and in 1864 an associate professor of "The Main School" (which later became Warsaw University), was the author of one of the best handbooks of psychiatry (28, 29) published at that time. On the basis of experience gained abroad and on his own observations and studies, he made a critical and objective analysis of contemporary scientific trends and views on mental diseases, their etiology, and their classiafication. He himself represented the materialistic approach to mental diseases. He looked for the pathogenesis of insanity in insufficient nutrition of nerve cells, in compression, degeneration, accumulation of fat corpuscles among nerve elements, insufficient circulation of arterial blood to the brain, infection, or effects of stupefying drugs. He attacked mysticism and doctrinarianism in psychiatry.

Adolf Rothe (1832-1903) was the author of *Psychopatologia Forensis (Science Dealing with Insanity in Jurisprudence)* (34) and *Psychiatry or the Science of Insanity* (35). He represents the following view of causes of insanity: ". . . The causes of insanity in general do not differ from those of other illnesses of the brain and of all diseases in general." Also: "A mad man is ill and madness is an illness in the strict sense, caused by illness of a certain organ of our body, hence madness is a bodily illness." Adolf Rothe belonged to the most outstanding group of Polish scientists of the 20th century.

3

DEVELOPMENTS AFTER 1900

Polish Psychiatrists Abroad

During the period following the partition of Poland, Polish scientists emigrated to various countries and were often able to work there. Of those who settled in Russia, Jan Baliński (1827-1902) was appointed to the first chair of psychiatry in Russia. He was a grandson of Jedrzej Sniadecki and is known as the "Father of Russian psychiatry." He was the representative of the first scientific psychiatric institution in Russia, and the organizer of modern psychiatric care in that country. Jan Mierzejewski (1838-1908), a scientist of Polish origin, was his follower. He represented the materialistic approach to mental diseases and believed in a somatic etiology. Stanislaw Danillo (1847-1897), Alfons Erlicki (1846-1902) and Otto Czeczott (1824-1924) were other links between Polish and Russian psychiatry (7).

Józef Babiński (1857-1932), a well known scientist, worked in France. The son of Polish emigrants who had to leave Poland in 1848, he completed his secondary education in the Polish School at Batignolles. He then studied medicine in Paris, where he was a pupil of Charcot.

Babiński worked independently in the Hôpital de la Pitié. He was one of the most outstanding innovators in the methodology of neurological examination. He maintained that the symptoms of hysteria are dependent on the psychical state and that they can be provoked or stopped by suggestion. Thus, he called hysteria *pithiatisme* (i.e., a state which can be removed by means of persuasion). Babiński pointed out similarities between hysteria and hypnosis and denied the widespread preconception of the time that anyone could be hypnotized aaginst his will.

Józefa Joteyko (1866-1928) worked in France and in Belgium. She exerted some influence on psychiatry as head of the psychophysiological laboratory of the University in Brussels for 14 years. In 1912, she organized the pedagogical faculty. After World War I, she was offered a chair in the College of France, but she returned to Poland and, in 1919, took the chair of General and Pedagogical Psychology in the National Pedagogical Institute (7).

The Period of Poland's Independence

In 1918, Poland regained her independence after nearly 150 years of occupation. After partition, the country inherited not only different systems of administration, but also a different psychiatric culture. The process of integration of the various regions of Poland was not easy and the difficulties were reflected also in psychiatry. In spite of lack of general directions and central planning, health services and psychiatric care gradually developed. The return of outstanding specialists from abroad greatly helped the development of psychiatry, assisted by new experts from five medical faculties of Polish universities. New forms of psychiatric care were introduced on a large scale and obvious progress was made. Expert consultants in psychiatry in the Ministry of Social Welfare and Health exerted a positive influence. The following were successively in charge of the consultations: Dr. Rafal Radziwillowicz (1860-1929), Dr. Jan Mazurkiewicz (1871-1947) and, for the longest period, Dr. Witold Luniewski (1881-1943).

Jan Mazurkiewicz (Plate LXVIII) was appointed professor at Warsaw University in 1919. He held the chair and managed the clinic there for 28 years, forming his own school and educating outstanding psychiatrists who succeeded him. During the period of Nazi occupation, he continued his psychiatric lectures in secret. He was the author of a number of works, among which *Introduction to Psychophysiology* was published after his death. The first volume of it, *Evolution of the Psychic Activity of the Cortex* (1950), dealt with normal psychophysiology, while the second volume, *Dissolution of the Psychic Activity of the Cortex,* dealt with pathological psychophysiology. In his research work, the author referred to the dynamic theory of Jackson, enriching it with the achievements of Semon, Monakov, Pavlov, Orbeli, Sherrington, and other scientists in the field of neurophysiology; he then undertook the task of creating his own theory of evolution and dissolution of human psychism. Mazurkiewicz's neo-jacksonism is an original conception, ingenious in all its details. The basis of the psychophysiological synthesis, he thought, is the preconception of the homo-

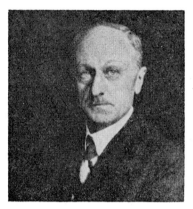

PLATE LXVIII.
Professor Jan Mazurkiewicz

genous growth, starting from the first manifestations of psychic life on the level of instinctive impulses and ending with its highest form, i.e. causal-logical and abstract thinking, as well as the higher sensitivity of a man. According to him the vegetative system was the background of human sensitive life. He discussed rapid prelogical dissolution and slow or prelogical schizophrenic dissolution as related to the conception of disintegration of personality and the division of schizophrenia into three groups: incoherent, hebephrenic, and paranoid and catatonic complexes. In his conclusions Mazurkiewicz discussed psychoneurotic dissolution, regression in dementia, and the role of manic and depressive states in dissolution.

Witold Luniewski (1881-1943), assistant professor of psychiatry at Warsaw University since 1932 and the head of the Psychiatric Hospital at Tworki since 1919, was a psychiatrist of great merit. During the period of Nazi occupation he prepared a manual of forensic psychiatry, published in 1950, and enlarged by Stanislaw Batawia (1898-   ), professor of criminology of the Department of Law at Lódź University and then at Warsaw University. The general part was published under the title *Outlines of Forensic Psychiatry* and was used by Polish physicians for ten years.

Meanwhile, the first professional journals were making their appearance: *The Psychiatric Annual* in 1923, *The Psychiatric News* in 1924, and *Mental Hygiene* in 1935. At the same time important institutions were founded: The Psychiatric Clinic at Warsaw University, in 1920, the Neurological-Psychiatric Clinic of the University of Wilno, in 1923, and also clinics in Lwów (1924), Poznań (1925), The State Institute for The Mentally Ill in Kobierzyn (1918), The State Psychiatric Hospital in Wilno (1927), The State Institute for Nervously Exhausted Women at Gościejewo (1927), The District Hospital for the Mentally Ill at Choroszcz (1930), The District Psychiatric Communal Hospital in Chelm Lubelski (1933), The District Hospital for the Mentally Ill at Gostynin (1933), The State Institute for Mentally Exhausted Men at Swiack (1933), and district hospitals for mentally ill prisoners at Grodzisk Mazowiecki (1928), in Grudziadz (1930), in Warsaw (1934), at Drohobycz (1934) and, for women, in Grudziadz (1934). A few psychiatric clinics, a civil and a military hospital, asylums for the mentally ill, and other special establishments should be added to this list. These, together with preventive care, medical services in industry, and so on, provided much-needed services on a national scale. At the outbreak of World War II there were 30,000 mentally ill patients and 17,000 permanent beds (7).

The Period of Nazi Occupation

The Germans, immediately after occupying Poland, started a movement aimed at the liquidation of the mentally ill in Polish hospitals. Patients in the following hospitals were murdered: Choroszcz, Dziekanka, Kochanówka, Obrzyce, Lubliniec, Owińska, Chelm Lubelski, Kobierzyn, Kulparków, Kocborowo, Wilno, and Swiecie. At least 400 patients from the Hospital of Jan Bozy were taken to the hospital at Choroszcz, where they were murdered; only 60 were left in the clinic. From among these 60, some were killed during the Warsaw Uprising, when they left the city with other civilians to seek refuge in nearby Pruszków.

During the German occupation, the Psychiatric Clinic of Warsaw University, the Neuro-Psychiatric Clinic of Poznań University, and other institutes ceased to exist. Nearly a thousand workers in the psy-

chiatric health service were murdered, among them 60 percent of
Polish psychiatrists (20). The occupation caused a complete disorganization of Polish psychiatry. Poland lost most of its technical, economic,
therapeutic, and scientific equipment. Most of the archives, libraries,
manuscripts, and works prepared for publication were destroyed. Organizational and professional life came to an end as well as all scientific
activity and education at university and secondary school level. Nevertheless, a small amount of scientific activity and education was carried
on in secret, thanks to the heroism of some individuals. The disasters
which overtook Poland during World War II obliged her sons, scattered all over the world, to unite in a collective effort to save their
culture. Their most important achievement was the founding of the
Medical Department at the Edinburgh University in Scotland. The
chair of neurology and psychiatry was taken by Jakub Rothfeld-Ros-
towski, assistant professor of neurology (1919) and titular professor
since 1928 at the University of Jan Kazimierz in Lwów (7).

After the Liberation

After the liberation Poland started an enthusiastic program of rebuilding in all fields. Polish psychiatrists took part, trying to rebuild
or reorganize whatever had survived after the war and establish a
material and spiritual basis for a health service and for psychiatric
care. In 1947, there were about 13,500 psychiatric beds for 24,000,000
inhabitants, served by 60 psychiatrists. Shortage of staff, especially of
physicians, was acute during the first years after the war; the slow
increase of staff could not, at first, satisfy the demands of a society that
was reawakening to a new life. Clinics and hospitals were obliged to
ease the shortage of beds by increasing the rate of discharge, made
possible by the modern methods of therapy which were introduced
on a large scale.

Under the new postwar conditions, formal legal frameworks for
the care of the mentally ill were arrived at; the organization of psychiatric affairs was centralized in the Ministry of Health, at first in the
Department of Social Medicine, and then in the Board of Prophylaxis
and Treatment. In addition a special organ came into being, the
Department for Diseases of the Nervous System. Central authority was
united with district administration and with special centers: the health
departments of the Voievodship National Boards, the sections of the
Institutes of Mental Hygiene, later changed to Dispensaries for Mental
Health, with consultants, and later country experts and voievodship
experts. This organization proved to be efficient and provided fruitful
results.

The majority of old hospitals and establishments started to function again and new hospitals and establishments came into being. Ten separate psychiatric clinics were established. The tragic postwar shortage of teaching staff was slowly being remedied. Due to the abundance of textbooks and the efforts of the teaching staff, psychiatric training reached an increasingly higher standard.

During the postwar period, a number of manuals of psychiatry were issued. The authors of these important works, aimed at qualified psychiatrists and at medical students, were Lucjan Korzeniowski, Andrzej Jus, Tadeusz Frackowiak, Zdzislaw Jaroszewski, Jan Jaroszyński, Stanislaw Cwynar, and Adam Bukowczyk.

Tadeusz Bilikiewicz wrote *Clinical Psychiatry,* a manual of psychiatry which is the largest psychiatric volume to have been published in Poland (4). It is based on the author's nosographic etioepigenetic system (3) (the principles of the etioepigenetic theory appeared in print in *Nova Acta Leopoldina,* 1970, entitled, *"Die Ätioepigenese in der Psychiatrischen Forschung"*) (6).

In more recent years the Polish Psychiatric Society has been engaged in evolving new forms of organization—therapeutic society, home hospitalization, day hospitals—and in the drafting of a Psychiatric Bill. The Bill, after discussion and examination in all its aspects, will become a basis for considering the complex problems involved in the care and the treatment of the mentally ill in Poland. In June 1971 the Minister of Health, Prof. Dr. J. Kostrzewski, presented the draft of the Bill in Parliament and decisions will soon follow concerning its acceptance and realization. The Psychiatric Bill, which is a great achievement of modern psychiatric thought in Poland, will greatly resolve the problems involved in the care and treatment of the mentally ill in Poland.

4

CLINICAL MANAGEMENT

In Poland, from antiquity onward, the mentally ill were treated in a gentle and humanitarian way. At first incantation, prayers, amulets, and herbs were used. Later, with the advent of the humoral theory, blood letting, purgatives, and enemas were employed. These remedies survived till the 18th century (22). "Physical treatment," i.e. whirl machines, the burning of heads in hot ovens, sudden throwing into water, skull helmets, etc., was not used in Poland (7).

In the 19th century Polish psychiatrists recommended the employment of patients and work in the open air (Bartlomiej Frydrych).
Physicians of that period maintained that a physician ought to be "an
eager guardian and a true friend" of the mentally ill (Klemens
Maleszewski). "Patience, forbearance, and most gentle treatment was
recommended" (Andrzej Janikowski) (24).

Among pharmacological remedies the following medicines were
recommended: digitalis, opium, belladonna, Peruvian bark, hops
(*humulus lupulus*), curare, and cocaine (Adolf Rothe). Electrotherapy
was also used (33).

Physicians of the 19th century continued to be interested in patients
after they had left hospital on completion of treatment. Adolph Rothe
tried to found an establishment which would provide employment for
patients leaving hospital and give them grants; the same organization
was to collect contributions for the ill, assure free medical care for
the poor insane, establish dispensaries, poorhouses, recreations, gardens, factories for the chronically ill, and, in general, fight against
the prejudices still rooted in society. Adolf Rothe's postulates were
realized in 1899, when the Warsaw Society for the Medical Care and
Protection of the Mentally Ill came into being. The society was a
charitable institution depending exclusively on the generosity of its
supporters (24).

Development of Psychotherapy in Poland

Information concerning the activity of Francis Mesmer (1734-1815)
and his concepts appeared relatively early, in 1784, in *Historical-
Political Memoirs,"* issued in Warsaw, but was read with reservations.
Three volumes of *The Magnetic Diary,* a work dealing with problems
of practical application of animal magnetism, appeared in Wilno, from
1816 to 1818. The constantly growing number of magnetizers caused
Józef Frank (1771-1842), professor and director of a clinic for internal
diseases in Wilno, to become interested in magnetism. In his paper on
animal magnetism he criticized the magnetizers and proved that their
activities were harmful.

Ludwik Perzyna, in his work, *A Physician for Peasants* (1793),
stressed the part played by "kind words" in the treatment of the mentally ill; it was the first concept of psychotherapy, although still undeveloped.

Józef Jakubowski (1796-1866), a professor of the Jagiellonian University in Craków, wrote a very interesting work on psychotherapy.
The dissertation "On the Method of Psychical Treatment" (13) was

published in *The Scientific Views,* in 1831. In this work he was pre-occupied with the character, behavior, and appearances of physicians and of the rest of the medical staff. He recommended relieving the distress caused by leaving home and going into hospital by engaging the patients' attention on other subjects; he wrote that "music is a wonderful psychical remedy," and that "employment is undoubtedly the most necessary and effective method of psychical treatment" (13). Jakubowski represented the views of Polish physicians of the 19th century, for whom humanitarian and gentle care in the treatment of the mentally ill was the most essential principle.

In 1863, the work of one of the most outstanding Polish scientists of the 19th century, Wiktor Szokalski (1811-1890), appeared as *Imaginary Sensory Symptoms,* in which the author wrote that various "moral influences" can be used to affect the body through the mind, and that they can be as effective as the physical substances used by the physicians directly on the organism. Thus, the author recognized the part played by magnetism and hypnotism in the treatment of the mentally ill. In the following 20 years physicians and scientists paid more attention to these problems due to the activities of Julian Ochorowicz (1850-1917), a philosopher and psychologist who was interested in hypnosis and telepathy. His experiments with magnetiza-tion caused controversy in the newspapers and gave rise to a series of clinical experiments. Although the experiments of Ochorowicz were a failure, they focused attention on the question of hypnotism and psychotherapy.

In 1899, an outstanding scientist, Edward Biernacki (1866-1911) wrote *The Essence and Limits of Medical Science* (1) in which he maintained that treatment, apart from material factors, contains also an immaterial, or psychical factor; he called this "the moral influence on the patient by those who offer him material help—the so-called suggestion."

Psychotherapy continued to attract interest. In the period, between the wars, Maurycy Bornsztajn (1874-1952), a representative of the psychoanalytical school of psychology, became interested in the prob-lems of psychoanalysis and wrote, in 1922, *Outlines of Clinical Psy-chiatry.* This manual was published again, in 1948, as *Introduction to Clinical Psychiatry.* In 1938, just before the outbreak of World War II, the first Polish manual of psychotherapy, entitled simply *Psychotherapy,* was written by Dr. Tadeusz Bilikiewicz in the third volume of the *Basic Encyclopaedia of a Medical Practitioner.* In 1948, the same author wrote *Psychology of Dreams,* basing his work on the oneiro-analytical method; this was followed by his *Psychotherapy in*

General Practice (5), in 1959. In the same year, Stanislaw Cwynar wrote *Introduction to Psychotherapy*.

At present the Section of Psychotherapy of the Polish Psychiatric Society and the Polish Society of Psychical Hygiene is concerned with matters pertaining to psychotherapy.

5

THE POLISH PSYCHIATRIC SOCIETY

The Polish Psychiatric Society came into being in 1920, but the first scientific clubs enabling exchange of ideas started in the 19th century.

In 1909, Dr. Rafal Radziwillowicz (1860-1929), an outstanding Polish psychiatrist, implemented the proposal of a nationwide congress of neurologists, psychiatrists and psychologists. Józef Babiński, from Paris, became one of the chairmen. The congress was held in Warsaw in October, 1909. Within the framework of the congress the psychiatric section conferred separately. The Second Congress of Polish Neurologists, Psychiatrists, and Psychologists was held in Cracow on December 20-23, 1912. At this Congress the Polish Neuro-Psychiatric Society was formed.

Up to 1939, the Polish Psychiatric Society held 19 congresses, discussing the most important scientific problems as well as problems connected with the organization and development of psychiatry in Poland.

With the regaining of independence, the first Congress of Polish Psychiatrists, this time without neurologists and psychologists, was organized by the Ministry of Public Health; the following subjects were discussed: principles of psychiatric legislation and organization of psychiatric care; the need for psychiatrists to be represented on the Codification Board; establishing university psychiatric clinics in Warsaw, Lwów, and Poznań; organizing psychiatric establishments for individuals with criminal predispositions and for mentally retarded children, and increasing the number of special schools for these children.

Right after the war, in 1945, the 20th Congress of Polish Psychiatrists was held at Tworki, on the 25th Anniversary of the Society, with 140 psychiatrists participating.

REFERENCES

1. BIERNACKI, E. (1899): *Istota i Granice Wiedzy Lekarskiej*. Warszawa.
2. BILIKIEWICZ, T. (1947): Z. Dziejów Medycyny Gdańskiej. *Sprawozdanie Polskiej Akademii Umiejetności*, XLVIII, 6.
3. BILIKIEWICZ, T. (1951): Próba Nozograficznego Układu Etioepigenetycznego w Psychiatrii. *Neurologia, Neuropsychiatria i Psychiatria Polska*, I, 1, 2, 3, 4. Warszawa.
4. BILIKIEWICZ, T. (1973): *Psychiatria Kliniczna*. PZWL. Warszawa (5th edition.)
5. BILIKIEWICZ, T. (1970): *Psychoterapia w Praktyce Ogólnolekarskiej*. PZWL. (4th edition in print).
6. BILIKIEWICZ, T. (1970): Die Atioepigenese in der Psychiatrischen Forschung. *Nova Acta Leopoldina*. J. A. Barth, 193, 35.
7. BILIKIEWICZ, T. & GALLUS, J. (1962): *Psychiatria Polska na Tle Dziejowym*. PZWL. Warszawa.
8. CZACKI, T. (1861): *O Litewskich i Polskich Prawach,o Ich Duchu Zródłach, Zwiazku i Rzeczach Zawartych w Pierwszym Statucie dla Litwy 1529 roku Wydanych, II*. W. Krakowie.
9. FRYDRYCH, B. (1845): *O Chorobach Umysłowych*. Warszawa.
10. GIEDROYC, F. (1908): *Zapiski do Dziejów Szpitalnictwa w Dawnej Polsce*. Warszawa.
11. GIEDROYC, F. (1911): *Zródła Biograf-Bibliograficzne do Dziejów Medycyny w Dawnej Polsce*. Warszawa.
12. GIEDROYC, F. (1913): *Rada Lekarska Ksiestwa Warszawskiego i Królestwa Polskiego (1809-1867)*. Warszawa.
13. JAKUBOWSKI, J. (1831): O Metodzie Leczenia Psychicznej. *Rozmaitości Naukowe*. W Krakowie.
14. JANIKOWSKI, A. (1845): *Zasady Dochodzeń Sadowo-Lekarskich co do Watpliwego Stanu Zdrowia*. Warszawa.
15. JANIKOWSKI, A. (1864): *Patologia i Terapia Chorób Umyslowych*. Warszawa.
16. KIENIEWICZ, S. & KULA, W. (1958): *Historia Polski*, II. Warszawa: PWN.
17. KOLLATAJ, H. (1905): *Stan Oświecenia w Polsce w Ostatnich Latach Panowania Augusta III* (1750-1764). Warszawa.
18. LUKASZEWICZ, J. (1850): *Historia Szkół w Krakowie i Wielkim Xiestwie Litewskim*. Poznań.
19. LUKASZEWICZ, J. (1858): *Krótki Opis Historyczny Kościołów Parochialnych* . . . Poznań. I.
20. LYSKANOWSKI, M. (1967): Los Psychicznie Chorych pod Panowaniem Ideologii Hitlerowskiej. *Przeglad Lekarski*, XXIII, 1.
21. LYSKANOWSKI, M. (1969): Procesy o Czary w Polsce w Wieku XVIII, *Psychiatria Polska*, III, 2.
22. LYSKANOWSKI, M. (1969): Leczenie Chorych Psychicznie w Wieku XVIII w Polsce i Zagranica. *Psychiatria Polska*, III, 2.
23. LYSKANOWSKI, M. (1970): Postepowanie z Psychicznie Chorymi w Polsce Centralnej w XVIII w. *Studia i Materiały z Dziejów Nauki Polskiej*, Seria B, 18.
24. LYSKANOWSKI, M. (In Print): Rozwój Postepowej Myśli Psychiatrycznej w Warszawskim Srodowisku Lekarskim w wieku XIX-ym. *Studia i Materiały z Dziejów Nauki Polskiej*.
25. MECZKOWSKI, W. (1905): *Stan i Potrzeby Szpitali Królestwa Polskiego*. Warszawa.
26. MECZKOWSKI, W. (1908): *Prowizorowie Szpitalni w Dawnej Polsce*. Warszawa.
27. MECZKOWSKI, W. (1936): *Szpitale Dawnej Rzeczypospolitej w Uchwałach Synodów Polskich*. Poznań.
28. PLASKOWSKI, R. (1868): *Psychiatrya. Część Ogólna*. Warszawa.
29. PLASKOWSKI, R. (1884): *Psychiatrya. Cześć Szczególowa*. Warszawa.
30. PRZYWIECZERSKI, W. RAKIEWICZ, F., & SIKORSKI, R. (1928): Rys Historyczny Szpitalnictwa Polskiego. *Warszawskie Czasopismo Lekarskie*, V. 31, 32.

31. ROTHE, A. (1864): *Krótki Rys Historii Psychiatrii*. *Tygodnik Lekarski*. Warszawa.
32. ROTHE, A. (1869): O Pilęgnowaniu Obłąkanych i Urządzaniu dla Nich Zakładów. *Pamiętnik Towarzystwa Lekarskiego Warszawskiego,* LXI. Warszawa.
33. ROTHE, A. (1871): O Leczeniu Obłąkanych w Czasach Dawniejszych i Teraźniejszych. *Gazeta Lekarska,* 39, 44. Warszawa.
34. ROTHE, A. (1879): *Psychopathologia Forensis*. Kraków.
35. ROTHE, A. (1885): *Psychiatrya czyli Nauka o Chorobach Umysłowych*. Warszawa.
36. ROTHE, A. (1892): Rys Dziejów Psychiatrii w Polsce. *Pamiętnik Towarzystwa Lekarskiego Warszawskiego,* LXXXVIII. Warszawa.
37. SMOLENSKI, W. (1949): *Przewrót Umysłowy w Polsce Wieku* XVIII. Warszawa.
38. STROJNOWSKI, J. (1968): *Psychofizjologia Jedrzeja Sniadeckiego*. PAN.
39. ZAWADZKI, J. (1917): Dobroczynność w Polsce. *Medycyna i Kronika Lekarska,* LII. Warszawa.

14

CZECHOSLOVAKIA

EUGEN VENCOVSKY, M.D.

*Head of the Psychiatric Clinic, Faculty of Medicine,
Plzen, Czechoslovakia*

1

MONASTERIAL HOSPITALS

The conversion to Christianity of the territory of the present Czechoslovakia in the 8th and especially in the 9th centuries provided the basis from which developed a system of philanthropic hospitals attached to the convents of various religious orders. The old and the sick were accepted in these monasterial hospitals, but people who could bequeath some possessions to the institution were preferred. The remaining places only were offered to the sick poor. Only a few mentally ill patients were accommodated in these hospitals, and they received no medical care; they were merely saved from the laughter and scorn that they would have had to bear outside the monasterial hospital. If there was any treatment it was limited to prayers and exorcism of the demons, who were said to occupy the bodies of the mentally ill. The church, the ruling knights, and later the Czech kings gave various privileges and liberties to the monasterial hospitals and supported them with money.

The first monasterial hospital was founded by the Czech knight Boleslav I in 929, in Prague, near the church of the Virgin Mary (the present church of the Virgin Mary called Tynská in the old Town Square). This so called Tynsky hospital was abolished in about 1274, when there were already some other monasterial hospitals in Prague.

The Czech king Vladislav I founded a hospital attached to the convent of the knights of Malta in 1159 (now there is a church of The Knights of Malta and Virgin Mary in the Old Town, Malá Strana). Princess St. Anežka founded a hospital attached to the church of St. František of the Order of Crusaders with the Red Star in 1234 (nowadays there is a church of St. František in Prague 2). In 1256, King Premysl Otakar II founded a hospital attached to the church of the Holy Cross of the religious order of Cyriak (nowadays there is a hospital run by the Brothers of Charity in Prague 2). The Prague Archbishop, Jan Očko of Vlašim, founded the monasterial hospital of St. Alžběta in 1364, on the site now covered by the railway bridge over the river Vltava.

In addition to those in Prague, monasterial hospitals run by various religious orders were founded in many towns: Brno, Olomouc, Opava, Jihlava, Klatovy, Plzen, České Budějovice, Cheb, et al.

The structure of the monasterial hospitals changed extensively during the Renaissance period. The change could be noticed in many towns. During this time the organizational and the administrative initiative was taken over by the public, the municipality, or the council.

2

PUBLIC HOSPITAL CARE FOR SOME MENTAL PATIENTS

The people living in larger towns, where industry and commerce were centered, called for an organized administration. This included the organization of medical care under the sponsorship of the ruling kings.

In 1484 the town council founded a public hospital in Prague, in Malá Strana, which was to serve people with no means of support. It was situated near the present Malostranské square. In 1505 another public hospital was founded for 50 indigent patients by the town council "Under Slovany." It was sited in the surroundings of the present rebuilt convent At Slovany. In 1512 the local board founded a public hospital in Brno and in the same year another hospital was established in Olomouc. The sick staying in these hospitals received occasional medical care and were looked after by guardians, who lived in the same hospital and were paid by the town council.

One cannot, however, speak of medical care of the mentally ill. If they were in this hospital, their presence was merely tolerated and they were kept in isolation in cellar rooms; on Sundays and on holidays they were put in iron cages and exhibited in the squares and public

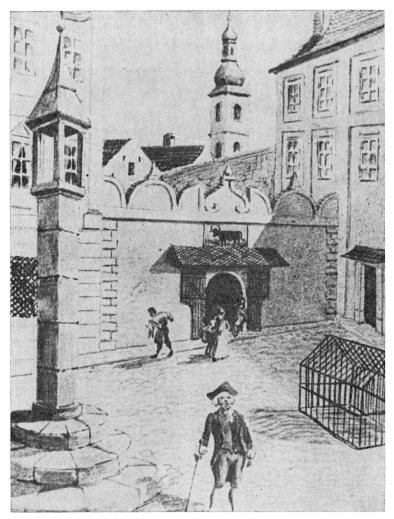

PLATE LXIX. An iron cage for exhibiting the insane. On the left is a "pillory of shame." From an etching dated 1768.

places, as a means of entertainment for the town citizens. The insane were very often kept in iron shackles or chained to the wall of cellars. In Brno the mentally ill were being shown to the public until 1770 (Plate LXIX).

The mentally ill in Moravia and in other countries in Europe were treated no differently from those in Bohemia; the trials and burning of the mentally ill, who were considered possessed by the devil,

witches, and sorcerers, took place all over the country. The last execution by fire of an insane woman occurred in 1782, not far from the
castle of Velké Losiny, near the town of Opava.

3

SYSTEMATIC CARE OF THE MENTALLY ILL

In the town of Znojmo, in Moravia, in 1458 the first "House" for the
mentally ill was founded. It was the *Hospitale hominum rationem
non habentium,* and it was built exclusively for the care of 5 to 15
mentally ill people. This house was financed by the public and by
municipal means, it was not supported by the church, and thus it
belonged to the system of public municipal care. It was the first independent asylum for the mentally ill in the territory of the present
Czechoslovakia (at that time in the territory of the Czech kingdom).

However, the systematic care of the mentally ill is supposed to have
started in the second half of the 18th century. The Order of the
Brothers of Charity began to establish their hospitals in the 17th
century (Valtice near Brno in 1605; Praha in 1620; Bratislava in
1672; and Brno in 1748). They were ordered to look after the mentally
ill as well as the physically sick. At first, only mentally ill priests were
accepted, but later they cared for many people irrespective of their
religion.

In the second half of the 18th century, the Order of the Brothers
of Charity started to establish special rooms for the mentally ill at
Brno and Bratislava. The wards, with a few adaptations, were used
for this purpose for more than 100 years.

Bohemia

In 1761 the hospital of the Order of the Brothers of Charity in
Prague became an integral part of Charles University in Prague and
patients suffering from internal disorders or requiring surgery were
transferred there, so that medical students could learn by direct contact with these patients. This hospital of the Order of the Brothers
of Charity had a great importance in the development of psychiatry
(Plate LXX). In 1783 an independent department for mentally ill
priests was established, and in the following year it was enlarged to
enable it to accept mentally ill laymen. Mentally ill women were
accommodated in a special department in the hospital of Alžběta in

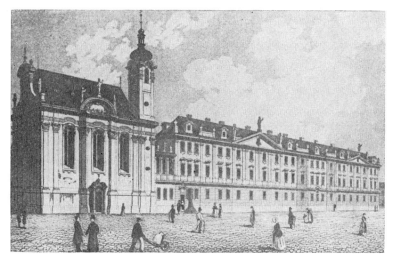

PLATE LXX. The hospital of the religious order of the Brothers of Charity. From an early 19th century illustration.

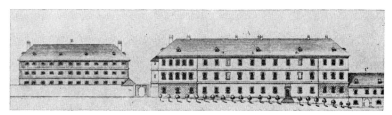

PLATE LXXI. The General Hospital in Prague, 1790. On the left (B) is the building of the Home for the mentally ill.

Prague (at present the At Slupi Hospital). However, both these hospitals for male and female patients functioned only until 1790. There was the disadvantage that the mentally ill and the physically ill were treated in the same hospital, although in separate wards.

At that time Prague had 80,000 inhabitants, and it was necessary to build a new hospital for its inhabitants. This was done in 1790 (Plate LXXI). A general hospital was reorganized and a separate home with 60 beds was established for the mentally ill. Taking into consideration the time, the Prague home was well equipped. It was situated in a garden surrounded by a wall, and the floors had a central corridor connected with 20 rooms for the patients and their guardians. At first, the home provided for 60 patients with a room for each of them. Later two patients were put into one room. The first floor was for male patients, and the second floor for female patients, while the third floor was in common divided by a lattice in two parts. This top ward was of a higher standard—the fees for treatment were higher and the patients were accepted incognito, if the family so wished. The condition for accepting a patient into the home required a written statement of a council set up by the authority and every patient had to be examined by an appointed doctor. The mentally ill, depending on the weather, spent their time in the garden or in a corridor sitting on benches, their guardians sitting among them.

The director of the newly built Prague general hospital was also the physician in charge of the home for the mentally ill; another doctor was appointed to care exclusively for the patients in the mental home. However, over-excited patients were still subjected to such treatment as the turning chair, which was used for calming them down.

In 1822 another home for the mentally ill was founded, as the old one was no longer sufficient to meet the needs of an increasing number of patients. Thus the former monastery of St. Katerina was adapted and rebuilt to accommodate 260 beds. In this institution, psychiatry was considered as a separate branch of medicine. In 1821 theoretical lectures on mental disorders were started and were made compulsory for all students.

J. Th. Held (Plate LXXII) (1770-1851) was a professor of internal medicine at the University of Prague, where he was dean and, from 1826 to 1827, chancellor of Charles University. Because of his influence on the development of psychiatry in the whole Czech territory he is regarded as the first Czech psychiatrist. He worked in the department for the mentally ill of the hospital of the Brothers of Charity, and was well versed in the theory and practice of psychiatry. Thanks to him, the Prague home for the mentally ill gained a very high reputation. He established a library and a music room, and recommended that the patients should work in the garden and be prescribed various exercises. He pointed out the importance of being kind, patient, and gentle to all the patients. Held respected Pinel's conceptions in psychiatry, and did his best to put them into practice. He worked at the St. Katerina Hospital for the mentally ill from 1822 until 1830, when the psychiatric department was closed down.

Josef Riedel (Plate LXXIII) (1803-1870), a pupil of Professor Held, began working in the home for the mentally ill and in 1838 was appointed director of this home, where he enlarged facilities and improved treatment. Thanks to him, St. Katerina was acknowledged as a very good mental home, as proved by the remarks in a surviving visitors' book, which includes comments by Skoda, Purkinje, Noel,

Dameron, van Leuwen, Moreau, Tuke, Charcot, Dubois-Raymond, Crédé, Griesinger, et al. Riedel introduced "the spa treatment," whereby chosen patients drank mineral water—especially that from the Mlynsky spring from Karlovy Vary—while walking in the garden, or, in bad weather, in the corridors. He also introduced music therapy, art therapy, hydro-therapy, and physical training. In 1840 he became the first associate professor of Prague University. In 1851 he left Prague to direct a newly built mental hospital in Vienna, where he died in 1870. Riedel established another home for the mentally ill,

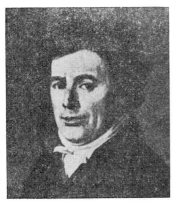

PLATE LXXII. Dr. Jan Th. Held (1770-1851), the first Czech psychiatrist.

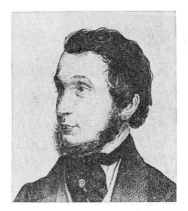

PLATE LXXIII. Dr. Josef Riedel (1803-1870), the first professor of psychiatry in Bohemia.

called New House, which is now the residence of the psychiatric clinic of the faculty of medicine in Prague. Founded in 1845, New House, with 240 beds, was exclusively for male patients, while the St. Katerina Home, with 260 beds, was exclusively for female patients. Lectures in psychiatry for the students were given in Dr. Riedel's New House (Plate LXXIV).

Moravia

The development of psychiatry in the second part of the former Czech kingdom, Moravia, and its capital, Brno, did not reach a standard comparable to that in Prague and Bohemia. From 1748 there was a small psychiatric department in the hospital of the Brothers of Charity and another in the general hospital of St. Anna, but the joint capacity of these psychiatric departments was only about 100 beds.

A large independent home for the mentally ill, with 350 beds, was built at Černovice, a suburb of Brno, in 1863. A former pupil of Riedel, Dr. Josef Cermak, who later became professor of psychiatry at the Austrian University in Graz, was responsible for establishing this home, which, after many adaptations, is still in use and has a capacity of about 1,000 beds.

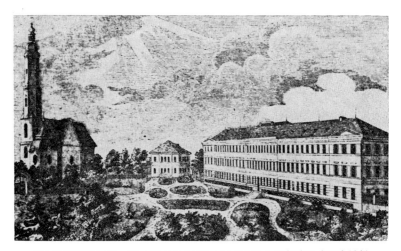

PLATE LXXIV. The New House in Prague. From a painting dated 1845.

Slovakia

From 1672 a very small department served the mentally ill in the hospital of the Brothers of Charity in Bratislava, the capital of Slovakia. A general hospital was also established there, in 1864, with a psychiatric department of 60 beds. A mental home of 450 beds was built in 1900. Nowadays the psychiatric clinic of the faculty of medicine in Bratislava occupies part of it and the remaining parts are used by other clinics.

4

FURTHER DEVELOPMENTS IN THE 19TH CENTURY

František Köstel (1852-1869) and Jakub Fischel (1869-1885) succeeded Riedel in the home for the mentally ill. They established branches of the home outside Prague. It was Fischel's idea to establish a large home for the mentally ill in West Bohemia, at Dobrany near Plzen, which started in 1881 with Alfred Pick as director. He was the author of a work on degenerate brain disorders later called *Pick disease.*

The years 1885 and 1886 are of the greatest importance for Czech psychiatry. Charles University was divided into two separate universities—one Czech and one German. Up to this time all the lecturing had been in German. This influenced the early foundation of the Czech psychiatric clinic at Charles University in Prague. Lectures in Czech enabled the professors to educate Czech doctors and Czech scientists in psychiatry also.

The first professor of the Czech psychiatric clinic at Charles University, Dr. Benjamin Čumpelík (1886-1891), established there a chemical histological laboratory, a scientific library, and archives. He was the first psychiatrist to describe visual hallucinations in *delirium tremens.* In 1891 he retired from his position of head of the clinic and accepted the office of director of the home for the mentally ill in Prague.

Dr. Čumpelík's pupil, Dr. Bohuslav Hellich, was the second professor of the Czech psychiatric clinic, from 1891 to 1895. After 1895 he was director of the home for the mentally ill at Dobrany, near Plzen.

During the last decade of the 19th century and in the first decade of the 20th century several branches of the home for the mentally ill were built in Bohemia and Moravia, and new psychiatric medical institutions were established.

In 1869 a branch of the Prague home was established at Kosmonosy for 280 patients; in 1875, another was established at St. Apolinarius in Prague, Karlov, for 300 chronic psychotics; in 1876, the Brno-Černovice home for the mentally ill established a branch for 120 patients in the newly adapted Brothers of Charity Hospital, at Brno; in 1887, a further branch of the Prague home for 210 patients was established at Oparany; in 1887, a branch of the same home for 100 patients was founded at Horní Berkovice; in 1889, a new home for 500 mentally ill people was established at Opava; and, in 1892, another new home of 450 beds was built at Šternberk. Further homes for the mentally ill were established at Jihlava (300 patients), at Kroměříž (1,100 patients) and in the suburb of Prague, Bohnice (1,800 patients).

5

THE 20TH CENTURY

Before World War I, in Bohemia and Moravia—parts of the former Czech Kingdom—there were about 7,000 beds in 18 psychiatric medical institutions. In all of them the chiefs and subordinate employers were of Czech nationality, educated at the faculty of medicine of Charles University in Prague.

Originally, Bohemia and Moravia had only one university—Charles University in Prague, founded in 1348—the first university in Central Europe. Since the Battle on the White Mountain, in 1620, near Prague, Bohemia and Moravia, although theoretically regarded as the Czech Kingdom, were in fact under the Austrian monarchy. In 1918, they became a sovereign nation and, together with Slovakia, created an independent and common country, Czechoslovakia.

October 28, 1918, marks the beginning of the historical development of Czech and Slovak psychiatry. In 1919 a new university was founded in Brno. It was named after the first president of the Independent Czechoslovakia, T. G. Masaryk.

In the capital of Slovakia, Bratislava, a new university was founded in the same year. It was named Komensky University, after a Czech philosopher and pedagogue, Jan Amos Komensky, or Comenius (1592-1670).

The psychiatric clinics established at these two universities were directed by Professor Kuffner's pupils: Zdeněk Mysliveček in Bratislava, and Karel Bělohradsky in Brno. Both of them continued to base their work on that of their teacher.

Between 1895 and 1929 the third professor at the Czech psychiatric clinic at Charles University, Dr. Karel Kuffner (Plate LXXV), directed the work there. He was the most important scientific psychiatrist in Czechoslovakia and the founder of the Czech psychiatric tradition. He was a follower of Meynert's psychiatric conceptions in Vienna. Kuffner's *Textbook of Psychiatry* (20) is one of the classic works of Czech psychiatric literature. Kuffner believed that an accurate examination of the somatic state of the patient was as important as the examination of psychopathological changes and symptoms. His pupil, Jan Jánsky (1873-1921), on the initiative of Karel Kuffner, undertook research in the blood groups of the mentally ill and discovered the IV blood group.

In 1926 Kuffner was one of the first to describe schizophrenia-like pictures. Kuffner had a large number of outstanding pupils during his long work at the clinic in Prague: Ladislav Haškovec, Antonín Heveroch, Jan Jánsky (1973-1921), Zdeněk Mysliveček (1881-1974), Leo Taussig (1887-1944), Karel Bělohradsky (1889-1929), and Hubert Procházka (1885-1935). Each of them, in an individual way, contributed to the development of Czech scientific psychiatry: Professor Heveroch as a clinical psychopathologist, Professor Haškovec as a neurologist, Professor Mysliveček as a neurophysiologist, and Professor Procházka as a forensic psychiatrist. The latter died serving his profession, shot dead by one of his patients. In 1940 Kuffner ceased to be a professor at the psychiatric clinic and died in the same year.

The period between the first and second world wars brought a great change in Czech psychiatry. In 1919 the Czechoslovak Psychiatric Society was founded. This society, one of the oldest scientific societies, published in its own journal, *Czechoslovak Psychiatry*, scientific papers

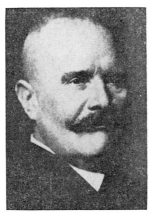

PLATE LXXV. Dr. Karel Kuffner (1858-1940), founder of scientific psychiatry in Czechoslovakia.

on mental diseases with summaries in foreign languages, which enabled the journal to be widely read abroad.

In 1929 Professor Karel Kuffner resigned and his pupil, Zdeněk Mysliveček, was chosen as the new head of the Prague psychiatric clinic. In this capacity, he worked at this clinic until 1956. At the age of 92, he was the Nestor of Czech psychiatry. He has contributed to the scientific and organizational development of Czech psychiatry. He trained many excellent psychiatrists: J. Krivy (1896-1942), J. Prokop (1903-1952), O. Skaličková (1906-1969), O. Janota (1898-1969), V. Vondráček (1895-   ), and many others, among them the author of this chapter (1908-   ).

The psychiatric medical institution, founded at Havlíčkuv Brod in 1934, is considered the most up-to-date Czech psychiatric institution.

World War II was a sad period in the history of Czechoslovakia and its psychiatry. Czechoslovakia did not exist any more. Hitler occupied the territories of Bohemia and Moravia and annexed them as a "protectorate" of Germany. All the universities and high schools were closed and many Czech psychiatrists were sent to concentration camps, where some of them died; among them were J. Krivy, professor at the university and head of the psychiatric clinic of the faculty of medicine at Brno, and L. Taussig, the assistant to the head of the psychiatric clinic in Prague. Hitler separated Bohemia and Moravia from Slovakia and formed the Slovak Republic, the representatives of which collaborated with him. In Slovakia, the universities remained open and Slovak students were allowed to continue their studies. However, the firm tie between Czech and Slovak psychiatrists was not broken and many Slovak psychiatrists joined the anti-fascist revolt. In fact many students took their degrees during the World War II in Slovakia, while in Bohemia and Moravia students had to wait until 1945 to resume their studies. Psychiatric clinics started to function again after the war. Two faculties of medicine were established—at Plzen and at Hradec Králové—which included psychiatric clinics and provided theoretical and practical teaching. A new university with psychiatric clinics was established at Olomouc, named after the Czech historian František Palacky. In Slovakia, a new university with a psychiatric clinic was established at Košice, named after a Slovak philologist, Pavel Šafarík. The faculty of medicine at Komensky University established another faculty of medicine at Martin.

By 1974 Czechoslovakia had five universities in Praha, Brno, Olomouc, Bratislava, and Košice, and eight university psychiatric clinics in Praha, Plzen, Hradec Králové, Brno, Olomouc, Bratislava, Martin, and Košice. Taking into consideration the number of inhabitants of Czechoslovakia—14,000,000—this is very satisfactory.

Mysliveček's pupils are in charge of almost all the newly established university psychiatric clinics; they continue his work and that of Kuffner, thus keeping alive the scientific tradition of Czechoslovak psychiatry, while adding new ideas of their own.

After the World War II, small psychiatric departments were established in regional and district hospitals, as well as special psychiatric institutions for children (Oparany, 500 beds; Běharov, 100 beds). In Slovakia, at Prešov, a new psychiatric hospital for 400 patients was founded and many older hospitals were adapted to serve as psychiatric institutions. There were 240 out-patient health centers; the number of beds reached about 19,000, and the number of psychiatrists was over 800.

A very important event was the foundation of the postgraduate school for psychiatrists in Prague, the director of which is J. Prokupek (1906-   ). A similar school was founded in Bratislava; the chief of the psychiatric clinic is also the director of this school. In 1961 an Institute for research in psychiatry was founded under the direction of L. Hanzlíček (1916-   ) in Prague.

6

CONCLUSIONS

The history of Czechoslovak psychiatry can be divided into five stages. From 1780 to 1830, independent homes for the mentally ill were established at general hospitals, and the Home at St. Katerina was founded in Prague. This period is linked with the name of J. Th. Held.

From 1830 to 1880 another home for the mentally ill, New House, was established, and the first two mental institutions were founded outside Prague, at Brno, Dobrany, near Plzen. This period is linked with J. Riedel, in Prague, and J. Čermak, at Brno.

From 1880 to 1920 the foundation of a separate Czech faculty of medicine took place, and the Czech psychiatric clinic was established in Prague. Many other psychiatric institutions were founded in Moravia and Bohemia after World War I, as well as further Czech psychiatric clinics at the newly founded universities at Brno and in Bratislava. This period is linked with the work of Kuffner and his pupils.

From 1920 to 1960 psychiatric clinics were established at the newly opened faculties of medicine at Plzen, Hradec Králové, Olomouc, Košice and Martin. The Czechoslovak Psychiatric Society and the postgraduate school for psychiatrists were founded during this period, which is linked with Zdeněk Mysliveček and his pupils.

The tradition of Czechoslovak psychiatry has always been enlightened and pioneering, within the limitations of each period, and has left posterity a rich inheritance of knowledge.

REFERENCES

1. BAYER, T. (1793): *Beschreibung der öffentlichen Armen-Versorgerungsanstalten der königl. böhmischen Hauptstadt Prag.* Praha.
2. BOGAR, J. (1932): *Milosrdní Bratri.* Praha.
3. ČERMAK, J. (1866): *Die mähr. Landes-Irrenanstallt bei Brünn.* Wien.
4. ELVERT, CRISTIAN, (1958): *Geschichte der Heil- u. Humanitäts-Anstalten in Mähren und Oesterr. Schlesien.* Brno.

5. FISCHEL, J. (1853): *Prag's Irrenstalt und ihr Wirken*. Praha.
6. FISCHEL, J. (1846): *Bericht über die k.k. Irrenanstalt zu Prag, Vierteljahrschr. f. prakt. Heilk.*
7. GUTHRIE, D. (1947): *A History of Medicine*. London.
8. HADLIK, J. (1961): *Rozvoj psychiatrie na Morave*.
9. HELD, J. T. (1823): *Kurze Geschichte der Heilanstalt der Barmherzigen Brüder in Prag*. Praha.
10. HELD, J. T. (1850): *Blick auf die praktische Medizin der Neuzeit*. Praha.
11. HEVEROCH, A. (1926): *O vyznamu pražského ústavu pro choromyslné pro pestování psychiatrie. Sborník zemského správního vyboru*, Praha.
12. HRASE, J. (1932): *Aktuality naší péče o duševne nemocné*, Praha.
14. JUNGMANN, A. (1840): *Skizzeirte Geschichte der medizinischen Anstalten an der Universität zu Prag*. Wien.
16. KIRSCHOF, J. (1929): *Deutsche Irrenärzte*. Berlin.
17. KLEBS, E. (1879): *Prager Kranken-und Heilanstalten, Medizinische Wochenschrift.*
18. KNEIDL, C. (1926): *Príspevek k dejinám péče o choromyslné. Sborník zemského správního vyboru*. Praha.
19. KÖSTL, F. (1863): *Vedecká zprava o kral. zem. blazinci v Praze. Čas. lék. čes.*
20. KUFFNER, K. (1897, 1900): *Psychiatrie I. a II. díl*. Praha.
22. LAEHR, H. (1907): *Die Anstalten f. psychisch Kranke*. Berlin.
23. MATOUSEK, M. (1937): *O vyvoji čsl. lékarství v 18. a 19. století*. Praha.
24. MYSLIVECEK, Z. (1929): *Professor Dr. Karel Kuffner, Sborník, prací, Haškovcova revue.*
25. NOWAK, A. (1835): *Notizen über die Prager Irrenanstalt*. Praha.
26. ODLOZILIK, O. (1948): *Karlova universita*. Praha.
27. PANDY, K. (1908): *Die Irrenfürsorge in Europa*. Berlin.
28. RIEDEL, J. (1830): *Prag' s Irrenanstalt und Ihre Leistungen*. Praha.
29. ROZSIVALOVA, E. (1951): *Dr. Jan Theob. Held. Čsl. nemocnice*. Praha.
30. SECKY, R. (1928): *Staropražské špitály*. Praha.
31. SCHÄFFNER, J. (1845): *Geschichte des Ordens und der Heilanstalt der Elisabethiner Klossterfrauen*. Praha.
32. SCHALLER, J. (1793): *Beschreibung der königl. Haupt- und Residenzstadt Prag*. Praha.
33. SCHLÖSS, H. (1912): *Die Irrenpflege in Osterreich in Wort u. Bild. Hall a S.*
34. SCHRUTZ, O. (1899): Prehled historiografie lékarství v Čechách. *Čas. lék. čes.*
35. TURCEK, J. (1966): Vyvoj psychiatrie na Slovensku. *Čs. psychiatrie No. 4.*
36. VENCOVSKY, E. (1966): *Od Hippokrata k Pinelovi*. Praha.
37. VENCOVSKY, E. (1957): *Počátky české psychiatrie XVIII. a XIX. století*. Praha.
38. VENCOVSKY, E. (1963): *Prehled historického vyvoje psychiatrického ústavnictví*. Brno.
40. WEITENWEBER, W. (1850): *Die Medizinal-Anstalten zu Prag*. Praha.
41. WEITENWEBER, W. (1847): *Aus dem Leben und Wirken des Herrn Dr. Joh. Th. Held s*. Praha.
42. WHITWELL, J. (1936): *Historical Notes on Psychiatry*. London.
43. ZAP, J. (1848): *Das historische Prag*. Praha.
44. ZAPLETAL, V. (1952): *Stredoveké počátky brnenskych špitalu. Lék. listy.*
45. ZILBOORG, G. (1941): *A History of Medical Psychology*. New York: W. W. Norton.

15

RUMANIA

V. Predescu, M.D.

Professor of Psychiatry, Dr. G. Marinescu Hospital,
Bucharest, Rumania

AND

D. Christodorescu, M.D.

Research Worker in Psychiatry, Institute of Neurology and
Psychiatry, The Academy of Medical Sciences,
Bucharest, Rumania

1

INTRODUCTION

The development of psychiatry in Rumania closely follows that of medicine in general, and has been influenced by the historical vicissitudes inherent to the geographical situation of the country.

The Rumanians are of Daco-Roman origin. The Rumania of today is made up of five provinces whose history each has run a different course. Moldavia and Wallachia, for many centuries under Turkish sovereignty, united in 1859 and became independent in 1877, when Dobrodgia was also joined to the country. After World War I, Transylvania and Banat, which had been under Austro-Hungarian rule, were also united to the rest of the country.

The harsh conditions of century-old oppression to which our country was subjected accounts for the slower development of science, technique, and medicine in the past.

2

EARLY PERIOD

The first documents referring to psychiatric patients belong to a period that is not so remote. Towards the end of the Middle Ages mental patients had begun to be cared for in the monasteries (Caldarusani, Balamuci, and Jitia in Wallachia; Adam in Moldavia). The "therapy" evidently consisted of exorcisms, prayers, and so on. The patients were treated gently, although the concept of the supernatural nature of the disease prevailed (divine punishment or possessed of the devil). This mildness, which impressed the Jesuits who came to visit our country, may be accounted for by the Rumanian's basic character and his revulsion for violent mysticism.

In 1652, in the *Pravila* (laws) of Matei Basarab (an enlightened prince, promotor of progress and prosperity), the first legal mentions of mental patients appeared. They stated that a judge and a physician had to establish whether the accused was or was not mentally alienated, and stipulated that an insane person could not be sentenced, also mentioning other aspects of their juridical status (. . . "For the judge to know whether he has to do with a madman he will have to call in a physician who will readily recognize the case. An insane person will not be punished but neither will he be let free to wander through the country; he will be constantly surveyed until he regains his reason.")

3

19TH CENTURY

In general the care given by the monks to the insane remained the same until the beginning of the 19th century. It then gradually began to improve following the sociopolitical and cultural changes in this part of Europe.

In 1838, in Wallachia, the mental patients were brought from various monasteries to the hermitage of Balamuci, where they were treated for the first time by a physician. In 1846 they were transferred to the asylum of Marcuta. Although within the precincts of a former monastery near Bucharest, this asylum was the first secular psychiatric hospital in our country, and one of its first head doctors—Dr. Protici—was the first qualified psychiatrist. Although the building was not ideal despite many improvements, Marcuta was used as an asylum until the Central Hospital was built. At first Protici alone, and then he together with Sutzu, opened workshops for occupational therapy (a carpenter's workshop for the male patients and handwork for the women).

Following the impulse given by Carol Davila, the great promotor of health organization in the United Principalities (the official name of Moldavia and Wallachia after their union in 1859), a statute was drawn up in 1864 providing not only for the administration of Marcuta but also stipulating the principles and treatment of the patients, revealing the strong influence of Pinel's ideas. At about the same time, asylums were opened in Moldavia at the monasteries of Neamtu, Golia, Galata, and Galati. The first correctional and re-habilitation homes were likewise founded in Vaslui, Dobrovat, Bise-ricani, and Pîngarati. In 1835, in Transylvania, a department for mental diseases was attached to the Carolina Hospital of Cluj. It was closed a few years later when an excellent psychiatric hospital was opened in Sibiu—still one of the most important psychiatric units in this part of the country.

In Wallachia, under the influence of Sutzu, a marked progress was made in psychiatry. He took over the Marcuta mental hospital in 1867 and was the first professor of psychiatry in Rumania. (The first School of Medicine was founded in 1859 and a few years later became the Bucharest Faculty of Medicine.) Sutzu's courses included both legal medicine and psychiatry, but the latter discipline initiated in 1867 became compulsory only in 1893. Sutzu was head of psychiatry at the Bucharest faculty of medicine until 1910 when Obregia succeeded him.

Sutzu (1837-1919) had a strong personality, a basic medical train-ing in many fields, and a liberal education. He was a promotor of new ideas and progress, belonged to the intellectual vanguard of those times, struggling for social and cultural development. Sutzu was also the author of the first Rumanian monograph on psychiatry. *The Mental Patient Confronting Society and Science* is a complex work which reveals his preoccupation with the legal aspects of the problem and his deeply humane views as a sociologist and psycho-logist. His book went far beyond the limits of mental pathology, and many of his views in the discussion of the problems evince a modern approach.

4

20TH CENTURY

Wallachia

Sutzu's collaborator, Alexandru Obregia (Plate LXXVI) (1860-1937), who continued his work, received a French and German university education, and specialized in histology. For 10 years he had been professor of histology at the faculty of medicine before taking up his

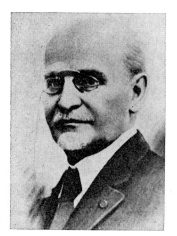

PLATE LXXVI. Professor Al. Obregia.

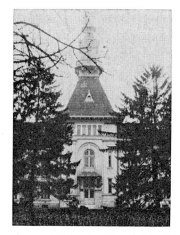

PLATE LXXVII. The central building of the G. Marinescu Hospital (formerly the Central Hospital for Nervous and Mental Diseases).

appointment as professor of psychiatry. Obregia was one of the most significant personalities of Rumanian psychiatry, due to his outstanding contribution as organizer, founder of psychiatric institutions, teacher, and scientist. Two of the main problems he studied were alcoholism and periodical psychic disturbances (within the framework of manic-depressive psychosis or outside it). He coined the term *cyclophrenia,* which he applied to all periodical psychic disturbances. This term is still used today by some Rumanian psychiatrists. Obregia's place in the history of medicine is marked especially by the use for the first time in the world of suboccipital puncture for analysis of the cerebrospinal fluid.

His major accomplishment was founding the Central Hospital for Mental and Nervous Diseases in Bucharest, to which he devoted many years of his life. Although building began in 1906, it was not opened until 1923. Many pavilions, with over 2,000 beds, mostly for mental patients, some for neurology, and later for neurosurgery and endocrinology, and numerous annex buildings, for occupational therapy, hydro-physiotherapy, and so on, were raised within a beautiful shady park, full of chestnut trees, creating a very carefully planned modern unit (Plate LXXVII).

The Central Hospital possessed fairly extensive domains outside the town of Bucharest, especially for the custodial care of chronic cases. Farmwork was introduced in the therapy of these patients, particularly for those from rural areas.

Remarkable in Obregia was his open-mindedness, his readiness to accept the initiative of his coworkers. He wanted to be up-to-date with the latest discoveries in psychiatry and promoted this idea among those he was working with. The Sakel cure and electroshock therapy were systematically applied shortly after their discovery. After malaria therapy for neurosyphilis was introduced in medical practice, he immediately reserved a whole pavillion for this treatment and the research work on malaria which started in his laboratory was continued until lately, with well known results.

Moldavia

The faculty of medicine in Iasi (the former capital of Moldavia) was founded in 1879, but the first chair of neurology and psychiatry was not established until 1912. C. I. Parhon (1874-1969) was appointed professor. He held this appointment until 1930 when he became professor at the Clinic of Endocrinology in Bucharest. At the beginning of his career he was the student and collaborator of the great Rumanian neurologist G. Marinescu, who himself had been preoccupied by several of the aspects of psychiatry, especially hysteria for whose etiopathogenesis he had a special concept of his own. C. I. Parhon had a vast medical culture and outlook, as a neurologist, psychiatrist, and endocrinologist. He distinguished himself especially in the field of endocrinology, publishing together with M. Goldstein, the first treatise of endocrinology in the world, in 1909. His main contribution in psychiatry was the study of endocrino-psychical relationships, particularly certain endocrine aspects and the endocrine etiology of certain psychical diseases. His report on these problems, read at the Congress of Neurology of Gand, in 1913, established this new domain of interdisciplinary studies.

Parhon was also the spiritual founder and leader of the Psychiatric Hospital of Socola, Iasi, similar in importance and function to the Central Hospital of Bucharest. Initially Socola had been a much simpler institution. It is likewise under his influence that *La Société de Neurologie, Psychiatrie, Psychologie Médicale, et Endocrinology de Iassy* was founded, publishing a bulletin in French. In Bucharest the Society of Neurology and Psychiatry, which also published its own bulletin, was founded in 1905 and separated into two independent societies in 1936.

In 1930, L. Ballif (1892-1968) took up his appointment as head of the Iasi Psychiatric Clinic. He received his education in Rumania and completed it in England, where he was the student and co-worker of Sherrington. His honest spirit is evident in all his studies, which clearly show the influence of his neurophysiological education. He was particularly interested in genetics, his concepts taking on a geneticist-constitutionalist note. He continued the tradition of his predecessor and was also preoccupied by the organosomatic aspects of psychical diseases and endocrinopsychiatry.

Transylvania

In Transylvania, in the 19th century psychiatric activity centered around the hospital of Sibiu which was founded with 200 beds and maintained its importance throughout the following century. One of the most important figures among its physicians was K. Pandy, who discovered the cerebrospinal protein flocculation test which bears his name. The Sibiu Hospital had a neuropsychiatric department where Pandy was neurologist between 1900 and 1919. This hospital owed its prestige to the civilized way in which the patients were cared for. It was here that a Society of Psychology was founded. A journal was published between 1936 and 1938.

In general, Transylvanian psychiatry differed from that in the Principalities, primarily due to political, administrative, and especially cultural influences. As they were under Austrian and then Austro-Hungarian rule and had no medical faculty of their own, many Transylvanian doctors studied in the Universities of Vienna and Budapest. Thus they were influenced by the Central European and German psychiatric concepts, whereas in the Principalities the influence of French psychiatry prevailed.

In Transylvania the first faculty of medicine and chair of neuropsychiatry were inaugurated in 1901, in Cluj. But the courses were held in Hungarian since the Austro-Hungarian government was partial to the dominant minority. Not until 1919, after Transylvania was united with Rumania, was a Rumanian faculty of medicine founded in Cluj. The first professor appointed to the clinic of psychiatry was C. Urechia (1883-1955), who worked there until 1945. He had a basic knowledge of psychiatry but was also a skilled neurologist and neuropathologist. He was particularly interested in the psychical disturbances of encephalitis, alcoholism, phacomatosis, and the borderline domain of neuro-ophthalmology. He not only was an honest and fecund investigator but also had remarkable didactic qualities. He was the first author, together with S. Mihalescu, of a Rumanian textbook on neurology and psychiatry that appeared in installments between 1924 and 1931.

Mid-century

On the eve of World War II the situation of Rumanian psychiatry was as follows:

The medical and scientific attainments of the psychiatrists of Rumania were equal to those of the psychiatrists throughout the continent. However, the material means, the equipment, and the number of hospital beds (in all 4,753 beds for a population of 18,000,000) were insufficient, and in this connection particularly deficient were the units for out-patient treatment. Apart from the consultations given in the large hospitals, ambulatory assistance depended on private medical practitioners only.

The control of psychiatric diseases was also hindered by the problems raised by the deplorable socio-economic and cultural situation of the great majority of the population. There was no specific psychiatric pathology of the Rumanian population, such as transcultural psychiatry described in other regions of the world, but because of the low standard of living mental disturbances due to puerperality, malnutrition (especially pellagra), neurosyphilis, and alcoholism were common.

World War II with the de facto occupation of the country by the Germans marked an important step back and resulted in disorder in all the compartments of Rumanian life including medicine and psychiatry. After the war there was a spectacular renewal connected with the radical political, economic, and social changes that occurred. The basic change consisted in the integral nationalization of medical assistance which became free for all. A vast network of out-patient units was created and the number of beds (almost 17,000 in 1970) and institutions of different specialties increased (sanatoria, hospitals for acute and chronic cases, institutions for oligophrenics, etc.). The number of psychiatrists likewise increased.

From the viewpoint of scientific concepts and the type of research after the war, especially during the first years, Rumanian psychiatry was strongly influenced by Pavlov. Rumanian psychiatry during the last quarter century has also kept up to date with the latest progress made, and American and English psychiatry is just as much studied as German, French, or Soviet psychiatry. Scientific curiosity has been open to all concepts, except the unilateral hazardous ones, and hence research work has been carried out or problems approached on a multilateral basis (electrophysiology, genetics, pure psychopathologic views, etc.). Impressive is the almost total eradication of certain mental diseases of social importance (neurosyphilis, pellagra).

Medical and psychiatric teaching was extended following the opening of the faculties and clinics of psychiatry of Timisoara (Banat) and Tîrgu-Mures (Transylvania). The clinics of psychiatry are also centers of scientific research, and this was further enhanced by the founding of a section in the Institute of Neurology and Psychiatry of the Academy of Medical Sciences, in 1971.

After the war Constanta Stefanescu Parhon was professor of psychiatry at the faculty of medicine and head of the department of psychiatry of the Central Hospital (now called the G. Marinescu Hospital). She centered her attention along traditional lines, especially in endocrinopsychiatry, psychical diseases of metabolic and infectious origin, and forensic psychiatry. When she withdrew in 1968 V. Predescu, associate professor since 1962, was appointed professor.

The Contemporary Scene

V. Predescu worked with a young and active team of assistants and research workers in a broad range of investigations: psychical diseases of the aged, drug therapy (in 1968 he wrote a voluminous monograph on psychotropic therapy), psychical disturbances in cytogenetic syndromes and the genetics of certain forms of oligophrenia, the pathologic anatomy of psychical diseases, and electroencephalography.

In Iasi, after the retirement of Ballif in 1966, Petre Brînzei became head of the clinic of psychiatry. He has an original concept of the nature of schizophrenia and is mainly occupied with the study of antisocial behavior and the rehabilitation of psychical patients. E. Pamfil, at first professor in Cluj and since 1960 in Timisoara, is primarily interested in psychopathology. He is the foremost authority in our country on the concepts of H. Ey, under whom he studied. After Pamfil, the clinic of psychiatry at Cluj remained under the direction of S. Rosu, a solid psychiatrist with great prestige and authority, and varied scientific preoccupations. He was deeply missed when he met an early death in 1971. At present Aurelia Sîrbu is head of the clinic.

The first to be appointed as head of the clinic of neuropsychiatry in Tîrgu Mures was the morphopathologist D. Miscolczy, of international repute. Subsequently, when psychiatric teaching was separated from neurologic teaching K. Csiki became head of the clinic. His major scientific interests are in psychical disturbances of organic origin and his contributions in the field of electrophysiology and psychopharmacology are well known.

After the war the Society of Neurology and Psychiatry was reopened and in 1958 separated into two societies. The National Society of Psychiatry, member of the Union of the Societies of Medical Sciences, with branches in the largest towns, publishes, together with the Society of Neurology, the journal *Neurologia, Psihiatria, Neurochirurgia,* which is now in its 17th year of existence. This Society, which has been a member of the World Psychiatric Association since 1965, also organizes national conferences every four years, which continue the tradition of the National Congresses of Neurology and Psychiatry that had been held between the two world wars.

REFERENCES

1. DOSIOS, A., PARHON-STEFANESCU, C. & PREDESCU, V. (1968): Some aspects of Rumanian psychiatry. In: *Psychiatry in the Communist World* Ari Kiev, (Ed.). New York: Science House.
2. BOLOGA, V. L., BRATESCU, G., DUTESCU, B. & MILCU ST. M. (1972): *Istoria Medicinei Rominesti, Editura Medicala, Bucuresti.*
3. PREDESCU, V. (1973): *Manual de Psihiatrie, Editura Didactica si Pedagogica,* Bucuresti.

16

BULGARIA

CHRISTO CHRISTOZOV, M.D.

Professor, Department of Psychiatry,
Medical Academy, Sofia, Bulgaria

1

INTRODUCTION

The geographical area which now constitutes Bulgaria was inhabited in ancient times by the Thracians, among others. The few documents of that period still in existence indicate that suggestion was then widely practised in the healing art. The Thracians used psychotherapeutic approaches for various ailments, basing their practices on tradition and empirical observation, though lacking in understanding of the mechanisms of interaction between mind and body. Masked or implicit suggestion was the method most frequently used, but there is evidence that the famous healer Zalmoxis in his "edifying discourses" applied direct suggestion as well (1).

There is little evidence about attitudes towards the mentally ill and about their treatment during the early centuries of the Bulgarian state, which was founded in 681. Little development is known to have taken place during the centuries of the Turkish Ottoman rule, which lasted until 1878. For five centuries the Bulgarian people existed in conditions of economic, political, and social backwardness, deprived of their essential rights under the despotism of the Turkish Empire. No medical science, and of course no scientific psychiatry, could evolve in such conditions. The then current ideas of the causes, nature, and manifestations of mental disorders had a demonological character.

The treatment of the mentally ill took place in monasteries and sanctuaries, as the sick were the traditional responsibility of the monks
(or of *hodjas,* or rabbis, for patients of Moslem or Jewish faith).
Similarly, folk medicine employed mainly magical rituals in the treatment of mental disorders.

The liberation of Bulgaria from Turkish rule in 1878 marked the
beginning of an era of national revival in the economic, cultural, and
social spheres, which made possible the development of scientific
medicine. Unfortunately, psychiatry was not in the forefront of that
rapid development, and the first psychiatric ward in a hospital was
not opened until 1888. The belated acceptance of psychiatry as a
branch of medicine resulted in a paucity of trained psychiatrists and
personnel. But despite this, soon after the first psychiatric wards had
been established a number of papers on mental health appeared in
medical journals and popular magazines. The following decade was
marked by the opening of psychiatric hospitals in Lovetch, Varna,
Karloukovo, and Byala.

2

THE 20TH CENTURY

Academic Developments

The acceptance of psychiatry by the medical profession and by the
general public was facilitated by the publications and public lectures
of the first Bulgarian psychiatrists, as well as by the many translated
articles by leading foreign authorities in the field. Among the pioneers
of psychiatry in Bulgaria during that period, special mention should
be made of S. Danadjiev (Plate LXXVIII), G. Payakov, V. Vladov,
D. Kalevich, D. Barakov, A. Golovina, N. Moskov, and M. Mikhaylov.
The leading figure among them was S. Danadjiev, who was the
founder of scientific psychiatry in Bulgaria. The monograph, *L'homi
cide en pathologie mentale* published in French by V. Vladov, in
1911, won him the award of the French Academy of Medical Sciences.

The main themes of the early research and publications in psychiatry in Bulgaria were: the organization of the psychiatric services, the
training of psychiatrists, the treatment and management of psychiatric
patients, forensic problems, case reports, and statistics.

In the early periods of the development of psychiatry in Bulgaria,
the pioneers of the profession had to overcome enormous obstacles in

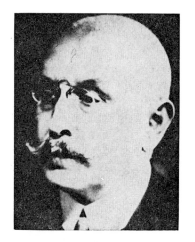

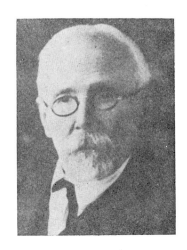

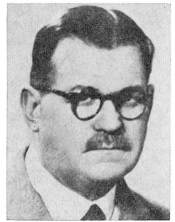

PLATE LXXVIII (upper left). Dr. S. Danajiev.
PLATE LXXIX (upper right). Professor N. M.
Popov. PLATE LXXX (left). Professor N. Krest-
nikov. PLATE LXXXI (lower left). Professor K.
Tcholakov. PLATE LXXXII (lower right). Pro-
fessor G. Usunoff.

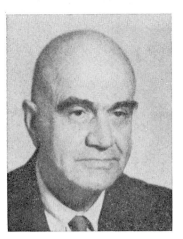

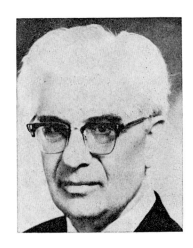

the face of the government's and health administration's indifference and neglect of psychiatry. In a setting of severe material limitations and administrative difficulties, those courageous men and women were in step with progressive developments abroad, creating occupational therapy units, regimes of non-restraint, and methods of active treatment of the psychoses.

In the years between the two wars, Bulgarian psychiatry was characterized by more sophisticated research and an improved level of clinical practice and teaching. Impetus for development was the opening of the Medical Faculty in Sofia, in 1918, where psychiatrists were, for the first time, on the academic staff.

Academic psychiatry in Bulgaria owed its first successes to the activity of Professor N. M. Popov (Plate LXXIX), the teacher of a whole generation of psychiatrists and the author of the first Bulgarian textbooks on psychiatry, *Foundations of General Psychopathology* (1923) and *Foundations of Special Psychopathology* (1925). Theoretically, the two textbooks were in the tradition of classical German psychiatry. The fine clinical erudition of Popov can be grasped from his papers on general paresis and schizophrenia.

Interesting contributions in the same period were made by A. E. Yanishevsky, a neurologist who also undertook clinical research in psychiatry; he was the first teacher who presented pavlovian ideas to medical students.

Psychopathology and Influence from Abroad

The 1930's were marked by the work of the most remarkable figure in Bulgarian psychiatry between the two wars, N. Krestnikov (Plate LXXX). He excelled in every area, as a clinician, teacher, and researcher. The influence of Bekhterev and Pavlov can be traced in his theoretically oriented works, but he attempted to construct his own conception of mental life and psychiatric disorders, which, despite its originality, suffered from speculative generalizations. Krestnikov believed that the reflex act was the basis of any form of mental life which could be reduced to elementary functional units ("psychones," analogous to the neurones in nervous activity). The functions of the mind could be divided into "centripetal" ones (e.g., sensations) and "centrifugal" ones (e.g., imagery, ideas), analysis and synthesis being performed by specialized, respectively receptor and effector, "psychones." Krestnikov postulated a central "self-psychone" which organizes the "processes of consciousness," with specialized centrifugal and centripetal psychones around it. Later he described subjective consciousness as a product of the reflex interactions between the "self-psychone" and the other psychones. Mental disorder was seen as a result of malfunction in either the centrifugal or centripetal psychones.

As a skilful psychotherapist, Krestnikov developed an original cathartic method, using an induced reproduction of the pathogenic experience. The method was described for the first time in a paper written in German in 1929, and was estimated by many to be the best about cathartic techniques. It is still very widely used in Bulgaria, in the psychotherapy of the neuroses.

Another prominent psychiatrist of the 1930's was K. Tcholakov (Plate LXXXI). He was influenced by the dualistic theory of the German philosopher J. Rehmke and by the psychobiological ideas of E. Kretschmer. Tcholakov was the author of another psychotherapeutic technique called by him "psychophysiological decapsulation for causal treatment of the neuroses." Later, in the 1940's and 1950's, Tcholakov tried to re-build his theory of psychopathology along pavlovian lines.

Toward the end of the 1930's another prominent Bulgarian psychiatrist, N. Schipkowensky, published his first works. Schipkowensky examined the psychopathological analysis of the clinical manifestations of the psychoses and neuroses in detail, and sharpened the tools of differential diagnosis. His publications cover such wide areas as forensic psychiatry, general psychopathology, the neuroses, and personality disorders. The method of psychological interpretation which was his main tool led him to generalizations which influenced psychiatric thinking: for example, the "dissolution of the links of the personality with the social and cosmic totality" in schizophrenia, or the "autochthonously emerging change of the general vital feelings" and the "improverishment of general drive" in hypochondriasis. Even before the last war, Schipkowensky was an active critic of Lombroso, Freud and Adler. In his later works, until the present day, he adhered to pavlovian nervism in psychiatry. His present activities are mainly in the fields of forensic psychiatry and gerontopsychiatry.

Developments after World War II

After the liberation of Bulgaria from fascism in 1944, the country was reorganized on a socialist basis. This period opened new perspectives for the development of psychiatry: the university department of psychiatry was reinforced, a new generation of psychiatrists went into training, a number of new psychiatric services—both in-patient and out-patient—were opened throughout the country. The most im-

BULGARIA 381

portant development was the institution of a network of psycho-neurological dispensaries which covered practically the whole of the population.

In parallel with these practical advances, much effort was given to the theoretical reconstruction of medical science in general, and of psychiatry in particular. Two major events in this respect were the open discussion on the state of psychiatry and neurology in Bulgaria (1949) and the session on medical theory and practice in Bulgaria in the light of the pavlovian theory (1951).

A leading figure during that period was G. Usunoff (Plate LXXXII). In his first well known work, *Atebrine Psychosis,* he tried to apply the principles of dialectical materialism in psychiatry, particularly with regard to the traditional dichotomy of endogenous and exogenous causation in psychiatric illness. Usunoff critically examined the theory of Bonhoeffer, who claimed that the central nervous system could re-act to external agents only in a limited number of ways which were non-specific and indirect (mediated by changes in other tissues and systems). Usunoff used his clinical material to show that a relative specificity could be found in the toxic psychoses caused by different agents, according to the temporal rate of involvement of the central nervous system and the localization of the pathological tissue changes. Apart from being a prominent psychiatrist, Usunoff took an active part in the International Peace Movement and in many national campaigns, such as the Committee for Sobriety.

Another psychiatrist of prominence in the contemporary scene is E. Sharankov, who made important contributions on ethno- and folk psychiatry. One of his outstanding works had as its theme the ancient religious ritual called *Nestinarstvo* (fire walking), in which he gave an interesting analysis of the social cathartic function of folk rituals. The neuroses and the personality disorders are also a field in which Sharankov made original contributions.

After 1956, medical schools were also opened in Plovdiv and Varna. The new schools have their own departments of psychiatry. Present-day Bulgarian psychiatry unites the efforts of many devoted workers from the academic departments and the hospital and dispensary network.

A number of national conferences on various problems, such as epilepsy, psychotherapy, and the organization of psychiatric care, have been held in the past two decades. Two national congresses of the Bulgarian neurologists, psychiatrists, and neurosurgeons have been important events. The Third International Symposium on Social Psychiatry, in 1971, the Fifth Danube Symposium of Psychiatry and the International Symposium on Electrosleep, in 1972, have been among recent international meetings taking place in Bulgaria.

Research in psychiatry is now largely directed toward social problems: epidemiology, effectiveness of night and day services, and so on.

Bulgarian psychiatry is eclectic. It eagerly accepts original and constructive ideas in psychopathology, clinical psychiatry, treatment, organization of psychiatric services, and sociology of mental disorders—wherever they may come from. As a science, Bulgarian psychiatry has a short history (2), but it has a good potential for growth and is open to progressive and fruitful ideas coming from various quarters of the world. Most Bulgarian psychiatrists agree that good foundations have been laid for the development of psychiatry in the service of society and of progress.

REFERENCES

1. Joncev, W. and Zaprianov, N. (1968): Suggestion in der Thrazischen Medizin. *Folia medica (Plovdiv)*, x, fasc. IV, 271-276.
2. Temkov, I., Ivanov, V. and Christozov, C. (1955): Development of Bulgarian psychiatry (Bulg.). *Nauchni Trudove na NIINP*, 1, 3-36.

17

TURKEY

Vamik D. Volkan, M.D.

Professor of Psychiatry, University of Virginia School of Medicine,
Charlottesville, Virginia, U.S.A.

1

INTRODUCTION

A bird's-eye view of the history of Turkey should precede any discussion of the development of psychiatry in that country. It is possible to divide Turkey's history into three periods: the time before the Ottoman Empire; the span of the Ottoman Empire, from 1299 to 1923; and modern Turkey, from the foundation of the Turkish Republic in 1923 to the present time.

The French historian Cahen (12) of the Sorbonne, who presented the research of a lifetime on the medieval Turkey in Asia Minor, states that it is virtually certain that "the earliest Turks known to history—although not called by that name—were the Huns," who were known to us from the Chinese Annals as early as the 3rd century B.C.

> Under the specific name of Turks (the meaning of which is uncertain), the Turks made their appearance, both in the Chinese sources in the East and in the Byzantine sources in the West, in the 6th century A.D. in the territory that is now Mongolia, but very soon also over a wide area, expanding towards the South and West (12).

Turks created two large empires in Central Asia, in Turkestan; their prosperity is attested to by inscriptions dating from the 8th

383

century (24). A western migration during the 9th and 10th centuries filled the vacuum left by the fall of the Arabic Islamic Empire with Turks, who adopted the faith of Islam. The migrants' adherence to Islam naturally exerted "a cohesive effect on otherwise disparate bodies of conquerors and conquered, and resulted in an almost invincible solidarity" (21). The expansion of Turkish power also coincided with the decline of Eastern Christendom.

During the 11th and 12th centuries Seljuk Turks settled in Anatolia and founded the Seljuk Empire, which at times reached as far as Afghanistan to the Mediterranean. With the disruption of this Empire the Ottoman Turks gradually came into power, and, in an ascendancy over rival Turkish dynasties in Anatolia, became undisputed leaders of the Moslem world. After being captured in 1453, Constantinople (Istanbul) became the capital of the Turkish Empire, the most powerful of its time. By the 16th century the Ottoman Empire covered the Balkan Peninsula, going all the way to Vienna from the Adriatic and Aegean Seas eastward into Persia, from the Crimea on the north of the Black Sea southward into the Arabian Peninsula, and in the northern part of Africa from Egypt to Algeria.

The decline of the Ottoman Empire began at the end of the 16th century and took more than 300 years to complete. When Turkey was to be left as a token territory at the end of World War I, the Turks fought their war of independence that was to mark the end of the Empire and the establishment of a Turkish Republic by 1923, attended by an effort under the leadership of Atatürk to achieve Turkey's speedy westernization.

2

PRE-OTTOMAN PERIOD

The Turks of Central Asia were originally animists, worshippers of the earth, sky, and water, but by the 7th century Buddhism spread among them. Manichaeism, Judaism, and Christianity made their way into Central Asia before the Turks turned to Islam. The beginning of Turkish psychiatry is undoubtedly connected with animism, mythology, and religion, as in other cultures (32) and the religious man was also a psychic healer. There is no documentation of Turkish behavior toward the mentally ill during the pre-Islamic period (1).

Passages in a book written in Turkish in 1069—*Kutadgu-Bilig* (the *Kudatkebilik*)—describe the *efsuncu,* who warded off jinns (demons) and occupied a role just below the *hekim* (physician) in the social hierarchy (17, 38). The same book gives an account of disagreements between *efsuncus* who treated their patients by "suggestion" and those medical men who scorned such methods. It states that within one Turkish group, the Uygurs, physicians limited their concept of treatment to treatment by physical means.

At the time Yusuf Hasi Hacib wrote *Kutadgu-Bilig,* Avicenna, the great Islamic physician, had been dead for 32 years. The ethnic origin of this eminent healer was disputed by Turks, Persians, and Arabs (10), but Turkish textbooks in psychiatry (1, 2, 5) refer to him as Turkish, as do writers (17, 36) who report the history of Turkish and Islamic psychiatry. Also known as Ibni Sina, Avicenna was born in Bokhara and only later settled in Ispahan. In his *Canon* (11) he refers to many psychiatric matters (his awareness that mania and depression constitute a recognizable clinical illness, for example). The following statements reflect his intuition and his perceptive observation and knowledge of child development:

> Children should be carefully attended and supervised regarding their behavior so that they do not exceed the limits of moderation. Outbursts of violent anger, fear, and anxiety should be checked. This is best ensured by considering the child's natural desires and inclinations, and keeping in view his aversions. The natural aptitudes of the child should be encouraged while the causes of irritation are removed. This type of training is good for body and mind both. The mind is benefitted because good habits and manners are permanently ingrained in the personality by early training. . . . When the child is six years old he should be sent to a teacher for education and training. Care should be taken to adopt a progressive system and not burden the child with books all at once. . . .

According to Avicenna, there were three types of psyche—plant, animal, and human. The plant psyche possesses nutritional and reproductive qualities, and the animal psyche has the additional qualities of motility and perception. The human aspect of the psyche is concerned with "high ideals" and morals (1, 5).

It is inappropriate to debate here the question of Avicenna's origin; it is possible that he was a Persian, but many Turkish scholars of the period wrote as he did in the Persian language. It is entirely clear, however, that Turkish medicine (and psychiatry) owes much to Islam, which demanded understanding and humane treatment for the mentally ill. Stories like the following attest to an understanding of the connections between anxiety and change in the human organism:

> A ruler's young kinsman fell ill, became anorexic, and withdrew from others. While examining him Avicenna "talked" to him as he checked his pulse. He noted that the pulse rate increased at the mention of a certain street in the city. Remarks about a house located on that street, and the name of a certain female occupant, evoked the symptom even more sharply, and the physician concluded that the young man's illness was caused by frustrated love for the young woman in question. Taking Avicenna's advice, the young man married the girl, and recovered from his illness (5, 9).

Avicenna's *Canon* was

> . . . a systematic attempt to correlate Aristotelian philosophy, Hippocratic observation, and Galenic speculations—as in Galen's writings, pages of excellent medical exposition are side by side with pages filled with medical trash (9).

However, it was "the most influential textbook ever written" (33) and not only influenced medicine in the Near East and Asia, but became a medical bible in Europe until the 16th century. It naturally had a definite influence on the Turkish mode of medical and psychological practice.

When the Seljuk Turks conquered Anatolia they inherited a land which had seen many great civilizations in the past. Anatolia had been the place of Aesculapian temples and other sanctuaries during the Hellenistic era. These places were used for the mentally ill, who were treated free of charge. The treatment method was based largely on suggestion; patients slept in the temple after receiving instruction from the priests concerning dreams, and the content of his dreams revealed to the patient what was necessary for his recovery. It may safely be assumed that the history and traditions of Anatolia, as well as the teachings of Islamic medicine, influenced the way in which the Seljuks treated the mentally ill, and that Aesculapian method "continued in changed but similar form during the reign of the Seldjukians and the Ottomans . . ." (18).

The Seljuk Turks were great builders, and their "principal innovation was the *madrasa* (medrese)" (12). Although certain precedents had already been set, the Seljuks

> . . . were the first to give them any real importance and to cause them to be put into practice on a large scale. The *madrasa* is an

establishment for instruction which . . . is specially organized for the teaching of the religio-judicial sciences (12).

The *madrasa* acquired great wealth through the establishment of pious foundations. Seljuk Turks (and later the Ottoman Turks) built urban communities that centered around these religious foundations and mosques. These included social and public institutions such as schools, libraries, and hospitals, and fountains and baths. Several hospitals built during the Seljuk period in Anatolia had sections for the care of the mentally ill, among them one built in 1205 in Kayseri, one in Sivas (1217), one in Kastamoni (1272), and still another in Amasya (1308) (5).

When the first organized hospitals were being erected in Anatolia, *tekkes* (houses of the sufitic belief) were being dispersed throughout the country. These were religious and philosophical establishments that offered treatment to the mentally ill. Koptagel (18) implies that they derived from the old Aesculapian temples.

> After the first acute stage of the illness the patient would be expected to work inside the establishment and would be gradually included in the small social circle of the inhabitants. The religious-philosophical atmosphere reigning in these establishments provided a means of sublimation for the patient. . . . The patients who failed to show adequate recovery remained in the institution and were made to work under control, as best they could. The patients who left the institution after their recovery were considered members of the union and retained a certain relationship with the institution all through their lives. The institution was a place of reliance for them where they could apply to any time in case of need (18).

In their basic plan of giving help these *tekkes,* which survived for many centuries, are strikingly like the community mental health centers recently developed in the United States.

3

THE OTTOMAN EMPIRE

It seems fitting to begin this account with a dream attributed to Osman Bey, who later became the founder of the Empire named after him, and its first ruler. In this dream a beam of light fell from the sky to the lap of a holy man and was then transferred to the lap of Osman Bey. A tree sprung out of the light, with a branch pointing to Istanbul and a shadow falling on the Caucasus Mountains and the Euphrates River. Then a wind scattered the leaves of this tree to distant lands. A ring rose from out the Black Sea and fitted itself to one of Osman Bey's fingers.

Adasal (1) describes this dream as a telepathic dream that forecast the expansion of the Empire. Its manifest content indicates Osman's preoccupation with the seizure of ever more widespread territories. There is, of course, no way to examine what deep psychic processes lay behind this dream nor what it meant to the dreamer in connection with his repressed childhood desires and conflicts (in spite of the rather open symbolism it contains), but the fact that this account of it has been passed from generation to generation of the Turkish people testifies to their sensitivity to the importance of psychic productions. The "dream" ascribed to their leader may have been indeed a common and shared dream that belonged to all Turks of the period—one reflecting their mood and embodying their goals. It is certain that they did conquer Istanbul in 1453 under the leadership of a 22-year-old Sultan.

In 1470 they opened a hospital for the exclusive use of the mentally ill in Istanbul. Both Aksel (5) and Adasal (1) refer, in their respective psychiatric textbooks, to the visit made by the famous French psychiatrist, Moreau de la Tours, to Istanbul in 1842; de la Tours inspected the ruins of this first of the Ottoman mental hospitals, and stated that it had a model hospital design, even for use in the 19th century.

During the reign of Bayazid II a smaller second mental hospital, still in existence although in ruins, was erected in Edirne. Lewis (21) describes it as follows:

> The great medical school founded by Sultan Bayazid II (1481-1512) in Edirne . . . had a mental hospital with individual rooms for the patients and a large hexagonal communal hall, acoustically perfect, with an open dome and a soothing fountain in the middle; at one end was a dais on which musicians sat and played to calm and distract psychopathic and melancholy patients. In most towns separate hospitals were provided for infidels, and these were also served by gifted and well-trained doctors and surgeons. The diet was always plentiful; if the hospital kitchens were found to be inadequate, food was brought in from the public kitchens.

It was usual in the Ottoman world to make their urban centers into large-scale agglomerations of buildings that were "impressive not only from an architectural point of view but also for the public and scientific spirit which they embodied" (8). For example, the famous 17th century Turkish traveler and writer, Evliya Celebi, wrote about Bayazid's foundation grant for the mental hospital in Edirne:

> . . . His majesty Bayazid II appointed three singers, as well as a flutist, a violinist, a flageolet player, a cymbalist, a harpist, and a lutanist to provide therapy for the sick, to improve the suffering, to strengthen the spirit of the insane and to reduce the bile. They come three times a week and play their music in front of the sick and insane. By the grace of the Almighty many of them feel relieved . . ." (8).

It is interesting that the contemporary books of psychiatric history written in English have almost no mention of the model psychiatric hospitals built by the Turks, or the "enlightened" treatment provided in them. Although Moslem Arabs had built insane asylums before the Turks did, it was the latter who, by becoming the champions of Islam, not only carried on with the Islamic tradition of benevolent treatment of the mentally ill, but made further improvements in their care, i.e. in music therapy and the design of mental hospitals. The contemporary historian of psychiatry, Mora (23), makes a brief reference to Bayazid's mental hospital and Evliya Celebi's description of it under the designation of "the enlightened view of the Arabs toward the mentally ill." Yet the truth is that Bayazid was a *Turkish* Sultan and the Turks and the Arabs are two different peoples.

Another mental hospital was built in 1539, in Manisa; this has been restored and is still in use. Still another, named after Süleyman the Magnificent (whom Turks prefer to call "The Lawgiver"), was built there by the great 16th century Turkish architect, Sinan. In his biography of Sinan, Stratton (34) describes it:

> . . . At the time of [the Sultan's] death this hospital was the finest in the world. The ill and the insane walked or were brought into the first courtyard. They were diagnosed in the surrounding domical rooms opening onto an arcade. Those with the ordinary maladies or fractures were put in bed in high and spacious rooms full of light and air. . . . Those found to be insane were led into the second courtyard . . . rectangular and arcaded like the other, with special rooms opening from it, open to the sky.
> . . . In the cells opening from this deep and rectified space, the worst of the insane were locked up—the powerful men, young or middle-aged or old, slaves or free men deranged by Holy War or by the conditions of peace; and likewise for their own safety, the women, too, all of them either slaves or ladies of the harem, to be married, already married, or widowed. Sinan understood

the diseases that we call paranoia and schizophrenia, and their complexes, vertigo, claustrophobia, delusions of grandeur and of persecution.

But make no mistake, Sinan did not design a Bedlam or a snakepit. Nor were the ill and the insane scanted in treatment and care by the best qualified and best trained medical practitioners and nurses in Europe, Asia, and Africa, which was the extent of the civilized world of those days. The patients were kept clean; they dined on game birds . . . delicate fresh fish . . . had flowers from the imperial gardens . . . heard the gentle splashing of the fountains and listened to the soothing music played by the court orchestra.

For centuries this was the main mental hospital in Turkey. Another, the Toptasi, was built to honor the mother of Murad III; his reign lasted from 1574 to 1595. When Süleyman's hospital eventually was no longer in use for mental patients, the Toptasi operated for their benefit until the establishment of the Turkish Republic. One of the early physicians-in-chief of this institution was an Italian psychiatrist, Mongeri Pere, who left documents indicative of the high degree of social awareness felt at the time, and the provision of humane treatment because of a commitment to help the mentally ill (1).

The Ottoman Empire, especially during its final three centuries of existence, declined in every aspect of medical care, including that of the mentally disturbed.

Cruel and punitive treatment of the mentally ill actually never existed to any recognizable degree in this part of the world, except probably in poor treatment in a few state hospitals during the latter stages of the Ottoman Empire (32).

During this period some of the Sultans themselves suffered from mental disorders. Sultan Abdülhamid II, whose reign spanned the years between 1876 and 1909, was afraid of the "insane," and required that the Toptasi Hospital become virtually a horrible prison for those confined there. The death rate of the inmates was high, and at one time it required the Sultan's permission to visit this hospital-prison. When Kraepelin visited Istanbul and asked to see it, he was unable to obtain permission to do so (1, 2).

Persian and Arabic were the original languages of Islamic medical science and continued to be used by Ottoman scholars. In the 18th century, Turkish scholars began writing in Turkish and translated Arabic and Persian classics into their own tongue. By the latter half of the 19th century, Western medicine exerted its influence and

French and German became the alternate languages of the educated, today largely replaced by English.

The first modern neuropsychiatric clinic in Turkey was opened in the late Ottoman period (1898) by Rasit Tahsin (Plate LXXXIII), who had studied with Kraepelin in Germany. In 1908, Tahsin became the first professor of neuropsychiatry in the Istanbul Medical School and gave the lectures on "modern" psychiatric issues. However, Turkish psychiatrists (1, 2, 3, 5, 7, 14, 15) agree that Mazhar Osman Uzman (Plate LXXXIV) was the founding father of modern Turkish neuropsychiatry.

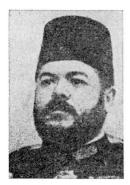

PLATE LXXXIII.
Rasit Tahsin.

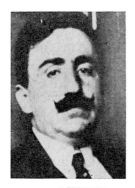

PLATE LXXXIV.
Mazhar Osman Uzman.

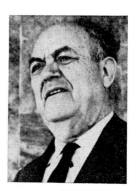

PLATE LXXXV.
Rasim Adasal.

It should be understood that details furnished here about psychiatric practice in the Ottoman period apply only to urban centers, since the rural population lived quite different lives from those of the city-dwellers, as to a great extent remains the case today. Turkish folk beliefs concerning mental illness will be discussed later.

4

MODERN TURKEY

Mazhar Osman Uzman was born in 1884 and graduated from the Turkish military medical school in 1904, later studying under Kraepelin and Ziehen in Germany (7). He held a variety of posts during his professional life, which spanned more than 40 years. He took over Tahsin's clinic in 1908, when its founder undertook his professorial duties, and remained there until 1918. After the War of Independence he became psychiatrist-in-chief of Toptasi Hospital. Uzman, often called the Pinel of Turkey, attempted to change and modernize what he found there, and was later instrumental in transferring all of the patients to a new and modern state hospital, the Bakirkoy Hospital (in 1927). This remains the most modern and progressive state hospital in the country, under the present leadership of Faruk Bayülkem.

After the establishment of the Turkish Republic and the reform of the educational system, psychiatric activities were separated from work in neurology, and Uzman became a professor of psychiatry and chairman of the psychiatric department at Istanbul University until his death in 1951.

The founder of modern Turkish psychiatry was influenced by Kraepelin, and was strongly oriented toward descriptive and organic psychiatry, which was not, in practice, a separate medical specialty from neurology in spite of the designation of a different chairman for each discipline. He made contributions to the study and understanding of multiple sclerosis and general paralysis as well as to work being done with obsessional neurosis. He wrote the first Turkish textbooks on neuropsychiatry; these were for their time excellent texts on descriptive and organic psychiatry. He published more than 220 papers, many in German or French, and a number were read at international congresses.

Between 1935 and 1937 Mazhar Osman Uzman concerned himself with mental deficiency in children (14), but formal establishment of modern child psychiatry in Turkey came after his death, when Sükrü Aksel succeeded him as chairman of the department of psychiatry. Turkish psychiatry tended for many years to reflect Uzman's emphasis on "descriptive" psychiatry and to stress nosology, and psychopharmacologic and somatic treatment. European study, often in Germany, was usual for the students of Uzman, who taught such leaders of Turkish neuropsychiatry as Aksel and Fahreddin K. Gökay, who was later to become a political figure, and, between 1949 and 1958, Governor of Istanbul. During the 1930's some of Freud's writings were translated into Turkish, and Turkish psychiatrists began somewhat hesitantly to refer to Freudian thought, although they did not delve deeply into it. Its psychodynamics were not truly integrated into Turkish psychiatry, which continued to be dominated by the classical German and French schools.

Rasim Adasal (Plate LXXXV) was foremost in promoting the assimilation into Turkish psychiatry of the psychodynamic approach and a social orientation; he can certainly be seen as a transitional figure. Becoming chairman of the psychiatric department of the new medical school opened at the University of Ankara in 1946, he remained there until his recent retirement. Active, and eager for knowledge, removed from the University of Istanbul's heavily traditional descriptive psychiatry, he began lecturing in the new school on aspects of psychoanalytic theory, human sexuality, etc. Although he did not abandon descriptive psychiatry, his lectures and textbooks added to their discussion of aspects of psychoanalytic theory, attention to behavior modification and the intimations of such systems as yoga, as well as illustrations of psychiatric processes and disorders by reference to both Turkish and Western Literature and films. Charismatic and able to communicate well with laymen, he fostered psychiatric awareness among educated modern Turks. Two of his assistants became the core personnel of the psychiatric department in Ankara's second medical school, Hacettepe Medical School, established in 1963. Dogan Karan, the department's chairman, was for some time dean of this new school, and another professor of psychiatry there is Orhan M. Öztürk, who received training in the United States and spent many years at the Austin Riggs Center, coming under the influence of Erik Erikson. Since the department's staff is largely psychoanalytically oriented, its teaching program, at both the undergraduate and graduate teaching levels, emphasizes the psychodynamic approach. It employs a somewhat unique teaching method: "By assigning each medical student to a family of low socioeconomic level from the first year on, the student is provided an opportunity to study the social and psychologic problems of the Turkish family" (32). An even newer medical school, in an eastern province, Erzurum, follows in its department of psychiatry the curriculum designed by the Hacettepe Medical School, and the publications from still another, the Aegean Medical School, indicate an emphasis on the social and cultural aspects of psychiatry.

Turkey now has a total of approximately 6,500 beds for psychiatric patients, distributed among university psychiatric centers, three state hospitals, 44 neuropsychiatric units of hospitals subsidized by the government and related organizations, and five private hospitals. The Ministry of Health and Social Welfare in 1971 listed 492 neuropsychiatric specialists, of whom 45 were women (32). Psychiatric clinics meeting community needs on an outpatient basis are increasing in number. In 1968, 23,000 outpatients were seen in the university clinics, and about 5,000 in Bakirkoy State Hospital. By 1971 Turkey had two outpatient departments for child psychiatry.

Three journals of psychiatry are published in Turkey. *Tip Dünyasi,* a monthly now in its 46th year, was founded by Gökay and serves as the official publication of the Turkish Society for Mental Hygiene and the Turkish Society of Social Psychiatry. *Nöro-Psykiyatri Arsivi,* published quarterly, serves as the archives of the Turkish Neuro-Psychiatric Society; it is now in its tenth year. The third journal comes from Bakirkoy Hospital.

5

FOLK BELIEFS CONCERNING MENTAL ILLNESS

Cahen (12) writes that the Islam that was introduced to the Turks

> . . . was of a particular kind. It was not the Islam of the great scholars, but that of the itinerant popular monks, of merchants of varying degrees of culture and of frontier soldiers, and was compounded as much of various practices, words, and charms as of true dogma (12).

Although there were Islamic scholars in the cities, in the traditional village religion was a system of quasi-religious beliefs and superstitions. Here the religious man was the center of community cohesion and at times a healer of its inhabitants. The hierarchical structure of the Ottoman Empire was based on the Islamic code, and religion and its attendant superstitions dominated the everyday life of the Turks (21). In 1925 the Atatürk revolution secularized the state, and all religious and quasi-religious educational and therapeutic institutions were abolished. Since that time the practice of folk healing has been outlawed and its practitioners prosecuted. Nevertheless, certain folk beliefs and practices persist in the more conservative segments of society.

A traditional villager's understanding of illness reflects his religious faith that all goodness and all suffering comes from God; the reasons for God's inflicting pain on mankind are beyond human understanding. The Moslem religion accepts the existence of spirits such as jinns, which are invisible, mobile, and usually aggressive beings living in ruins, among rocks and deserted houses, and in chimneys, and which are capable of seducing humans; these are traditionally blamed for any illness, particularly for mental illness (21, 27, 32). Another example of externalized power can be found in the belief in the "evil eye"—a belief that Turks share with Greeks, and other groups in the Middle East. The "evil eye" is held accountable for sickness, particularly the sickness of children. Successful and attractive people are considered particularly vulnerable to its malign influence, and persons with blue or green eyes are suspected of enjoying its unique power. Countermeasures have been developed to foil it; eye-shaped blue beads and amulets are supposed to guard against it. Many places of pilgrimage and veneration, most considered holy since early times, continue to be visited by those who bring candles and pray to petition for help or to unburden themselves of guilt. Some of the holy spots are tombs, the graves of honored spiritual leaders, or those traditionally connected with the mythology of the locality.

The religious man still acts at times as a healer.

> Many of them have no religious training or function but are able to find a means of introducing themselves as men of religion and wisdom; they use a good deal of quackery (32).

Öztürk describes (25) the "folk treatment" of mental illness in Turkey, and gives (27) the details of the "treatment" given a 13-year-old schoolboy in a remote village on the Black Sea in today's Turkey. The boy suffered from attacks of acute anxiety, for which he was treated for two weeks by a "religious" man. In the "treatment" the religious man drew a broken circle on a piece of paper and commanded that the boy see jinns inside it. The boy produced certain images, while crying and showing great fear and excitement. He was then asked to cut the jinns into pieces and burn them. After getting rid of each jinn during the continuing daily sessions it was possible to close the "exit" where the circle was incomplete, and although the child improved when this was accomplished, his symptoms returned after a month.

Lewis (21) describes in detail the practice of another traditional exorcist, the "lead-pourer" during the Ottoman period. His tools were a melting-ladle, a bowl of water, a towel, and a lump of lead. Such beliefs and rituals are in many ways adaptive-defensive; they help to guard against felt anxiety.

6

CURRENT DIRECTIONS

Turkey is a country in the midst of continuing modernization and industrialization, as it has been since the great Atatürk Revolution. Many problems remain, however—among them problems of mental health. So many dynamic changes are going on there that one can no longer speak in terms of any prototype of the Turkish family, but must consider that the Turkish family structure in undergoing change Although as recently as 1958 Lerner (20) reported that the traditional Turkish villager would never dream of leaving his village and would prefer death to leaving it behind, such reluctance is no longer usual (32). Turkish workers now flood the European countries, especially Germany; contact with the Western world in the past was available only to the elite of Turkey.

The Republic's psychiatrists, the majority of whom still basically practice "descriptive psychiatry" with emphasis on somatic treatments, besides learning, teaching, and researching modern psychiatry, are greatly involved with the psychological aspects of these changes in the Turkish scene, and are obliged to study external dynamic factors in human psychology, and to go beyond the descriptive-organic approach. However, psychological insights into the Turkey of today require a grasp of the life style of the traditional Turkey. All too frequently the American psychiatrist writing about Turkey either gives a brief statistical summary of Turkey's mental health activity (19), or draws hasty and unscientific conclusions on the basis of hearsay, against the background of a travelog. For example, Masserman (22) questions the existence of the classical Freudian castration complex on the basis of information given him that few Turkish children are traumatized during the rites of circumcision that occur at the height of the oedipal stage of psychosexual development. And the account of Gardner's (16) four-day diagnostic-therapeutic home visit in Turkey is criticized by Öztürk (30) as containing "loose socio-cultural generalizations."

Öztürk himself is the leading student of Turkish psychology. A psychiatrist, he has scrutinized child-rearing practices customary in the Turkish village, and has tried to demonstrate their intrapsychic consequences (26, 29). Öztürk and Volkan (32) have studied the stresses faced by the traditionally reared Turk from infancy to the end of his life. Circumcision practices in Turkey have had special attention from Öztürk (28, 31) and Cansever (13).

E. A. Sumer (35) uses the terms *transitionals* and *moderns* when describing those present-day Turks who have turned from the traditional ways, and Lerner (20) found such classification useful in his writings. Transitionals make up half the population, and moderns a minority of perhaps 15 per cent. The latter are typically born in large metropolitan centers, are well-educated, and come from well-to-do families. "They have wholly integrated Western thoughts and ways in their personalities and lives, and are chiefly responsible for shaping the character of contemporary life in Turkey" (35). Sümer sees restlessness among all generations as the search for a new Turkish identity takes form, and says, in reference to Freud's statement that dissolution precedes any new construction: "It is, perhaps, a little exaggerated to say that Turkey has entered a stage of mass neurosis which is the price one is said to pay for civilization" (35). Koptagel (18) speculates about how to apply modern methods of psychiatric treatment to those segments of Turkish society that remain in the traditional mold. Those bound to the old ways still see mental illness in metaphysical terms, and Koptagel, noting how greatly such beliefs contribute to a sense of security, is concerned with what may be substituted for them. She insists on taking into account the social fabric of the country in any attempted solution of its mental hygiene problems, and on developing cultural values that will take the place of the old traditions the Turkish people are being asked to give up. Öztürk and Volkan (32) report a movement within the universities toward more dynamic and socially oriented psychiatry, and observe that universities have considerably more responsibility for the direction medicine will take than do government organizations.

Certain specific aspects of the contemporary social scene in Turkey are reflected in Turkish psychiatry: industrialization (37), temporary emigration to the labor market of Europe for employment (4, 6), and the trouble in Cyprus. Volkan (39, 40) has written of the latter and pointed to the way in which Cypriot Turks dealt with the psychological stress of being surrounded by their enemies and confined within a limited space by adopting a mass hobby—the rearing of parakeets in captivity. This dramatization of the simile "free as a bird" represented the response of those whose freedom was severely limited and who felt threatened over long periods of time.

Like many other countries, Turkey has undergone a "brain drain" and many Turkish scholars, physicians, and other specialists have sought rewards outside their homeland. No history of Turkish psychiatry would be complete without reference to the large number of Turkish psychiatrists now living in the United States. In 1971 two of them who are now U.S. citizens (Volkan and Ismet Karacan of Baylor University in Texas) attempted to organize their psychiatric compatriots at the annual meeting of the American Psychiatric Association, and located approximately 100 Turkish graduates practicing psychiatry in the States or in Canada. This is the largest number of Turkish psychiatrists practicing outside Turkey; since among the approximately 500 neuropsychiatrists in the homeland a number are neurological specialists or psychiatrists also engaged in neurology, the North American group is of significant size. The distribution is continent-wide; indeed, two Turkish psychiatrists practice in Hawaii. There are many university professors in the American group, and one is on the faculty of a psychoanalytic institute; it is interesting to note that there are enough in academic psychiatry to operate a fair-sized department of psychiatry with an exclusively Turkish faculty. In recent years Turkish psychiatrists in the States have contributed much to sleep research, psychopharmacology, child psychiatry, psychotherapy and psychoanalysis, and such special fields as the study and treatment of bereavement, and have published extensively.

The Turkish group has met twice at annual meetings of the American Psychiatric Association, with 54 present at the most recent occasion; it plans to formalize its organization at the 1974 annual meeting. This step may initiate further communication with the national psychiatric organization in Turkey, and affect psychiatric developments there. Already many young psychiatrists now practicing in Turkey have had training in the United States, and some of them have moved to positions of leadership in the universities of their homeland.

REFERENCES

1. ADASAL, R. (1964): *Medikal Psikoloji* (Medical Psychology), Vols. I and II. Ankara: Ankara Üniversitesi Yayinlarindan.
2. ADASAL, R. (1969): *Klinik Psikiyatri, Ruh Hastaliklari* (Clinical Psychiatry, Mental Illness). Ankara: Ankara Universitesi Yayinlarindan.
3. ADASAL, R. (1971): Mazhar Osman Hocayi anarken (Remembering Mazhar Osman). *Nöro-Psikiyatri Arsivi*, 8, 185.
4. ADASAL, R., EGE, I. & KÖKSAL, C. (1969): Dis ülkelerdeki yurtdaslarimizda ortaya çikan psikiyatrik sendromlar (Psychiatric syndromes among our countrymen who live in foreign countries). *Nöro-Psikiyatri Arsivi*, 6, 19.
5. AKSEL, I. S. (1959): *Psikiyatri* (Psychiatry). Istanbul: Ismail Akgün Matbaasi.
6. AKSEL, I. S. (1968): Some remarks on psychosomatic diseases. *Nöro-Psikiyatri Arsivi* 5, 68.
7. AKSEL, I. S. (1971) Mazhar Osman Hoca (Mazhar Osman, The Teacher). *Nöro-Psikiyatri Arsivi* 8, 181.
8. AKURGAL, E., MANGO, C. & ETTINGHAUSEN, R. (1966): *Treasures of Turkey, The Earliest Civilizations of Anatolia, Byzantium, Islamic Period*. Geneva: Skira.
9. ALEXANDER, F. G. & SELESNICK, S. T. (1966): *The History of Psychiatry: An Evaluation of Psychiatric Thought and Practice from Prehistoric Times to the Present*. New York: Harper & Row.
10. AMMAR, S. (1965): *En Souvenir de la Medicine Arabe*. Tunis: Imprimerie Buscone et Muscat.
11. AVICENNA (1966): *The Canon of Medicine*, transl. and ed. by M. H. Shah. Karachi: Naveed Clinic.
12. CAHEN, C. (1968): *Pre-Ottoman Turkey*, transl. by J. Jones-Williams. New York: Taplinger.
13. CANSEVER, G. (1965): Psychological effects of circumcision. *Brit. J. Med. Psychol.*, 38, 321.
14. CEBIROGLU, R. (1971): Mazhar Osman ve Cocuk Sorunlari (Mazhar Osman and pediatric issues). *Nöro-Psikiyatri Arsivi*, 8, 188.

15. DOGULU, S. (1971): Mazhar Osman Uzman. *Nöro-Psikiyatri Arsivi*, 8, 191.
16. GARDNER, R. A. (1970): A four-day diagnostic-therapeutic home visit in Turkey. *Family Process*, 9, 301.
17. GÖKAY, F. K. (1969): Ruh hekimligi sahasinda Türklerin çalismalari (Turks' studies in the field of psychiatry). *Tip Dünyasi*, 42, 526.
18. KOPTAGEL, G. (1971): Rehabilitation of the mentally handicapped in Turkey: past and present. *Soc. Sci. Med.*, 5, 603.
19. LAUGHLIN, H. P. (1960): European Psychiatry: England, Denmark, Italy, Greece, Spain, and Turkey. *Am. J. Psychiat.*, 116, 769.
20. LERNER, D. (1958): *The Passing of Traditional Society-Modernizing the Middle East.* Glencoe, Ill.: The Free Press.
21. LEWIS, R. (1971): *Everyday Life in Ottoman Turkey.* London: B. T. Batsford. New York: G. P. Putnam Sons.
22. MASSERMAN, J. H. (Ed.) (1968): *Psychiatry East and West.* New York: Grune & Stratton.
23. MORA, G. (1967): From demonology to the narrenturm. In *Historic Derivations of Modern Psychiatry*, Iago Galdston, (Ed.). New York: McGraw-Hill, Inc.
24. MULLER, H. J. (1961): *The Loom of History.* New York: American Library, a Mentor Book.
25. ÖZTÜRK, O. M. (1964): Folk treatment of mental illness in Turkey. In: *Magic, Faith and Healing*, A. Kiev (Ed.). New York: Free Press of Glencoe, Div. of Macmillan.
26. ÖZTÜRK, O. M. (1965): Child-rearing practices in the Turkish village and the major area of intrapsychic conflict. *Turkish J. Ped.*, 7, 124.
27. ÖZTÜRK, O. M. (1965): Folk interpretation of illness in Turkey and its psychological significance. *Turkish J. Ped.*, 7, 165.
28. ÖZTÜRK, O. M. (1968): Psycho-social effects of ritual circumcision in Turkey performed during the phallic and latency stages. *Proc. Fourth World Congress of Psychiatry, 1966*, J. J. Lopez-Ibor, ed. Amsterdam: Excerpta Medica Foundation.
29. ÖZTÜRK, O. M. (1970): Anadolu topumunda Θedipus Kompleksi Teorisinin Geçerligi (The applicability of the theory of Oedipus complex in the Anatolian society). *Cocuk Sagligi Ve Hastaliklari Dergisi*, 13, 1.
30. ÖZTÜRK, O. M. (1970): Commentary on a four-day diagnostic-therapeutic home visit in Turkey by R. A. Gardner. *Family Process*, 9, 318.
31. ÖZTÜRK, O. M. (1973): Ritual circumcision and castration anxiety. *Psychiatry*, 1, 49.
32. ÖZTÜRK, O. M. & VOLKAN, V. D. (1971): The theory and practice of psychiatry in Turkey. *Am. J. Psychother.* 25, 240.
33. ROBINSON, A. (1972): *The Story of Medicine.* New York: The New Home Library.
34. STRATTON, A. (1972): *Sinan.* New York: Charles Scribner's Sons.
35. SÜMER, E. A. (1970): Changing dynamic aspects of the Turkish culture and its significance for child training. In: *The Child in His Family*, E. James Anthony and C. Koupernick, (Eds.). New York: Wiley Interscience.
36. SÜMER, M. C. (1970): Iran'da psikiyatri (Psychiatry in Iran). *Tip Dünyasi*, 43, 476.
37. SÜMER, M. C. (1971): Sosyal psikiatrik açidan endüstrilesmenin dogurdugu problemler (From a social psychiatry point of view—the problems arising from industrialization). *Tip Dünyasi*, 44, 132.
38. ÜNVER, A. S. (1943): *Tip Tarihi* (History of Medicine). Istanbul: Istanbul Universitesi Yayinlarindan.
39. VOLKAN, V. D. (1972): The birds of Cyprus, a psychopolitical observation. *Am. J. Psychother*, 26, 378.
40. VOLKAN, V. D. (1973): Externalization among Cypriot Turks. *World J. Psychosynthesis*, 5, 24.

18

CANADA

Indian and Eskimo Medicine, with Notes on the Early History of Psychiatry Among French and British Colonists

EDWARD L. MARGETTS, M.D.

*Professor of Psychiatry and Lecturer in the History of Medicine,
University of British Columbia, Vancouver,
British Columbia, Canada*

1

THE BEGINNINGS—FOLK MEDICINE OF THE CANADIAN INDIAN AND ESKIMO

Medicine in Canada had its origins in the medicine of its two aboriginal groups, the indian (44, 49, 60, 76, 91, 92) and the eskimo (2, 43, 49, 53, 60, 99). The name "indian" is a misnomer which can be traced back to Columbus, who, in 1493, thinking he had reached the Indies when he "discovered" America, named the aborigines he contacted "Indios," meaning inhabitants of India. "Eskimo" probably comes from indian names meaning "eaters of raw flesh" (Abenaki *eskimantsic*, Ojibwa *ashkimeq*). The eskimos call themselves *inuk* or *inyuit*—the people. Both of these groups had, within their cultures, systems of healing based on magic, superstition, religion, suggestion, and deception in addition to physical treatments, surgery, and a *materia medica* of sorts.

There are, as in the magical-religious-medical beliefs and practices of all primitive cultures, common threads between the indian and the eskimo, but with a few differences primarily in quantity rather than quality and in practice rather than belief. Our sources of information about traditional Canadian aboriginal medicine are from tribal myths and legends passed down by word of mouth, from the anecdotes and writings of early explorers, traders, missionaries, and settlers, and from the recent work of anthropologists and others (33). Indian medicine, in general, has been touched upon in Chamberlain (20), Ciba (23), Clements (24), Corlett (26), Coury (27), Eliade (31), Harris (33), Hrdlicka (38), Jenness (49), Konig (53), Maddox (67), Rogers (79), Stone (87), Swanton (89), Vogel (98), Whitbread (100), and eskimo in Ackerknecht (2), Balikci (3), Boag (7), Boas (8, 12), Jenness (43), Radin (75), Stefansson (85, 86), and Weyer (99).

The Mental Mechanisms and Psychopathology of the Canadian Aborigines

Father François de Peron said of the Hurons, "The nature of the Savage is patient, liberal, hospitable; but importunate, visionary, childish, thieving, lying, deceitful, licentious, proud, lazy; they have among them many fools, or rather lunatics, and insane people" (95).

From what can be pieced together from historical accounts, archaeological and anthropological findings and conversations with presently living indians and eskimos, it seems true that they always had qualitatively the same mental mechanisms and psychopathology as anyone else. They believed in a soul and a life hereafter and in spirits, demons, and animism.

Their instincts of sex and aggression, their emotionality and affectivity are as in all peoples. Differences would appear to be quantitative, not qualitative, depending on the particular environment and culture and the time epoch of evolution along with the time period of acculturation. All the phylogenetic mechanisms were there, but the primitives incorporated more credulity and magical belief, the submersion, recession, and control of which takes place only with time and scientific learning and with the advances of technology.

Shaman and Medicine-Man

"Medicine-man" is perhaps the best general term to describe the individual in primitive cultures whose function is to diagnose and treat disease and injury. The details of his—or her—functions and titles often vary from culture to culture and even within the same culture. His functions would sometimes merge with those of other practitioners, particularly the seer, medium, or priest and sometimes the "chief," since disease was so often connected with supernaturalism, demonology, and infraction of taboo or tribal law.

Anthropologists have utilized the word *shaman* (61, 89) as a generic word to signify or to include medicine-man, particularly of the North American indians. The Siberian Tungu *samân* (excited, moved, raised), from which the word *shaman* is apparently derived, was primarily a spirit-medium who derived supernatural powers during trance and who saw visions and became possessed. He was not a medical doctor, though he may have had a partial function as such. The *samân* was much the same as the Central eskimo *angakok*. The indian medicine-man usually had a much more generalized and more complicated expertise. While he, too, could be a medium and oracle, he relied more on patient or client-centered action, such as the directive psychological methods of suggestion mixed up with deception, and also of physical methods (wound dressings, hydrotherapy, diaphoresis, massage, blowing, sucking), herbal *materia medica,* and of surgery (bleeding, blistering, burning, cauterizing, cutting, setting fractures, sewing up wounds). The Canadian indian medicine-man even employed trepanation of the skull, perhaps for the removal of foreign bodies or spirits, or for the relief of headaches, epilepsy, insanity, and other conditions relating to the head (29, 52, 58, 68). Trepanation is of particular significance, since it might support the contention that primitive man localized the "mind" in the skull and that he might even have thought of it as part of brain function.

One must not oversimplify the classification of magical and ritual practitioners. The medicine-man was only one type of several, as in most cultures. Some of these can be determined in the indian and eskimo. Magic is "good" or "evil," white or black, and all practitioners in all present cultures or reported in history can be divided into two groups:

A. *Practitioners of good intent ("white" magicians)*

1. Medicine-men or healers or folk doctors (an archaic term for healer still used sometimes is "leech"):

(a) Surgeons (who use cutting procedures, and would include midwives, obstetricians, genital operators—circumcisers, excisers, and infibulators—bone-setters, trepanners, tribal-mark scarifiers).

(b) Physicians (who do not ordinarily use cutting procedures and include herbalists, exorcisers, psychologists, hypnotists, religious healers, undertakers, midwives.)

2. Other magicians:

Diviners, seers, soothsayers, mystics, mediums, priests, prophets, oracles, dance masters, conjurors, finders or "smellers-out" of evil magicians, rainmakers and other weather-controllers, blacksmiths, garden, fishing and hunt magicians, amulet makers.

B. *Practitioners of evil intent ("black" magicians)*

1. Witches and wizards or sorcerers (casters of spells, charmers, necromancers, etc.).
2. Zoanthropists (vampires, werewolves, etc.).
3. Ghouls (human living or spirit devourers of corpses).

There is, of course, considerable overlap between "good" and "evil" intent ("white" and "black" magic) and good and evil practitioners, but this division has much to commend it because it indicates *motive*. The indian and eskimo medicine men were usually "white" magicians. They were highly respected, sometimes feared, because of their powers, and their services commanded high fees.

It has been proposed that the medicine-man might be mentally sick or deficient (31, 51). Many no doubt were, and the closer they were to being spirit mediums, the more likely it is that they were unbalanced. The average indian or eskimo medicine-man was probably not mentally ill. It is true, however, that in many cultures, including the indian and eskimo, the medicine-man might go through a *maladie-initiation* or *maladie-vocation* (31) of pseudosickness, vision, etc., but this was temporary and may have been culture-determined, not illness-determined. Both the indians and eskimos, by isolation, fasting, and so on, sought "purification" in order to experience visions and commune with spirits, in what is termed a spirit, vision, or dream quest (46). There is no support for the claim that alcohol was used to hasten a dream quest. Indians drink to get drunk, not to seek visions. They sometimes spent several years seeking such a "call"—for instance, Old Pierre during four years sought his enlightenment and finally obtained the "power" at the age of 14 years (48). It is true, however, that mentally or physically sick people and psychopathic personalities, cunning and good at deception, could also become medicine men.

Detailed topical studies of indian and eskimo medicine are many, and available in the anthropological reports of the National Museum of Canada and of the provincial museums (e.g., Barbeau (5), Duff (30), Jenness (41, 42, 45, 46, 47, 48, 49), Leechman (59), Ravenhill (76), etc.) and, of course, in other media (e.g., Beardsley (6), Boas (9, 10, 11, 14, 15, 16, 17), Darby (29), Gunn (32), Harrison (34), Hodge (36),

Hoffman (37), Jilek (51), Mac Dermot (63), Macdonald (66), Miles (70), Parker (72, 73), Riddell (77), Saindon (81), Sapir (83), Strath (88), Van Wart (97), Whitbread (100), etc.). There is a huge and scattered literature, much of it second-hand and not well documented or interpreted.

The mixture of magic and materialism and of magician, "priest" and physician, as in most primitive races throughout history and today, was apparent in both groups. The culture of the indian was a good deal more complicated than that of the eskimo. The indian had an animistic and highly complicated mythology with levels of spirits. The eskimo had a simpler "religion" with fewer protective spirits. He did, however, have a demonology and invoked ghosts of the dead. The eskimo did not usually adhere to a hierarchy of gods. They did believe in the old woman who lived under the sea—their life centered on the sea for food, and usually the earth was covered with snow or ice, or at least was frozen hard, so it is reasonable that the eskimo "great mother" lived in the sea instead of on the land, cf. "earth" mother in most other cultures. Both the indian and the eskimo had a high degree of material technology, but the indian applied it much more to healing than did the eskimo.

Psychiatric Illnesses in Canadian Aborigines

All indian and eskimo tribes have equivalent or descriptive names for discrete mental illnesses such as "madness," "confusion," "epilepsy," etc., and they have crude nomenclatures. The native syndromes have not been adequately investigated by Canadian psychiatrists; much of the information we have is anecdotal and sensational, often second-hand, inaccurate, incomplete, and reported not by doctors but by others who had limited understanding of mental medicine. Early written descriptions of madness in the Eastern indians may be found in the Jesuit relations (95).

The indians would very frequently kill their insane, particularly if they feared they were dangerous. Hudson's Bay Company agents have left records. William Falconer in 1774 from Severn House, Hudson Bay, reported with much sympathy,

> *(29 September)* . . . The poor man deprived of reason was inhumanly murther'd last night by those Indians that came from Beaver river, one of whom is the deceased's wife's brother, who, (after they had attempted to strangle him) bruised his scull in a shocking manner with a Hatchet. I enquired why they had put him to death as there was no danger from him when fast in irons? To which they answered he was so furious in the night they were

afraid he would have broke the irons, and entreated us to continue them on, otherwise he would get out of his Grave and come
back and kill them, and frighten trading natives from coming
to the place. Their Superstition leads them so far as to imagine
People deprived of reason stalk about after death, and prey
upon human flesh; such they say are Witiko's (i.e.) Divils. In the
month of February an. 1772 the above unhappy man was so
distress'd for food that he kill'd his own Sister and her child. . . .
(H.B.C. Arch.B. 198/a/19).

Joseph Colen, of York Fort, Hayes River, Hudson Bay, in 1798 wrote
also with considerable human feeling,

> *(26 April)* . . . Four set up with the manic last night—and ap-
> pointed two to attend him during the day; but as he appeared
> much better this morning after being bled—he was allow (ed)
> the liberty to walk about the Inner yard—but he found means
> to elude the care of his attendants and run off up the River. One
> of the Men caught by the outer garment which he soon threw off
> and left the House with only a shirt—a pair of Indian Stockings
> and Shoes.—Dispatched three Men in pursuit of him.—His flight
> so much alarmed the Natives at the Goose Tent one and all came
> to the factory.—Its astonishing the Dread they have of being near a
> person Insane—even the Idea of having a madman on the Coast—
> will alarm all the Natives for many Miles—and the very name
> of one being within several days Journey from their Hunting
> Ground will occasion that quarter to be deserted for some years—
> and my fear is that our Goose Hunt will suffer in consequence of
> this Man's escape—about Midnight the men sent after the poor
> man returned. . . .

John Jewitt, a prisoner of the Nootka Indians in 1803, taken prisoner from the trading ship *Boston,* described madness in Tootoosch,
the brother-in-law of Chief Maquina. Tootoosch was violent and was
persecuted by the ghosts of two men he had killed during the massacre
of Jewitt's shipmates. He was treated, at Jewitt's suggestion, by whip-
ping, but the punishment was terminated by the sympathetic Maquina and Tootoosch remained mad (50).

The Algonquian-speaking indians of northeastern Canada (Ojibwa,
Cree) believe in a giant monster, the *windigo* (variously spelled),
who has a heart or skeleton of ice and who feeds on human flesh (18,
25, 35, 72, 80, 94). A person of this tribal background, if he becomes
mentally ill, may believe he is possessed by the *windigo* and develop
cannibalistic tendencies. This "*windigo* psychosis" is in fact a culturally determined delusional symptom complex which might be classified as a schizophrenic, depressive, or other delusional psychosis.

Both the indian and the eskimo on occasion are said to suffer from "thanatophobia" (fear of death) which is an archaic European diagnostic term, but still occasionally employed to denote psychogenic death or death by suggestion—the fixed belief, in the absence of apparent physical illness, that one is going to die.

The most confused syndrome is the eskimo "arctic hysteria" or *piblokto* (various spellings*). Admiral Peary described *piblokto* during his arctic explorations (74), and his wife, Josephine, reported a case as early as 1893. This condition has been reviewed by many (73). *Piblokto* would appear to be a non-psychotic, short-lived mental disorder with a varied symptomatology including tremors, fits, emotional outbursts and histrionic acting-out.

Alcohol and drugs are today a considerable problem in the Canadian indian group and to a lesser extent in the eskimo. It has been said many times that alcoholic beverages did not exist before the white man introduced them, but this is based on very few occasional and anecdotal reports of the early explorers. Grains and berries were included in the staple diets of the aborigines of Canada. It is, in fact, known that the Hurons drank a repulsive concoction made from fermenting corn, and the Western eskimos had wines made from berries. They did not know about distillation, and it was not until brandy was introduced to them by the French traders and whisky by the English that intoxication became a problem for the indians as it has now become also for the eskimos.

Primitive Ideas about Causation of Disease

There are insufficient facts collected about the ideas of the Canadian aborigines concerning the causes of disease (10-17, 24, 26, 90, 93, 96, 98, 99). Occasionally, hereditary or natural etiology was inferred for certain illnesses. Except for trauma, this was the exception rather than the rule. In almost all cases, supernatural causes were presumed. Disease was related to the infraction of a taboo, to witchcraft malevolence, to possession, or intervention by harmful demons or spirits, or to soul-loss. The evil eye mechanism, based on referential and paranoid thinking, was rarely reported. Witchcraft manifested itself usually in the form of what is sometimes called "object intrusion." This is the "throwing" or "sending" of material substances into the body of the patient—perhaps a bird's beak, a hair, a stone,

---

* According to a personal communication (unpublished, 1957) from Vilhjalmur Stefansson, a more accurate spelling would be *pi-luktok,* which means "something wrong with him/her/it." According to Stefansson's account, the condition might better be called *isumaluktok* (*isuma,* the mind; *luktok,* spoiled, worn out, evil) .

an arrowhead, some dirty liquid, a worm, snake, or small animal, etc. "Spirit intrusion" is a related mechanism, a spirit or demon getting into the body and perhaps even "possessing" it. In the British Columbian indians particularly, illness was most commonly attributed to "soul loss." There were many different concepts of soul, from immaterial vapors to birds which would fly away, to tiny man-forms which could wander from a person, or be blown out during sneezing. They would often go to some faraway, mythological place, which only a shaman of all mortals could reach.

The Activities of the Medicine Man

Nicolas Denys, a French pioneer of Acadia, in 1672 wrote of the indians:

> If they were ill and dying of old age, or by some accident happening through trees or other object falling upon them, or where there was no apparent cause, there were old men who claimed to speak to the *manitou,* that is to say, the Devil, who came to whisper to them. These fellows put many superstitions into the mind, of which I have mentioned several in the foregoing. They were men who had some cunning more than the others, and made them believe all they wished, and passed for their physicians. These fellows came there to see the sick man, and asked of him where his ill was. After being well informed in all, they promised health, by blowing on him. For this purpose they set themselves a dancing, and speaking to their *manitou.* They danced with such fury that they emitted foam as big as the fists on both sides of the mouth. During this performance they approached the patient from time to time, and at the place where he had declared he felt the most pain, they placed the mouth upon it, and blew there with all their might for some time, and then commenced again to dance. Following this, they returned again to the sick man to do just the same as before. Then they said it was the *manitou* which had possession of him, and that he (the sick man) had passed through several places where he had not rendered the accustomed homage, or some other similar follies. And (they said) that in time they hoped to make him get out. This lasted sometimes seven to eight days, and finally they made a pretence of drawing something from his body by dexterously showing it, saying—"There, there, he has gone out; now he is cured." And often in fact the man got well through imagination. And if the patients did not grow well, they found some other excuse, such as that there were several *manitous,* that they had been unwilling to go out, and that they had too far ignored them. They always made out a good case for themselves. One never omitted to give them something, though not so much as if he had been entirely cured. Those medicine-men were lazy old fellows who would no

longer go hunting, and who received from others everything they needed. If there were any fine robes, or other rarity in a wigwam, that was for Monsieur the Medicine-man. When animals were killed, all the best parts were sent to him. When they had cured three or four persons, they never lacked anything more. This it was not difficult for them to do, since the greatest malady of the Indians proceeded only from their imagination. This being removed from the mind, immediately they became well (29a) .

This early description is probably of sucking (*infra*) rather than "blowing." Other 17th century descriptions of Eastern indian medicine men, by De La Hontan, Hennepin, and Marquette have been cited by Hoffman (37), and by De Dièreville by Riddell (77).

The medicine-man's power and prestige in primitive societies is undisputed, and sometimes their manipulations may be of some curative usefulness. However, natives and naïve outside observers were apt to be uncritical and wax romantic about them. Here is an extract from the 1884 diary of the Rev. Joseph Nicolaye:

Edward Nasmakshitl died after a short illness, which started by a slight headache. Doctor Hamishinathl sucked blood through the lad's ear, who shortly after turned lunatic, and died at the age of 16. A slight rheumatic headache caused Dr. Hamishinathl to bite three big gashes in the boy's head, and to pour boiling oil into the open wounds. The poor lad lost his senses; and as he in his reveries sang now and then a church song, and repeatedly uttered a few words of English, learned in school, the blame of the boy's death was put on the priest's shoulders by saying that too much study was the original cause of this fatal end. Such is the life in the far West (71).

Indian and eskimo ethnomedicine has probably not changed much since the time of Denys, Champlain, and other early explorers and travelers, but we now know a great deal more about it as a result of archaeological, anthropological and medical research.

The Diagnostic Methods of the Medicine-Man

The "diagnostic" methods of the medicine-man are of infinite variety, since his medicine is based largely on magic and the supernatural and he is relatively free to originate any "technique" he wants, without recourse to scientific reasoning. Of course there were sensible methods when based on obvious situations such as trauma, pregnancy, lack of food, disrupted social relations, etc.

There were, then, many different diagnostic techniques depending on the kind of ritual practitioner, whether he be visionary, spirit medium, herbalist, or surgeon. Whatever the practitioner was depended largely on his spiritual endowment, reasoning intelligence, honesty, integrity, manual skills, and also (to a large degree) on what was expected of him by the people within his culture. Frequently, all these criteria were combined in a free-enterprise system which depended on self-confidence, trial and error, success and failure. Then, as now!

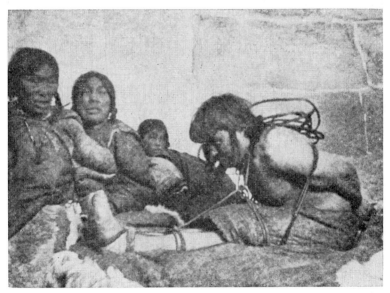

PLATE LXXXVI. Bondage. Aivilirmiut eskimo *angakok* tied up, to aid dissociation during seance and to impress by escape.

At the extreme end of the spectrum stands the visionary and spirit-medium, who would, by psychic detachment aided by rhythmic movement, sound, sensory isolation, immobilization, etc., go into a state of dissociation which could be manifested as violent activity, ecstacy, convulsive movement, or automatic behavior. He might obtain a vision and commune with spirits or a deity. To assist in experiencing a vision or otherwise dissociating himself, a medicine man would often aid the process by rhythmic movement and sensory perception, e.g., by dancing and swaying and by drumming, rattling and singing. He also could aid dissociation by bondage and immobilization (eskimo) and by blocking out visual sensation by closing the eyes tightly or by putting a basket over his head (Salish, Stalo (30)) (Plates LXXXVI

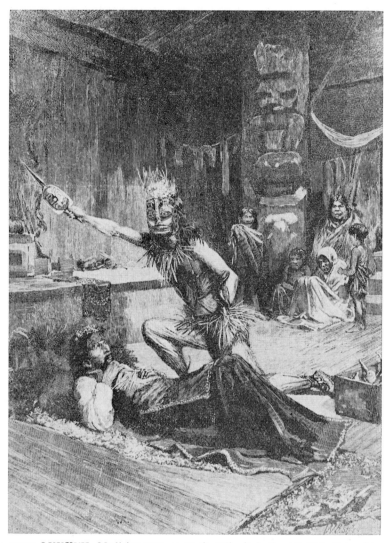

PLATE LXXXVII. Medicine-man at work. Tlingit indian, British Columbia. Note mask, rattle in right hand, rattle (?) also in box, boughs, dressing (?) on patient's head; carved house-post behind onlookers. Old illustration, source unknown, signed W. B. Styles.

and LXXXVII). He might locate the illness—the immaterial lost soul or intruded spirit or demon and the material intruded foreign body by palpating for it in the patient or by listening here and there.

Treatment Methods of the Medicine-Man

A classification of primitive treatment methods employed by Canadian aborigines would be under the headings of magical, psychological, physical, herbal, and surgical. All methods were in fact usually incorporated into healing procedures.

To treat the sick, the medicine man can employ one or all of the three methods of classical magic (oral rites, manual rites, and accessory observances). By oral rites is meant psychological activity based primarily on language (incantation, suggestion). By manual rites is meant activity in which there is bodily contact or the use of intermediary apparatus. By accessory observances is meant ritual which takes account of time of day, place, taboos, manner of preparation for and conclusion of the magical act, etc.

Magical oral rites merge with the psychological, which can in fact be considered as a more rational extension of magical. Magical activity included the trance, dream, and other dissociation states in which the practitioner would seek spirits and commune with them or see hidden things and recover souls lost in the supernatural worlds. He might be possessed and speak as an oracle; he might talk gibberish as we see clinically in the syndrome of *glossolalia* (*xenoglossia*) or "speaking in tongues." He could often exorcise subjects who had become possessed of demons by frightening them, cursing them, propitiating them, blowing them away, and so on. Occasionally, in some western tribes, the medicine-man during his ritual might place his twisted cedar rope collar under the neck of the reclining patient and pull up the head to indicate spirit intervention or raise the patient out of illness (Plate LXXXVIII). Boas in 1888 reported "head lifting" in the Central eskimo (8). The *angakok's* spirit was questioned; if the spirit's answer was yes, the head was easily lifted; if no, the head was heavy and immovable.

Much of the medicine of the indian and eskimo depends on the recovery of a lost soul. The psychology of the belief in a soul—or souls—is varied; Crawley (28) summarized some of the literature to 1909 (see also Hultkrantz (39)). After locating the soul in a dream, in a trance, or by palpating the patient, the medicine-man might have used his cupped hands (Kwakiutl (15); Stalo Salish (30)), or a hollow bone or wood tube (Haida, 9, 34); Ojibwa (37)) in which

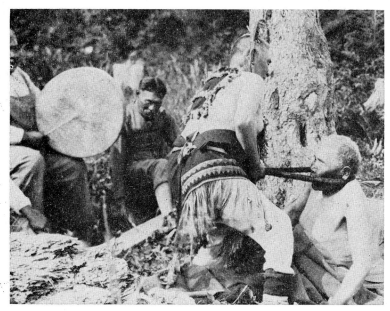

PLATE LXXXVIII. Head lifting. West coast indian medicine-man pulling up patient with plaited cedar rope.

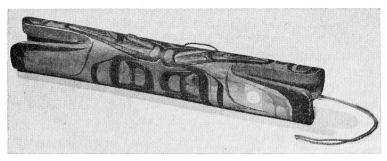

PLATE LXXXIX. "Soul catcher." West coast indian soul trap; carved head at each end of cedarwood tube.

to capture the soul. In the latter case sometimes the ends of the tube were plugged up so the soul, once trapped, could not escape. Occasionally, a stopper-like cork was inserted into a hole cut through to the lumen of the tube. Soul capture could be for good purposes as in medicine, or for evil purposes as in witchcraft. The soul after capture was then returned to the owner or was retained prisoner by the magician. The Tlingit, Haida, and Tsimshian "soul catchers" were sometimes carved with various designs (34) (Plate LXXXIX). One type of tube, usually of hollow bone such as femur, had a carved animal head with open jaws at each end, the lumen of the tube being the mouth. The double head is usually identified as a two-headed snake, serpent, or dragon. It may appear more like a double-headed wolf, as stated by Darby (29). Rarely, the soul catcher may be in the form of a killer whale. A face or entire crouched human form was usually carved on the convex surface between the two animal heads. Occasionally, the human figure was carved in the round on top of the tube, and the head might be movable. One wonders if this human figure might have represented the soul, or perhaps the shaman seeking it. We know little in fact about these curious soul traps. Sometimes the tube was hung around the neck of the medicine man and acted as a talisman, the symbol of his power. It should not be confused with the tube sometimes used in blowing away illness or sucking it out. The Salish magician might form a symbolic canoe from boards stuck in the ground and in drama paddle to the land of the dead seeking a lost soul. To aid in capturing lost souls, the Western indian frequently had a "spirit-helper" or "guardian-spirit," somewhat comparable to the "familiar," or "imp" or "familiar spirit" of the European witch. The "spirit-helper" was generally inhuman, i.e. an animal, bird, or fish.

Apart from the stories passed on by word of mouth, and by the writings of explorers and anthropologists, indian and eskimo mythology and legend have come to us through "art," from pictographs and petroglyphs to "long houses." Most indian and eskimo "art" is "folk" art, of anthropological interest; some of it is fine art in the usual sense, and much of the rest of it may be pleasing and skillfully executed from the technical aspect. There is a considerable literature and beautifully illustrated books on the artwork of Canada's aborigines, particularly of the West coast indian. Northwest indian art is highly symbolic and of stylized design. The most striking traditional art comes to us from the great carved cedar totem poles, house-posts and beams, and graveyard monuments (4, 49). The art of the West coast is of particular interest to medicine in that the wood and argillite carvings sometimes depict the medicine-man and the occasional medicine woman (5). The indicators of this calling seen in the carvings of the Haida might include: dance apron, rattle, drum or tambourine, wand, twisted cedar bark collar, magic crystal or other talisman, hair tied up in top-knot, spike through the nasal septum, and spirit helper.

There were all kinds of deceptive tricks employed by the medicine men, both indian and eskimo. Illness, evil spirits, and demons could be blown away, brushed away, massaged out, washed away in a stream, transferred to an animal, or burned. Objects believed to have been projected into a person were removed by faking. The medicine man would pretend to suck out such foreign bodies as stones, splinters worms, arrowheads, etc. Blood sucked out was from the medicine man's own mouth; the objects were previously hidden in the mouth or palmed there during the procedure. By conjuring tricks, bodies were opened up, fictitious wounds closed, and the dead were revived.

Magical images were sometimes employed in various ways during healing rituals. These would act as intermediaries between patient, spirits and magician. "Marionette" or puppet type images with movable parts were used in ritual and magical procedures and sometimes even ventriloquism would be employed to help animate them (Plate XC).

Amulets of various kinds to protect against misfortune or illness were used, some of these beautifully carved wood or bone, others plain stones and odd bits and pieces of material. Talismans to impart magical power were a significant accoutrement of the medicine man; they "enabled" the practitioner to receive inspiration and to find lost souls. In the Western indian, the "magic crystal" of the Haida and neighboring tribes was such a talisman. The spike through the nasal septum was also a shaman's talisman.

True psychological methods included, of course, suggestion, though this is also largely magical. Explanation, persuasion, and command no doubt were occasionally helpful. Frightening the patient or the disease or demon was as often as not as magical as it was psychological. Many writers have claimed that hypnosis as we understand it is or was much used by traditional healers. This, in fact, is not so, though hypnosis could occasionally result, usually by chance. The error would seem to come from two sources: the credulous need to believe in it and ignorance, i.e. the confusion of hypnosis, which is a technique, with hysterical trance, which is a condition, a syndrome. The latter, though it sometimes can be induced by hypnosis, is quite a different phenomenon.

Monotonous singing, drumming, whistling, or rattling and dancing by the medicine man and suppliants were and are common in the indian and eskimo. Participants would be relieved of possession or would "get the spirit" (become one with the spirit); this was observed as abreactive hysterics—trance, convulsion, shouting, automatism, etc. Jenness (44) reported this procedure by drumming and whistling in a

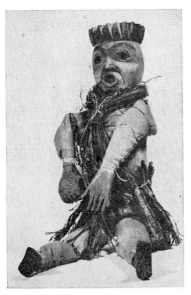

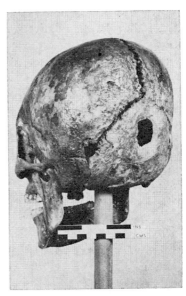

PLATE XC. Medicine-man's puppet. Kwakiutl tribe, British Columbia; used as intermediary ritual appliance between shaman and patient.

PLATE XCI. Trepanned skull. Occipital trepanation in indian skull from Eburne kitchen midden shell mound, Marpole, copper burial, presumably Salish, dated prior to about 1450 A.D.

Carrier indian afflicted by the "dreaded mountain spirit." Dream interpretation by magic inference was commonly practiced by indian and eskimo magicians.

Confession as a psychological "treatment" is no doubt sometimes useful in cultures which have developed a conception of good and evil and of conscience and sin. It is said to have been encouraged by the eskimo and by the Déné (61).

Physical methods of treatment were employed considerably. The "sweat houses" indicated a belief in the efficacy of raising the temperature and of causing diaphoresis. Bathing of various kinds in sea and rivers was a common form of hydrotherapy and of purification, sometimes accompanied by flagellation with branches. Manipulation and massage were somewhat developed. Enemas were used in some tribes. Pressure bands were used for headaches, and could have been physiologically useful if the headache happened to be the right kind. There is little written on the indian and eskimo physical treatment of the insane—isolation, restraint, and beating no doubt were employed. If too troublesome the mentally deranged might be killed.

The indian had a relatively limited *materia medica*. While he included a considerable number of herbs (roots, leaves, bark, seeds, flowers), most of them were non-specific or had magical significance only, i.e. the shape, smell, or color was of importance, not the pharmacological action. There were exceptions, e.g. emetics (sea-water was naturally the most common one utilized by the coast-dwellers), cathartics, haemeostatics (charcoal and ashes are the simplest examples), a few poisons, astringents, soothing balms, mild sedatives, and pain-killers. Animal and mineral remedies were less employed and even less specific than the herbs. The eskimo had little in the way of herb lore, since there was little vegetation in the Arctic land. He did not practice much "surgery." His effectiveness was largely "psychotherapeutic" —by suggestion, command, confession, recapturing lost souls, and so on.

Surgical procedures included trepanation of the skull, which was practiced by the West coast indians (Plate XCI). It was known within human memory at the time Kidd wrote his article (1946), but so far as we know it is no longer practiced. The motives for it were unclear, but we infer that the operation might have been used for insanity, epilepsy, headache, spirit intrusion, and the like. Excellent specimens of trepanned skulls have been collected from British Columbia (52, 58, 68).

2

FROM EARLY HOSPITALS, PATIENTS, AND SETTLER DOCTORS TO "PROVINCIAL ASYLUMS"

There are very few references to mental illness by the early settlers. Those who became unmanageably insane were usually guarded in jails. If they did not recover, they were often sent back to France or to England. In the Jesuit relations of 1660, the case was mentioned of one Barbe Halé of Beauport, who had been "possessed with a

Demon of Lunacy for five or six months" (95). Considering the risks
from indians and the terrible death-dealing epidemics of the time
(smallpox, influenza, dysenteries, plague, cholera, typhus, yellow
fever, etc.) and the ravages of scurvy, pneumonia, and tuberculosis,
it is not surprising that mental illness and hysterics were not considered priorities. For a decade or two, from 1773, there was an unpleasant epidemic *mal de la baie St. Paul,* which is usually considered
to have been syphilis. The local people had to blame the contagion
on somebody, so they blamed it on a Scotsman and called it for a
while the *mal écossais.* Others blamed it on the indians (1, 21, 22).
Dr. Phillippe Louis Badelart, surgeon-major of the French army, was
commissioned by the British government to investigate the disease.
In 1785 his report, *Direction pour la guérison du mal de la Baie
St. Paul,* was distributed to all parishes of Canada. It was said to
be "the first known Canadian medical publication" (1). The Hudson's Bay Company had its own doctors. Dr. Giles Wills at Port Albany
on James Bay in 1730 had compiled a drug list which included *pulvis
ad guttetam* ("epileptic powder"), an anticonvulsant composed of
pulverized wild valerian and peony roots (40). Dr. William Smellie
at York Factory in 1847 left good notes on one Frederick Frost, a clerk
who had become insane (H.B.C. Arch B239/a/166). There are other
references to insanity in the H.B.C. Archives.

The early settlers and later immigrants (German, Russian, Japanese,
Chinese, Czechs, "American" Negroes, and others) all had their own
cultures and their own superstitions and folklore. There is a relatively
limited literature on this subject, but as an example, for review of
folklore, magic, demonology, and witchcraft in the early French
Canada, see Séguin (84).

3

THE EARLY HOSPITALS

L'Hôtel Dieu, Quebec City

It was not long before the settlers recognized the need for hospitals.
The first institution which can be called a hospital was l'Hôtel Dieu
in Quebec (Plate XCII), founded by the charity of Madame de Com-
balet, la Duchesse d'Aiguillon, née Marie-Madeleine Wignerod de
Pontcourlay, the niece of Cardinal Richelieu. The hospital was to be
staffed by les Augustines Hospitalières de Dieppe, who arrived at
Quebec in 1639. The foundations were started in 1638, but work was

discontinued in 1640. The Hospitalières had been lodged in a house which temporarily served as their hospital, but in 1640 they moved to Sillery, about four miles away. There, another house was placed at their disposal and functioned as a hospital. However, since it was dangerous in Sillery because of attacks by the Iroquois, in 1644 they moved back to Quebec and were accommodated temporarily, until the building started in 1638 was completed, in 1644. The original direction of the hospital was to treat indigents, crippled, and idiots.

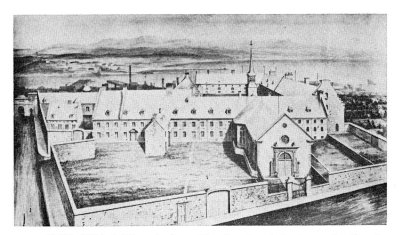

PLATE XCII. L'Hôtel Dieu, Québec. The first hospital of note in Canada, started in 1638. A general hospital which also received the insane. This picture is dated 1877.

It may be inferred that the latter included the insane. Actually, the hospital was a general one, and cared for indian and settler alike, taking in all cases, including smallpox and other infections and serious illnesses. The first attending physician was Robert Giffard, Seigneur de Beauport. This hospital was burned twice, and most of the old archives are lost. The Hôtel Dieu had four locations prior to the temporary quarters necessitated by fire, but it still stands and functions on the original 1638 site in the modern city of Quebec (57). It may be noted here for interest that the first hospital in continental North America was established not by the French in Canada but apparently by the Spanish in Mexico City. This was *Nuestra Señora de la Concepción,* or *Jesús Nazareno,* opened in 1524, and still in use; a charming place with a central courtyard.

L'Hôpital Général, Quebec City

The next hospital of particular interest to psychiatry is l'Hôpital Général de Québec (Plate XCIII) close by l'Hôtel Dieu, which also has been in continuous operation since its foundation. The Recollet monastery, built in 1621 and transferred to Monseigneur de Saint Vallier, the Bishop of Quebec, in 1692, was opened as a hospital in

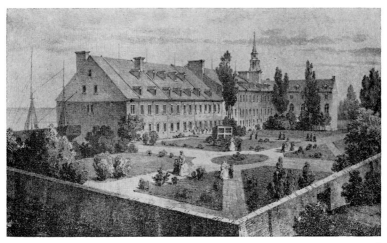

PLATE XCIII. L'Hôpital Général, Québec. Old Recollet monastery, opened as hospital in 1693. In 1717, the "loges" (not shown; on the other side behind the steeple) housed insane women; a "separate but adjacent" unit of a general hospital. St. Charles river, ship, to left.

1693. In 1717, Saint Vallier added a small house containing six cells on the grounds for the housing of insane women. In 1723, another six-cell house was erected for insane men (69, 82). Thus, the first special accommodation for the insane in Canada was really a "separate but adjacent" part of a general hospital. The facility was no doubt crude, unsanitary, and inadequate, but probably little worse than other institutions of the time. The house adjacent to the east facade of the hospital across the brook, named *"loges"* in the plan by Mlle. St. Ours in 1785 and the *"maisons de force"* in the annals of the day, would be the location of the cells where the insane were confined. These loges, and additions, were demolished after the insane were moved to Beauport Asylum in 1845. At that time there were the original six cells plus 18 built later at public (government) expense.

It must be pointed out that the first hospital in continental North America devoted to the care of the insane was not the Hôpital Général de Québec, as is sometimes stated, but apparently the Hospital de San Hipólito in Mexico City, established in 1566. This ancient hospital operated for 344 years, until 1910, when patients were transferred to a new state mental institution. The San Hipólito building, near the church of the same name, was still in use as domestic housing in 1961 when visited and probably is still standing—one would hope that it will be preserved as a national monument.

The Grey Nunnery, Montreal

In 1694 there was opened an institution called l'Hôpital Général de Ville-Marie in Montreal, but it did not flourish. In 1747 it was handed over to the Seminary of St. Sulpice and under Madame Youville's order, the Grey Nuns (*Soeurs Grises*), or Sisters of Charity, it flourished as the "Grey Nunnery," caring for the sick, aged, incurable, orphaned and insane. The order erected special accommodation for the insane, which remained in use until 1831. This was perhaps the first "hospital" for the insane in Montreal. The facility was destroyed by fire in 1765. A new structure was built and occupied in 1871 on the site of the present "Grey Nunnery."

In the Richardson report of 1824 it is mentioned that there were 24 cells for the care of the insane in l'Hôpital Général de Québec, six in the Ursuline Nunnery at Three Rivers, and eight in the Grey Nunnery at Montreal (19).

Lunatic Asylum, St. John, New Brunswick

Later on in Canada, as the population increased, the general hospitals were unable to cope with the insane, and special facilities apart from residences, general hospitals, and jails became necessary. This led to the building of the government insane asylums housing only the insane and retarded. Apparently the first one in Canada was in the province of New Brunswick, not in Quebec as would have been expected. A small building in St. John, which had been erected as an isolation hospital in 1832, was converted and opened as a lunatic asylum in 1835 (Plate XCIV). George Matthew, overseer of the poor, was placed in charge, and George P. Peters was named the visiting doctor. This hospital continued to function under difficult circumstances, with the usual government lack of understanding, inertia, and inadequate funding, until it was abandoned in 1848, when the 90 patients residing there were transferred to a new Provincial Lunatic Asylum on the

west bank of the St. John River, with Peters as medical superintendent. He remained in charge of it for about a year until 1849 when
John Waddell succeeded him. Waddell remained until 1875, when
James T. Steeves took over; then came George A. Hetherington from
1896-1903 and James V. Anglin from 1904.

Thus was launched the age of "provincial asylums." Most of these
were government institutions, the primary exceptions being those in
Quebec, which were run by religious orders or private enterprise with

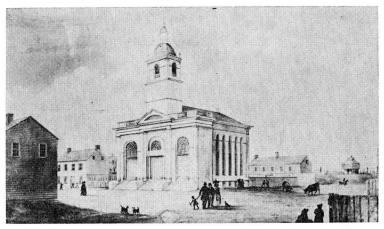

PLATE XCIV. Lunatic Asylum, St. John, New Brunswick. Main building is
the Centenary Church; building to the right of it with smoking chimney,
behind the cows, is Canada's first government or "provincial" asylum for the
insane, 1835.

or without government assistance. From 1850 to 1950, most of the
psychiatry in Canada was centered on custodial care and in-patient
treatment within the mental hospitals.*

With the advent of electrotherapy from 1938 and of chlorpromazine
and other psychopharmaceuticals from 1952, and a more enlightened
society, psychiatry in Canada, as elsewhere, has emerged as a major
specialty of general medicine and drawn somewhat away from special

---

* The history of the later government mental hospitals and the private hospitals
for the insane should be described in some detail but this article is limited in length
and it is impossible to offer here the complete story. The interested reader may
refer to the monumental reference edited by Hurd (39 a), written in 1916-17, where
much of the mental hospital history of Canada to that date was documented, largely
by Dr. Thomas Joseph Workman Burgess (1849-1926) of the Verdun asylum in
Montreal.

"mental hospitals." Treatment of many patients has become possible in places less restrictive for the patient, such as general hospitals, outpatient clinics, the private psychiatrist's office and the home.

4

LATER TIMES

Medicine in Canada, as elsewhere in the world, began with folk medicine, first practiced in the community and then in the "general hospitals." Most of the mentally ill were perhaps treated in general hospitals and, in the old days, many died there. If they were too troublesome, noisy, or violent, they may have been shifted to jails. One must always keep in mind the difficulties doctors often have in controlling psychotic patients, even with good facilities and treatment methods. In the days before modern physical and psychotropic drug therapies, keeping patients clean, safe, quiet, and comfortable and separating them from an intolerant society must have been a trying task.

When the numbers of lunatics became so great that they overflowed the ordinary hospitals and jails, thinking and planning men, both medical and lay, soon realized that additional, and government-financed, facilities would be required. And so they planned special mental asylums, as existed in Europe. There was, as now, much difficulty in convincing government of the need for additional facilities, even when the need was obvious and sometimes acute. The care of the insane has always been of low priority, primarily because madness rarely kills and because of ignorance, denial, and political expediency. At any rate, New Brunswick led the way in setting up special hospitals. The rest of Canada followed within several decades. The need was no doubt greatest in the east of Canada, where the population was concentrated.

In the sparsely populated far north, hospitals were not provided; there are none there even now which can provide special care for the insane. The first North West Mounted Police Surgeon, Major George Kittson, in a report from Fort Walsh in the North West Territories, wrote in 1880:

> I would respectfully call your attention to that questionable guardroom at Fort Walsh which serves the triple purpose of guardroom, jail and lunatic asylum. The whole structure measures about 16 x 12 on the inside. Half of the space is taken up by three cells, in which I have seen as many as five and six prisoners

incarcerated, and the other half is usually occupied by a guard of four to six men. . . . Within the last two years we have had the care of two lunatics. The first one was an old squaw, somewhat inclined to cannibalism; she was completely maniacal and very difficult to manage. Her filthy habits infected the guard-room to such an extent that she had to be removed to a small building by herself. Under kind treatment and good food she completely recovered her mind. The second was a young half-breed, who was said to endanger the lives of his young nephews. He was found perfectly harmless and obedient, and was released last summer (78).

The federal general hospitals, which were military during wartime, were given over primarily to the care of veterans and to several other groups in peace time, those who were the responsibility of the central government—armed service personnel, R.C.M.P., mariners, etc. These hospitals in general have given first-class clinical and rehabilitative care and in addition many of them have been excellent teaching centers for medical students, nurses and orderlies. One of the notable advantages of these institutions has been the detailed clinical and social case records which may in individual cases go back more than 75 years.

A mental health service does not consist only of government facilities and service. In the most comprehensive and practical viewpoint, it includes also non-government facilities and free-enterprise clinical practice. Government's main responsibility is to provide money for the provision and maintenance of the service. A mental health service is an intricate, organized system of prevention, treatment, rehabilitation, and support set up to maintain the best possible mental health of the population. Such a system would include sub-systems or processes involved in a complicated network involving education, clinical practice, and facilities and research, allowing free and easy flow of information, aid, and patient and personnel movement between all these activities. The sub-systems consist of contact (case finding), ingress, diagnosis, distribution, psychological, biological, and social treatment, egress, administration, maintenance, and support (personnel, hospital and out-patient facilities, and funding), internal development (improvement), teaching and research, including evaluation and operational research.

After the pioneering days, and after the development of modern scientific medicine, not all general hospitals were disposed to care for the mentally ill on their wards. The famous teaching hospital, the Montreal General, was not very sympathetic, and could not "get rid of" the insane (to the asylums) quick enough in the old days. "The German is deranged and could not be kept in the ward with the other patients" (1825) (62). The hospitals had their troubles in those times. There were no electrotherapy and no strong psychopharmaceuticals such as we have now. An entry of 1847 read that a seaman admitted with typhus "died by hanging himself to a tree in the garden" (62).

Until recent times, most of our great hospitals had not been partial to the admission of psychiatric patients. The Royal Victoria in Montreal had a Rockefeller grant from 1921 to further psychiatry, but it was not until 1944, with the opening of the Allan Memorial Institute of Psychiatry, that psychiatric in-patients could be adequately cared for at this hospital which had long been a leader in general medicine and surgery.

Since World War II there has been a great deal of thought about the usefulness, size, location, and function of mental hospitals, psychiatry in general hospitals, mental health centers, and "community psychiatry," whatever that is (all mental health and psychiatry services are part of community psychiatry). There is no question that more psychiatric hospital facilities are required, particularly psychiatric beds in general hospitals and mental health clinics and centers, preferably polyclinics where all specialties contribute. Inexpert planning, mixed with politics, bureaucratic control, and lack of interest and sympathy of governments have not helped advance psychiatric services in the country. The medical-political bickering and power-playing is nothing short of unbelievable.

However, psychiatric facilities may not be as wanting as some promotional movements maintain. The main problem would seem to be that services, particularly manpower, are inclined to be concentrated in the cities, leading to patchy coverage. Moreover, there is an imbalance between mental hospital as compared with general hospital and private hospital facilities. Psychiatry can be overdone, and it is not rational that services should be offered to all those who *want* them. Services should be offered to those who *need* them. People should try to learn by themselves to live happily and in mental equilibrium. This is a matter of life adjustment. Adequate services naturally should be available to anyone with incapacitating mental illness, but an emphasis on the improvement of society and education in living and self-reliance would no doubt prevent a lot of minor incapacitation leading to the overburdening of services, including manpower, which is apparent at this time.

There has been much recent criticism of mental hospitals being far removed from the "community," and particularly from friends and relatives of the patients. As a matter of fact, most patients probably do not care how far away from home they are, and most relatives think that the farther away the patient is the better. How far is far? Anyway, for those who throughly believe in "togetherness" it may be mentioned that as early as 1866 the American, Edward Jarvis, wrote on *Influence of distance from and nearness to an insane hospital on its use by the people,* referring to Canada West and Nova Scotia. He had previously written on this subject as early as 1850, but did not mention Canada.

The Mental Health Division of the Department of National Health and Welfare in Ottawa was established in 1945. It functions as a national agency. Treatment services and facilities are the responsibility of the provincial governments. The budget, personnel and accommodation of this Division are far too small for a country like Canada. Much of the Division's work has to do with the arranging and distribution of grants to the provinces for improvement of services, education, and research. The Division also produces *Canada's Mental Health,* which is a helpful, multi-disciplinary promotional and news medium. Without adequate operating money, it is impossible for the Division to obtain adequate staff and expertise to accomplish more active promotional consultation and preventive work and to institute national cultural and international affairs programs relating to service, education, and research.

The government of Canada is imposing medicare throughout the country; each province at the present time may have its own scheme in cooperation with the federal government. There are good and bad aspects to such government control of medicine, and this is not the place to argue pro and con. The province of Saskatchewan was the first to impose socialized medicine, and this caused an unpleasant confrontation between government and medical profession. The history of the Saskatchewan situation has been documented by MacTaggart (65), and further psychiatric references are Lawson (54, 55, 56), and McKerracher (64).

The problems and the faults in Canadian psychiatry lie not so much in the shortage of skilled manpower as in the inadequacies of provincial or government subsidized hospitals and the status gap between university departments and these facilities. The problem is an economic, political, and status problem between these two power structures. Caught between these are the highly skilled and experienced clinicians in private practice. There is good reason to return to the "clinical" with less emphasis on the "academic" structure which is now so much promoted. The university and government positions could be occupied by more brilliant minds than now fill many of them if the jobs offered better income. Many of the very capable physicians take to private practice in order to avoid the bureaucracy and politics and to earn more money.

There are about 1,500 qualified active psychiatrists in Canada, as estimated from recent figures of the Canadian Psychiatric Association and the Royal College of Physicians and Surgeons of Canada. For a small population in a big country with a short history, and inadequate financial support for services, education, and research, Canadian doctors have nevertheless made a remarkable contribution to the advancement of medical and psychiatric services.

According to the statistics presented by the government of Canada, at the end of the year 1971 there were 34,584 men and 27,908 women "on the books" in 274 mental, general, and other hospital units (or on probation) for the treatment of mental illness or mental retardation. These figures are limited in that they do not include the non-hospitalized patients under extramural care. If 1,000 psychiatrists each had 20 patients under treatment, this would mean 20,000 more patients. Counting the population at 22 million, this means one Canadian in about 250 might be in psychiatric treatment at one point in time.

NOTE

In conclusion, the author can only apologize for leaving out so much material available about the history of mental health and psychiatry in Canada. The hospital history was barely touched. There is much to write on the history of different types of facilities and services, on administration, planning, manpower, and surveys. One would like to have included material on teaching and research, on nursing, psychology, the social and cultural milieu, minority groups, social action, philanthropy, extramural care, voluntary and professional organizations, technical journalism, on forensic, child and geriatric psychiatry, on the curiosa of psychiatry, and so on.

All this cannot be covered in an abbreviated book chapter. Time permitting, the author could present it in book form.

It was the editor, who, with the author's agreement, decided to include most of the submitted text which concerned the indian and eskimo since this is unusual material and probably far more "interesting" then much of the rest of it, which unfortunately had to be left out.

REFERENCES

1. ABBOTT, M. E. S. (1931): *History of Medicine in the Province of Quebec*. Montreal: McGill University.
2. ACKERKNECHT, E. H. (1948): The eskimo. *Ciba Symposia*, Vol. 10, No. 1 (four articles).
3. BALIKCI, A. (1970): *The Netsilik Eskimo*. Garden City, New York: The Natural History Press.
4. BARBEAU, M. (1950): *Totem poles*. Bulletin no. 119. Anthropological series no.

30. Department of Resources and Development, Development Services Branch. National Museum of Canada. Ottawa: Cloutier, 2 vols.

5. BARBEAU, M. (1958): *Medicine-men on the north Pacific coast.* Bulletin no. 152. Department of Northern Affairs and National Resources, National Museum of Canada. Ottawa: Cloutier.

6. BEARDSLEY, G. (1941): Notes on Cree medicines, based on a collection made by I. Cowie in 1892. *Papers of the Michigan Academy of Science Arts and Letters*, 27, 483-496.

7. BOAG, T. J. (1970): Mental health of native peoples of the Arctic. *Canadian Psychiat. Ass. J.*, 15 (2), 115-120.

8. BOAS, F. U. (1888): *The central eskimo.* Sixth annual report of the Bureau of Ethnology to the Secretary of the Smithsonian Institution 1884-85. Washington: Government Printing Office.

9. BOAS, F. U. (1890): *First general report on the indians of British Columbia.* Report of the fifty-ninth meeting of the British Association for the Advancement of Science . . . 1889. London: Murray. Pp. 801-900.

10. BOAS, F. U. (1893): The doctrine of souls and of disease among the Chinook indians. *J. Am. Folklore*, 6 (20), 39-43.

11. BOAS, F. U. (1897): *The social organization and the secret societies of the Kwakiutl indians based on personal observations and on notes made by Mr. George Hunt.* Report of the U.S. National Museum, under the direction of the Smithsonian Institution . . . 1895. Washington: Government Printing Office. Pp. 311-738.

12. BOAS, F. U. (1901): I—The eskimo of Baffin Land and Hudson Bay. *Bull. Am. Museum of Natural History*, 15, part I; vi-xviii, 1-370.

13. BOAS, F. U. (1907): II—Second report on the eskimo of Baffin Land and Hudson Bay. *Bull. Am. Museum of Natural History*, 15, part II; 371-570.

14. BOAS, F. U. (1916): *Tsimshian mythology based on texts recorded by Henry W. Tate.* Thirty-first annual report of the Bureau of American Ethnology to the Secretary of the Smithsonian Institution 1909-1910. Washington: Government Printing Office.

15. BOAS, F. U. (1921): *Ethnology of the Kwakiutl based on data collected by George Hunt.* Thirty-fifth annual report of the Bureau of American Ethnology to the Secretary of the Smithsonian Institution 1913-1914. Washington: Government Printing Office. 2 parts.

15a. BOAS, F. U. (1930): The religion of the Kwakiutl indians. *Columbia University contributions to anthropology*, volume X. New York: Columbia University Press. 2 vols.

16. BOAS, F. U. (1938): *The Mind of Primitive Man.* New York: Macmillan.

17. BOAS, F. U. (1966): *Kwakiutl Ethnography.* Codere, H. (Ed.). Chicago: University of Chicago Press.

18. BROWN, J. (1971): The cure and feeding of windigos: a critique. *Am. Anthropologist*, 73 (1), 20-22.

19. BURGESS, T. J. W. (1898): A historical sketch of our Canadian institutions for the insane. *Proc. Transact. Roy. Soc. Canada*, 4 (4), 3-122.

20. CHAMBERLAIN, A. F. (1911): Disease and medicine (American). In: Hastings, J. (Ed.), *Encyclopaedia of Religion and Ethics.* Vol. 4. Edinburgh: Clark. Pp. 731-741.

21. CHARLTON, M. R. (1923): Outlines of the history of medicine in Lower Canada under the French régime, 1608-1759. *Ann. Med. Hist. O. S.*, 5 (2), 150-174; 5 (3), 263-278.

22. CHARLTON, M. R. (1924): Outlines of the history of medicine in Lower Canada under the English régime. *Ann. Med. Hist.*, 6 (2), 222-235; 6 (3), 312-354.

23. Ciba Symposia (1939): Medicine among the American indians. *Ciba Symposia*, Vol. 1, no. 1. (four articles).

24. CLEMENTS, F. E. (1932): Primitive concepts of disease. *University of California Publications in American Ethnology*, 32, 185-252.

25. COOPER, J. M. (1933): The Cree witiko psychosis. *Primitive Man*, 6 (1), 20-24.

26. CORLETT, W. T. (1935): *The Medicine-Man of the American Indian and his Cultural Background*. Springfield: Charles C Thomas.

27. COURY, C. (1969): *La médecine de l'Amérique précolombienne, appendice sur les codices mexicains par M.D. Grmek*. Paris: Dacosta.

28. CRAWLEY, A. E. (1909): *The Idea of the Soul*. London: Black.

29. DARBY, G. E. (1933): Indian medicine in British Columbia. *Canad. Med. Ass. J.*, 28 (4), 433-438.

29a. DENYS, N. (1908): *The Description and Natural History of the Coasts of North America* (Acadia). Translated . . . by W. F. Ganong. Toronto: The Champlain Society.

30. DUFF, W. (1952): *The upper Stalo indians of the Fraser valley, British Columbia*. Anthropology in British Columbia memoir no. 1. Victoria: British Columbia Provincial Museum.

31. ELIADE, M. (1951): *Le Chamanisme et les Techniques Archaïques de l'Extase*. Paris: Payot.

32. GUNN, S. W. A. (1966): Totemic medicine and shamanism among the northwest American indians. *J. Am. Med. Ass.*, 196 (8), front cover, 700-706.

33. HARRIS, W. R. (1915): *Practice of medicine and surgery by the Canadian tribes in Champlain's time*. Annual archaeological report 1915. Toronto: Wilgress. Pp. 35-57.

34. HARRISON, C. (1925): *Ancient Warriors of the North Pacific, the Haidas, their Laws, Customs and Legends with some Historical Account of the Queen Charlotte Islands*. London: Witherby.

35. HAY, T. H. (1971): The windigo psychosis: psychodynamic, cultural, and social factors in aberrant behavior. *Am. Anthropol.*, 73 (1), 1-19.

36. HODGE, F. W. (Ed.) (1906, 1910): *Handbook of American indians north of Mexico*. Smithsonian Institution Bureau of American Ethnology bulletin 30. Washington: Government Printing Office. 2 vols.

37. HOFFMAN, W. J. (1891): *The mide'wiwin or "grand medicine society" of the Ojibwa*. Seventh annual report of the Bureau of Ethnology to the Secretary of the Smithsonian Institution, 1885-86. Washington: Government Printing Office.

38. HRDLICKA, A. (1906): Medicine and medicine-men. In: Hodge, F. W. (Ed.), (1906, 1910). *Handbook of American indians north of Mexico*. Smithsonian Institution Bureau of American Ethnology bulletin 30. Washington: Government Printing Office. Part 1, pp. 836-839.

39. HULTKRANTZ, A. (1953): *Conceptions of the soul among North American indians, a study in religious ethnology*. The Ethnographical Museum of Sweden, Stockholm (Statens Etnografiska Museum). Monograph series, publication no. 1. Stockholm.

39a. HURD, H. M. (Ed.) (1916-1917): *The Institutional Care of the Insane in the United States and Canada*. Baltimore: Johns Hopkins Press. 4 vols.

40. JARCHO, S. (1971): Drugs used at Hudson Bay in 1730. *Bull. N. Y. Acad. Med.*, 47 (7), 838-842.

41. JENNESS, D. (1922): *The life of the copper eskimos*. Report of the Canadian Arctic expedition 1913-18. Vol. XII. Southern party—1913-16. Ottawa: Acland.

42. JENNESS, D. (1924): *Myths and traditions from northern Alaska, the Mackenzie delta and Coronation Gulf*. Report of the Canadian Arctic expedition 1913-18. Vol. XII. Southern party—1913-16. Ottawa: Acland.

43. JENNESS, D. (1928): *The People of the Twilight*. New York: Macmillan.

44. JENNESS, D. (1933): An Indian method of treating hysteria. *Primitive Man,* 6 (1), 13-20.
45. JENNESS, D. (1935): *The Ojibwa indians of Parry Island, their social and religious life.* Canada Department of Mines and Resources. National Museum of Canada, bulletin no. 78, anthropological series no. 17. Ottawa: Patenaude.
46. JENNESS, D. (1937): *The Sekani indians of British Columbia.* Canada Department of Mines and Resources. National Museum of Canada, bulletin no. 84, anthropological series no. 20. Ottawa: Patenaude.
47. JENNESS, D. (1938): *The Sarcee indians of Alberta.* Canada Department of Mines and Resources. National Museum of Canada, bulletin no. 90, anthropological series no. 23. Ottawa: Patenaude.
48. JENNESS, D. (1955): *The faith of a coast Salish indian.* Anthropology in British Columbia, memoir no. 3. Victoria: British Columbia Provincial Museum.
49. JENNESS, D. (5th ed. 1960): *The indians of Canada.* Bulletin 65, anthropological series no. 15. National Museum of Canada. Ottawa: The Queen's Printer and Controller of Stationery.
50. JEWITT, J. R. (1816): *A narrative of the adventures and sufferings of John R. Jewitt, only survivor of the crew of the ship Boston during a captivity of nearly three years among the savages of Nootka Sound with an account of the manners, mode of living, and religious opinions of the natives.* New York: Fanshaw.
51. JILEK, W. G. (1971): From crazy witch doctor to auxiliary psychotherapist— the changing image of the medicine man. *Psychiatria Clinica,* 4, 200-220.
52. KIDD, G. E. (1946): Trepanation among the early indians of British Columbia. *Canad. Med. Ass. J.,* 55 (5), 513-516.
53. KÖNIG, H. (1936): Schamane und Medizinmann. *Ciba Zeitschrift,* 4 (38), 1294-1301.
54. LAWSON, F. S. (1958): Mental hospitals: their size and function. *Canad. J. Publ. Hlth.,* 49 (5), 186-195.
55. LAWSON, F. S. (1959): Program of the Department of Public Health, Province of Saskatchewan, Canada. In: *Progress and Problems of Community Mental Health Services.* New York: Milbank Memorial Fund. Part I, pp. 200-211.
56. LAWSON, F. S. (1965): I. Saskatchewan's first regional mental health facility. *Mental Hospitals,* 16 (2), 85-86.
57. LE BLOND, S. (1949): History of the Hôtel-Dieu de Québec. *Canad. Med. Ass. J.,* 60 (1), 75-80.
58. LEECHMAN, J. D. (1944): Trephined skulls from British Columbia. *Trans. Roy. Soc. Canad. Series III,* 38, Sect. II, 99-102, pl. I-IV.
59. LEECHMAN, J. D. (1954): *The Vanta Kutchin.* National Museum of Canada Bulletin No. 130, Anthropological Series No. 33. Department of Northern Affairs and National Resources, National Parks Branch. Ottawa: Cloutier.
60. LEECHMAN, J. D. (1966): *Native Tribes of Canada.* Toronto: Gage.
61. MAC CULLOCH, J. A. (1920): Shamanism. In: Hastings, J. (Ed.), *Encyclopaedia of Religion and Ethics.* Vol. 11. Edinburgh: Clark. Pp. 441-446.
62. MAC DERMOT, H. E. (1950): *A History of the Montreal General Hospital.* Montreal: Southam Press.
63. MAC DERMOT, J. H. (1949): Food and medicinal plants used by the indians of British Columbia. *Canad. Med. Ass. J.,* 61 (2), 177-183.
64. MCKERRACHER, D. G. (1966): *Trends in Psychiatric Care.* Royal Commission on Health Services. Ottawa: Duhamel.
65. MAC TAGGART, K. (1973): The first decade the story of the birth of Canadian medicare in Saskatchewan and its development during the following 10 years. Ottawa: Canadian Medical Association.
66. MACDONALD, E. (1959): Indian medicine in New Brunswick. *Canad. Med. Ass. J.,* 80 (3), 220-224.

67. MADDOX, J. L. (1923): *The Medicine Man, a Sociological Study of the Character and Evolution of Shamanism.* New York: Macmillan.

68. MARGETTS, E. L. (1967): Trepanation of the skull by the medicine-men of primitive cultures, with particular reference to present-day native East African practice. In: Brothwell, D. R. and Sandison, A. T. (Eds.), *Diseases in Antiquity, a Survey of the Diseases, Injuries and Surgery of Early Populations.* Springfield: Charles C Thomas. Ch. 53, pp. 673-701.

69. MARTIN, C. A. (1947): Le premier demi-siècle de la psychiatrie à Québec. *Laval Médical,* 12 (7), 710-738.

70. MILES, J. E. (1967): The psychiatric aspects of the traditional medicine of the British Columbia coast indians. *Canad. Psychiat. Ass. J.,* 12 (4), 429-431.

71. MOSER, C. (1926): *Reminiscences of the West Coast of Vancouver Island.* Victoria: Acme Press.

72. PARKER, S. (1960): The wiitiko psychosis in the context of Ojibwa personality and culture. *Am. Anthropol.,* 62 (4), 603-623.

73. PARKER, S. (1962): Eskimo psychopathology in the context of Eskimo personality and culture. *Am. Anthropol.,* 64 (1), 76-96.

74. PEARY, R. E. (1910): *The North Pole.* New York: Stokes.

75. RADIN, P. & GRAY, L. H. (1912): Eskimos. In: Hastings, J. (Ed.), *Encyclopaedia of Religion and Ethics.* Vol. 5. Edinburgh: Clark. Pp. 391-395.

76. RAVENHILL, A. (1938): *The Native Tribes of British Columbia.* Victoria: Banfield.

77. RIDDELL, W. R. (1934): Medicine of the indians of Acadia two and a quarter centuries ago. *Medical Record,* 140, 95-96.

78. RITCHIE, J. B. (1957): Early surgeons of the North West Mounted Police. II. Dr. John George Kittson: first surgeon. *Historical Bulletin . . . Calgary Associate Clinic,* 22 (1). 130-144.

79. ROGERS, S. L. (1942): Shaman and Medicineman. *Ciba Symposia,* Vol. 4, No. 1 (three articles).

80. ROHRL, V. J. (1970): A nutritional factor in windigo psychosis. *Am. Anthropol.,* 72 (1), 97-101.

81. SAINDON, J. E. (1933): Mental disorders among the James Bay Cree. *Primitive Man,* 6 (1), 1-12.

82. ST. FELIX, SOEUR, (NEE O'REILLY, H.) (1882): *Monseigneur de Saint-Vallier et l'Hôpital Général de Québec. Histoire du monastère de Notre-Dame des Anges.* Québec: Darveau.

83. SAPIR, E. (1921): Vancouver Island indians. In: Hastings, J. (Ed.), *Encyclopaedia of Religion and Ethics.* Vol. 12. Edinburgh: Clark. Pp. 591-595.

84. SEGUIN, R. L. (1961): *La Sorcellerie au Canada Français du XVIIe au XIXe Siècles.* Montréal: Ducharme.

85. STEFANSSON, V. (1908): Notes on the theory and treatment of diseases among the Mackenzie river eskimo. *J. Am. Folklore,* 21, 43-45.

86. STEFANSSON, V. (1913): *My Life with the Eskimo.* New York: Macmillan.

87. STONE, E. P. (1932): Medicine among the American Indians. New York: Hoeber.

88. STRATH, R. (1903): Materia medica, pharmacy and therapeutics of the Cree indians of the Hudson Bay Territory. *St. Paul Med. J.,* 5, 735-746.

89. SWANTON, J. R. (1910): Shamans and priests. In: Hodge, F. W. (Ed.), (1906, 1910). *Handbook of American indians north of Mexico.* Smithsonian Institution Bureau of American Ethnology, bulletin 30. Washington: Government Printing Office. Part 2, pp. 522-524.

90. SWANTON, J. R. (1910): Witchcraft. In: Hodge, F. W. (Ed.), (1906, 1910): *Handbook of American indians north of Mexico.* Smithsonian Institution Bureau of American Ethnology, bulletin 30. Washington: Government Printing Office. Part 2, pp. 965-966.

91. SWANTON, J. R. (1953): *The indian tribes of North America.* Smithsonian Institution Bureau of American Ethnology, bulletin 145. Washington: Government Printing Office.

92. SYMINGTON, F. (1969): *The Canadian Indian, the Illustrated History of the Great Tribes of Canada*. Toronto: Maclean-Hunter/McClelland and Stewart.
93. TEICHER, M. I. (1954): Three cases of psychoses among the eskimos. *J. Ment. Sci.*, 100 (419), 527-535.
94. TEICHER, M. I. (1960): Windigo psychosis a study of a relationship between belief and behavior among the indians of northeastern Canada. Seattle: American Ethnological Society.
95. THWAITES, R. G. (Ed.) (1896-1901): *The Jesuit Relations and Allied Documents Travels and Explorations of the Jesuit Missionaries in New France, 1610-1791*. Cleveland: Burrows.
96. VALLEE, F. G. (1966): Eskimo theories of mental illness in the Hudson Bay region. *Anthropologica N. S.*, 8 (1), 53-83.
97. VAN WART, A. F. (1948): The indians of the maritime provinces, their diseases and native cures. *Canad. Med. Ass. J.*, 59, 573-577.
98. VOGEL, V. J. (1970): *American Indian Medicine*. Norman: University of Oklahoma Press.
99. WEYER, E. M. (1932): *The Eskimos, their Environment and Folkways*. New Haven: Yale University Press.
100. WHITEBREAD, C. (1925): The indian medical exhibit of the division of medicine in the United States National Museum. *Proceedings of the United States National Museum*, 67 (10), pl. 1-2, 1-26.

19

UNITED STATES OF AMERICA

JEROME M. SCHNECK, M.D.

*Attending Psychiatrist, Division of Psychiatric Training and
Education, St. Vincent's Hospital and Medical Center,
New York, New York, U.S.A.*

1

INTRODUCTION

In colonial days, American practice and belief relating to mental illness bore European influences—French, German, and British among them. But ideas and actions were modified by the colonists so that, for example, witchcraft delusions existed, yet apparently never to the degree encountered in France and Germany (124). Asylums for the mentally ill were established early and their nature was influenced by those abroad. They increased in number and may have become more significant in the American scene than their counterparts in Europe. Evidence is not available, however, to indicate any noteworthy change in the amount of mental disease arising during the American colonial era.

Treatment of the mentally ill was essentially similar in the colonies to that in the mother countries. Some of the sick remained at home; those without families wandered about; and still others entered almshouses or jails and were dealt with mildly or badly as people and circumstances dictated. They were flogged or placed in stocks or incarcerated and treated according to the discretion of their custodians. When a town was large enough to maintain a jail or almshouse, it might serve concurrently as a small hospital, a workhouse, and a penal institution. Early examples are those set up in Philadelphia in 1732 and in New York City four years later. But the mentally ill did not enjoy any special services. Particular attention was eventually given to them when in 1752 the Pennsylvania Hospital became the first establishment catering to the sick in the English colonies.

Prior to colonization of the eastern seaboard and concurrently as well, the American Indian tribes flourished over the vast expanse of territories that would eventually become part of the United States. As among similar peoples elsewhere, concepts of disease incorporated the influence of spirits and the power of offended gods. Medicine was magico-religious and pervaded with supernaturalism. The world of spirits reflected men's anxieties and the violation of a taboo was a powerful psychological force. Physical and psychological measures merged therapeutically. Magic, medicine, and religion were one. The loss of the soul was important as a cause of disease; this has been so among American Indians of the Northwest as among primitive groups in Siberia, among the Eskimos, in Polynesia and Melanesia (127).

2

THE BEGINNINGS

Benjamin Rush (Plate XCV) is generally regarded as the father of American psychiatry. Much is known about him through his letters and autobiographical works as well as his professional publications, and much has been written about him (25, 33, 50). His life and activities spanned the late colonial period, the Revolutionary War, and the early years of the newly formed United States. He was the most famous physician of his time in America, a signer of the Declaration of Independence, and the holder of the highest medical positions in George Washington's military forces during the War of Independence. He was in the forefront of battles waged in support of public welfare, an opponent of slavery, a fighter for prison reform, a proponent of expanding opportunities for good education. His name is linked with courageous efforts to fight yellow fever, but his great stress on bleeding and purging attracted many critics and it is not a minor point to note that some accused him of probably killing more patients than he saved. Rush was certainly a controversial figure—religious, dogmatic, moralistic—the determined man with perhaps as many enemies as friends. He insisted on his ideas of truth, at times to the point of

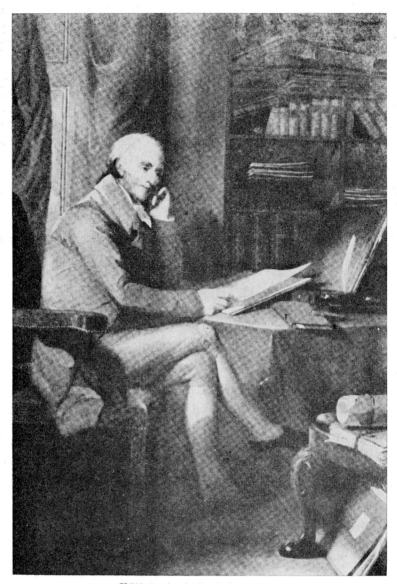

PLATE XCV. Benjamin Rush, by Thomas Sully.

arrogance, and certainly on occasions with an absence of tact. He was not given to compromise.

The humanitarianism of Rush, while associated with his devotion to all patients, is seen to be reflected especially in his concern for the mentally ill. Kind though he may have been, he accepted intimidation of some psychiatric patients for therapeutic purposes as did some European doctors at that time (141). He was a clinician of broad experience and he was compared to Sydenham, whom he admired. Rush's friend in London, John Coakley Lettsom, the well known physician, felt he even surpassed Sydenham (1). And while Rush loomed large as the first significant American psychiatrist, opinions about him differ even on this score. He has at times been given lukewarm estimates as a medical psychologist (98). At the same time, another historian recognized Rush's interest in personality and his anticipation of a modern orientation in psychiatry (125). Furthermore, Rush's perception of personality functioning has been evaluated in apparently opposing ways. His approach to psychological issues has been regarded as dualistic by the latter historian, while a distinguished psychiatrist, basing his views on Rush's lectures on the *Institutes and Practice of Medicine,* in addition to his other writings, has said that Rush saw "mind and body as a unit" and that he was aware of "the unity of dynamics of disease" (83).

Rush continued to be productive through the late 18th century and into the early 19th century, and his major psychiatric work, *Medical Inquiries and Observations upon the Diseases of the Mind* was published in 1812 (105). This book is often regarded as his most important scientific contribution. It was the first general volume on psychiatry in America and the only textbook of its kind which continued to be of influence for more than half a century. Two publications by Englishmen were issued in the United States before Rush's book. One was *View of the Nervous Temperament,* by Thomas Trotter, reprinted in Troy, New York in 1808, and the other was *Practical Observations on Insanity,* by Joseph Mason Cox, issued in Philadelphia in 1811.

Rush had taken a good medical apprenticeship during the colonial period and had then traveled abroad, receiving an M.D. from Edinburgh. When he returned to Philadelphia, he became a professor in the first medical school in the English-American colonies. He served many years on the staff of the Pennsylvania Hospital, the period recognized as the true beginning of American psychiatry (73).

It should be noted that Rush was not simply interested in psychiatric patients. He tried to place the study and treatment of mental

disease on a scientific basis which it had not been accorded previously
in America. Some of his treatment measures, such as the tranquilizer
chair for immobilization of the patient and the gyrator, are felt to
have been "shock techniques" with punitive implications, and Rush
has been criticized for this. By the time he was using such mechanical
devices several physicians had already achieved reputations for their
attempts to remove or ease mechanical restraints. Among them were
Vincenzio Chiarugi, the famous Italian who put his ideas into practice at St. Boniface in Florence in the 1770s and 1780s, and soon
thereafter Philippe Pinel at the Bicêtre and the Salpêtrière in Paris,
whose name and work have overshadowed Chiarugi in most historical
writings (37). And there were similar movements in the British Isles
when, for example, William Tuke played an important role in establishing the famous Retreat at York, where the humane treatment
included removal of fetters and manacles, although the whirling
chair, plunge baths, and similar measures were still in use in England,
Scotland, and Ireland well into the 18th century (91). Whereas Rush
was a strong adherent to bloodletting, Pinel objected to the manner
in which it was often used. The "moral treatment" in which Pinel
was engaged has been compared to the 20th century "total push" concept with its incorporation of psychotherapy, occupational therapy,
and recreational therapy (75).

On the positive side of the ledger for Rush and his influence should
be noted a significant transition between Sydenham and Rush in their
views on psychological medicine. Sydenham had been aware of the
considerable significance of psychological issues in medical practice
and Rush was indebted to him for this. But he went beyond Sydenham
in stressing the importance of psychology in general medical training
and he focused concretely on the study of the patient as an individual, combining psychological and physiological functioning into a
holistic pattern with the view that has been acquiring increasing emphasis in medical education (112).

Turning from Boerhaave with an emphasis on humoral pathology
and moderate treatment which appealed to leading physicians of his
time, Rush moved in the direction of William Cullen of Edinburgh,
stressing tension pathology. The vascular system assumed a position
of central importance in disease. John Brown of Edinburgh was known
for the stress on two pathological conditions, vascular tension and
laxity, and the historian who viewed Rush's outlook as dualistic in
his psychiatric opinions saw him as reducing everything in medical
theory to tension alone, in contrast to the popular Brunonian system of which Rush denied he was a follower. This interest in somatics

in any case did not prevent him from preparing a textbook that revealed wide-ranging interest in, and observations of, psychological forces impinging on personality well-being. This apparently influenced the opinion that the longstanding prestige of *Diseases of the Mind* could be explained reasonably by the view that Rush's psychiatry could be adapted to the somatic emphasis of the 19th century and the psychological approaches of the 20th as well (126).

Aggressive in his personal animosities, Rush in his military days saw his arch rival William Shippen, Jr. facing a court-martial, and it was evident that accusations and counter-accusations had as much to do with his personality clash with the well known sociable, more extraverted obstetrician and teacher of anatomy than with medical and administrative differences (32). It is not surprising that from the military historian's point of view, Rush was a poor subordinate (10). Rush and Shippen, when studying at St. Thomas' Hospital in London, had encountered poet-physician Mark Akenside, and their impressions of him did not coincide either (121). But on some fronts his perseverance was devoted to social causes where he left his imprint, causes centering around the issue of intemperate drinking and the movement for abolition of slavery (114, 89). It is not surprising that his interest in various aspects of the relations between the black and white populations was pointed up again only recently in view of the present focus on racial tensions and associated realignments.

It is of interest that apart from recognition of Rush's efforts to classify psychiatric disorders, to teach through lectures and publications, and to make his mark on the broad social scene, little has been said about his awareness of some fine points in personality functioning which would perhaps negate some claims of deficiencies as a medical psychologist. A careful reading of his textbook reveals that he commented on the influence of buried memories, and while others may have been aware of this it was nevertheless 80 years later that the "original causes" which had "perished in the memory" were fervently sought and revived by Josef Breuer and then in his collaboration with Freud (113, 22). In addition it may be noted that Rush furnished an example of the early recognition of denial of illness when he supplied an account of his work in the Philadelphia yellow fever epidemic of 1793 (116, 104). These specific points are important in taking the full measure of the man. At the same time one can easily generalize and point out that Rush's medicine focused on the notion of a tension system. And the latter fact is true in its way. The view has been expressed that Rush offered a variation of John Brown's system by reducing the number of diseases from two to one so that he was more of an 18th century systematist than a follower of Sydenham (2). At the same time it can be claimed that his psychiatric methods were consistent with his theories, and blood-letting was in keeping with his idea that the cause of mental illness was related to the blood vessels of the brain. When the brain was overcharged with blood, it was right to deplete the body of it, even to the point of inducing faintness and debility (24).

If it appears that Rush has been accorded disproportionate attention, it should be reiterated that not only was he the leading and most controversial physician of his time but that, according to one assessment, his influence on his colleagues may have exceeded that of Sir William Osler on his fellow physicians a century later (45). Of parenthetical interest is the fact that one of Benjamin Rush's children was James Rush (1786-1869), who is described as an original thinker and labelled the first behaviorist. He opposed metaphysical thinking and authored a system of psychology based on objectivistic principles (99).

3

EARLY 19TH CENTURY

Beginnings of the American Psychiatric Association

The 19th century was for psychiatry a great period for description, classification, and study of reaction types. It was a period of hospital construction, founding of societies, publishing of books and periodicals. Psychiatry developed as a medical specialty and became an important item of cultural development in Europe and in the United States. The Association of Medical Superintendents of American Institutions for the Insane was founded in 1844. The influence of Benjamin Rush had been great prior to this. For the remainder of the century the history of psychiatry coincided with the development of the Association which became known as the American Medico-Psychological Association in 1892 and finally the American Psychiatric Association in 1921. The founders of the organization, many of whom achieved a fair measure of fame in their day and some of whom remain important in the history of American psychiatry, are still known as The Original Thirteen (Plate XCVI). Their names are Samuel B. Woodward, Isaac Ray, John S. Butler, Samuel White, Charles H. Stedman, Pliny Earle, Thomas S. Kirkbride, Luther V. Bell, William M. Awl,

John M. Galt, Amariah Brigham, Francis T. Stribling, and Nehemiah Cutter. The birth of the American Psychiatric Association followed that of the Medico-Psychological Association in England. The latter was already on the scene in 1841.

The forerunner of the present day *American Journal of Psychiatry* was the *American Journal of Insanity.* Its publication began in 1844,

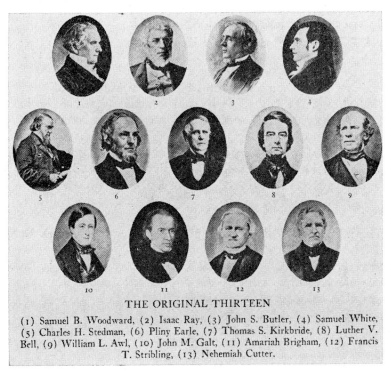

THE ORIGINAL THIRTEEN

(1) Samuel B. Woodward, (2) Isaac Ray, (3) John S. Butler, (4) Samuel White, (5) Charles H. Stedman, (6) Pliny Earle, (7) Thomas S. Kirkbride, (8) Luther V. Bell, (9) William L. Awl, (10) John M. Galt, (11) Amariah Brigham, (12) Francis T. Stribling, (13) Nehemiah Cutter.

PLATE XCVI. The Original Thirteen.

the same year as the founding of the parent organization, and the same year in which appeared the *Allgemeine Zeitschrift für Psychiatrie,* and one year later than the *Annales Médico-Psychologiques.* It was fully 30 years later, in 1874, that another well known American publication, *The Journal of Nervous and Mental Disease,* first appeared.

Early Hospitals and Patient Management

Psychiatry in 19th century America fostered a humanitarian theme. The Bloomingdale Hospital, the Hartford Retreat, and the Friends'

Asylum of Frankfort were part of this development in the change from madhouse to asylum and in growing efforts at treatment of patients. The groundwork had been started elsewhere. The development of private and state hospitals in the United States incorporated a type of occupational therapy involving use of patients' labor on farms and in dairies and in workshops. Such activities for patients were already on hand and Guillaume Ferrus, who was associated with Pinel at the Salpêtrière in 1818, had pioneered these measures. He visited hospitals in France and England, observed the poor living conditions of patients and the paucity of hospitals, and noted the merging of criminal and psychiatric patient populations. When he became physician-in-chief at the *Bicêtre* in 1826 he was already interested in criminology, legal psychiatry, and prison reform on which so much attention is centered periodically in the United States and again at present following an all too familiar series of conflicts and catastrophes. And while John Conolly was moving in England toward the elimination of mechanical restraints, his views were seen as purely idealistic by some experienced psychiatrists. Ferrus described his viewing a patient held down by four strong guards in a padded cell of Conolly's hospital. But the non-restraint movement was propagated throughout Europe and America.

The reforms of William Tuke and the milieu of the York Retreat which he founded in 1792 in England influenced the tone of American mental hospitals that were established later. In time, the careful observations, methodical procedures, and professional involvements regarded as enlightened eclecticism by layman Tuke's great-grandson, Daniel Hack Tuke, had counterparts in the lives and careers of 19th century American psychiatrists. The activities of psychiatrists and their work in hospitals reflected complex trends, and differences of opinion were much in evidence. With the passage of time Daniel Hack Tuke, publishing in 1885 a study on *The Insane in the United States and Canada,* saw the well known American psychiatrist John P. Gray as a strong defender of mechanical restraint and recognized the fact that many British psychiatrists regarded the views of John Conolly and Robert Gardiner Hill, a strong opponent of restraint, as "pious opinion" (111, 137).

Trends in attitudes toward restraint may be traced historically, but it is important that certain difficulties in evaluations be recognized (109). There are different types of restraints and varying degrees of restraint. The term "non-restraint" does not have a simple meaning and significance. The Friends' Asylum in Frankfort has been regarded as the second oldest dedicated to the mentally ill in the United States and the first in which a chain was never used for confining a patient. But elimination of restraint was not implied because leather was substituted for the iron. At Friends' Asylum and in other hospitals there was a trend toward substituting solitary confinement for direct, mechanical, body restraint.

During the early 19th century considerable optimism emerged and blossomed in mental hospitals in the United States (72). And about the time of the meeting of Samuel B. Woodward of Worcester State Hospital in Massachusetts with Francis T. Stribling of Western State Hospital in Staunton, Virginia, a number of psychiatrists, many of them founders of the psychiatric organization which grew out of the Woodward-Stribling meeting, made significant contributions. A study of Woodward himself has shown that his ideas about the etiology of insanity grew out of his somatic definition of it. He felt too that while insanity was a somatic illness it could have psychological causes. The abnormal behavior of a person was the primary cause of insanity. The individual possessed free will. Abnormal behavior led to brain impairment and the brain was the organ of the mind. In a certain sense insanity was, therefore, self-inflicted. Woodward was a strong advocate of moral treatment while relying heavily on "medical therapy" at the same time (52). In fact, with the view that Woodward relied so much on drug therapy. Thomas Kirkbride of the Pennsylvania Hospital, when visiting Woodward at Worcester, claimed that Woodward prescribed medicine three times a day "even when it was required but twice" (19). Kirkbride was well known in connection with the type of hospital construction bearing his name and prevalent in mental institutions throughout the country.

Treatment, Statistics and the Cult of Curability

Pliny Earle, in 1848, published his *History, Description and Statistics of the Bloomingdale Asylum for the Insane.* Until then, statistical records and reports had not been of great concern in hospital administration (106). The merits and conclusions have been debated, but this is a point not uncommon in connection with statistical evaluations (90). Five years prior to the appearance of Earle's treatise and in the year before the founding of the American Psychiatric Association, Amariah Brigham became the first superintendent of the first New York State Asylum for the Insane in Utica. The first report of this institution included statistical data relating to movements of patients, monthly admissions, ages on admission, their condition, occupations, nativity, and residences. The causes of their mental illness were included. This material established a pattern followed by other institutions. The history of state hospitals constitutes a significant part of the history of psychiatry in the United States, and special studies have appeared on regional areas (of which California is one example) (69). Brigham himself serves as an example of an American psychiatrist stressing humanitarian efforts that characterized the work of other psychiatrists in England and France. He too is credited with supervising patient activity programs which were eventually referred to as occupational and recreational therapy. This meritorious work is believed to have been duplicated only in relatively recent times (27). And it was Brigham who founded and edited the *American Journal of Insanity,* now the *American Journal of Psychiatry.*

Woodward, the first president of the American Psychiatric Association, originally organized as an association of medical superintendents, was succeeded by William M. Awl who served also as vice-president of the American Medical Association. It is believed that Awl was the first to suggest that schools be established in the United States for idiots and imbeciles, following the pioneer studies in France by Itard and then by Séguin (102).

Although Benjamin Rush had been one of the first Americans to recommend bibliotherapy, John Minson Galt II of Williamsburg, Virginia, was the first American to write an article on the subject and to supply an overall picture of libraries in the asylums for the insane. His material was presented first as a lecture in 1848. Reading was regarded as one of the most desirable therapeutic measures for mental patients. By the middle of the 19th century, every major mental hospital had a library for patients. Galt presented in some detail the theory and practice of bibliotherapy, first in the annual reports of the Eastern Lunatic Asylum of Virginia, and afterwards in his book on treatment of insanity. The history of psychiatry incorporates the efforts of several generations of a few families on behalf of the mentally ill. Various members of the Galt family were associated with the administration of the Eastern Lunatic Asylum of Virginia (Plate XCVII) from its founding in 1773 as the first hospital in the United States to be used solely for the care of mental patients. Galt's father had been a physician at this hospital. The superintendents had usually been laymen, and in the case of John Minson Galt II, the appointment of a new superintendent was actually delayed until he could finish his medical studies. He assumed office in 1841 when he was 22 years old, and he was the youngest of the 13 founders of the American Psychiatric Association (132). Interest in bibliotherapy and mental hospital libraries, as reflected in Galt's work, grew and diminished from time to time and was stressed again in the middle of the present century (108).

During this era of developing and expanding care for psychiatric patients in the United States, an aura of optimism pervaded the mental hospitals between 1800 and 1850, when a "cult of curability" appeared. It was reflected in the enthusiasm of William Maclay Awl of Ohio. The point has been made that he was so terribly optimistic that he became known as Dr. "Cure-all" Awl. Assertions were put

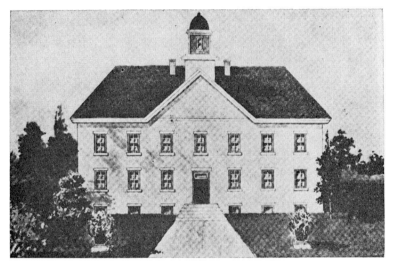

PLATE XCVII. An early print of the Eastern Lunatic Hospital at Williamsburg, Virginia—the first public hospital in America exclusively for the treatment of the mentally ill.

forward of 90 to 100 per cent cures, and while the figure may seem remarkably exaggerated, it is not unusual to encounter similar claims today in relation to at least special treatment techniques and their application to some types of mental illness. Initial claims are generally reduced in time by more sober investigators.

Isaac Ray

In recent years, Isaac Ray has received attention greater than that accorded other founders of the American Psychiatric Association, largely, perhaps, because of concerns with forensic psychiatry. He not only saw the deficiencies in the social order of his day, but possessed

the ability and determination to act on them (128). He published
a classic work, *Treatise on the Medical Jurisprudence of Insanity*
(Plate XCVIII) in 1838 (93). This is his best-known work; it still
attracts attention, and is regarded as a curious achievement of a
physician who was engaged in rural practice with only occasional
contact with psychiatric patients. The treatise contains reformist ideas

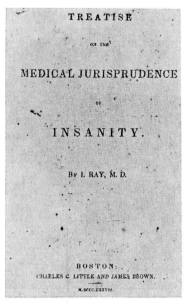

PLATE XCVIII. Title page of *Treatise on the Medical Jurisprudence
of Insanity* by Isaac Ray, M.D.

and an unusual presentation of medico-legal problems (88). Many
years later, when Ray published *Mental Hygiene* in 1863, it was one
of the earliest uses of this term (94). The expression "Ray's mania,"
is encountered only occasionally. It pertains to the condition called
"moral insanity" which has been described by others (17).

Ray's *Treatise* of 1838 was well used five years later in the famous
M'Naughten trial (39). In 1843 Daniel M'Naughten was tried at the
Old Bailey, London, for the murder of Edward Drummond, secretary
to Sir Robert Peel, the British Prime Minister. The influential
M'Naughten Rules emerged from this trial and maintain their impact
today. The assassination of Drummond had actually been intended

for Peel. M'Naughten was found not guilty on the ground of insanity and there was much opposition to this verdict. It is of interest that in 1830, eight years before Ray's treatise appeared and 13 years before M'Naughten was tried, relevant legal-psychiatric issues were presented in the well known novel by Stendhal (Henri Beyle), *Le Rouge et le Noir*, a book proclaimed by its admirers as the first psychological novel (120). Apart from such assertions, the relevant sections as far as Ray's psychiatric interests are involved are at the end when Julien Sorel, after shooting his former mistress, awaits trial and faces death by the guillotine. Five years after Stendhal's novel appeared, Prichard published *A Treatise on Insanity and Other Disorders Affecting the Mind*. Here, the concept of "moral insanity" is pertinent to the issues surrounding the fictional Julien Sorel, a paranoid psychopath. It seems that Ray's work carried more weight at the time of the M'Naughten trial than did Prichard's ideas which, when published, did not meet with immediate or easy acceptance in England (92).

The "moral" (seen as emotional or psychological) treatment of early 19th century psychiatrists has been defined as measures which made the patient comfortable, aroused his interest, invited his friendship, encouraged discussion of his troubles, and helped to fill his time with purposeful activity (18). At the Hartford Retreat, Eli Todd fostered such attentions as did Woodward at Worcester. When Todd presented his results to the public he claimed 90 per cent recovery of first-admission patients. When criticisms were leveled elsewhere at Pliny Earle for his assertions promoting the idea of a cult of curability, he was reluctant, it has been said, to face any evidence which did not support the view that claims of recovery rates were artificially exaggerated by repeated recovery of readmissions.

Moral Treatment, Somatic Treatment, and Hospital Reform

The events in Massachusetts during the first half of the 19th century have been regarded as fairly representative of the entire country as far as the establishment of a system of public mental hospitals was concerned. Other states appeared to follow its lead and toward the end of the century the therapeutic features of the hospitals gave way to the custodial. Moral treatment emerged from humanitarian and religious interests of the time. Social, economic, psychological, and intellectual influences were brought to bear on mental hospital activities. A point of view significant for such developments is that moral treatment related to the assumption that a close therapist-patient relationship probably stemmed from similarities in ethnic, economic, and religious backgrounds and environment with a shared, common cultural heritage (53). Moral treatment apparently was less effective after 1850 when more and more hospital patients came from diverse ethnic, economic, and religious backgrounds. The psychiatrists made the point that funds were insufficient for their needs, and made claims of inherent character defects in this new urban and industrial population of a heterogeneous type with which they were evidently unprepared to deal. In any case, psychiatrists now saw mental disease no longer as curable as they once had seen it. The psychological features of etiology and treatment accepted by many during the first part of the 19th century gave way to the somatic in the second part. An era of confinement and custodial care set in. This incorporated a professionalism in psychiatry which increasingly excluded the role of laymen who had played effective roles in caring for the mentally ill during earlier decades. The hospitals grew larger and larger. Personal attention decreased. A feeling of adequate contact with patients from poor, immigrant families lessened. And it has been suggested that racial prejudice was involved in the breakdown of moral treatment and of ordinary decent hospital living standards.

While medical men moved to the forefront and the somatic emphasis began to triumph, some laymen continued to play a helpful role. Among them Dorothea Lynde Dix was an important example. Instrumental in the significant movements associated with attempts to improve the lot of the mentally ill, this New England school teacher struck out at public indifference and directed her efforts toward legislative groups. She was influential as early as the 1840's and eventually was credited with having played an important role in the founding and development of more than 30 state institutions for the mentally ill. Her investigations of the abuse and neglect of psychiatric patients in particular took her through almshouses and local jails with their lack of attention and defective care. She had a searching curiosity and possessed firm determination. She has also been described as imperious and rigid. From the small, inadequate quarters of the almshouses and jails, the sick were shifted to small local institutions, then to county hospitals newly constructed, and finally to the larger state hospitals that replaced them, a trend which has been reversed in more recent years with the establishment and growth of community mental health centers and psychiatric divisions in general hospitals, again hopefully with the goal of better care and treatment. Differences of opinion on this score existed then as they do now.

4

LATE 19TH CENTURY

Hospitals and Hospital Care

Large numbers of patients could be cared for with greater economy in this 19th century phase of large hospital construction, but such economy often took precedence over the actual welfare of patients, and the clashes began to appear between patient-minded physicians and economy-minded legislative bodies. There were some advantages claimed for the big institutions, such as greater uniformity in administration and treatment, but these were counterbalanced by increasing absorption by doctors in administrative duties which precluded adequate contact with the patients they were to aid. Because of this, colonization was again considered for its possible advantages, and Gheel is usually thought of as a fine example for this purpose. But Gheel itself had already come in for criticism and this colony, the pride of Belgium, had been found fault with by Ferrus, owing to cruelties he had observed there. In any case the idea of the plan opposed to large hospitals was one for placing public and private patients in cottages and homes in which extensive personal liberties could be granted and arranged. Placement in the villages of homes and special cottages would follow initial reception of patients in small hospitals. Patients would be visited by supervisors under the jurisdiction of physicians in charge. Concerns about such a system related to risks of suicide and improper treatment of patients stemming from insufficient watchfulness and control. Despite opposition on this score, such plans were put into operation in various parts of the United States. They were also employed, incidentally, in Canada, and a cottage system had already been used with alleged success in Scotland.

During the second half of the 19th century, pyschopathic hospitals captured attention, and in 1879 one was associated with Bellevue in New York City. Stress in such hospitals was on observation of patients and temporary detention. Gradually, as the focus of attention centered less on division of patients into curable and incurable, and when separations among them developed more in accordance with their therapeutic requirements, the trend toward independent psychopathic hospitals gained pace. In addition to such hospitals, additional attention was given to the development of psychiatric wards within general hospitals, a trend which has been accorded renewed interest in recent years. The psychopathic hospital associated with

Bellevue was not the first to appear. Credit for this has been given to the institution of this type which opened one year earlier in Heidelberg.

Many other hospitals of this nature were established. The main feature ascribed to them was an interest in research and in treatment of early cases of mental disease. Yet the interest in early treatment of patients by no means awaited the establishment of such separate psychopathic hospitals. In 1751, for example, stress was placed on treatment of patients ill for less than one year, and this special focus of attention occurred in St. Luke's Hospital in England. Furthermore, the belief in setting up psychiatric wards in general hospitals had long been present in various places at various times. A general hospital of the 13th century in Cairo had this arrangement, and in 1728 special wards of this type existed in Guy's Hospital in London. The New York Hospital had this arrangement in 1792. The Psychopathic Hospital idea favored a trend toward intensive observation and short-term treatment of patients with acute personality disorders, and these hospitals were frequently affiliated with medical centers which furnished opportunities for instruction of medical students in psychiatry as well as for research. Developments that followed the establishment of these facilities included rapid growth of mental health or psychiatric clinics connected with various hospitals.

George Miller Beard and Silas Weir Mitchell

George Miller Beard and Silas Weir Mitchell are linked intimately with the second half of 19th century American psychiatry. Mitchell was a distinguished neurologist who had much to say about psychiatric issues. But when it was claimed of Beard that he was the first to introduce psychological medicine to America, it was an unwarranted exaggeration (28). Beard is identified with the concept of neurasthenia, and while it has been said that Beard centered attention on nervous exhaustion as a practical problem for neurologists to deal with instead of an issue of diagnosis only, the fact remains that its therapeutic aspects had not actually been ignored and elements inherent in this theme can be traced at least to John Brown and William Cullen. In the Brunonian system, life is based on stimulation from brain and emotions and the external stimuli of food and other elements. The two categories of disease are the sthenic, with increased excitability, and the asthenic, with decreased excitability. But these views have been regarded as an oversimplification of those proposed by Cullen (62). Life is maintained, according to Cullen, by brain energy extending from the central nervous system to muscles and solid organs, with the muscles seen as continuations of the medullary substance of the nervous system. Energy to nerve endings is transmitted by a hypothetical fluid which is not really a liquid. The energy supported a healthy state of excitement. Lack of such excitement resulted in disease. Such a view, not remarkably different from others stated in various ways before Cullen, is a reminder of still others that came later, including some ideas concerning libidinal processes representative of certain conventional psychoanalytic constructs.

Beard's popularization of the notion of neurasthenia earned him an international reputation. He has been regarded on the one hand as a brilliant and courageous pioneer in psychosomatic medicine, and on the other as neither a profound nor a critical thinker. His presentations have been called a mixture of fashionable and influential ideas of his time, and one historian has claimed that it was the familiarity rather than the novelty of Beard's theories which made them easily and rapidly accepted (103, 15). In Beard's time, neurasthenia was a fashionable diagnosis. E. H. Van Deusen has been credited with having described the essentials of this condition before Beard, a condition which evidently incorporated, in accordance with succeeding diagnostic labels, features not only of hysterical but of psychophysiological reactions. At the same time, the notion of neurasthenia was counterbalanced by that of cerebral hyperemia proposed by William A. Hammond, but the latter never achieved the popularity and acceptance of the former. Hammond was one of the prominent neurologists of his day, achieving distinction also as a specialist in mental disease. And he is known also for his role as Surgeon General of the United States Army during the Civil War.

This was a period when the practicing neurologist served the role of non-institutional psychiatrist, and the personality of the doctor as psychotherapist was, then as now, deemed to be of considerable importance. So Weir Mitchell has been evaluated with Thomas Salmon and Austen Riggs, who were to make their mark later, specifically in connection with this theme (49). As neurasthenia is linked with Beard, the Rest Cure is identified with Mitchell. Its ingredients consisted of rest, proper food, and isolation. Since contact with relatives was prohibited, the patient was separated completely from the setting in which his illness developed. The Rest Cure became very popular in the second half of the 19th century, overlapping the popularity of electrotherapy associated with Wilhelm Erb in Europe. Electrotherapy was in fact part of the Rest Cure for some patients, and the method went through various modifications over a period

of time. It incorporated exercise and massage. Kindness with firmness, isolation from relatives, special attention, and above all the
personality of the physician and the implications of the doctor-
patient relationship, as has often been regarded of crucial importance,
have been seen as most important ingredients of the Rest Cure method.
Mitchell was a versatile man, probably the foremost neurologist of
his time. He contributed not only to neurology and psychiatry, but
to toxicology and to American literature (115, 57, 43). He was a
popular writer, an author of poems, short stories, novels, and biographies. His clinical psychiatric experiences and insights found their
way into his literary productions (95). There are at least three different accounts of the origin of the Rest Cure, and one of them is contained in a memorandum by Osler who related his conversation with
Mitchell about the patient involved in its beginnings. One of his
biographers said that Mitchell was "almost" a genius, that his contemporaries regarded him as such, and that this opinion was one
which Mitchell came to share. One additional fact worth mentioning
about Mitchell related to his long remembered criticism of the American Medico-Psychological Association when it was celebrating its 50th
anniversary in 1894. He took the group to task on its scientific status
at that time. A later reassessment of the issue held that the scientific
status of psychiatry did not properly reflect the contemporary level
of scientific investigation. The decades to follow highlighted studies
along psychological lines emphasizing interpersonal relations rather
than neurologically based research (136).

Two years after Mitchell addressed his criticisms to the national
audience of psychiatrists, the Pathological Institute, later to be known
as the New York State Psychiatric Institute, was established. It is
believed to have been the first multidisciplinary organization to incorporate research sections in biological, psychological, and social
sciences in the field of medicine, and the first of its kind to concern
itself with etiology, prevention, and treatment of mental disease (123).
Ira van Gieson conceived and established this first research institute
of its type in the United States. It had research departments in
anatomy, bacteriology, cellular biology, comparative histology, anthropology, psychology, and pathology. Van Gieson developed a new
staining method for blood vessels, proposed structural-functional
correlates, and pioneered in neuropathological studies of the central
nervous system. He was regarded as an unusually imaginative and
scholarly man (100). Four years after the founding of the Institute,
van Gieson was succeeded as director by Adolf Meyer who started
clinical teaching in the state hospitals and suggested affiliation with

a medical school in order to develop further the educational and research programs. Adolf Meyer and the Commissioner of Lunacy of the State of New York, Frederick Peterson, after the turn of the century aimed for a relationship between the Institute and a small hospital, again to facilitate clinical research. Similar institutes were to be established afterwards in various parts of the United States and abroad.

5

EARLY 20TH CENTURY

Morton Prince and Psychopathology

While these developments were taking place in New York, the distinguished physician Morton Prince was active in his studies of psychopathology in Boston during the late 19th and early 20th centuries. His descriptions of psychological disturbances and his attempts to fathom their significance coincided with the productive period of Freud's work in Vienna. Studies of Prince's work and interests reveal him to have been an investigator with views in line with those of famed psychopathologist Pierre Janet rather than Freud. Janet had made meritorious studies of hysteria and observations on dissociation, and he continues to have strong supporters although there has been a lessening of claims regarding significant influences of Janet on Freud's formulations (11, 85).

Prince studied mental processes which he labelled co-conscious, examined manifestations of hysteria, absorbed himself in evaluations of hallucinations, and is very well known for his remarkable descriptions and observations of multiple personalities. He went beyond the psychopathology of Charcot and was stimulated in his researches by the influence of physician-psychologist-philosopher William James. In 1905, Prince published *The Dissociation of a Personality*, which attracted enormous attention, and in 1914 he put out *The Unconscious*, based on his extensive researches. He was viewed by some at that time as the most outstanding experimental psychiatrist in the United States. There was considerable emphasis on somatological concerns during his years of efforts, and psychological disease, seen as brain disease, the 19th century view much associated with Wilhelm Griesinger, had considerable influence in psychiatry. Prince's work contributed much to advancing the importance of psychogenesis of many personality disorders in the midst of the emphasis, then and at present, on dividing concepts of malfunctioning into somatic and psycho-genic categories.

Morton Prince's unusual evaluations of multiple personality high-lighted an area of study which continues today, especially in inves-tigations involving hypnotic techniques. The latter played an im-portant role in Prince's work. His understandings of unconscious pro-cesses were evidently not consistent with meanings propagated by Freud. Among others who thought in similar but not identical terms was von Hartmann. His concepts were more in line with those of Prince, who has at the same time been regarded as a "psychical monist" and a proponent of purposive psychology. It is evident now that Prince's contributions, regardless of their interest and place in the historical development of psychiatry, were overshadowed by the impact and rapid growth of psychoanalysis. Prince founded the in-fluential *Journal of Abnormal Psychology* in 1906, and he also founded the American Psychopathological Association and the Harvard Psy-chological Clinic.

About this time, Austen Fox Riggs was involved with therapeutic work, and it has been stressed recently that as early as 1913, before Freud turned his attention to such concerns, Riggs had developed a conceptual system of ego psychology. He organized a therapeutic com-munity in Stockbridge, Massachusetts, and between 1913 and 1940 prepared groundwork for the re-educational treatment of the psycho-neuroses and allied states. During the course of this effort he devel-oped specialized services which are discernible in areas of student mental health, child guidance, community psychiatry, and in the teaching of psychosomatic medicine (84).

The Impact of Freud and Psychoanalysis

At the turn of the century, Freud published *The Interpretation of Dreams*. He had been involved before that in neurological studies and also in psychopathological studies including those on hysteria. He had been associated with Josef Breuer in the latter, and for a while had incorporated hypnotic techniques. A recent assessment of his abandonment of hypnosis ascribes it as having been linked most prob-ably to his personal and professional ambitions rather than to specific clinical issues. The point is of historical interest in that a continua-tion of his original explorations might well have led to the amalgama-tion of additional hypnotic methods and analytic concepts leading to forms of hypnoanalysis which have emerged in the United States during the past few decades (117, 118). From his theoretical formula-tions centering on his concepts of a dynamic unconscious, and from his clinical work with patients, there flowed an enormous body of writings. Many of his analytic views became and still remain much a part of psychotherapeutic practice in the United States and an integral part of what has generally been called dynamic psychiatry, even though much of what he had to say remains controversial. The perspectives he stressed have, in any case, influenced activities for several decades in the fields of sociology, anthropology, literature, and history, in addition to psychology and psychiatry. Freud's life and work have been studied meticulously and meritoriously, though often with considerable bias, and the history of psychoanalysis in the United States has been traced and published (63, 86).

While the main thrust of psychoanalysis was powered by Freud in Vienna, the acceptance and utilization of it was greater in the United States than in Europe. Certainly it is not unusual for recognition, at least initial recognition, of creative efforts to occur first in foreign lands. Among the forces operating on behalf of psychoanalysis were the rapid growth of private practice of psychiatry in the United States and the flow of psychoanalytically oriented psychiatrists to this country for social and political reasons, as developments in Europe pressed on to the outbreak of World War II. While psychoanalysis was being accepted more readily in America than in Europe by psychiatrists, at the same time that it was often viewed as cultist or akin to the spread of a new religion, it has also been regarded in its early 20th century spread in America as part of a general reform or progressive movement concerned with the public good, even though basic Freudian tenets were not fully grasped (23). The fascination with multiple fine points in the growth and impact of psychoanalysis on individuals, psychiatry, and society in the United States still continues among some historians (55, 56).

Freud visited the United States in 1909 to deliver his lectures on psychoanalysis at Clark University at the invitation of G. Stanley Hall, known for his work in genetic psychology (107). Hall was the first president of the University and of the American Psychological Association as well. He launched the *American Journal of Psychology,* which is usually regarded as the first psychological journal in the English language, though it was preceded by a short-lived publication which consisted only of seven numbers in 1883 and 1884. This magazine, the *Journal of American Psychology,* was intended to further the goals of the National Association for the Protection of the Insane and the Prevention of Insanity, and the core of its activities appears to have been primarily medical, the contributors to the publication mainly people in the private practice of psychiatry and mental hospital administrators in the United States and abroad. Continuing support, however, was lacking (44).

Although Freud's life spanned the 19th and 20th centuries, his productive work appeared so much during the latter that he is regarded basically as a 20th century figure (142). At the same time, growing criticisms of Freud's views, as time passed, often incorporated the claim that they were geared to the thought and conventions of a Victorian age and the milieu of Viennese culture and society. Certain aspects of his early work involving hypnosis do relate more to 19th century endeavors, and present day contributions to this field are more attuned to his achievements in the first part of the 20th century. Despite claims of cultist and religionist attributes leveled at psychoanalysis, its proponents gradually obtained a strong hold on the psychiatric educational structure through independent institutes and many medical schools throughout the country. Having achieved strength, it was maintained as a psychiatric political force at the same time that the psychoanalytic tenets were under attack. During the past few years there has been some diminution in the percentage of young psychiatrists interested in affiliation with, and accreditation by, psychoanalytic institutes (139). A forceful claim made recently is that psychoanalysis has fallen upon evil days and that the period of daring innovation and creativity has given way to limited refinements and suffocation of spirit (122).

One medical historian, when comparing Freud to Charcot, said essentially that Charcot saw neuroses whereas Freud heard them—Charcot dramatized them whereas Freud employed auscultation of patients' verbalizations with a concern similar to that of Laennec, who listened to the chest sounds of his patients (80). In the course of his work, Freud modified some of his ideas. While his own modifications were usually accepted by his followers, at least during his lifetime, the changes suggested by others generally gave rise to bitter controversies over theory and technique.

To the extent that psychoanalysis flourished in the United States more than abroad, these controversies raged all the more. The differences of opinion centered on a variety of issues including efficacy of psychoanalytic treatment as a whole and in relation to certain personality types, criteria of improvement, problems about length of therapy and its intensity, and frequency of analyst-patient contact. There have been differences over treatment methods, psychoanalytic and others, in terms of which is better, at times with regard to types of patients who might be better served by one method rather than another. Controversial issues have included claims of "transference cures" and their stability, and this has been part of the argument over long-term versus short-term treatment. The extent and duration of beneficial change, no less than the limitations in types and numbers of patients amenable to help by relatively conventional psychoanalytic methods, were problems which gradually gave rise to a growing feeling in the psychiatric community and among other interested groups that psychoanalysis had been oversold in the same way that various aspects of psychiatry in general, with its several treatment measures, have tended to be oversold, especially when modifications of treatment or new treatment methods are in their early states of application.

With psychotherapy weighted heavily in psychoanalytic principles as an increasingly dominant influence in the United States, it became fashionable to discredit apparent beneficial changes stemming from non-analytic therapy or explorations in psychoanalytic therapy on a short-term basis. Their representation by critics as transference cures with pejorative connotations had to give way to recognition of the fact that favorable personality changes in short-term treatment were often stable and significant, at least as much as if not more so than the long-term treatment so often claimed, often unwarrantedly, to be superior. Eventually a number of therapists, who had previously adhered to conventional points of view, acknowledged benefits through modified and short-term treatment ventures which others had long recognized and described before them (6). During the past two decades, at least, it has also become clear that modifications in psychoanalytic procedures were practiced far more in psychotherapy than had been evident and acknowledged in published writings. The actual practice of what is often called classical psychoanalysis was seen to be less prevalent then ordinarily believed (71).

The many differences of opinion about method and theory had grown considerably by the middle of this century in the United States. Cleavages occurred and enclaves developed among those identified with psychoanalysis, so that several separate groups were established and functioned as self-contained units. While some premises were shared, usually the differences were stressed. Yet at the same time the basic principles of psychoanalytic thought became integrated into the broad practice and development of psychotherapy within psychiatry as a medical specialty.

The Influence of Deviations from Freud

Two early major defections from the Freudian circle during the second decade of this century were those of Carl Jung and Alfred Adler. Jung had been interested in word association studies and schizophrenia, and had discussed concepts of extroversion and introversion. The idea of a collective unconscious is closely identified with him. Various differences in addition to the personal have been mentioned to account at least in part for the separation of Freud and Jung, among them the latter's disagreement with basic Freudian sexual theories, a greater concern with ego functioning, more interest in spiritual components of personality functioning, an inclination toward mystical ideas, a basic family medical tradition and Protestant influence, the influence of Eugen Bleuler and Pierre Janet, experimental and clinical psychology, and a special concern with the psychoses rather than the neuroses (64). It is of interest that many people concerned with psychoanalytic issues and psychotherapy are aware of Jung, but not of the details of his work. The latter are not nearly as widely known and understood in depth, and in the United States it is details of his reputation more than his contributions that are grasped. His followers in America have been comparatively few, and if any one comment were offered by those who have not been his adherents, it would often be that Jung and his ideas are too mystical.

Circumstances surrounding the second major break with Freud in the second decade of this century were somewhat different. Alfred Adler was concerned with general feelings of inferiority, ideas of organ inferiority, strivings for superiority, and drive toward power in its various forms. He was much involved with problems of children (5). Most of his major contributions were made before he visited the United States in the 1920's and his subsequent travels between the United States and Europe. After 1926 and until his death in 1937 he spent the academic year in the United States and the months of June to September in Vienna (4). Hall, who had invited Freud and Jung to lecture at Clark University, became a student of Adler's writings and regarded the idea of compensation for feelings of inferiority as the most important key for psychology. He felt sex anxieties were symbolic of this deeper sense of abatement of the will to live. In some areas Hall had anticipated Adler's views. They had interests in common in order of birth, early recollections, pampering and neglect of children, attention seeking, the frequent wish of girls to be boys. Hall wished to have Adler deliver a series of lectures five years after Freud had done so, but the outbreak of World War I prevented this (8).

Adler's views faded into the background for a while, but by midcentury they gained attention increasingly. Clinic and teaching centers focusing on Adlerian concepts were built in several major cities in the United States, but while the designations "individual psychology" for Adlerian ideas and "analytical psychology" for the Jungian are known to professional people, they are less familiar to the general public than is psychoanalysis. Strong supporters of individual psychology have contended that so-called neo-Freudians should more properly be called neo-Adlerians (9). Assertions have been made, for example, about the influence of Adler on the outlook of Karen Horney, the leading figure in another psychoanalytic faction. She recognized the claims regarding this link as far as some of her proposals were concerned. But in one of her works she said that despite some similarities, her interpretations rested fundamentally on Freudian grounds and saw Adler's views as somewhat one-sided (59). Yet it has also been said that after additional work on her own ideas, the debt to Adler was eventually acknowledged (134). Points that come through in Horney's writings are that Freud's outlook was basically pessimistic in contrast to her own optimism, and that the focal point in her view of neurosis is often reflected in the idea of a struggle toward self-realization (60). Concurrently, Harry Stack Sullivan was making an impression on segments of American psychiatry by stressing the fundamental importance of interpersonal relations and their disturbances as influences on neurotic development. An assessment of the man and his work emphasizes that Sullivan's thinking differed from that of Freud by its avoiding seeing man and his culture as opposed to one another. His greatest contribution may have been in the demonstration that schizophrenics could be helped by psychotherapy consisting of modifications of classical analysis (35).

Another interesting figure in the early 20th century American scene was Paul Schilder, who emigrated from Europe to the United States and spent a decade in research at Bellevue Psychiatric Hospital in New York. He had described *encephalitis periaxialis diffusa* when he was but 26 years old. Although he published, among others, books on psychotherapy and the brain and personality, he apparently considered, as did others, his most important book to be *The Image and Appearance of the Human Body* (3). He seemed to be strongly anchored in a biological organismic orientation on a psychoanalytic basis and is quoted as having often said that it would be a mistake to believe that phenomenology and psychoanalysis could be separated from brain pathology—that there was no gap between the organic and the functional (67).

Adolf Meyer and Psychobiology

While the names of psychiatrists identified with psychoanalysis and its deviating factions have been especially well known in the United

States because of the considerable impact the subject itself had on psychiatric thought and practice in addition to the general publicity, Adolf Meyer (Plate XCIX) was mentioned often as the leading psychiatrist in America during the first half of this century. He was born in Zurich and emigrated in 1892. He served as a pathologist in mental hospitals in Kankakee and Worcester, and became Director of the New York State Psychiatric Institute. As one study of him put it, he went to Kankakee frankly to obtain brain material and departed two and a half years later with a professional commitment to the

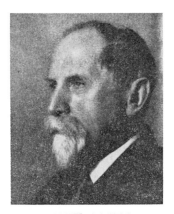

PLATE XCIX. Adolf Meyer.

hospitalized patient (138). From 1910 to 1941 Meyer served as professor of psychiatry at The Johns Hopkins University. He thought of mental illness in terms of an amalgam of biological, historical, social, and psychological forces. For him illness was divided into reaction types, rather than diseases. He introduced a technical terminology involving *"ergasias,"* but it was short-lived. The "common sense" concept is identified with him. The life history of the patient was for Meyer the important focus of attention in any study of personality development, and schizophrenia, for example, was seen as the outgrowth of progressive maladjustment, poor adaptations, and uneven personality growth (130). The views of Adolf Meyer were subsumed under the term "psychobiology," and these ideas were influential in the development of psychiatric education in American medical schools, also favorably influencing hospital organization. The psychobiological outlook fused structural and psychological elements in the investigation of the total patient, stressing a holistic orientation with the patient seen as a unitary, functioning individual within his social matrix. In his time, Meyer was the strongest link between the medical psychology of Europe and America. It is probably correct to say that his teachings became so firmly a part of American psychiatric theory and practice that in time the range of his influence was often overlooked (77).

Mental Hygiene, Psychosomatics, and Insulin Therapy

Other developments important for the enrichment of American psychiatry were taking place concurrently. Clifford Whittingham Beers, who had experienced at first hand the plight of severe mental illness, was at the forefront of the growth and expansion of the mental hygiene movement early in the 20th century, and his autobiography was widely read (16).

Adolf Meyer was credited with applying the term "mental hygiene" to this development. In the realm of psychiatric and psychoanalytic publication, Smith Ely Jeliffe, whose interests were identified in part with "psychosomatic medicine," edited *The Journal of Nervous and Mental Disease* and *The Psychoanalytic Review* for many years. He was concerned with the integration of psychoanalytic concepts into a dynamic psychiatry and has also been referred to as the father of American psychosomatic medicine (82). Jeliffe's co-editor was William Alanson White, prominent in the development of American psychiatry during the first part of this century and for many years superintendent of Saint Elizabeth Hospital in Washington, D.C. A record of some aspects of the psychiatric scene comes through in White's *Outlines of Psychiatry*, first published in 1908. It was favorably received, and frequently reappeared in new editions (74). This record is found also in White's autobiography (135). He was regarded as the type of psychiatrist capable of getting along with others of divergent thought and practice, an ability not always to be taken as routine and widespread.

The early introduction and growth of psychoanalysis in the United States was much identified with A. A. Brill, who translated many of Freud's writings into English. Brill was often involved in the controversies of that time.

But it was not just psychoanalysis which engendered considerable controversy on the American scene. Manfred Sakel introduced insulin shock treatment for schizophrenia in 1927 in Europe. It then made an impact on the hospital practice of psychiatry in the United States, and in a way that paralleled arguments about psychoanalytic technique, there were differences of opinion regarding insulin shock. These centered not only on the treatment in general but on claims about greater effectiveness of the original methods of application versus various modifications of the original techniques, the classical or traditional procedures as opposed to deviations from them. Thus in assessing claims and achievements there is reason to believe that what innovators bring to their therapeutic endeavors technically and psychologically has important implications, and these implications pertain to excessive claims as well as to truly effective results. Not only did some psychiatrists feel that the atmosphere of despair in psychiatric hospitals was changed, but it was felt that insulin shock as a turning point in psychiatric treatment supplied the impetus for the introduction of subsequent physiological measures such as electric and metrazol shock (58).

6

MIDDLE 20TH CENTURY

Electroshock Therapy and Psychosurgery

It was electroshock therapy that turned out to have significant, widespread, and more lasting appeal than insulin or metrazol therapy. Electroshock was generally felt to be particularly effective with some types of depressions. While in Vienna, for example, the "classical procedure" for insulin shock in schizophrenia still remained in favor, it was rapidly losing its following in the United States along with its modifications. The time, effort, and proper facilities required undoubtedly had their share in the discouragement, but there were questions also about theoretical issues, the problems of recurrences, and concern about failure to incorporate psychotherapeutic measures for maintenance of stability at a time when psychotherapy itself was gaining in popularity and a secure place in the theoretical and practical aspects of psychiatric practice. While studies were done and conjectures supplied on the neurophysiological basis for the effectiveness of electroshock treatment, there was concurrent emphasis in the United States among psychotherapy enthusiasts on the possible psychological implications of electroshock that could account for its results. This stress on conjectured psychodynamics did not necessarily play a role, however, in the psychotherapy that at times accompanied electroshock. In any case the concurrent psychotherapy was not used as often by some as it was encouraged by others. Again, the stress on a formal or structured psychotherapy in this instance was in keeping with the widespread emphasis on psychotherapy in the United States in mid-century. And this influence played a role too on the insistence in some quarters that insulin coma and its variations had to be evaluated in terms of the entire psychological milieu in which it was applied, and in terms of the psychodynamic implications of the procedure itself for the patient.

The situation was different as far as psychosurgery is concerned. Various surgical procedures were introduced into the United States and employed after Egas Moniz, the Lisbon neurologist, in collaboration with the surgeon Almeida Lima, presented in 1936 their work with leucotomy (46). The frontal lobes were a focus of attention following which several operative sites were explored as additional operative techniques were devised. The diversified means of destroying areas of brain tissue, and the irreversibility of the effects produced, played a significant role in the hesitancy of many psychiatrists to regard such measures favorably. The usual disagreements arose over benefits achieved versus harm produced. Although psychological studies were done on patients experiencing psychosurgical procedures, the main interest in such operations was to be found largely among those psychiatrists described as neurologically oriented. It could be expected that considerable criticism would be generated largely among psychiatrists favoring psychological methods of treatment, but condemnation of the tissue destroying approach was voiced also by others (12). By late mid-century, with increasing public concern about, and pressures on, medical practice, psychosurgery drew attention again, not only in terms of its continuation rather than demise, but with anxiety over its potential abuse for political and social controls (7). Surgery for control over violence and aggression in patients came under attack in an effort to fend off possible undesirable control and limitation of an individual's freedom, just as the issue of involuntary hospitalization and treatment without consent grew to be a major issue in hospital practice. In any case, while psychosurgery was approaching its height of application in mid-century, it was predicted that if chemotherapeutic measures proved to be significant, they might lead to a lessening of surgical interventions. This evidently did occur.

While surgical procedures can be traced back to trepanations performed as part of magico-religious systems in very ancient times, the more recent psychosurgical techniques are not quite the only surgical methods of modern times. In the United States, for example, Henry Cotton, starting about 1922, centered attention on focal infection and its alleged role in the etiology of mental illness. He advocated removal of teeth, tonsils, and finally colons. Choosing optimistically to see what he believed to be a relatively bright side of this picture, an observer claimed that at least one achievement in such treatment was its encouragement of some interest in mental disease among doctors who were not specialists in psychiatry.

Psychology, Social Work, and Psychotherapy

It has been possible to trace certain aspects of the development of psychiatry, with its advances and recessions, including divergent points of view and treatment methods, in the records of individual hospitals (131). There have been intuitive predictions during the course of this development. One example is the awareness of the neuropathological laboratory as a fundamental unit in many hospitals at the turn of the century, followed in 1907 by William A. White's focus of attention in an annual report of Saint Elizabeth Hospital on the establishment of a psychology department. He considered this one of the advanced trends in psychiatry at that time, and he predicted that it would be as necessary a part of the psychiatric unit as the pathology laboratory had been up to that point (61). Growth in the relationship between psychology and psychiatry went far beyond that. Not only did psychology become integrated into research and diagnostic activities in hospital settings, but it moved beyond hospital walls into clinics. With the advances in clinical psychology, especially after World War II, it surged into the field of therapy, at first under the control and guidance of psychiatrists, and then more and more on its own course, parallel to or overlapping the psychotherapeutic field of operation of the psychiatrists. As the number of clinical psychologists increased, there came the establishment of organizations, clinics, and training institutes, and the assumption of a significant place in the sector of mental health services offered to the general public. In the United States, as a result, the conflicts, differences of opinion, and complex problems associated with the acceptance of this role for clinical psychologists and its significance for psychiatry as a medical specialty have become very much a part of the recent history of psychiatry. To a lesser degree this path has applied to social workers participating in private practice as psychotherapists, following their role of service in hospitals and as part of the psychiatrist-psychologist-social worker team in the operation of expanding mental hygiene or psychiatric clinics which functioned within hospitals or under local governmental auspices, or independently, and more and more so after World War II. The move in the direction of the role of psychotherapist has, in any case, played a significant part, undoubtedly, in organization of a newer team approach such as in crisis therapy groups, in which the "primary" therapist may be a doctor, psychologist, social worker, nurse, or a member of some other ancillary group. Historically, the concept of psychiatric social work in the United States is believed to have been introduced with the publication in 1922 of *The Kingdom of Evils,* by Elmer E. Southard and Mary C. Jarett (38). It is difficult to conceive of the emergence of present-day community mental health centers and community psychiatry without the psychiatric social worker trend as forerunner. The impetus for the psychiatric social work movement apparently emerged from World War I, during which a course of lectures on psychiatry was given to social workers at Smith College by Southard, who was Director of the Boston Psychopathic Hospital.

Psychiatry and the General Public

The expansion of the mental hygiene movement and the mounting interest of the general public in psychiatric issues were accompanied by a flood of books on psychological themes for the general reader. Most were and are now of questionable value. A few have been of definitely good quality and influence. Two examples are *The Human Mind* and *Discovering Ourselves,* the latter by Edward A. Strecker, a former president of the American Psychiatric Association (20, 81). By mid-century such books often stressed concepts of dynamic psychiatry, which was mentioned in the past as a term never defined precisely, but which began to be used more and more from about 1915 onward (79). Eventually, however, it was generally assumed to imply an incorporation of some of the basic premises of psychoanalytic theory. It might be added parenthetically that "psychiatrist" had been used before the middle of the 19th century and was often encountered by 1895, although "alienist" was a designation frequently acceptable in the United States during the second half of the 19th century.

An important book not of the popular variety, but on the contrary a scholarly work, was *The Mentally Ill in America,* carrying the subtitle, *A History of Their Care and Treatment from Colonial Times.* It appeared initially in 1937 and was reprinted several times. Albert Deutsch, its author, was a well known writer who, while capable of preparing studious research of this type, was also able to serve influentially as an intermediary between experts in the mental health field and the general public. He accomplished this through magazine articles and newspaper columns. In this respect he was an important figure in the field of social psychiatry and the mental health movement, and he contributed to the drive for better care and understanding of the emotionally ill (68). William A. White wrote the introduction to Deutsch's book, and felt that his approach to his subject as a social historian rather than as a psychiatrist added an objective view "free from the temptations of professional partisanship." Deutsch's work was seen as an extension of the types of contributions, incorporating social conscience, of prime movers such as Dorothea Dix and Clifford Beers.

World War II and Subspecialization

During World War II the need for psychiatric services increased enormously and the armed forces had to utilize the abilities of, and to train, non-psychiatric physicians to fill the demands. Psychiatry as a specialty received a great deal of attention. At the same time there was pressure for recognition of its full value. William C. Menninger had an important part in these developments, placing psychiatry on an equal footing with medicine and surgery when he became Director of the Neuropsychiatric Consultant's Division in the Surgeon General's office (14).

After World War II, psychiatry became increasingly subspecialized. One major division, child psychiatry, started with the care and training of the mentally retarded, an area of concern especially emphasized during the years 1846 to 1909 (78). There was concurrent interest in child study with stress on education, and then from 1909 to 1919 attention turned to problems of delinquency among children. The Chicago Juvenile Psychopathic Institute was founded by William Healy in 1909. It pioneered child guidance clinics and has been regarded as the first clinic for children which incorporated psychiatric, psychological, and social disciplines, although there was a Psychological Clinic at the University of Pennsylvania which was started in 1896 by Lightner Witmer (21). Child guidance clinics were formed rapidly from about 1919 onward. In addition in-patient and out-patient services in psychopathic, state, and general hospitals developed as well as various types of schools and institutions for children with psychiatric problems. Although there was often a major emphasis on psychopathology, some centers engaged in intensive evaluations of normal development. The latter is well represented by Arnold Gesell, who directed the Clinic of Child Development at Yale (48).

During the 1950's psychopharmacology experienced a steadily increasing growth. In mid-century American psychiatry became essentially tripartite. The three-fold pattern consisted mainly of a physical approach characterized by psychosurgical measures and electroconvulsive treatments, a chemical approach reflected in psychopharmacology, and a psychological orientation reflected in various forms of psychotherapy. There was some overlapping in theory and practice, but practitioners tend to adhere largely or exclusively to their favored methods. Extremists among them possess little or no interest in the thinking, investigation, and clinical activities of others, while the more moderate favor their own interests, but observe the work of others and maintain a measure of professional contact with them. The physicians stressing physical methods find their origins among the 17th century iatrophysicists, known also as iatromechanists and iatromathematicians (among whom Giovanni Alfonso Borelli and Giorgio Baglivi were prominent). The iatrochemists were represented by Franz de le Boë. Then, as now, adherents to such views were at times more so in theory than in practice, where greater flexibility was displayed (119). The term iatropsychology, recently introduced, parallels iatrophysics and iatrochemistry, and iatropsychologists deal mainly with psychological concepts in medicine (110). Iatropsychology appears to have reached its height in the United States in mid-century, with its presence felt mostly in psychiatry and its influence most evident in the attention to psychosomatics. A precursor of the iatropsychologists is George Ernst Stahl, the late 17th and early 18th century proponent of animism, perhaps the predecessor of vitalism. Following Stahl was Franz Anton Mesmer, whose animal magnetism was basically a psychotherapeutic technique, regardless of its theoretical foundations. Then there was Sigmund Freud, whose work set the stage for the most extensive advance of iatropsychology in theory and practice. The compartmentalization into iatropsychology, iatrophysics, and iatrochemistry became most marked in mid-century psychiatry, while the fusing of chemical, physical, and psychological measures was probably greater among psychologically oriented general physicians than among many subspecialized psychiatrists. A trend toward merging of two of the components of psychiatric practice was discernible when iatropsychologically inclined psychiatrists rejected some physical treatment measures because of their adverse psychological implications and discovered the ease of incorporating some of the chemical measures into psychological treatment settings. The latter was accompanied by the more recent directions of research with its focus on neurochemistry. A greater unitary quality in psychiatry may yet supplant the aforementioned tripartite image with even greater stress on the holistic view of medicine.

The term "psychosomatic medicine" had been mentioned early in the 19th century, but it became increasingly popular after 1935 (41, 133). Stanley Cobb, however, saw psychiatrists persisting in giving lip-service to a monistic concept of the human organism while retaining dualistic views (30). Promoting the idea of health and illness as reactions of an organism to complex internal and external environments, he recognized the worth of Walter B. Cannon for his investigations into the physiology of the emotions (26). Cobb felt that 20th century psychosomatic medicine was a reaction against the emphasis on laboratory medicine during the second half of the 19th century (29). In clinical areas, Sir William Osler had been singled out as more interested in the "organic" than the "functional" diseases of the nervous system by Lewellys Barker, his successor in Baltimore. Barker believed Osler's views were consistent with his pathological-anatomical rather than pathological-physiological background, and Barker made a point of his own interest in propagating the importance of psychotherapy (13). While Sir Clifford Albutt and medical historian Fielding H. Garrison stressed what they regarded as the unfortunate separation of medicine and surgery centuries ago, a similar issue existed in the opinion of many others as far as the separation of psychiatry from medicine was concerned (47, 65, 101).

Additional Treatment Methods and Modifications

Psychiatry is deluged at present with countless treatment methods and modifications. Some of them are questionable, since their proponents are doubtfully "therapists" in the true or traditional sense— within the context, at least, of medical disciplines. Controversy on this score is expanding. Varieties of group therapy are implicated. "Group therapy" may first have appeared as a special term according to one account only as recently as 1931 (34). Its modern beginnings, however, are ascribed frequently to the activities, at the turn of this century, of internist Joseph H. Pratt in his work with groups of patients whom he was trying to help with emotional problems connected with tuberculosis. While its original intent may have been as a time-saving measure primarily, its psychological potentialities in a broader sense were recognized and investigations were encouraged by William Alanson White after the first World War. A psychoanalytic orientation was of interest to Paul Schilder (54). The issue of appropriate controls is of much concern. A familiar declaration of such concern is evident in claims to the effect that participation in T-groups or their derivative encounter, sensitivity, confrontation, and marathon groups can predispose to psychopathological reactions, including psychoses (66). Such predispositions may be relevant to countless treatment measures and the stress on caution had long been placed on hypnotherapeutic involvements. It is worth noting, incidentally, that from a historical point of view it was not the application of hypnotic methods during World War II which led to its scientific growth, because narcoanalysis and narcosynthesis were in far greater use in keeping with their amenability to the training of physicians who had to be prepared rapidly for wartime emergencies (51). It was after the war that clinical and experimental hypnosis attracted widespread scientific interest and the significant broader involvement of psychiatrists and psychologists under the motivating force of the founding of The Society for Clinical and Experimental Hypnosis in 1949. After a long history of assessment by investigative commissions of official bodies, the best known of which was the French Royal Commission of 1784 (which included Benjamin Franklin among its members and which rendered an essentially unfavorable report on mesmerism), the American Medical Association issued a favorable official statement in 1958 after the British Medical Association had already done so three years earlier. In the midst of the wrangling over what is or is not valid therapy or good therapy or properly trained and functioning therapists, the reforms of Dorothea Dix and those who came before her and after seem at times to melt away in the face of a continuing wasting away of countless mentally ill in ill-equipped and ill-cared for mental hospitals and other facilities as daily newspapers reveal to the public, periodically and often sensationally, today as they did in former times.

New Opinions, Problems, and the Social Scene

After the 1950's, with the expansion of psychopharmacology, much publicity was given to the decrease in size of hospital populations. Patients were given maintenance dosages of medications while attending after-care clinics or while securing medications privately without recourse to hospitalization at all. But the social climate was changing too, and especially among young adults enclaves were developing in various parts of the country in which behavior regarded as bizarre or eccentric and abnormal by others was accepted by peers and not labelled in psychiatric diagnostic terms. The point at issue then is the attitude and point of view adopted toward statistics of hospital populations and incidence of mental disorder. To complicate matters further, with greater stress on the individual's rights and liberties, and a questioning of the medical model in assessments of behavior, the very existence of "mental illness" was questioned in some quarters (97). To some extent the issue may be a matter of preference in labelling apart from matters of personal freedom and involuntary incarceration. In addition, matters of practical expediency may be involved insofar as rights and restrictions of professional functioning are concerned. The following appears to be greater among psychologists, for example, than among psychiatrists in support of the notion of "the myth of mental illness."

At mid-century an assessment was made of psychiatric treatment under the auspices of the Association for Research in Nervous and Mental Disease. While recognizing that therapy must encompass the individual, his family, and his social environment, various psychological, social, pharmacological, electrical, and neurosurgical procedures were evaluated (140). During the past two decades there has been additional stress on the first three areas and a falling off of interest in the last two, especially the neurosurgical approaches, although in some quarters efforts in the latter have not waned. While vogues in therapies have come and gone, an underpinning of ancillary services has stayed on. Apart from the professional field of psychiatric nursing, one major area, for example, has been occupational therapy, the complex features of which were presented by William Rush Dunton, Jr. (42).

Prior to the recent emphasis on community psychiatry there was much talk of social psychiatry. Thomas Rennie emphasized a few decades ago that it certainly did not imply a new kind of psychiatry. It reflected a greater attention to contributions by sociologists, anthropologists, and psychiatrists to the interrelationships of their problems and disciplines, converging on issues of psychiatric care and evaluations. These cross-disciplinary evaluations have continued to develop (70, 87). This has affected increasingly and appropriately even the very special, structured doctor-patient relationship which is influenced by the cultural matrix with respect to acquired orientation to disease, treatment, and cure (129). The more extensive and intensive explorations of these issues have not replaced the parallel studies of genetic substrates epitomized, for example, in the work of Franz Kallman, known for his studies using the "twin family methods" which he developed, and for his publications which included *The Genetic Theory of Schizophrenia*. A former director of the New York State Psychiatric Institute, with which Kallman was associated, pointed out that there was very little activity in the field of genetics in American psychiatry in 1936, and with the arrival of Kallman, who was born in Germany, it was possible to start the first full-time medical genetics department in a psychiatric institution in the United States (76).

Concern about economic as well as cultural influences on behavioral problems has affected attitudes toward hospitalization and imprisonment. The point stressed is that people in better economic and social circumstances are less likely to be subject to both. Furthermore, the serious limitations in availability of proper treatment facilities have highlighted the issue of patients' rights and the entire question of involuntary hospitalization. The outmoded M'Naughten Rules of 1843 are still adhered to widely, but they have been questioned and attacked more and more (although there is no general agreement on replacements). In 1954 one of the leading contenders emerged as a result of the *Durham* v. *United States* case which was commented on by William O. Douglas, of the United States Supreme Court. The point involved was that the "right and wrong" as well as the "irresistable impulse" tests of insanity as defenses in criminal cases be replaced by the view that an unlawful act does not carry with it criminal responsibility if it is the product of mental disease or defect (40). This concept did not attract universal support. While there were attempts in the past at cooperation between the legal and medical professions (and in another area, physicians and clergymen), such efforts have grown in recent years. But with a mountingly complex society, the problems at issue have become more and more difficult to fathom and work out.

Psychiatry, A Problem in Perspective

Some points mentioned in my book, *A History of Psychiatry,* published more than a decade ago, probably still apply in the opinion of many historians. It was said then that the scientist and educator James B. Conant stressed the high degree of empiricism in the practical application of sciences dealing with human behavior. At midcentury, according to Conant, the future appeared to be promising, but psychologists and anthropologists must concede that available conceptual schemes were the equivalent of those within grasp of chemists and physicists of the late 18th century (31). Relevant also to any historical account is Sir William Dampier's observation that such accounts stress successes and theories that survive for a time, but that an impression of a series of triumphs is misleading. The many failures match the successes (36). And the view expressed in my book about the development of psychiatry still applies. It reflects advances and retrogressions and periods of relative light and relative darkness, with evaluations of such periods changing to lesser or greater extent from time to time because much depends on perspective, the perspective conditioned in turn by leading opinions and fashions of the time. And it is no easy task to rise above the tides and pressures of contemporary conformity.

Many psychiatrists would probably agree essentially with remarks concerning the current status of the mental health field regarding its encompassing an expanse of studies that include genetics; molecular, general, medical and neurobiology; psychology, social psychology, and psychoanalysis; sociology and anthropology; and administrative sciences (96). At the same time, taking into consideration the best in the development of psychiatry and its growth amidst other fields of medical specialization, psychiatry is presenting for many of its researchers and practitioners a blurred image of the place it now holds and may hold in the future as a medical specialty within the broad area of mental health groups and in the context of the widespread pressures and surge of diverse mental health activities. Like all else, however, it will have to meet the challenge of changing times and adapt itself as well as possible to them.

REFERENCES

1. ABRAHAM, J. J. (1933): *Lettsom*. London: William Heinemann.
2. ACKERKNECHT, E. H. (1955): *A Short History of Medicine*. New York: Ronald Press.
3. ADLER, ALEXANDRA (1965): The work of Paul Schilder. *Bull. N. Y. Acad. Med.*, 41, 841.
4. ADLER,, ALEXANDRA (1970): Recollections of my father. *Amer. J. Psychiat.*, 127, 71.
5. ADLER, ALFRED (1931): *What Life Should Mean To You*. New York: Grosset and Dunlap.
6. ALEXANDER, F. (1955): Discussion of Paul H. Hoch: aims and limitations of psychotherapy. *Amer. J. Psychiat.*, 112, 321.
7. Anonymous (1972): Two views of neurological surgery clash at meeting. *J. Amer. Med. Assn.*, 220, 17.
8. ANSBACHER, H. L. (1971): Alfred Adler and G. Stanley Hall: correspondence and general relationship. *J. Hist. Behav. Sci.*, 7, 337.
9. ANSBACHER, H. L. AND ANSBACHER, R. R. (1956): *The Individual Psychology of Alfred Adler*. New York: Basic Books.
10. ASHBURN, P. M. (1929): *A History of the Medical Department of the United States Army*. Boston: Houghton Mifflin.
11. BAILEY, P. (1956): Janet and Freud. *A. M. A. Arch. Neurol. Psychiat.*, 76, 76.
12. BAILEY, P. (1956): The great psychiatric revolution. *Amer. J. Psychiat.*, 113, 387.

13. BARKER, L. F. (1942): *Time and the Physician*. New York: G. P. Putnam's Sons.
14. BARTON, W. E., BROSIN, H. W. AND FARRELL, M. J. (1966): William Claire Menninger 1899-1966. *Amer. J. Psychiat.*, 123, 614.
15. BEARD, G. M. (1880): *A Practical Treatise on Nervous Exhaustion (Neurasthenia), its Symptoms, Nature, Sequences, Treatment*. New York: William Wood.
16. BEERS, C. W. (1910): *A Mind That Found Itself* (2nd ed.). New York: Longmans.
17. BETT, W. R. (1957): Isaac Ray (1807-81) of "Ray's Mania." *Med. Press.*, 237, 62.
18. BOCKOVEN, J. S. (1963): *Moral Treatment in American Psychiatry*. New York: Springer Publishing Company.
19. BOND, E. D. (1947): *Dr. Kirkbride and His Mental Hospital*. Philadelphia: J. B. Lippincott Company.
20. BOND, E. D. (1959): Edward A. Strecker, M. D. 1886-1959. *Amer. J. Psychiat.*, 115, 959.
21. BORING, E. G. (1950): *A History of Experimental Psychology* (2nd ed.). New York: Appleton-Century-Crofts.
22. BREUER, J. AND FREUD, S. (1895): *Studies on Hysteria* (new ed.). New York: Basic Books.
23. BURNHAM, J. C. (1967): *Psychoanalysis and American Medicine, 1894-1918: Medicine, Science, and Culture. Psychological Issues*, Vol. 5, No. 4, Monograph 20. New York: International Universities Press.
24. BUTTERFIELD, L. H. (1946): Benjamin Rush: a physician as seen in his letters. *Bull. Hist. Med.*, 20, 138.
25. BUTTERFIELD, L. H. (1951): *Letters of Benjamin Rush*. Princeton: Princeton University Press.
26. CANNON, W. B. (1929): *Bodily Changes in Pain, Hunger, Fear and Rage*. New York: D. Appleton and Company.
27. CARLSON, E. T. (1956): Amariah Brigham: 1. life and works. *Amer. J. Psychiat.*, 112, 83; (1957) 2. psychiatric thought and practice. *Amer. J. Psychiat.*, 113, 911.
28. CASAMAJOR, L. (1943): Notes for an intimate history of neurology and psychiatry in America. *J. Nerv. Ment. Dis.*, 98, 600.
29. COBB, S. (1948): One hundred years of progress in neurology, psychiatry, and neurosurgery. *Arch. Neurol. and Psychiat.*, 59, 63.
30. COBB, S. (1957): Monism in psychosomatic medicine. *Psychosom. Med.*, 19, 177.
31. CONANT, J. B. (1951): *Science and Common Sense*. New Haven, Conn.: Yale University Press.
32. CORNER, B. C. (1951): *William Shippen, Jr., Pioneer in American Medical Education*. Philadelphia: American Philosophical Society.
33. CORNER, G. W. (1948): *The Autobiography of Benjamin Rush*. Princeton: Princeton University Press.
34. CORSINI, R. J. (1955): Historical background of group psychotherapy: a critique. *Gr. Psychother.*, 3, 219.
35. CROWLEY, R. M. (1971): Harry Stack Sullivan: his contributions to current psychiatric thought and practice. Nutley, N. J.: Hoffman-La Roche.
36. DAMPIER, W. C. (1944): *A Shorter History of Science*. Cambridge: Cambridge University Press.
37. DEUTSCH, A. (1944): *The Mentally Ill in America*. New York: Columbia University Press.
38. DEUTSCH, A. (1944): A history of mental hygiene. In: Hall, J. K. (ed.), *One Hundred Years of American Psychiatry*. New York: Columbia University Press.

39. Diamond, B. L. (1956): Isaac Ray and the trial of Daniel M'Naughten. *Amer. J. Psychiat.,* 112, 651.

40. Douglas, W. O. (1956): *Law and Psychiatry.* New York: William Alanson White Institute of Psychiatry.

41. Dunbar, H. F. (1935): *Emotions and Bodily Changes, A Survey of Literature on Psychosomatic Interrelationships.* New York: Columbia University Press.

42. Dunton, W. R., Jr. and Licht, S. (eds.) (1950): *Occupational Therapy, Principles and Practice.* Springfield, Ill.: Charles C Thomas.

43. Earnest, E. (1950): *S. Weir Mitchell, Novelist and Physician.* Philadelphia: University of Pennsylvania Press.

44. Evans, R. B. (1971): *The Journal of American Psychology:* a pioneering psychological journal. *J. Hist. Behav. Sci.,* 7, 283.

45. Flexner, J. T. (1939): *Doctors on Horseback.* New York: Garden City Publishing Company.

46. Freeman, W., and Watts, J. W. (1950): *Psychosurgery in the Treatment of Mental Disorders and Intractable Pain.* Springfield, Ill.: Charles C Thomas.

47. Garrison, F. H. (1929): *Introduction to the History of Medicine.* Philadelphia: Saunders.

48. Gesell, A. (1952): Autobiography. In: Langfeld, H. S., Boring, E. G., Werner, H., and Yerkes, R. M. (eds.), *A History of Psychology in Autobiography,* Vol. 4. Worcester, Mass.: Clark University Press.

49. Gildea, M. C.-L., and Gildea, E. F. (1945): Personalities of American psychotherapists, Mitchell, Salmon, Riggs. *Amer. J. Psychiat.,* 101, 460.

50. Goodman, N. G. (1934): *Benjamin Rush.* Philadelphia: University of Pennsylvania Press.

51. Grinker, R. R. and Spiegel, J. P. (1943): *War Neuroses in North Africa.* New York: Josiah Macy, Jr. Foundation.

52. Grob, G. N. (1962): Samuel B. Woodward and the practice of psychiatry in early nineteenth-century America. *Bull. Hist. Med.,* 36, 420.

53. Grob, G. N. (1966): The state mental hospital in mid-nineteenth century America: a social analysis. *Amer. Psychol.,* 21, 510.

54. Hadden, S. B. (1955): Historic background of group psychotherapy. *Int. J. Gr. Psychother.,* 5, 162.

55. Hale, N. G., Jr. (1971): *James Jackson Putnam and Psychoanalysis: Letters Between Putnam and Sigmund Freud, Ernest Jones, William James, Sandor Ferenczi, and Morton Prince, 1877-1917.* Cambridge, Mass.: Harvard University Press.

56. Hale, N. G., Jr. (1971): *Freud and the Americans, 1876-1917,* Vol. 1. New York: Oxford University Press.

57. Haymaker, W. (1953): Silas Weir Mitchell (1829-1914). In: Haymaker, W. (ed.), *The Founders of Neurology.* Springfield, Ill.: Charles C Thomas.

58. Hoff, H. (1958): Foreword. In: Sakel, M., *Schizophrenia.* New York: Philosophical Library.

59. Horney, K. (1937): *The Neurotic Personality of Our Time.* New York: W .W. Norton.

60. Horney, K. (1950): *Neurosis and Human Growth.* New York: W. W. Norton.

61. Ives, M. (1957): Fifty years of hospital psychology. *Amer. Psychol.,* 12, 150.

62. Johnstone, R. W. (1959): William Cullen. *Med. Hist.,* 3, 33.

63. Jones, E. (1953-57): *The Life and Work of Sigmund Freud,* 3 Vols. New York: Basic Books.

64. Jung, C. G. (1961): *Memories, Dreams, Reflections.* New York: Pantheon Books.

65. Kagan, S. R. (1929): *Life and Letters of Fielding H. Garrison.* Boston: Medico-Historical Press.

66. Kane, F. J., Wallace, C. D., and Lipton, M. A. (1971): Emotional disturbances related to T- group experience. *Amer. J. Psychiat.,* 127, 954.

67. KAUFMAN, M. R. (1962): Schilder's application of psychoanalytic psychiatry. *Arch. Gen. Psychiat.*, 7, 311.
68. KENWORTHY, M. E. (1962): Albert Deutsch (1905-1961). *Amer. J. Psychiat.*, 118, 1064.
69. KLOTTER, A. S. (1957): California mental hospitals. *Bull. Med. Libr. Assn.*, 45, 159.
70. KLUCKHORN, C., AND MURRAY, H. A. (eds.) (1948): *Personality in Nature, Society, and Culture.* New York: Alfred A. Knopf.
71. KNIGHT, R. P. (1953): The present status of organized psychoanalysis in the United States. *J. Amer. Psychoanal. Assn.*, 1, 197.
72. LEBENSOHN, Z. M. (1962): American psychiatry—retrospect and prospect. *Med. Ann. D. C.*, 31, 379.
73. LEWIS, N. D. C. (1942): *A Short History of Psychiatry.* London: Chapman and Hall.
74. LEWIS, N. D. C. (1956): Review of the scientific publications from Saint Elizabeths Hospital during the past 100 years (centennial papers). Washington, D.C.: Saint Elizabeths Hospital.
75. LEWIS, N. D. C. (1958): Historical roots of psychiatry. *Amer. J. Psychiat.*, 114, 795.
76. LEWIS, N. D. C. (1966): Franz Joseph Kallman 1897-1965. *Amer. J. Psychiat.*, 123, 105.
77. LIDZ, T. (1966): Adolf Meyer and the development of American psychiatry. *Amer. J. Psychiat.*, 123, 320.
78. LOWREY, L. G. (1944): Psychiatry for children, a brief history of developments. *Amer. J. Psychiat.*, 101, 375.
79. LOWREY, L. G. (1955): The contribution of orthopsychiatry to psychiatry: brief historical note. *Amer. J. Orthopsychiat.*, 25, 475.
80. MARTI-IBANEZ, F. (1956): The historical and philosophic background of psychobiology. *J. Clin. Exp. Psychopath.*, 17, 360.
81. MENNINGER, K. A. (1930): *The Human Mind.* New York: Alfred A. Knopf.
82. MENNINGER, K. A. (1956): Freud and American psychiatry. *J. Amer. Psychoanal. Assn.*, 4, 614.
83. MEYER, A. (1945): Revaluation of Benjamin Rush. *Amer. J. Psychiat.*, 101, 433.
84. MILLET, J. A. P. (1969): Austen Fox Riggs: his significance to American psychiatry of today. *Amer. J. Psychiat.*, 125, 120.
85. MURRAY, H. A. (1956): Morton Prince: sketch of his life and work. *J. Abnorm. Soc. Psychol.*, 52, 291.
86. OBERNDORF, C. P. (1953): *A History of Psychoanalysis in America.* New York: Grune and Stratton.
87. OPLER, M. K. (1956): Cultural anthropology and social psychiatry. *Amer. J. Psychiat.*, 113, 302.
88. PASAMANICK, B. (1954): An obscure item in the bibliography of Isaac Ray. *Amer. J. Psychiat*, 111, 164.
89. PLUMMER, B. L. (1970): Benjamin Rush and the negro. *Amer. J. Psychiat.*, 127, 93.
90. POLLACK, H. M. (1945): Development of statistics of mental disease in the United States during the past century. *Amer. J. Psychiat.*, 102, 1.
91. POWER, D'A. (1930): *Medicine in the British Isles.* New York: Paul B. Hoeber.
92. PRICHARD, J. C. (1835): *A Treatise on Insanity and Other Disorders Affecting the Mind.* London: Sherwood, Gilbert and Piper.
93. RAY, I. (1838): *A Treatise on the Medical Jurisprudence of Insanity.* Boston: Charles C. Little and James Brown.
94. RAY, I. (1863): *Mental Hygiene.* Boston: Ticknor and Fields.
95. REIN, D. M. (1952): *S. Weir Mitchell as a Psychiatric Novelist.* New York: International Universities Press.

96. REISER, M. F. (1972): Training for What? *Amer. J. Psychiat.*, 128, 118.

97. REISS, S. (1972): A critique of Thomas S. Szasz's "Myth of Mental Illness." *Amer. J. Psychiat.*, 128, 71.

98. ROBACK, A. A. (1952): *History of American Psychology.* New York: Library Publishers.

99. ROBACK, A. A. (1961): *History of Psychology and Psychiatry.* New York: Citadel Press.

100. ROIZIN, L. (1970): Van Gieson, a visionary of psychiatric research. *Amer. J. Psychiat.*, 127, 98.

101. ROLLESTON, H. D. (1929): *The Life of Sir Thomas Clifford Allbutt.* London: Macmillan.

102. ROND, P. C. (1955): Ohio psychiatric pioneer—William Maclay Awl (1799-1876). *Ohio St. Med. J.*, 51, 882.

103. ROSENBERG, C. E. (1962): The place of George M. Beard in nineteenth-century psychiatry. *Bull. Hist. Med.*, 36, 245.

104. RUSH, B. (1794): An Account of the Bilious Remitting Yellow Fever as it Appeared in Philadelphia in the Year 1793. In: Rush, B. *Medical Inquiries and Observations*, Vol. 3 (1819 ed.). Philadelphia: Anthony Finley.

105. RUSH, B. (1812): *Medical Inquiries and Observations upon the Diseases of the Mind* (5th ed., 1835). Philadelphia: Grigg and Elliot.

106. SANBORN, F. B. (1898): *Memoirs of Pliny Earle, M.D.* Boston: Damrell and Upham.

107. SARGENT, S. S. (1944): *The Basic Teachings of the Great Psychologists.* Philadelphia: Blakiston Company.

108. SCHNECK, J. M. (1950): Bibliotherapy in neuropsychiatry. In: Dunton, W. R., Jr., and Licht, S., *Occupational Therapy.* Springfield, Ill.: Charles C Thomas.

109. SCHNECK, J. M. (1960): *A History of Psychiatry.* Springfield, Ill.: Charles C Thomas.

110. SCHNECK, J. M. (1961): Iatrochemistry, iatrophysics and iatropsychology. *Dis. Nerv. Syst.*, 22, 463.

111. SCHNECK, J. M. (1962): An historical outline of psychiatric non-restraint. *Dis. Nerv. Syst.*, 23, 87.

112. SCHNECK, J. M. (1962): The Thomas Sydenham—Benjamin Rush transition in the history of psychiatry. *Med. Hist.*, 6, 389.

113. SCHNECK, J. M. (1963): Benjamin Rush on the influence of buried memories. *Dis. Nerv. Syst.*, 24, 173.

114. SCHNECK, J. M. (1963): Benjamin Rush, intemperate drinking, and the Common Council of the City of New York. *Bull. Hist. Med.*, 37, 377.

115. SCHNECK, J. M. (1963): William Osler, S. Weir Mitchell, and the origin of "the rest cure." *Amer. J. Psychiat.*, 119, 894.

116. SCHNECK, J. M. (1964): Benjamin Rush on denial of illness. *Amer. J. Psychiat.*, 120, 1129.

117. SCHNECK, J. M. (1965): *The Principles and Practice of Hypnoanalysis.* Springfield, Ill.: Charles C Thomas.

118. SCHNECK, J. M. (1965): A reevaluation of Freud's abandonment of hypnosis. *J. Hist. Behav. Sci.*, 1, 191.

119. SCHNECK, J. M. (1965): Tripartite psychiatry—iatropsychology, iatrophysics, and iatrochemistry. *Psychosomatics*, 6, 145.

120. SCHNECK, J. M. (1966): Legal insanity, moral insanity, and Stendhal's *Le Rouge et Le Noir*. *Med. Hist.*, 10, 281.

121. SCHNECK, J. M. (1969): Benjamin Rush, William Shippen, Jr., and Mark Akenside. *N. Y. St. J. Med.*, 69, 1108.

122. SHERMAN, M. H. (1971): Theodore Reik and the crisis in psychoanalysis. *Psychoth. Social Sci. Rev.*, 5, 15.

123. SHERVERT, H. F. (1971): Milestone in research and education: PI's 75th anniversary symposium. *Bull. N. Y. St. District Branches, A. P. A.*, 14, 5.

124. SHRYOCK, R. H. (1944): The beginnings: from colonial days to the foundation of the American Psychiatric Association. In: Hall, J. K., Zilboorg, G., and Bunker, H. A. (eds.), *One Hundred Years of American Psychiatry*. New York: Columbia University Press.

125. SHRYOCK, R. H. (1945): The psychiatry of Benjamin Rush. *Amer. J. Psychiat.*, 101, 429.

126. SHRYOCK, R. H. (1971): The medical reputation of Benjamin Rush: contrasts over two centuries. *Bull. Hist. Med.*, 45, 507.

127. SIGERIST, H. E. (1951): *A History of Medicine*, Vol. I, *Primitive and Archaic Medicine*. New York: Oxford University Press.

128. STEARNS, A. W. (1945): Isaac Ray, psychiatrist and pioneer in forensic psychiatry. *Amer. J. Psychiat.*, 101, 573.

129. SZASZ, T. S., KNOFF, W. F., AND HOLLANDER, M. H. (1958): The doctor-patient relationship and its historical context. *Amer. J. Psychiat.*, 115, 522.

130. WALL, J. H. (1956): Problems in schizophrenia. *N. Y. St. J. Med.*, 56, 2864.

131. WARNER, J. D. AND MOSS, C. S. (1958): A century of medical treatment at State Hospital No. 1, an historical perspective. *Amer. Psychol.*, 13, 120.

132. WEIMERSKIRCH, P. J. (1965): Benjamin Rush and John Minson Galt, II: pioneers of bibliotherapy in America. *Bull. Med. Libr. Assn.* 53, 510.

133. WEISS, E. (1956): The origins of psychosomatic medicine. *Philad. Med.*, 52, 620.

134. WHITE, R. W. (1957): Is Alfred Adler alive today? *Contemp. Psychol.*, 2, 1.

135. WHITE, W. A. (1938): *The Autobiography of a Purpose*. New York: Doubleday, Doran.

136. WHITEHORN, J. C. (1944): A century of psychiatric research in America. In: Hall. J. K. (ed.), *One Hundred Years of American Psychiatry*. New York: Columbia University Press.

137. WINKLER, J. K. AND BROMBERG, W. (1939): *Mind Explorers*. New York: Reynal and Hitchcock.

138. WINTERS, E. E. (1966): Adolf Meyer's two and a half years at Kankakee. *Bull. Hist. Med.*, 40, 441.

139. WITTKOWER, E. D. (1971): Psychoanalysis: world view. *Psychiatric Spectator*, 7, 19.

140. WORTIS, S. B. (ed.) (1953: *Psychiatric Treatment*. Baltimore: William and Wilkins.

141. ZILBOORG, G. AND HENRY, G. W. (1941): *A History of Medical Psychology*. New York: W. W. Norton.

142. ZILBOORG, G. (1951): *Sigmund Freud*. New York: Charles Scribner's Sons.

20

LATIN AMERICA

CARLOS A. LEON, M.D., M.S.

Professor and Chairman, Department of Psychiatry,
Universidad del Valle Medical School
Cali, Colombia

AND

HUMBERTO ROSSELLI, M.D.

President, Colombian Psychiatric Association
Bogotá, Colombia

1

ABORIGINAL BELIEFS AND PRACTICES

It is estimated that no less than 200 different Indian groups existed in Latin America during pre-Columbian days. Their cultural levels were quite variable, extending from tribes who lived in a truly primitive state to those who built great empires and attained a very high stage of socio-cultural development—the Mayas, the Aztecs, and the Incas. The sources for exploring the indigenous notions and practices related to medicine during this period are scarce. Information is available only from monuments and archeological findings, a few Mayan, Aztec, and Inca codexes, writings of the Spanish chroniclers, and anthropological studies on the surviving customs and beliefs which are still to be found in the regional folklore of present tribes.

The aboriginal practices included magical and shamanistic medicine, priestly rituals, and a more or less advanced state of botanical knowledge. All these types of practices taken together do not seem to have been less advanced than the contemporary European medicine at the time of the Spanish conquest.

For most of the aboriginal Americans, and certainly for the ancient Peruvians, disease was attributed to several different sources: the malevolent power of witches or sorcerers, the ill will of deities angered by sin or neglect of worship, the accidental contact with evil spirits (such as those found in winds, springs, ravines, caves, mountains), the intrusion of foreign objects in the body, and the loss of the soul which was frightened out of the body. Even to this day, a number of popular myths are related to these notions which still may be found in Peru, Ecuador, and Bolivia where *jani, susto* (fright), *kaika* and *sonco-nanay* (heart ailment) are quite prevalent, the same as *aire* and *espanto* are present in all the Mayan zones of influence, and *daño, gualicho,* or *huacanque* are known in the southern part of the continent (20, 21, 25, 39, 40).

Mental disorders were well known by the ancient Mexicans, who used different terms for agitated syndromes (*Tlauililocayotl*), and non-agitated syndromes (*Xolopiyotl*) (7). Among the Mayas, the epileptics were described as "men who fall down to earth among the plants." Those who committed suicide were supposed to have their own heaven; they were regarded as sacred and had a private deity, the goddess *Ixtab,* also called "the lady of the rope" (47).

It is difficult to ascertain what factors or elements were regarded as specific causes of mental disorders. Among the Mayas, diseases originated in a mystic cause; he who cured diseases was the same one who produced them. "Medicine men and sorcerers are the same thing," says the chronicler Bishop Diego de Landa (47). The Aztecs regarded as a frequent cause poisoning by the leaves of the *Tolcatzin*—but only when more than four were taken (7). For the Guaraníes in present Uruguay and Tucumán, insanity was attributed to *padrejon* (male principle) or *madrejon* (female principle), which had invaded the head (15). Depression and consumptive illnesses were attributed by the Aymara in Bolivia to the action of the *Kharisiri,* evil spirits who sucked the fat from the bodies of their victims through a small wound in the abdomen (35).

Among the Peruvians, popular religion was dominated by the notion of the *huaca,* which is anything holy, filled with spiritual force, or the dwelling place of a spirit. *Huacas* ranged from household fetishes to temples, trees, caves, or springs (34). A parallel notion to that of the *huaca* was the *Achachila,* which applied to geographic elements such as mountains, lakes, and waterfalls, regarded by the Indians as sacred ancestors through whom entire nations were born (35). Any deliberate or inadvertent offense against a *huaca* would bring about a commensurate punishment, usually in the form of disease. Apart from this and the general causes mentioned above, there was a belief in the *Yaguas,* or illnesses produced by the action of the mother on the fetus (15). Individual or collective sin was regarded as an ubiquitous cause for disease. Ritual ceremonies for "confession of sins" were scheduled at certain periods of the year. It is said that even the Inca had to submit to this ritual (confessing to the Sun), aided by the main guardian of the temple where the virgins of the Sun were kept. Whispering in the ear of the sovereign during the ceremony, he helped him to remember his surreptitious entries into the sacred precinct.

A feature which scandalized Incas and Spanish chroniclers alike was the existence of regions in the New World where the "nefarious sin" of sodomy was rampant and deeply ingrained in the population. The Mochica and Chimú are said to have been strongly inclined to anal copulation with both men and women. "Incas when they finally conquered them (1460-70) regarded the practice as abominable and tried to stamp it out, destroying families and even tribes, but it persisted" (46). According to Bernal Díaz del Castillo (10), sodomy was also common among the Mexicans. A well known tradition in Paraguay says that in remote times an Indian nation, where the "nefarious sin was practiced recklessly," was flooded and converted into Lake Yupacaray (21). As noted by the Spanish chronicler Bustamante, the Pampa Indians were also fond of sodomy and "when they were not at war they always rode pillion with their concubines or even more often with their homosexual partners" (21).

Medicine-Men

The prototype of the medicine-man in most of the early American populations had the characteristics of the shaman. Besides being a healer, he was a psychopomp, the spiritual guide of souls to the netherworld, the intermediary between men and supernatural powers and a worker of miracles and sorceries which produce disease or damage to his enemies. According to Haro (23), the magic healer is essentially a "blower," as it is suggested by the etymological meaning of most of the aboriginal terms used to designate him. Many of the healing rituals seem to be aimed at blowing away the evil principle (demons, spirits, wind) sometimes with the aid of water, tobacco, herbs, etc. On the other hand, Granada (21) quotes several sources to demonstrate that the method most frequently used by aboriginal healers was sucking (in order to extract the material causes of the disease).

In view of the close connection between the magical notion of illness and supernatural phenomena, people showing abnormal characteristics were regarded as exceptionally apt to practice shamanism. Unusual phenomena such as hallucinations or seizures were an omen of the connection between the future shaman and the extraterrestrial spirits, determining his profession and future life in an inevitable way.

Among the Incas, diagnosis and treatment for royal persons were performed by high priests, while ordinary people were tended by priests of low rank. Secret sorcerers were not members of the priesthood. Mayta Capac, the fourth Inca in the dynasty, legitimized the practice of soothsayers and medicine-men, who before then had to practice their profession in a clandestine manner (28). At the height of its development, the Inca civilization had, aside from the priests, three kinds of doctors: the master curers, or *Hampi-camayoc,* who used mostly botanical remedies; the *Camasca,* who made sacrifices to effect the cure; and the *Soncoyoc,* who used suction to suck off the disease (46). Among the Mochica, doctors, *Oquetlupuc,* "were very respected, enjoyed great favors and social privileges, but if they killed their patients through ignorance, they themselves were killed" (46).

The generic name *Laikha* was used by the Aymaras to designate sorcerers in general; however, they had several special kinds, such as the *Chamacani,* fearsome characters who dealt with black magic and evil incantations through communication with demons and the dead; the *Thaliri* who worked through tricks and sleight of hand; and the *Yatiri,* or wise-men, who in addition to magic used their botanical knowledge (35).

In the Aztec empire there was a sort of exchange of functions between priests and authorities since priests were intimately related to official and civic life, playing a leading role in government while chiefs directed the most important ceremonies. Priests were regarded as interpreters of the divine and healing was one of their prerogatives (41). Among the Mayas, the high priests were called *Ah-Kin.* During the Mayapan period there were 12. They were the highest healers and had the *Chilam,* the *Chac,* and the *Nacom* under them (47). The *Chilam* was a kind of visionary shaman, who received messages from the gods while in state of trance, his prophecies being interpreted by the assembled priests (12). The *Chac* were elders who helped the priests in their rituals. The *Nacom* were in charge of opening the chests of the sacrificed victims and plucking out their hearts (47).

According to one source, the Aztecs had an "elite group of physicians," the *Teixtomani,* who were trained for several years at the temples (*Calmecac*) of the goddess *Tlazolteotl,* "eater of impurity."

They supposedly "had an amazing grasp of psychology; translations of their documents show that they developed concepts about ego formation and psychic structure not unlike Freudian ones. Those concepts appeared in an Aztec document about dream interpretation. These physicians knew how to recognize persons who were maniac, schizoid, hysterical, depressive, or psychopathic. Such persons were treated at Calmecac by a variety of methods, including trephination, hypnosis, and specific herbal potions for specific disorders" (4).

Four kinds of witch-doctors or sorcerers are said to have existed in the kingdom of Quito as recorded in the proceedings of the first synod held in 1570, according to the historian Vargas (23). These were the *Omos, Hambicamayocs, Condeviecas* and *Achicocs*. The *Omos* would correspond to priests of traditional deities who would be in communication with the gods and make oracular pronouncements and ritual cures; the *Hambicamayocs* cured with herbs; the *Condeviecas* or *Caviacoc* were charlatans and jesters; and the *Achicocs* practiced divination through instrumental means.

The medicine-men of the Mapuche or Araucanians were the aboriginal American healers who most closely resembled in their practices the Siberian shamans. These healers, called *Machis,* acted as sorcerers and intermediaries between men and spirits through the phenomenon of trance. The faculties for divination were reserved to another type, the *Dunguve*. Originally most of the *Machis* were male transvestites, but they were gradually replaced almost totally by women who assumed the role not only of sorcerers, but also of advisers of tribal leaders in matters of war and peace (27).

The Chibcha priests (*Ogque, Jeque*) were supposed to undergo a prolonged training period of up to 12 years. This time was spent in seclusion in a seminary or *Cuca* ruled by an old priest in charge of teaching the neophytes, who were submitted to a very rigorous diet and a multitude of hardships. They were instructed in the art of healing and acquired knowledge about the medicinal properties of plants, in addition to religious and ritual teachings. Another variety of healers among the Chibchas included the *Mohans*: sorcerers, magicians, and interpreters of dreams, who also performed cures by inducing a state of trance through smoking or chewing tobacco (17).

The Guaraní sorcerers also had to submit to ordeals in order to acquire magical powers. They went through severe fasting, had to submit to strenuous physical punishment, and never bathed. They lived naked in remote, dark, and cold places and their appearance inspired horror to anyone who met them by chance (21).

Healing Practices and Methods

In regard to forms of treatment, there is great variation between the different Indian tribes of pre-Columbian America. According to the Spanish chronicler Cieza de León (11), coca leaves were used by the wise men, or *Amautas,* in ancient Peru for divination and healing and were burned as a sacred offering before religious ceremonies and to purify suspected places from evil spirits. They were also offered to *Pachamama* (the mother earth) to insure her favor in crops. Cieza de León was told in the province of Callao about how the hero *Wiracocha* healed all who were sick and restored sight to the blind "by words alone." The ancient Peruvians used as specific treatment for mental diseases balneotherapy, blood-letting, and individual and collective confession. A kind of collective psychotherapy was enacted at the *Situa* festival which was celebrated at Cuzco every year in the months of August or September. Either individuals or entire communities were submitted to a period of fasting which lasted up to five days, after which the priests listened to the penitents in confession; then they proceeded to strike their backs lightly with stones; and finally priest and penitent together spat on a handful of grass which was thrown into a river. This might have been a symbolic way of washing away the sins (30).

Among the Mayas, the goddess *Tlazoltleotl* seems to have played a very important role for collective confessions, since she was regarded as the "eater of filth," as well as the "goddess of dirt," "the earth mother," and the "mother of the gods." "By eating refuse, she was supposed to consume the sins of mankind, leaving them pure" (41). Aztecs treated psychopaths and persons who committed misdemeanors or had sexual disorders by a technique of "transformation of hearts" (4). This technique required fasting and very rigorous emotional and mental disciplines (33).

The Maya priests (*Chilam*) in a collective ceremony purified the audience with copal and tobacco smoke and asked people to "confess their sins," according to the interpretation given by Bishop Diego de Landa (47). If one of those present confessed to having committed an obscene act, he was cast out of the circle. For the primitive Mayas, confession was compulsory. If there were someone who was impure and did not confess, then he would become a social outcast, but confession erased the offense. When someone was ill the *Ahmen* was called. He diagnosed the illness by means of divination and invoked the goddess of medicine *Ixchel* (who was also the goddess of pregnancy), placing her image in front of the patient. Afterwards, copal incense was burned and the *Ahmen* smoked tobacco, blowing the smoke in the face of the patient; then he used medicines. Stones were roled in front of the patient in order to divine the prognosis. For epileptics, the powdered horns of a deer or the macerated testicles of a crocodile were mixed in cold water and drunk. If this proved to be ineffective, the patient was asked to take off one of his sandals, urinate in it, and drink the urine (47).

According to Father Simon, the Chibcha priests chewed tobacco in order to communicate with the devil; coca was also used to communicate with the spirit world (18). Even in our day the Araucanian Machis pretend to contact the spirit world and talk with the spirits. They undergo possession by the high spirit *Hoinguenechen.* The Machi, when possessed, falls in ecstasy, speaks and acts under the influence of the spirit (27).

Among the ancient Peruvians, both patient and healer drank *Ayahuasca* together. Out of the hallucinations produced by it, instructions as to the cause and cure of the illness were given (45). The surgical ability of the Incas is regarded as exceptional. Cranial trephination and cauterization were performed in a great number of cases and with sophisticated techniques (48). However, it is not exactly known whether these procedures were used for decompression following trauma or for exorcistic rituals. Graña and Rocca (22), who replicated these operations using the original instruments, remark on the very high degree of technical competence displayed by the ancient Peruvian surgeons.

The Badiano codex, written in Mexico in the 16th century by the Indian physician Martin de la Cruz and his translator Juan Badiano, is an important source of information about methods of treatment. The book recommends a poultice made of different plants which if used with cold water "stops the heat in the head," and with hot water, "holds the coolness inside the head." Several plants and flowers were prescribed for fatigue of those who administer the government and public offices. For melancholy, called by Badiano "black blood," a potion of herbs and juices obtained from flowers with nice fragrances was prescribed. Epilepsy, which was called by Badiano *morbus comitialis* according to the terminology used by Pliny, was treated with emetics and ritual spells. Shyness and fear should be treated with a hypnotic potion and with an ointment made of animal ingredients, which suggests the desirability of acquiring some of the characteristics of the animals involved (7).

The Chocó Indians of Panama and Colombia placed insane people in special booths covered with figures and symbols and "so small as if they were fit for dogs," in order that the evil spirits of insanity would feel uncomfortable and fly away from the patient" (3). In Guarani and Araucan territories, collective dancing was used as a therapeutic resource of first order in the treatment of mental disturbances. However, agitated patients were tied down, given emetics, and submitted to intense sweating, together with exorcisms and vigorous dancing (15).

Intoxicants and Psychoactive Plants

A cultural fact of great importance was the medicinal use of several American plants known to the aborigines, which have been progressively incorporated into the official pharmacopoeia. Francisco Hernández, in his *Historia Natural de las Indias* written in 1577, estimated that Mexico alone had about 3,000 species of medicinal plants (36). Father Bernardino de Sahagún (47) enumerates dozens of plants used for divination. The psychotropic properties of plants were used specially in ritual ceremonies by the shamans to induce trance and hallucination. The use of these plants was restricted to the high authorities, the priests, or the shamans. Through their use, they were able to interpret dreams, discover the cause of illness, prophesy, and communicate with the spirit world. For the non-initiated, they were regarded as dangerous and conducive to insanity of a chronic nature. The ancient Mexicans used *Ochtli* or *Pulque,* a fermented beverage made from the *Maguey* plant whose goddess was called *Mayahuel.* It was believed that persons who were born under the sign *2-Rabbit* of the Aztec Calendar were predestined to use alcoholic beverages (8). The Aztec government took several measures to restrict the use of *pulque,* ranging from admonitions voiced by the emperor at the time of his election to social repudiation of alcoholics, physical punishment such as jailing, and even death. Old people were the only members of the community who were allowed to drink without restrictions (8). *Chicha,* a fermented beverage made out of maize, was used profusely in all Inca territories, especially for collective rituals and offerings to the deity. To prepare *chicha* the boiled corn was chewed and spat into a large pot, where the saliva enzymes converted the malt sugar into dextrose and later alcohol. The chewed corn was mixed with water, poured into vessels for fermentation, and set aside for a day. During the Inca era it was exclusively prepared by women. According to Cieza de León (11), "It is amazing how much beverage or chicha these Indians can drink, for the cup is never out of their hand." Vessels of *chicha* were always placed beside the dead in the burials. *Chicha* was also made with the addition of a resinous plant called *Molle,* and this variety was especially appreciated for ritual purposes.

Out of the immense variety of plants used by the aboriginal Americans for intoxicant, medical, or magico-religious purposes, the following stand out, because of both their widespread use and the great ceremonial value attached to them.

Coca (*Eritroxilon coca* L. and other varieties), also known as *Hayo,* was used extensively in Bolivia, Peru, Chile, Ecuador, and Colombia. The dried leaves were chewed together with lime, powdered calcinated shells, or ashes (*Mombe*). It was burned as an offering to the gods, mixed together with llama fat. Its use was preserved initially to priests and chiefs and then became widespread during the demoralization which followed the conquest and destruction of the Inca empire. It was chewed for divinatory purposes and communication with the deity. Because of its inhibitory properties on hunger and thirst and a mild euphoric effect, it was regarded as a sacred food and a gift of the gods to mankind. During colonial days, great plantations of *coca* were exploited by Spanish landlords, who became rich trading with this crop. The use of *coca* became so prevalent after the collapse of the Inca empire, and was such a necessary element for the subsistence of the aboriginal population, that Cieza de León (11) said "If *coca* didn't exist, neither would Peru."

Ayahuasca, Yage, Pilde, Caapi, Natema (several species of Banisteriopsis, especially *Banisteria caapi* and *Banisteria inebrians*), is a vine, widely distributed and used throughout the Amazonic and Orinoquian basins of Peru, Ecuador, Colombia, and Venezuela, as well as in Central America. It could be prepared fresh, chopped to bits, ground, and mixed with cold or boiling water; but most often it was used as a concentrated potion with the appearance of a red syrup, with bluish or greenish hues. It was drunk individually or in groups, the ceremony being usually directed by a priest, *Curaca* or *Piache*. It induced a state of intoxication with convulsions, vomiting, diarrhea, delusional and hallucinatory experiences such as traveling to heaven and hell, weightlessness, micropsia, colored hallucinations, dreams, telepathy, and clairvoyance. The vines have been found to contain psychotropic alkaloids such as *Harmine* (32). The term *Ayahuasca* refers to the belief that ancestors (*aya*=death, *huasca*=vine) appear in visions and make prophetic pronouncements or advise the person on a crisis. When used for medicinal purposes, both healer and patient drink the potion in order that the nature of the illness be revealed to them, together with its prognosis and treatment.

Yopo, Cohoba, Parica, Hatax, Vilca Cevil, Epena (several species of Acacia, including *Piptadenia peregrina, P. macrocarpa, P. colubrina*). The seeds or bark of these plants were usually toasted and powdered and used as snuff aspirated through a hollow bone of a bird. In Peru, it was usually inhaled into the nose through the shank-bone of the oil bird. It was used for shamanistic practices, in order to induce ecstasy or trance, and for divination. Extensively used in Peru, Ecuador, Colombia, Venezuela, Central America and the Caribbean, these plants are rich in Metiltriptamine, an active psychotropic compound from the *indol* series (32).

Borrachero, Huantug, Floripondio, Tonga, Chamico (several species of *Datura,* especially *Datura arborea, D. suaveolens, D. sanguinea*). These are plants rich in scopolamine, hyosciamine, and atropine. The powdered seeds were mixed with a drink, usually *chicha*. They were widely used throughout the territories of the Inca empire and Central America.

Tobacco (*Nicotiana tabacum, N. rustica, N. undulata*) was used particularly in the Caribbean region. For shamanistic practices, it was either chewed, smoked or snuffed (inhaled through the nose).

Yerba mate, Caa, Yerba del Paraguay (*Ilex paraguayensis*) was regarded as a gift to mankind of the *guarani* culture-hero Pay Zume. It is a mild euphoriant and stimulant and was used heavily in Paraguay, Argentina, Southern Brazil, and Uruguay for ritual purposes of communication with the deity, divination, healing practices, and other ceremonies.

Peyote, Peyotl, Mescal, Jiculi (*Lophophora Williamsii*) was first described by the Spanish priest Bernardino de Sahagún in 1560 as a narcotic cactus used ritually by the Chichimeca. "Those who eat or drink it see visions either frightful or laughable; this intoxication lasts two or three days and then ceases" (24). It is widely used by several Mexican aboriginal tribes, especially the Toltec, the Chichimeca, and the Aztec. Its use has survived, mostly among members of the Huichol tribe in northern Mexico and also in the southern United States. The dried buttons of the cactus are soaked in water and eaten. It produces hallucinations, depersonalization, and distortion of body image. The cactus is rich in mescaline and other alkaloids.

Aguacolla or *Sanpedro,* another species of cactus (*Tricocerens pachamoi*), is rich in mescaline and still widely used in Peru and Chile.

Teonnacatl (*Psyloscibe mejicana*) was extensively used in Mexico and Central America. These are mushrooms which are ingested or smoked for ceremonial and healing purposes. They contain the active principle psyloscibine.

Ololuqui (Ipomea violacea), an ornamental plant, was used by the ancient Mexicans for its hallucinatory properties. The seeds were ingested or smoked. They have been found to contain lysergic acid diethylamide and related principles.

2

THE CONQUEST

It seems as if the psychotropic plants used by the Indians became at certain times weapons for political warfare, as happened in May, 1537, to the troops of Gonzalo Jiménez de Quesada, who had invaded the kingdom of the Chibcha. The chronicler Joaquin de Acosta (1) describes the episode thus: "40 of Quesada's soldiers who marched from Bogotá to Chocontá temporarily went out of their minds when they arrived at a place where some Indian women had mixed their food with the seeds of a plant called *borrachero (Datura arborea)*." Another chronicler, Juan de Castellanos (9), mentions that eating wild mandioc made some soldiers "walk around as if drunk or insane."

Several members of the Spanish army and government became psychotic, as shown by the following narratives: Pedro Alcón, a soldier of Pizarro and one of the members of the group of 13 at Isla del Gallo, on returning from an expedition in 1528 suffered an episode of wild agitation, for which it was "necessary to tie him down and keep him in prison on a board" (42). The governor and general captain of Venezuela, Enrique Rembolt, on being informed about a disaster which befell his army, became ill with a "mortal melancholy" in 1544 (3). In 1575, the Andalucian Andrés de Valdivia, conquistador and governor of the province of Antioquia (Nueva Granada), became insane upon receiving an anonymous letter in which his wife was accused of adultery. During his derangement, he committed all sorts of deplorable acts against the aborigines, who in revenge assassinated him (38).

Most of the conquistadores succumbed to the collective insanity of a compulsive search for gold. The myth of *El Dorado* inflamed their minds and led them to the wild chase of a chimera which often ended in disease, starvation, and violent death. Because of *El Dorado* the conquistadores fought, killed, became alternatively rich and poor, turned greedy, callous, and cruel, and forgot all their traditions and beliefs. Particularly poignant in this respect is the history of Don

Pedro de Mendoza, a wealthy Spanish nobleman who, motivated by greed and deceived by the fantastic stories concocted about the fabulously rich Rio de la Plata, organized and financed on his own a big expedition, which after many hardships ended in failure. On his voyage back to Spain, ruined, depressed, and crippled, he died, supposedly "because of a great discomfiture produced by eating dog meat for lack of fresh food aboard" (21).

The Clash of Cultures

Several chroniclers have recorded the state of shock that some of the mores and practices of the aboriginal tribes produced in the conquistadores.

The soldier chronicler Bernal Díaz del Castillo, who arrived in Mexico in 1514, describes how the conquered territories were "full of [human] sacrifices and evil deeds" (in Mexico City and neighboring villages alone 2,000 persons were said to have been sacrificed in one year). He also relates how in some ceremonies they cut off "foreheads, ears, tongues, lips, breasts, arms, buttocks, legs, and even genitals." He goes on to curse the multitude of temples and shrines which were filled with "demons and diabolical figures," and expresses bewilderment at the widespread homosexuality particularly prevalent among those who lived in the coasts and warm climate. "There were boys who walked around in women's dress, earning money through the practice of such a diabolic and abominable endeavor." He was also shocked by cannibalism and narrates that in all towns they had "jails made up of thick wood resembling houses where many women, men, and adolescent Indians were kept to get fat, and once they became fat they were sacrificed and eaten." Incestuous practices are also described and condemned, being partially attributed to drunkenness. He remarks about the "unheard of vileness" of a practice he witnessed at Pánuco, where people "funneled wine into their ass-holes through a reed until their bellies were swollen with it." He ends by saying "Our Lord Jesus Christ willed that with his holy support, we the conquistadores, who escaped from wars and battles and dangers of death, plucked [all these vices and evilness] out from them and we put them under a good living policy and we taught them the holy doctrine" (10).

It is not hard to imagine what must have been the reaction of the conquistadores when they found that the favorite sacrifice the Aztecs offered the sun-god *Toniatuh* was performed by "four priests who spread-eagled the victim while a fifth opened his breast to tear out the [still palpitating] heart as an offering to the god" (41). In the sacrifices to *Xipe Totec* the victims were flayed and scalped alive in order that the god might wear their skins as a garment, according to the description of the chroniclers Francisco Hernández and Bernardino de Sahagún (17). Even more hideous, however, was the ritual offered to *Huehueteotl,* the god of fire, in which: "After preparing a great fire, each priest seized a captive and, binding him hand and foot, lifted him onto his back. A macabre dance took place around the burning coals, and one by one they dumped their burdens into the flames. Before death could intervene to put an end to their suffering the priests fished out the captives with large hooks and wrenched their hearts from their blistered bodies" (41).

On the other hand, the Spanish missionaries were ready to identify some of the culture heroes of the aboriginal tribes with figures of the Christian pantheon. In this way *Wiracocha, Quetzalcoatl, Bochica,* and *Zumé,* were at different times identified with the apostle Saint Thomas.* Bishop Diego de Landa marveled at witnessing rituals which he identified as confession and baptism among the Mayas and the same occurred to father Pedro de Aguado (2).

The psychological impact of the conquest, experienced by American aborigines as an apocalyptic destruction of their world, has never been adequately assessed. But in all probability the prolonged and hazardous war, the unendurable hardships of slavery, and the cruelly repressive regime imposed by the conquerors for several centuries during colonial days may have generated intense feelings of frustrated anger, hopelessness, and inferiority among the Indians, who took refuge in isolation and restriction of contacts with the white population. Besides, with the vanishing of the traditional order, the disorganization of the system of beliefs and precepts brought about a wave of abuse of intoxicants such as *coca, chicha, pulque,* or *peyotl.* This, together with suicide and a pathetic refusal to participate in agricultural work, could very well be regarded as the futile depressive mechanisms of a subdued race.

The Spanish chroniclers Gonzalo Fernández de Oviedo and Bartolomé de las Casas (16), although disagreeing on several matters, are concordant on the description of mass suicides of entire populations, such as the Arwak in the Antilles, because of the cruelties of the Spanish *encomenderos.* The vigorous defense of the Indians by Father Las Casas was instrumental in bringing to Latin America the black slaves from Africa.

---

* In the present atomic era the fantasies inspired by the conquest of outer space and interplanetary travel see these same heroes as cosmonauts who came to earth from the sidereal realm to accomplish a transcendental civilizing mission (44).

3

THE COLONIAL PERIOD

Background and Early Stages

It is a well known fact that Spain at the time of the discovery already had a tradition of humanitarian concern for the treatment of the insane. The first psychiatric hospital of the Western world was founded in Valencia in 1409 through the good offices of the mercedarian monk Juan Gilabert Jofré. This was followed by the creation of other institutions in Spain which used "moral treatment" for insanity. Worthy contributions to the incipient field of psychology were made by the humanist Juan Luis Vives (1492-1540), the physicians Andrés de Laguna (1499-1560), and Juan Huarte de San Juan (1503-1600). However, perhaps with the exception of Mexico, this influence did not extend to the Latin American colonies. Colonial psychiatry, as well as medicine, was very poor indeed in these regions of the New World. With the Spanish colonization, a number of botanists, physicians, and pharmacists traveled to America. Hospitals began to be established and a new kind of medicine was born (albeit smothered in its beginnings by witchcraft, ritual healing, and other magical practices of the aborigines). The first university medical teachings began at the universities of San Marcos de Lima (1571) and Mexico (1580). However, most of the health needs of the population were invariably covered by the work of sorcerers or native healers.

In 1566, only 45 years after the conquest of Mexico by Cortez, the Spaniard Bernardino Alvarez (1517-1584), who in his youth had been one of the soldiers of Cortez, "adventurer, gambler, and escaped convict," founded the *Hospicio de San Hipólito,* the first psychiatric hospital of the New World. He devoted himself to the care of the mentally ill with the same zeal he had displayed in his youthful adventures. The following year, he founded in Oaxtepec a colony for the custodial care of chronic patients. He was also the founder of the religious order of San Hipólito dedicated to the care of the ill, which survived until the first years of the Mexican Republic. In addition, he built six general hospitals, including the hospitals of La Habana and Guatemala on which he spent all of his fortune (31).

In 1687, José Sayago, a carpenter, and his wife founded in Mexico City the *Hospital Real del Divino Salvador,* for female mental patients. In the 18th century it was said that "no hospital in the world offered a better care than this" (31). In 1747, the first Society for

Help to the Mentally Ill was created in Mexico under the name of *Real Congregación de Nuestra Señora de los Dolores y Socorro de Mujeres Dementes.*

An institution for senile and mentally ill priests was created in Mexico in 1689 called the *Hospital de la Santísima Trinidad,* which existed until 1905.

In most of the other countries in Latin America, the mentally ill were secluded in cells, or jailed and chained to the floor. They were submitted to all sorts of abuse such as whippings and cold showers. If not secluded, they walked around the streets, as objects of amusement and derision for the populace. Unfortunately, these conditions prevailed in some cities as late as the middle part of the present century.

Some of the general hospitals maintained *loquerías* (insane quarters), such as those in the hospitals of *Santa Ana* (women) and *San Andrés* (men) in Lima. A royal edict allocated the sum of 2,000 pesos a year to take care of the "insane" at this latter hospital (15). Similar sections were founded in *Hospital de Misericordia,* Rio de Janeiro (1582), *Hospital San Martín,* Buenos Aires (1611), *Hospital San Juan de Dios,* Bogotá (1564), which in 1759 was given a generous grant by Viceroy Solis to improve the condition of the inmates, and *Hospital General de Montevideo* (1782). The *Hospicio de Pobres* was founded in Quito in 1785, but not until 40 years later did it begin to admit mental patients (13).

The Holy Office in the New World

One of the possible reasons for the incipient development of psychiatry during colonial days was that a substantial proportion of the mental and moral health of the population was entrusted to the three Tribunals of the Inquisition founded in Lima in 1570, in Mexico in 1571 and in Cartagena de Indias in 1610, all strategically distributed to offer coverage to all the provinces of Spanish America. Since 1599, Archbishop Zapata de Cárdenas had requested the creation of a Tribunal for the New Kingdom (Colombia), with the argument that "of all territories His Majesty owns, this is the most wicked in customs and all sort of vices, being inhabited by altered and quarrelsome men" (29). According to a chronicler, "what startled the inquisitors more than anything was the infinite number of witches and sorcerers who swarmed in the New Kingdom . . . in the task of extirpation of such a pitchblack evil (*mal carboniento*) their lordships employed such commendable eagerness that very soon the whole kingdom was greatly edified at their zeal and activity" (38).

The Tribunals of the Inquisition in America were noticeably more lenient than those of the preceding centuries in Europe. They had already been forewarned to "proceed with temperance, smoothness, and much consideration" with the aborigines. In two and a half centuries of activity, there only were 15 executions in Lima, 39 in Mexico, and 6 in Cartagena.

The inquisitors recognized mental diseases of natural causes as distinct from phenomena produced by witchcraft. However, quite often an error in diagnosis surely brought some clearly psychotic people to the stake. Although in the inaugural *auto-da-fé* of the Inquisition in Cartagena it was suggested that many women could be hallucinated or alienated by the use of "certain beverages made out of herbs or roots," this would not reduce the punishment, since it was considered that if the accused had reached such extremes of wickedness it was because of their "concupiscence and dealings with the devil" (29).

The cases of epileptic seizures, psychotic episodes, and suicides were rather frequent in the secret jails of the Holy Office. Inquisitor Varela in Cartagena stated that "soon after the accused enter the prisons, they become ill and many lose their wits." This was attributed to the narrowness of their jails and to the hot climate. The use of *coca, chamico* and *peyote* were among the habits condemned by the Inquisition. Since this attracted the attention of authorities in Spain, the inquisitors explained that these plants were used by "women of easy life and corrupt customs, in order to work divination and amatory sortileges" (29).

In their zeal, the inquisitors got involved with the ecclesiastic authorities, and ended up by indicting each other with faults very similar to those they punished in their victims. This contamination may perhaps be better explained by postulating that the antithetic pair, witch-inquisitor, forms a dynamic system which reinforces itself, in the sense that the presence of one element facilitates the emergence of the other. An inspecting visitor in Cartagena, using a mechanism of rationalization, attributed most of the faults of the inquisitors to the adverse influence of the environment, describing ". . . in these provinces, full of stupid negroes, raised amidst superstition and sorceries, men and women who did not fit in Spain, and who, if good when they left, were later prevaricated by the land (which as its own fruit does not offer more than stupid and vile Indians)" (38).

In the absence of truly important matters against the faith, inquisitors kept busy trying to punish sensuousness and lust, which was supposedly "bewildering in its intensity and variety" (29). It is well known that for repressed people a common fantasy consists in linking exotic countries with instinctive liberation. In traveling to the New World, both colonizers and inquisitors probably increased their contradictory fantasies of erotic acting-out and accompanying guilt, which was subsequently dealt with through projection.

The Printing Press

The first printing press in America was set to work in Mexico City in 1534, and from 1570 to 1727, several books on medicine, surgery, and hygiene were published. As pioneers of the psychiatric bibliography in Latin America during the colonial period, the following books should be mentioned: *Primera Parte de la Miscelánea Austral,* by Don Diego D'Avalos y Figueroa, Lima, 1602, which deals, among other things, with love, jealousy, shame, and dreams; *Manías Particulares,* by Father Francisco González Laguna, Lima, 1791; and *Crónica Moralizadora de la Orden de San Agustín en el Perú,* by Father Antonio de la Calancha, Lima, 1653, in which interesting descriptions of cases of neuroses and psychoses are to be found. Incidentally, two of the greatest colonial painters suffered with mental disorders: Miguel de Santiago (?-1673) from Quito, who supposedly wounded his model mortally in order to copy the expression of agony and ever since suffered with frequent "cerebral hallucinations" (13), and Gregorio Vásquez Arce y Ceballos (1638-1711), the celebrated painter from Bogotá, who died in a state of dementia (38).

On the eve of independence, the neo-granadian naturalist and mathematician Francisco José de Caldas included interesting notes on social psychology of several regions of the New Kingdom (Colombia) in his book, *Del Influjo del Clima sobre los Seres Organizados,* published in 1808. In this valuable essay on human ecology, the author states that "climate and food influence the physical fabric of man, his character, his virtues, and vices." Almost concomitantly, Hipólito Unanue published in Lima his *Observaciones sobre el Clima de Lima y sus Influencias en los Seres Organizados, en Especial en el Hombre* (1806). He recognized the influence of physical environment on man, but also pointed out the existence of a psychological force which regulates human behavior. In his psychiatric thinking, he followed the ideas of Benjamin Rush (42).

4

THE REPUBLICAN PERIOD

The French Influence

The subject of interrelation between climate and behavior continued to be the center of interest for several years among scientists and practitioners in the newly established Latin American republics. Abel Brandin, a French physician who between 1820 and 1840 practiced variously in Chile, Peru, Ecuador, and Mexico, published many books and is regarded as a precursor in Peruvian psychiatry (42). He published a book on the influence of climate on man with particular attention to the climates of South America, and edited the Medical Annals of Peru, Ecuador, and Mexico, through which he spread current psychiatric knowledge. He also advised the use of the Rush tranquilizer, was the first physician who talked about occupational therapy, and published the first legal psychiatric expertise in Ecuador (13).

The presence of Brandin brought the influence of Paris to Latin America, an influence which lasted more than a century. Cosme Argerich and J. M. Fernández de Agüero brought to Buenos Aires the teachings of Pinel and Cabanis in 1822. José Félix Merizalde, professor of legal medicine and hygiene, gave lessons on psychiatry at the school of medicine in Bogotá in 1826 and translated Pinel. Simultaneously José Maria Vargas (1786-1854), an outstanding physician and political figure, taught the vitalist theories of Bichat in Caracas and performed the first dissections of the nervous system.

The first Latin American thesis on psychiatry was written by Diego Alcorta (1807-1842) in Buenos Aires in 1827 under the title of *Disertación sobre la Manía Aguda* in which he supported the thesis of Pinel on hospital reform and postulated the "moral treatment of the mentally ill" (19). In 1841, at the request of the Brazilian Emperor Pedro II, Luis Napoleao Chernoviz edited the *Formulario o Guia Medica* based on the French *Codex,* issued in several countries of Latin America until the last part of the 19th century (37). Augustin Cueva Vallejo (1820-1873) was a pioneer of psychiatry in Ecuador. He founded a school of medicine in Cuenca, where he followed the teachings of Pinel and Esquirol (13). In 1851 Manuel Ancízar published the *Lecciones de Psicología* in Bogotá.

In 1850 Francisco Carassa, director of the Beneficencia de Lima, ordered that the treatise by Pinel be copied by hand, for the physicians working at the *Casas de Locos* (Houses for the Insane) in Lima (42).

The "Enlightenment"

Throughout the 19th century there was a growing interest in the mental patient, reflected in the progressive development of psychiatric institutions, by an increase in the number of publications, the beginning of teachings on psychopathology, and the promulgation of several laws aimed at protecting the mentally ill.

Velasco Alzaga (43) states that there was a concordance between the socio-political changes in Latin America countries, the establishment of specialized hospitals for the treatment of the mentally ill, and the development of programs and organizations for mental health. In 1828, the *Hospital San Dionisio* (later called the *Mazorra*) was founded in Havana. A society to improve the status of the mentally ill was started in 1861. José Joaquín Muñoz, director of the *Mazorra,* and the pioneer of Cuban psychiatry, published the translation of a textbook on mental alienation by Baillarger (6).

The psychiatric *Hospicio Pedro II* was inaugurated in Rio de Janeiro in 1852, thanks to the efforts of the physicians José Clemente Pereira and José Da Cruz Jobim. On this occasion the statutes for the first law on care of the mentally ill were approved. Philippe Rey, a French psychiatrist who visited the Hospicio in 1875, said that "despite its imperfections it could be envied by more than one great city in Europe. Thus the *asyla* in Italy, just to mention those which we have had the opportunity to visit, specially those of Milan, Florence, and Rome, are far behind if compared with Hospicio Pedro II" (5). José Pereira Das Neves, a psychiatrist working at the Hospicio, who trained in Europe, is considered to be the first Brazilian psychiatrist.

The *Hospicio Sao Joao* in Sao Paulo, administered by the Alvarenga family, was also inaugurated in 1852. The *Asilo de San Juan de Dios* in Bahia was inaugurated in 1874, and the *Hospital San Pedro* in 1879 in Rio Grande do Sul. The national law for assistance to the mentally ill was promulgated in Brazil in 1890.

The first psychiatric hospital in Puerto Rico called *Hogar de Beneficencia de San Juan* was founded in 1844. The *Casa de Orates* (house for the insane) was inaugurated in Santiago de Chile in 1852, under the aegis of Doctor Laurent Sazie, a French physician. His successor, the Argentinian Ramón Elquero, gave some lessons on psychopathology and wrote the first psychiatric book in Chile, *Memorias de la Casa de Orates.* Manuel Beca compiled the first statistics about mental disorders in Chile in 1891.

Juan N. Navarro, Director of *Hospital de San Hipólito* in Mexico in 1853, is considered as the reformer of the care of the mentally ill and the founder of puericulture in Mexico. The Mexican public health code was implemented in 1891.

The *Hospital de la Misericordia* was inaugurated in Lima in 1859. Its director, José Casimiro Ulloa (1829-1891), is regarded as an innovator in psychiatric care in Peru. He started ward rounds, kept an accurate system of statistics and classification of patients, started work-shops, and enforced humanitarian rules. He is also known for his active campaigns against alcohol, his interest in hygiene, and for several civic and welfare activities. His successor, Manuel Muñiz, abolished all means of restraint, continued the use of statistics, recommended for the first time the creation of psychiatric services in the general hospitals, and showed interest in cultural psychiatry.

In Montevideo, the mental patients had been kept in a section of *Hospital Maciel* up until 1860 when they were moved to a country house which later became the *Manicomio Nacional del Uruguay,* inaugurated in 1880 under the direction of the psychiatrist Enrique Castro.

La Casa de Locos in Buenos Aires was opened in 1863 and 20 years later became the *Hospicio de Las Mercedes.* In 1884, the psychiatric colony for chronic patients, *Melchor Romero,* was founded in La Plata. The Argentinian psychiatrist Domingo Cabred is regarded as the leading figure of Argentinian psychiatric care, "which, in his time, was the most advanced in Latin America" (5). He started the open-door type colonies of Lujan (1899), Oliva (1908), and Torres (1915). Statistical studies were initiated in 1879 by Samuel Gache, who published *La Locura en Buenos Aires.*

The *Asilo de Locos* (Asylum for Insane Men) in Bogotá was founded by the Beneficencia de Cundinamarca in 1870. It was followed by the *Casa de Locas* (House for Insane Women) in 1874. Antonio Gómez Calvo at the beginning of this century compiled the first statistics and used a classification system following that of Morel. The *Manicomio de Antioquia* was inaugurated in Medellín in 1878, and the first statistics were compiled by Ricardo Escobar Ramos.

The *Asilo Nacional de Enajenados* (National Asylum for the Alienated) in Caracas was inaugurated by Enrique Perez Blanco in 1876. It was reformed in 1892 and later in 1926 by Francisco Torrealba, the first Venezuelan psychiatrist. The *Manicomio José Vélez* was founded in Guayaquil in 1881 by Emilio Gerardo Roca. In 1909, it was transferred to the present *Hospital Lorenzo Ponce.* The first clinic for alcoholics was started in Cuenca, Ecuador, in 1886 under the name of *La Temperancia* (13).

The *Manicomio Nacional Pacheco* was founded in Sucre, Bolivia, in 1884 under Nicolás Ortiz, who gave lectures on psychiatry until 1898.

Starting in the last decade of the 19th century, the rest of the Latin American countries continued to create new psychiatric institutions, among which the following should be mentioned in chronological order: Santo Domingo, 1886; Costa Rica, 1889; Guatemala, 1890; San Salvador, 1896; Paraguay, 1898; Panama, 1933; Nicaragua, 1946; and Honduras, 1956.

5

CONTEMPORARY DEVELOPMENTS

Teaching, Research, Academic, and Clinical Interests

The first chair of psychiatry in Latin America was inaugurated in Buenos Aires in 1888 where José María Ramos Mejía was appointed Professor of Nervous Diseases. He "set the basis for neurology and scientific psychiatry" (19). Among his publications, two are particularly important: *Las Neurosis de los Hombres Célebres en la Historia Argentina* (1878), and *Estudios Clínicos sobre las Enfermedades Nerviosas y Mentales* (1893).

The chair of clinical psychiatry and nervous diseases was created at Universidad de Rio de Janeiro in 1887 where Nuño de Andrade was appointed professor and psychiatrist at Hospicio Pedro II. One of his successors, Teixeira Grandao, is regarded as the founder of scientific psychiatry in Brazil. He published numerous papers and was the initiator of research in experimental psychiatry.

Psychiatric teaching was started in Santiago de Chile in 1891 by Augusto Orrego Luco, who occupied the chair until 1906. In Havana the first chair of psychiatry was given to José Antonio Valdés Anciano in 1907. In Montevideo, psychiatric teaching was started in 1912 by Bernardo Etchepare; in Quito, in 1913 with Carlos Alberto Arteta. Julio Endara (1899-1970), appointed professor in Quito in 1926, performed outstanding work in teaching, research, mental hygiene, anthropology, criminology, and forensic psychiatry; he was one of the leading figures in Latin American psychiatry for several decades. In Colombia the first course of psychiatry was given by Juan B. Londoño in Medellín in 1914. In Bogotá, psychiatric teaching was started in 1916 by Miguel Jiménez López (1875-1955).

The initiator of psychiatric teaching in Peru was Hermilio Valdizán (1885-1929), who was appointed professor in 1916. He is regarded as one of the most outstanding figures in Peruvian medicine. An excellent clinician, a brilliant lecturer and a prolific writer, he produced valuable works on the history of Peruvian medicine, folkloric psychiatry, mental hygiene, and forensic psychiatry. He was succeeded by Honorio Delgado (1892-1969), another great figure in

Latin American psychiatry, who introduced psychoanalysis to South America and was the first Latin American to become a member of the International Psychoanalytic Association, although he later abandoned this orientation. He published textbooks on psychiatry and psychology, was a member of several academies and scientific societies, and a public figure in government. He founded associations and journals and "emerged as an outstanding leader for many years in the course of Peruvian psychiatry" (42).

The present century has seen great expansion of psychiatric teaching in Latin America evidenced by the large number of medical schools where psychiatry is taught as an independent subject. At present there are 154 schools of medicine in Latin America, of which 73 are in Brazil. Psychiatry is taught throughout the medical career rather than as a single course in several of these medical schools. Currently, there are 68 departments of psychiatry in Latin America, most of which offer teaching at both the undergraduate and the graduate level. It is estimated that there is a total of about 90 institutions for the training of psychiatrists (26). A seminar for the teaching of psychiatry in medical schools was organized by the Pan-American Health Organization in Lima in 1967. Another, on the teaching of psychiatry to graduate students, was sponsored by the same agency in Bogotá in 1972.

In 1908, Franco Da Rocha created in Sao Paulo the first system of foster home care for the mentally ill in Latin America. The first outpatient clinic for psychiatric patients was created at Hospital Santa Ana in Lima in 1915. Baltasar Caravedo Prado, the initiator of the medical mental health movement in Peru, started the first private psychiatric clinic in partnership with Hermilio Valdizán in 1919. In Bogotá, the first private psychiatric clinic was started in 1902 by the Sisters of Charity at El Campito. The first private clinic in Chile was inaugurated in 1920. The first non-profit organization for private care of the mentally ill was organized in Bogotá in 1952 under the name of Instituto Colombiano del Sistema Nervioso.

In 1941, Carlos A. Seguín inaugurated at Hospital Obrero in Lima the first psychiatric service in a general hospital. Seguín gave a very strong impulse to the development of psychosomatic medicine, psychotherapy, teaching and folkloric psychiatry; he created the first institute of social psychiatry in Lima in 1967 and publishes extensively. The Mexican Social Security Institute, the first of its kind in Latin America, was inaugurated in 1943. The director of psychiatric services for this institution was Raúl González Henríquez (1906-1952), a brilliant teacher, researcher, and organizer, one of the precursors of the psychoanalytic movement in Mexico and one of the initiators of the Asociación Psiquiátrica de America Latina (APAL).

Forensic medicine and psychiatry had reached a parallel stage of development during the 19th century, at the time when the theories of Lombroso were in vogue. However, in later years psychiatry made a more rapid progress. Several textbooks on forensic psychiatry were published towards the end of the last century, in particular those by Gerónimo Blanco (Venezuela, 1881), Leoncio Barreto (Bogotá, 1890) and Carlos E. Putnam (Bogotá, 1896). In 1900 Francisco Veyga started in Buenos Aires a series of works on medico-legal psychopathology.

Criminology was a common ground for psychiatric and medico-legal studies. The journal *Archivos de la Psiquiatría y Criminología* was founded by José Ingenieros (1877-1925) in Buenos Aires in 1902. Ingenieros is also regarded as a philosopher and sociologist. He was a champion for the social and cultural development of the Latin American countries. His versatile studies embraced psychological, medico-social, historical, philosophical, and criminological themes. He is popularly known throughout Latin America by his book, *El Hombre Mediocre,* an essay which was influential for several generations of Latin Americans. He founded in 1907 the Instituto de Criminología in Buenos Aires, the first of its kind in South America.

The Instituto de Medicina Legal was founded in Bogotá in 1914 and has been quite active through the efforts of Professor Guillermo Uribe Cualla, author of several works on forensic psychiatry. The textbook by the Argentinian Nerio Rojas, *Psiquiatría Medico-Legal,* (1932) was for several years a standard reference book for students, as was *Psiquiatría Clínica e Forense* (1940), by the distinguished Brazilian psychiatrist Antonio Carlos Pacheco e Silva. The Instituto de Criminología was founded in Quito by Julio Endara in 1936, and the Instituto de Ciencias Penales in Santiago in 1937.

In regard to influential orientations in psychiatric thought and practices in Latin America, 19th century psychiatry was influenced by the theory of degeneracy as proposed by Morel and developed by Magnan, Moreau de Tours, Krafft-Ebing, and Lombroso. In addition to the well known work by Ramos Mejía in Argentina, this theory inspired studies such as those of Lisandro Alvarez, *Neurosis de Hombres Celebres de Venezuela* (1893), and by Diego Carbonell, *La Psicopatología de Bolívar* (1916). These works provoked very heated polemics in academic circles as late as the first decades of this century.

The subject of hypnosis, known through the works of Mesmer, Charcot, and Bernheim, was also enthusiastically taken up by several

Latin-American clinicians of the last century. Antonio Uribe Silva published in Colombia in 1875 his *Ensayo Sobre Magnetismos*. Proto Gomez, Nicolas Osorio, and Juan David Herrera practiced hypnosis in Bogotá in 1890 and wrote on the subject. Mariano Peñaherrera, professor of forensic medicine in Quito, published in 1902 his book, *Hipnotismo y Terapeutica*.

Hypnosis seems to have regained some of its former prestige after World War II. Several articles began to appear in the journals and two societies were organized: Federación Latinoamericana de Hipnosis Clínica (1959), and Confederación Latinoamericana de Hipnosis Clínica y Experimental (1960), both established in Argentina. The term *sofrosis*, coined by the Colombian Alfonso Caicedo in the early 1960's, led to the establishment of the Sociedad Internacional de Sofrología.

Psychotherapy was publicly acknowledged in academic circles in Latin America with the presentation of the doctoral thesis, *Psicoterapia*, by Juan A. Agrelo in Buenos Aires in 1908. In 1910 German Greve, a disciple of Freud who practiced in Chile, presented to the Interamerican Congress of Medicine and Hygiene in Buenos Aires his work, *Sobre Psicología y Psicoterapia de Ciertos Estados Angustiosos*, which received flattering comments by Freud. In 1915, the Peruvian psychiatrist Honorio Delgado published his thesis *Psicoanálisis*. He later traveled to Vienna, participated in the Congresses of Berlin (1922), and Innsbruck (1927), and made the first Spanish translation of *Técnica del Psicoanálisis* (1929). Gregorio Bermann (1896-1972) began to apply techniques derived from psychoanalysis around 1920 and published articles on the psychodynamics of paranoia and obsessive states. He visited Freud in Vienna in 1930 and founded the journal *Psicoterapia* in 1936. However, like Delgado, he later abandoned his interest in psychoanalysis. Julio Pires Porto-Cabello, the first Brazilian disciple of Freud, started to work in Belo Horizonte in 1935. Angel Garma, an outstanding Spanish psychoanalyst and member of the Berlin Psychoanalytic group, arrived in Buenos Aires in 1938. Together with Celes Ernesto Cárcamo, Arnaldo and Luis Rascowsky, Enrique Pichon-Riviere, and Marie Langer he founded the Asociación Psicoanalítica Argentina in 1942. This has been for many years the leading group for the psychoanalytic movement in Latin America, exercising a strong intellectual influence through its journal *Revista de Psicoanálisis* founded in 1943, the first of its kind in Latin America.

The Argentinian psychoanalytic association was soon followed by similar groups in Montevideo, Rio de Janeiro, Santiago, Porto Alegre, Mexico, Bogotá, and Caracas. The first Latin American Congress of

Psychoanalysis took place in Buenos Aires in 1956. A coordinating organization of Latin American psychoanalytic associations (COPAL) was founded in Santiago in 1960.

Numerous schools and tendencies of contemporary psychotherapy are represented in Latin America such as the reflexological, behavioristic, existential, phenomenological, cultural, anthropological, etc.

The development of the neo-analytic movement in Mexico was due to the initiative of Raúl González Henríquez and Guillermo Dávila, who were able to secure the residency in Mexico of Erich Fromm, who started a vigorous and productive school in 1952.

Apparently stimulated by the success of Fromm in Mexico, two other leaders decided to travel to Latin America to start local branches of their schools: Victor Frankl visited Argentina in 1954 and founded the Sociedad Argentina de Logoterapia; likewise, Igor Caruso stayed for some time in Bogotá in 1964, presided over a Latin American Symposium on Depth Psychology, and founded the Círculo Colombiano de Psicología Profunda.

Group techniques have had a considerable development in Latin America. One of the pioneers was Arnaldo Rascowsky in Buenos Aires in 1947. The Asociación Argentina de Psicoterapia de Grupo was founded in 1947 and a journal has been published since 1961. The first Latin American Congress was held in Buenos Aires in 1957. The Asociación de Psicodrama y Psicoterapia de Grupo was founded in Buenos Aires by Jaime Rojas Bermúdez in 1965.

The era of psychotropic drugs had a brilliant precursor in the Peruvian psychiatrist Carlos Gutierrez Noriega (1906-1950), whose untimely death deprived Latin America of an outstanding researcher and clinician.

Publications

According to Valdivia Ponce (42), who conducted a compilation of the literature, a total of 1,234 works on psychology and psychiatry were written in Latin America during the period 1794-1962. In the Medical School of Bogotá alone, 128 doctoral theses dealing with neuropsychiatric themes were accepted during the period 1889-1954.

During the present century psychiatric journals have been published in almost every country of Latin America. Unfortunately not many of them have been able to survive for a long time. The first periodical publication in Latin America was *Archivos de Criminología y Psiquiatría,* founded in Buenos Aires in 1902 by José Ingenieros, as mentioned before. It was followed by *Archivos Brasileros de Psi-*

quiatría, Neurología y Ciencias Afines, founded by Juliano Moreira in 1905. The *Revista de Psiquiatría y Disciplinas Conexas* was founded by Honorio Delgado and Hermilio Valdizán in Lima in 1920, and the *Revista de Psiquiatría del Uruguay* appeared in Montevideo in 1924, followed in chronological order by: *Archivos Brasileros de Higiene Mental* (1925), *Boletín de Higiene Mental* (Lima, 1932), *Revista Mexicana de Psiquiatría, Neurología, y Medicina Legal* (1933) *Archivos de Criminología, Neuropsiquiatría, y Disciplinas Conexas* (Quito, 1937), *Neuropsiquiatría* (Lima, 1938), *Revista de Psicoanálisis* (Buenos Aires, 1943), and *Anales Neuropsiquiátricos del Frenocomio de Mujeres de Bogotá* (1942).

Gregorio Bermann and Claudio de Araujo Lima founded in 1951 the *Revista Latinoamericana de Psiquiatría,* which unfortunately did not last long; it was succeeded in 1954 by *Acta Psiquiátrica y Psicológica Argentina* which later became *Acta Psiquiátrica y Psicológica de América Latina.* This journal not only has been able to survive for almost two decades but also enjoys a wide circulation. Under the dynamic direction of Guillermo Vidal, well known author, teacher, and ex-president of the Argentinian Federation of Psychiatrists, it has become a forum for diffusion of psychiatric ideas and knowledge in Latin America.

Professional Associations and Meetings

Psychiatric societies in Latin America have run a course parallel to that of psychiatric journals and their names and orientations follow the evolution and prevalent tendencies of psychiatry. As a rule, in early years, they included joint groups of psychiatrists, neurologists, psychologists, forensic doctors, criminologists, and similar professionals, but gradually they became independent and restricted to only one type of specialty.

The Sociedad de Psicología, the oldest in Latin America, was founded in Buenos Aires in 1908. The Sociedad Brasilera de Neurología, Psiquiatría and Medicina Legal was founded the following year (1909). The Sociedad de Psiquiatría y Medicina Legal de Lima was founded in 1916 by Hermilio Valdizán. Honorio Delgado founded the Sociedad de Neuropsiquiatría y Medicina Legal del Perú in 1938. The Asociación Psiquiátrica Peruana was founded in 1954.

The Sociedad de Psiquiatría del Uruguay was started in 1924; the Sociedad de Neurología, Psiquiatría y Neurocirugía de Chile in 1937, the same year as the Sociedad Mexicana; the Sociedad Colombiana de Neurología, Psiquiatría y Medicina Legal in 1940. Similar psychiatric societies were founded in Ecuador (1942), Venezuela (1942), and Bolivia (1954). The Federacion Argentina de Psiquiatras was founded in 1959, the Sociedad Colombiana de Psiquiatría in 1961 and the Asociación Brasilera do Psiquiatría in 1966.

The first Latin American conference on neurology, psychiatry, and forensic medicine was held in Buenos Aires in 1928. The Jornadas Rioplatenses de Neuropsiquiatría, which annually bring together Argentinian and Uruguayan psychiatrists, were started in 1930. The First Interamerican Conference of Mental Hygiene took place in Rio de Janeiro in 1936. The following year (1937), the Primeras Jornadas Neuropsiquiátricas Panamericanas met in Santiago de Chile. The system of classification of mental disorders used by the American Psychiatric Association was recommended at this meeting, which, in a way, seems to have been an acknowledgment of the North American influence on Latin American psychiatry.

The International Congress of Mental Hygiene took place in Rio de Janeiro in 1940. The Fourth Congress of the World Federation for Mental Health was held in Mexico in 1951, and the 15th and 20th Congresses in Lima in 1962 and 1967, respectively. The First International Congress of Neuropsychiatry took place in Santiago de Chile in 1952. The First Interamerican Congress of Psychology was held in Santo Domingo in 1953 and the First Ibero-American Medico-Psychological Congress met in Buenos Aires in 1956.

A series of Latin American Congresses on Mental Health was started in Sao Paulo in 1954 and continued in Buenos Aires (1956), Lima (1958), Santiago de Chile (1960), Caracas (1963), and again in Buenos Aires (1966).

A group of prominent Latin American psychiatrists attending the First World Congress of Psychiatry in Paris (1950) conceived the idea of creating the Asociación Psiquiátrica de la América Latina (APAL). It was through the untiring efforts of Gregorio Bermann, José Angel Bustamante, Guillermo Dávila, Raúl González-Henríquez, Antonio Carlos Pacheco e Silva, and Carlos A. Seguín that this association, which brings together 14 national psychiatric societies in Latin America, was formed. There have been congresses in Caracas (1961), Mexico City (1962), Lima (1964), Buenos Aires (1966), Bogotá (1968), Sao Paulo (1970), and Punta del Este (Uruguay, 1972).

The Inter-American Council of Psychiatric Associations (IACPA), which coordinates the Latin American Psychiatric Association with the American Psychiatric Association and the Canadian Psychiatric Association, was founded in 1965 under the aegis of Daniel Blain, Guillermo Dávila, and Carlos A. Seguín. Under the auspices of IACPA, the first Conference for Mental Health in the Americas took place in San Antonio, Texas, in 1968, attended by an enthusiastic group of psychiatrists from the hemisphere. This was a unique opportunity for assessing the present and future of psychiatry in terms of existing services, needs, resources, education, research, and planning.

The Fourth Congress of the World Psychiatric Association was held in 1971 in Mexico City with an attendance of more than 6,000 professionals. The Mexican psychiatrist, Professor Ramón de la Fuente, a distinguished teacher, therapist, and author, was elected vice president of WPA.

The Pan American Health Organization (PAHO), the western hemisphere branch of the World Health Organization, started the Regional Program for Mental Health in 1960. The directors of this program, Jorge Velasco Alzaga and René González Uzcátegui, have accomplished valuable work in promotion and development of plans to improve the levels of service and training activities in the continent. The meeting of three Latin American seminars on mental health in Cuernavaca (1962), Buenos Aires (1963), and Jamaica (1964) afforded excellent opportunities for exchange of information and analysis of problems. Later on, PAHO sponsored seminars on the undergraduate teaching of psychiatry (Lima, 1967), administration of public mental health (Viña del Mar, Chile, 1969), and the training of psychiatrists (Bogotá, 1972). It was also instrumental in organizing the First Conference for Mental Health in the Americas in San Antonio (1968).

Perspective Views

Honorio Delgado and Oscar Trellez (14) were of the opinion that, although Latin American psychiatry was making a rapid progress, there were still countries in which the mentally ill were regarded as nothing more than diagnostic cases rather than as human beings in need of understanding and help. The separation of psychiatry from other disciplines had just started, psychiatry still being particularly dependent on neuropathology and forensic medicine. However, psychiatrists were striding forward to promote changes in psychiatric practice and teaching, engaging in an active fight against the resistances from both the community and official bodies.

From a more recent vantage point, Velasco Alzaga (43) distinguishes the following chronological stages in the development of different types of social actions towards the mentally ill: destruction of the mentally ill; seclusion of patients, which began in Latin America in 1566 and lasted for almost 300 years; systematic study of the patient, which began with the creation of the first psychiatric chairs in the medical schools; scientific research on mental illness, which started with the inauguration of the first laboratory of experimental psychology in 1899; and, finally, prevention of mental disorders. Although this latter development started with the Leagues for Mental Health and the passing of special laws, only recently has it begun to reach the consciousness of society and the government.

A summary view of the current state of psychiatry in Latin America, its needs, trends, and future perspectives has been outlined elsewhere (26). What seems to be clear at present is that, in spite of an arduous and protracted course, psychiatry in Latin America is not only attaining maturity, but also widening its horizon through a search for solutions congruent with the historical, social, and cultural characteristics of this part of the world.

REFERENCES

1. ACOSTA, JOAQUIN DE (1848): *Compendio Histórico del Descubrimiento y Colonización de la Nueva Granada en el siglo decimosexto*. Paris.
2. AGUADO FRAY PEDRO DE (1956): *Recopilación Historial*. Tomo I, Biblioteca de la Presidencia de Colombia, Editorial A.B.C. Bogotá.
3. ALVAREZ, RICARDO (1942): *La Psiquiatría en Venezuela desde la época precolombina hasta nuestros días*. Caracas.
4. BELSASSO, GUIDO (1969): The history of psychiatry in Mexico. *Hosp. & Community Psychiatry*, 20, 342-344.
5. BERMANN, GREGORIO (1960): *Nuestra Psiquiatría*. Bs. Aires: Paidós.
6. BUSTAMANTE, JOSE ANGEL (1958): Tres Precursores de la Psiquiatría en Cuba: José Joaquín Muñoz, Gustavo López y José A. Valdés Anciano. *Arch. de Neurol. y Psiq.*, 8, 168-180.
7. CALDERON-NARVAEZ, GUILLERMO (1964): Conceptos psiquiátricos en la medicina azteca contenidos en el Código Badiano escrito en el siglo XVI. In: Seguín C. and Ríos-Carrasco R. (Eds.), *Anales del Tercer Congreso Latinoamericano de Psiquiatría*. Lima.
8. CALDERON-NARVAEZ, GUILLERMO (1968): Consideraciones acerca del Alcoholismo entre los pueblos pre-hispánicos de México. *Rev. del Inst. Nal. de Neurol.*, 11, 5 (México).
9. CASTELLANOS, JUAN DE (1956): *Elegías de varones ilustres de Indias*. Biblioteca de la Presidencia de Colombia, Editorial A. B. C. Bogotá.
10. CASTILLO, BERNAL DIAZ DEL (1970): *Historia verdadera de la Conquista de la Nueva España*. México: Editorial Porrúa.
11. CIEZA DE LEON, PEDRO (1932): *Parte primera de la Crónica del Perú* Madrid: Espasa-Calpe.
12. COE MICHAEL D. (1966): *The Maya*. Harmondsworth: Penguin Books.
13. CUEVA-TAMARIZ, AGUSTIN (1966): *Evolución de la Psiquiatría en el Ecuador*. Cuenca: Casa de la Cultura.
14. DELGADO, HONORIO & TRELLEZ J. O. (1939): La Psychiatrie Dans L'Amérique du Sud. *Ann. Med-Psychol.* (Supplement, April 1939).
15. DELGADO ROIG, JUAN (1948): *Fundaciones Psiquiátricas en Sevilla y Nuevo Mundo*. Madrid: Edit. Paz Montalvo.
16. DIETSCHY, HANS (1960): Rasgos depresivos en el arte de los indios de América. *Documenta Geigy*, 1960.

17. DUQUE-GOMEZ, LUIS (1965): Etno-Historia y Arqueología. In: Academia Colombiana de Historia (Eds.), *Historia Extensa de Colombia*, Vol. I, Part I. Bogotá: Ediciones Lerner.

18. DUQUE-GOMEZ, LUIS (1967): Tribus indígenas y Sitios Arqueológicos. In: Academia Colombiana de Historia (Eds.), *Historia Extensa de Colombia*, Vol. I., Part II. Bogotá: Ediciones Lerner.

19. ETCHEGOYEN, RICARDO HORACIO (1963): Estado actual de la psicoterapia en la Argentina. *Acta. Psiquiat. Psicol. Arg.*, 9, 93.

20. GILLIN, J. (1956): El temor mágico. In: *Cultura Indígena de Guatemala, Ensayos de Antropología Social.* Guatemala: (Edit.) Ministerio de Educación Pública.

21. GRANADA, DANIEL (1947): *Supersticiones del Río de la Plata*. Buenos Aires: Editorial Guillermo Kraft.

22. GRAÑA, FRANCISCO, ROCCA, ESTEBAN, & GRAÑA, LUIS (1954): *Las trepanaciones Craneanas en el Perú en la época prehistórica*, Lima.

23. HARO, SILVIO LUIS (1967): *La magia en la medicina primitiva del Reino de Quito*. Quito: Edit. Minerva.

24. LA BARRE, WINSTON (1959): *The Peyote Cult*. Camden: The Shoe String Press.

25. LEON, CARLOS A. (1963): "El Espanto" Sus implicaciones psiquiátricas. *Acta Psiquiat. Psicol. Arg.*, 9, 207-217.

26. LEON, CARLOS A. (1972): Psychiatry in Latin America. *Brit. J. Psychiat.*, 121, 121-136.

27. MARIANI-RAMIREZ, CARLOS (1964): Personalidad del hechicero indígena. El Machi o hechicero Mapuche. In: Seguín, Carlos A. and Ríos-Carrasco, Rubén (Eds.), *Anales del Tercer Congreso Latinoamericano de Psiquiatría*. Lima.

28. MASON J. ALDEN (1960): *The Ancient Civilizations of Peru*. Harmondsworth: Penguin Books.

29. MEDINA, JOSE TORIBIO (1952): *Historia del Tribunal de la Inquisición de Cartagena de Indias*. Bogotá: Ediciones de la Biblioteca Nacional de Colombia.

30. METRAUX, A. (1962): *Les Incas*, p. 133. Paris: Editions du Seuil.

31. MURIEL, JOSEFINA (1956): *Hospitales de la Nueva España*, Vol. I. México: Edit. Jus.

32. NARANJO, PLUTARCO (1970): *Ayahuasca: Religión y Medicina*. Quito: Editorial Universitaria.

33. NICHOLSON, IRENE (1968): *Mexican and Central American Mythology*. London: Paul Hamlyn.

34. OSBORNE, HAROLD (1968): *South American Mythology*. London: Paul Hamlyn.

35. PAREDES, M. RIGOBERTO (1963): *Mitos, supersticiones y supervivencias populares de Bolivia*. La Paz: Ediciones Isla.

36. PEREZ DE BARRADAS, JOSE (1957): *Plantas Mágicas Americanas*. Madrid.

37. PEREZ-FONTANA, VELARDE (1967): *Historia de la Medicina en el Uruguay*, Vols. I-II. Montevideo: Edit. Ministerio de Salud Pública.

38. ROSSELLI, HUMBERTO (1968): *Historia de la Psiquiatría en Colombia*, Vols. I-II. Bogotá: Edit. Horizontes.

39. RUBEL, A. J. (1964): The epidemiology of a folk illness: susto in Hispanic America. *Ethnology*, 3, 268-83.

40. SAL Y ROSAS, F. (1958): El mito del Jani o Susto de la Medicina indígena del Perú. *Rev. Sanid. de Policía*, 18, 167-89.

41. VALIANT, G. C. (1965): *Aztec of Mexico. Origin, Rise and Fall of the Aztec Nation*. Baltimore: Penguin Books.

42. VALDIVIA PONCE, OSCAR (1964): *Historia de la psiquiatría peruana*. Lima.

43. VELASCO-ALZAGA, JORGE M. (1967): Actitudes sociales y legales ante el enfermo mental. Evolución Histórica. Reunión Nal. de la Asociación psiquiátrica Mexicana A. C., México (Mimeographed).

44. VON DÄNIKEN, ERICH (1971): *Chariots of the Gods*. New York: Bantam Books.
45. VON HAGEN, VICTOR W. (1957): *Realm of the Incas*. New York: Mentor Books.
46. VON HAGEN, VICTOR W. (1964): *The Desert Kingdoms of Peru*. New York: Mentor Books.
47. VON HAGEN, VICTOR W. (1970): *El mundo de los Mayas*. México: Editorial Diana.
48. WEISS, PEDRO (1958): *Osteología Cultural—Prácticas Cefálicas*. Part 1. Lima: Imprenta Universidad de San Marcos.

21

THE WEST INDIES

M. H. Beaubrun, M.D., P. Bannister, M.D.,
L. F. E. Lewis, G. Mahy, K. C. Royes,
P. Smith and Z. Wisinger

1

INTRODUCTION

A short-lived political federation united the islands of the British Commonwealth Caribbean and the nearby mainland territories in 1957, but in 1962 the federation broke up. Jamaica and Trinidad became independent from Britain, followed soon afterwards by Guyana and Barbados.

The University of the West Indies, with campuses in Jamaica, Trinidad, and Barbados, remains federal in structure, serving 14 separate governments. The medical school is located in Jamaica, with clinical teaching facilities in Trinidad and Barbados.

2

JAMAICA

The treatment of the mentally ill by the aboriginal Arawaks of Jamaica was described by a Spanish settler in 1531. In the earliest known record of psychiatry in the island he stated: "Lunatics they call 'mind-riven' and attend with lavings and unguents while singing and with salvent herbs which also they blend with food and leave hung on fruiting trees for those that wander." The results of these measures seem to have been so good that the colonists attributed them to sorcery; the Arawaks' use of indigenous herbs was adopted, however, and became one of the sources of local folklore about mental illness to the present day.

In the 1570's, some 60 years after colonization by Spain, the local council designated a four-room building for the care of mentally ill persons, which was adjacent to the monastery in the main town, Santiago de la Vega (the "Spanish Town" of today). This innovation was largely due to the efforts of Beniamo da Caceres who was very highly esteemed for his devoted medical services during the frequent epidemics of fevers. Having prominent influential members of the clergy and the laity suffering from febrile deliria, he was able to point out that "where ardent fevers abound other demons are rare." Although nothing is known of this first institution it is noteworthy that da Caceres, who was of Jewish parentage, was responsible for its operation, and that exorcism and trial for witchcraft of mentally ill persons are not known to have taken place in Jamaica.

The monastery and annex were abandoned when the island changed hands in 1655. An increase in the number of mentally ill persons occurred with the influx of British sugar planters "unassimilated to the climate" and of enslaved Africans "reft of language and rite." The former were placed in rooms in general hospitals and the latter in dungeon-like "hot houses" on the estates (Plate C). Treatment followed the prevailing British lines and for two centuries this consisted of restraint and confinement. The slaves were not permitted to practice any of their native customs and African thought did not influence local psychiatric methods.

There was no dearth of sound medical talent or medical literature in the island in these sugar-rich years. John Quier in 1774 wrote about the unhappy consequences of maternal deprivation and of unstable parental relations. He also described psychotic symptoms (encephalitis) associated with measles in African slaves, and mentioned the "white aphthous specks on the gums" which Koplik noticed 122 years later. Apart from this much of the psychiatric observations tended to be speculative and to give rise to such persisting misconceptions as tropical neurasthenia (15).

When the end of slavery came in 1838, with the closing of estate hospitals for slaves, the annex of the public hospital in Kingston was enlarged and officially designated the Lunatic Asylum for the reception of all mentally ill persons from the population of 400,000. Visits were made by doctors from the public hospital with the care of the patients left largely to the matron, close confinement being the rule for all, and immersion in a Rush tank of water for the more unruly.

A significant improvement in psychiatric care resulted from the efforts of Lewis Bowerbank, a physician in private practice in King-

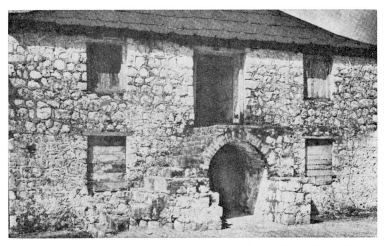

PLATE C. Remains of a building believed to have been a Sugar Estate Hospital for Slaves, the Lower Floor or "Hot House" being used for those mentally ill.

ston who campaigned for many years for medical reforms, which led eventually to the British Commission in Lunacy. Its wide powers were used to ensure the completion of a new hospital on ample grounds. Bowerbank pressed successfully for the appointment of a competent full-time psychiatrist and for the enactment of the Lunatic Asylum Law of 1861.

In 1863 the new Jamaica Lunatic Asylum, built on 28 acres by the sea in eastern Kingston, began operations with 172 patients from the former asylum. Thomas Allen, who came from Suffolk Infirmary at the age of 27 to be the medical superintendent, introduced an efficient system of asylum management on British lines and actively pioneered humane moral treatment in the institution in its first 23 years, with mechanical restraint abolished from that time and individual case records started. With nurses by their example "inducing the patients in groups" in many interesting and rewarding activities —which included seine fishing—high standards were maintained. Allen also helped to draft the revised Lunatic Asylum Law of 1873 that remained in force for 99 years, and to reorganize the Barbados Asylum in 1875, but his plea for extension of psychiatric services throughout Jamaica was not implemented.

During the past 60 years when the island's population doubled to 1,200,000, the number of patients and the size of the asylum increased considerably and the name was changed to Mental Hospital. New diagnostic classifications were adopted on English lines. Various sedative medications were introduced, including chemo-convulsive injections.

In 1948, insulin coma and electro-convulsive therapy were initiated, psychiatric nurse training was organized, and an out-patient clinic was started at Kingston Public Hospital; this clinic later helped in the teaching program of the new University of the West Indies. Out-patient services were extended to major population centers in the island, and with the introduction of the phenothiazines in the late 1950's the population of the Mental Hospital (Bellevue Hospital) began for the first time to show some reduction (1)—from 3,123 patients in 1959 to 2,800 in 1965—but the hospital was still overcrowded and understaffed (9). Recruitment of psychiatrists was slow and the rate of attrition high.

In 1964 a comprehensive plan for a National Mental Health Program was produced for the government by Alex Richman, a WHO consultant, but was not immediately implemented (28). In November, 1964 the first Professor of Psychiatry was appointed at the University of the West Indies and came to Jamaica in January, 1965. The new department provided a new image for psychiatry and the focus for improved recruitment, the story of which is told in the last section of this chapter.

3

TRINIDAD AND TOBAGO

The first available evidence of official concern for the mentally ill in Trinidad was reflected in 1844 by the passage of an ordinance for the safe custody of insane persons charged with offenses, and of persons suspected to be insane. The ordinance authorized the keeping of such persons in custody at the Royal Gaol. Another major step was taken in 1858 with the opening of the Belmont Lunatic Asylum in Belmont Circular Road, Port of Spain. This asylum was at first supervised by a succession of medical officers who had no special training in the treatment of mental illness. The inmates were housed in three separate buildings with open galleries, with accommodation for 80 persons. The buildings contained padded cells for very disturbed cases. A dispatch from the Secretary of State to Governor Keate, dated July 1, 1864 stated: "I find on examination that the reports, returns, and regulations of the Lunatic Asylum in Trinidad are remarkably minute and complete; and I fully recognize the care and attention given to the asylum by Dr. Murray and Mr. Pashley." Thomas Murray was then the medical attendant, and the resident superintendent was Mr. Pashley. In 1863, 24 patients were admitted, 12 discharged, "7 relieved and taken away by friends," and 4 died, 54 remaining in hospital. The total budget for 15 staff members for 1863 was £1,945. 16s. 8d.

Conditions at the asylum deteriorated over the next few years and did not improve again until the appointment as medical superintendent in 1882 of Seccombe, who "had acquired wide experience in the management and treatment of the insane in England." He found conditions in the asylum so primitive that he remarked it was behind the age, and that one would have to go back 40 years in the history of the insane to find another such institution in Britain. The defects were many and varied; "the site was unsuitable and did not lend itself to major improvements; the buildings were in a state of disrepair and badly arranged; the water supply was inadequate; the sanitary arrangements presented a sad spectacle; the two sexes were not sufficiently kept apart; the bath rooms and closets were shared alike by males and females; supervision was lacking and the overcrowding was deplorable; industrial employment as a means towards mental restoration was absent; and there was little or no amusement which is generally useful in the cure of some forms of lunacy" (29). Seccombe effected many improvements. An English-trained female head attendant was appointed and plans for a new institution were prepared in 1883, but the construction had to be delayed for some years. In 1900 the new buildings were completed and the patients removed to the more spacious St. Ann's Asylum as the new institution was called. By then, the number of patients in daily residence had risen to over 400. An assistant medical superintendent was appointed in 1900. Seccombe retired in 1908 after 26 years of devoted service. It was agreed that under his regime, and with the help of his assistant, Rake, the institution had been brought to a high level of efficiency.

There is a dearth of recorded information about the history of the institution during the next 25 years. The name of the institution was changed in 1935 from Lunatic Asylum to St. Ann's Mental Hospital, and in 1961 the name was further changed to St. Ann's Hospital. From 1908 to 1940 there were several medical superintendents including Samuel, Vincent, and Smith. The first Trinidadian medical superintendent—E. P. L. Masson—was appointed in 1940, though his period of service at the hospital dated from 1935. During his regime a systematic attempt was made to diagnose the illness of every patient. L. F. E. Lewis joined the staff in 1943 as assistant medical superintendent and served under Masson for the next 12 years.

In 1943 some cases of general paralysis of the insane were treated with malaria therapy. In 1944 all patients at the hospital were given a serological test for syphilis and the practice of routine serological tests for all new patients on admission was instituted. ECT was introduced by Masson in 1945, and two cases of neuro-syphilis were successfully treated by the induction of artificial fever by the Kettering Electric Hypertherm.

Prior to 1943 and for some years afterwards most of the patients admitted to St. Ann's had been certified. Most of the patients from the capital city of Port of Spain and its environs were admitted via an observation ward at the General (then Colonial) Hospital, where they had been observed for from one to seven days or longer before being certified. During their period of observation, they were kept in separate cells little better than horse stalls, and were attended by doctors and nurses with no training in psychiatry. Many were noisy and restless and some were dehydrated by the time they reached St. Ann's. The treatment in 1943 and for some years before was to put new admissions routinely on a bromide mixture. Very disturbed patients were given injections of morphia and hyoscine while paraldehyde was used for night sedation. Restless new admissions might be given a course of veronal, while the most restless were given 90 grains of sulphonal spread over a week. Not surprisingly, cases of bromism occurred (26). With the introduction of ECT and an increase in medical staff in 1947, bromide, barbiturate, and sulphonal sedation on a thrice-daily basis was discontinued.

In the decade of the 1940's, there was still considerable stigma attached to admission to St. Ann's Hospital, and relatives and patients alike often delayed such admission for as long as possible. Mentally ill patients were taken to consult priests, "science men," *obeah* men, Shango priests (30), spiritual Baptist elders, or "mothers," before they were finally brought for medical attention. Belief in spirit possession as a cause of mental illness was common.

The era of aggressive physical treatments which commenced at St. Ann's in 1945 was intensified after 1949. In that year insulin treatment was introduced. Electronarcosis was started in 1951 but results proved to be no better than those from ECT, which was less time-consuming. Transorbital leucotomy was first performed by L. R. Wynter of Antigua on a visit to the hospital in 1951 following a paper presented at the Conference of Caribbean Branches of the British Medical Association in January, 1951 (35). Between 1951 and 1955, 103 patients were leucotomized by a general surgeon, Henry Pierre.

Chlorpromazine and reserpine were first used at St. Ann's in 1954 (18). The introduction of the phenothiazines and other psychotropic drugs brought many changes. Insulin coma and leucotomy were gradually abandoned, though the former treatment was continued on the female side up to the end of 1960. Newly admitted patients remained in hospital for a shorter period and after 1957 an active program of treatment was carried out on the long-stay wards, resulting in the discharge of many patients who had hitherto been regarded as likely to remain in hospital for the balance of their lives. Some of these results at that time seemed little short of miraculous. Many patients were referred to out-patient clinics for follow-up treatment after discharge. These clinics, which had been started in 1950, began to be badly overcrowded after 1956. The number of clinics per week in Port of Spain increased from two in 1955 to six in 1971. During this period, clinics were also started in the towns of San Fernando, Sangre Grande, and Arima, and on the nearby island of Tobago.

An active program of treatment of alcoholism using mainly a combination of emetine aversion treatment and group psychotherapy was commenced in May, 1956 by Beaubrun, and has been continued up to the present. In 1956, the number of cases thus treated was 17, but admissions for alcoholism rose steadily especially after 1961, when a separate alcoholism treatment unit was set up. In that year the number of cases of alcoholism admitted for treatment rose to 332, including 22 women, and the growth of A.A. groups was stimulated throughout Trinidad (8).

In 1958 the Minister of Health appointed a committee under the chairmanship of Lewis to produce a comprehensive mental health plan for the territory. This report was submitted in 1959 and was accepted in principle by the government. One recommendation adopted from the report was the creation of a psychiatric unit as a ward at the General Hospital, Port of Spain. The unit was opened in March 1965 and has done valuable work. Since 1967 an attempt has been made to use the unit for psychiatric residency training. Residents have been sent from the U.W.I. Medical School in Jamaica and from the Clarke Institute, Toronto, to do a year of their training in Trinidad (10). The University of the West Indies also uses the unit for some undergraduate teaching. One result of the functioning of the psychiatric unit at the General Hospital, Port of Spain, and later the provision of beds under the charge of a full-time psychiatrist at the General Hospital, San Fernando, was to reduce drastically the number of new patients seen at St. Ann's Hospital.

Up to the end of 1964, the practice of psychiatry in Trinidad was influenced preponderately by the philosophy and teaching of psychiatry as practised in Great Britain. The influence of the Maudsley Hospital, London, was greatest in the period from 1940 to 1964, when three of its trainees, E. P. L. Masson, L. F. E. Lewis, and M. H. Beaubrun occupied in succession the post of Medical Superintendent of St. Ann's Hospital and worked together on the staff of the hospital for part of this period. The title of the post was later changed from Medical Superintendent to Psychiatric Hospital Director, and the Acting Director since August, 1971 is John Neehall, who is also Maudsley-trained. During the years 1966 to 1970, when a Canadian Technical Aid Program was in operation, the influence of Canadian psychiatric thought and practice was in evidence.

Little information is available about the early history of the training of mental nurses in Trinidad. Originally young men and women were recruited as attendants and, until the late 1930's, they received little formal training; they were supervised by trained nurses recruited from the United Kingdom. After some sporadic effort in formal training, a four-year period of theoretical and practical training for students was begun in 1955.

Psychiatric social work was first started in Trinidad in 1952; after 1965 nurses from the staff of St. Ann's Hospital were attached to the social workers department to assist with the visiting of homes and the follow-up of discharged patients.

Originally, large numbers of patients were kept occupied in maintenance work, growing vegetables and other crops, keeping the grounds clean, working in the laundry, kitchen, and bakery, or assisting at the quarters of the senior staff. In the early 1950's, several factors combined to alter this pattern which had continued unbroken for 50 years; occupational therapy became part of a more active treatment program, and new patients had shorter periods in hospital, thereby reducing the number available for hospital maintenance work.

The First Caribbean Conference for Mental Health in Aruba in 1957 provided the impetus for the formation of the Trinidad and Tobago Association for Mental Health in November, 1958, with Ray Lange as its first president. The Trinidad and Tobago Association for the Retarded was founded in the same year. The Lady Hochoy Home and School for Retarded Children was opened in March, 1961, followed by a second home opened more recently in San Fernando. Mentally retarded children and adults are also admitted to St. Ann's Hospital where the first School for the Mentally Handicapped was opened in 1958 (5).

Reference has already been made to the first ordinance in 1844 dealing with the mentally ill. The Petitions in Lunacy Ordinance and the Rules were passed in the year 1863. They provided for an enquiry as to whether a person was of unsound mind and incapable of managing his affairs. The Lunacy and Mental Treatment Ordinance—an ordinance relating to the custody of persons of unsound mind—came into operation on March 1, 1878. There have been subsequent additions and revisions. In the 1930's there was an ordinance to permit the admission of voluntary and temporary patients to St. Ann's Hospital. Other ordinances in 1940 dealt with the naming of "colonial mental hospitals" where persons suspected of being of unsound mind could be detained for observation. In the same year St. Ann's Mental Hospital was declared to be a criminal lunatic hospital for purposes of the ordinance. Ordinance No. 12 of 1946 Section 5 dealt with the transfer of patients from a colonial hospital to a colonial mental hospital for observation. In the same year, a Mental Hospital Board was established to review twice each year the cases of all mentally ill prisoners detained at St. Ann's Mental Hospital and to make recommendations about their discharge, or their further detention. The last revision of the Lunacy and Mental Treatment Ordinance Chapter 12 No. 10 was published in 1950 when all the laws of Trinidad and Tobago were revised. A draft Mental Health Bill has been in preparation since 1960 and it received its first reading in the House of Representatives in August, 1962. Since then it has been the subject of several minor revisions but has not yet received its second reading.

4

BARBADOS

The early history of psychiatry in Barbados prior to the building of the Mental Hospital in 1893 is obscure except for the occasional reference made in government papers and in land transactions of that period.

During the 1880's, most of the "lunatics" of that time were housed in dilapidated buildings on Constitution Road before being moved to an even more dilapidated structure on Powder Lane opposite Glendiary Prison. This latter building was always apparently crowded and the overflow of female patients was accommodated in the District "B" Police Station close to that area.

The discussions in the 1880's concerned the building of new and proper accommodation to house these inmates, and many sites were suggested. Land was actually bought near Codrington on the East Coast, but this site was excluded on the basis of poor sewerage; indeed throughout these times, it is clear that the main objectives in psychiatric care were to prevent the patients from dying of yellow fever and typhoid which were endemic diseases at that time. The final choice of site was of a small plantation named Jenkinsville on the Black Rock Road close to the West Coast of the island, and this purchase included about 70 acres of arable land. It was felt at that time that its proximity to the Lazaretto would mean that one doctor could administer both these institutions.

The reports of the first superintendent, Albert Field, at the opening of the hospital in 1893, are of great interest. He wrote, "Most of the patients walked over and some came in carriages while the more violent or respectable ones came at night." A few days later he comments, "The male patients appear to like the change and seem to be somewhat quieter but the female patients just the reverse." Field's report, written in perfect copper plate, shows from his conscientious comments that he perhaps was one of the first and most humane doctors to deal with these early lunatics. There were problems with management of kitchen and laundry, but by the time Field retired in 1902, the hospital seems to have established itself in an active, albeit custodial, way.

C. J. Manning, who succeeded him, was notable for his efforts to develop the "farm" and to produce, insofar as was possible, a self-supporting institution. One of the returns for the Mental Hospital's produce from 1904 includes 54,060 pints of milk at £337. 17s. 6d.; 102,500 pounds of sweet potatoes for £128. 3s. 9d.; and 18 coffins at 1/8d each. Clearly the efforts of the authorities then concerned to maintain the place and the health of the inmates were successful, for in that same year the death rate among the 368 patients was the lowest on record at 29. However, there is again a comment which shows that the outlying parishes were having to "pack off" their cases of psilosis to the asylum as lunatics—*Plus ca change, plus c'est le meme chose*. Pellagra was also occasionally diagnosed and many of these old patients were admitted in a moribund state.

Efforts to build up the "farm" were amply rewarded and it became known as a center for pedigreed cattle and pigs. Some were even exported to Trinidad and the smaller islands. During this period, the facilities of the hospital were improved by the addition of airing courts and shady trees, but nonetheless, from the visitor's book of that period, the then Colonial Secretary could still write "This is . . . the first and I hope the last time that I visit this institution." Very little medicine must have been available to those who worked here and in addition the standard of the staff, paid at $10.00 per month, was that of purely custodial keepers. It takes little imagination to conceive of the bedlam that must have existed.

In 1922 for the first time advertisements were made for recruitment of female "wardresses," and clearly, size and weight were the important criteria for their selection. It was shortly after this that W. S. Birch became Medical Superintendent in 1927, although Manning continued to assist at the hospital and was apparently a popular figure, since in those days the tramway was opposite the hospital gate and it was a regular event to see Manning, who always wore frock coat and top hat, travel down to Bridgetown in a tram to visit the General Hospital.

Birch was superintendent for nearly 20 years and, slowly but consistently, with a humane approach to his problem, he managed to change the asylum from a purely custodial institution to a hospital in itself, by gradually improving the physical sanitation and adding new buildings. Indeed, during this period, the hospital acquired a good name for itself among the islands and there was a considerable pride in Barbados of the institution which had been built as a farsighted venture in the 1890's.

During this year, Birch was clearly in touch with what was happening in other countries in the field of psychiatry. He managed to abolish all restraint by using modified insulin treatment, magnesium sulphate purges, and cold showers. This latter does seem a bit barbarous but we must remember that in that era no other effective medications were known; such physical treatments were tried often in a spirit of desperation.

Birch died in 1947, and his post was taken by Robert Lloyd Still, who remained until 1965. This was again a period of active expansion within the hospital and although it was initially the pre-phenothiazine era, Lloyd Still set about knocking down the walls with great zest and succeeded in opening all the wards within the hospital with the exception of one on the male side. As the phenothiazines came in, the general feeling was that there would be no more long-term patients, and an open-door policy was more actively pursued. Particularly for this reason, and because of the general shortage of land in the island, the Ministry of Health agreed to the transfer of most of the agricultural land to be used as a housing estate. This in a way was a sad decision since it has subsequently been shown that far from admitting fewer chronic patients, the numbers in fact continue at about the same rate.

No mention of nurses was made until 1940, when the first matron, Kathleen Walker, was appointed. Her standing order as matron carried many responsibilities for kitchen, laundry, and sewing room. She was the supreme authority on mental nursing. She changed the uniform from ankle length to 14 inches above the ground, panama hats to caps, and began alterations on an organized basis. She left a small booklet of 101 points which is still used in the Nursing School today. She intensely disliked the term "attendant" and addressed them as "nurses."

The early 1960's saw the introduction of ministerial government and the responsibility for the management of the hospital was transferred from the governor to the Ministry of Health. Finally in 1966 Barbados itself achieved independence. By that time, the Nursing School was thriving and producing its own registered nurses. This school successfully acquired full reciprocity with the Royal College of Nursing in London in 1966, issuing its own Registered Mental Nurse qualification.

This brief history is of interest in view of contemporary experience. There is a sense of *deja vu* in much of the present plans to provide extensive rehabilitation. What remains of the "farm" area has been opened up again and horticulture together with animal husbandry and sheltered workshops, offering employment on light industry lines, have all been established successfully. These activities of yesteryear do still clearly fulfill some need that is relevant to the community. More and more treatments over the years eventually find their own level and so in a salutory way, it is useful to see this historical perspective as something that can both temper one's enthusiasm and bridle one's pessimism.

5

THE WINDWARD ISLANDS

Grenada, St. Vincent, St. Lucia, and Dominica make up the Windward Islands, so called because of the prevailing trade winds. Table 1 shows comparative data for hospital beds and psychiatrists as of 1971/72:

TABLE 1

Island	Population	No. of Mental Hospital Beds	Psychiatric Beds in General Hospital	Psychiatrists
Grenada	95,136 (1970 census)	200+	8	1
St. Lucia	110,142 (1966 census)	120	0	1
St. Vincent	89,100 (1970 census)	96	0	0
Dominica	70,177 (1967 census)	60	8	1

Grenada

Grenada, with a population of 95,136, has one mental hospital a little less than 100 years old and, since 1971, an eight-bed psychiatric unit at the General Hospital.

In 1779, the site of the present mental hospital was a plantation called Mount George Estate, owned by the Hon. William Lucas. The French successfully wiped out the British in July of that year by an inland approach through this estate. This site, about 700 feet above sea level, was suitable for defense, so a fort was erected immediately after forcibly appropriating the land. When the British got it back four years later through the Treaty of Versailles, they named it Fort Matthew after Lt. Governor Edward Matthew.

After 24 years of planning and minor alterations, in 1879 "lunatics" from Grenada and all the other "Islands of Government," except Barbados, were brought to Fort Matthew. To this date this is still the only mental hospital in Grenada (Plate CI).

The first Mental Hospital Ordinance was written on March 27, 1895 with revisions in 1934, 1940, 1947, 1956, and 1958. The existing law provides for the admission and discharge of voluntary patients, but is outdated in many ways; e.g. when any patient dies at the mental hospital the coroner must be informed and an inquiry made. A new Mental Health Act prepared in 1971 is now awaiting final approval.

From 1879 to about 1960, in-patient care at the mental hospital was the only mental health service in Grenada. There was no follow-up

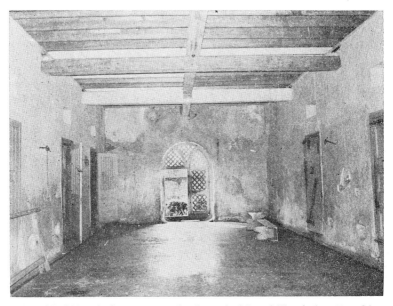

PLATE CI. Old seclusion room at the Grenada Mental Hospital at Fort Matthew. The use of such rooms was abandoned in 1968.

after discharge. Little concern was shown for the hospital by government, and the only recorded improvements over 93 years were minor alterations like asphalting the cells in 1904 and the installation of a new toilet system about 1913.

In the 1940's conditions were so bad at the mental hospital, the "house of refuge," and the tuberculosis hospital that a young medical officer, L. M. Commissiong, published a booklet of poems about the "Bedlam-like" conditions, drawing attention to the neglect of these institutions. He later became the chief medical officer of Grenada and helped to bring about much-needed change.

The hospital commenced in 1879 with 32 patients, closed with 36, 16 admissions for the year and a daily average in-patient population of 31.8 per cent. The population of Grenada at this time was about 42,200. For the next 25 pears the admission rate continued to rise yearly, reaching its peak in 1904 with a total of 40 admissions for the year. The in-patient population rose steadily, again peaking around 1906 with 135. There was a dysentry epidemic in 1906, and with an island population of 70,505 the death rate was 24.53 per cent. At the hospital there were 22 deaths and a peak death rate of 16.29 per cent.

At the end of the first year of the hospital there were 10 discharges; 25 years later this was unchanged. Even in 1949, 70 years later, with a five-fold increase of in-patients, the number discharged was just about three times what it had been at the start of the hospital.

There were four attendants at the outset but this number was soon increased to eight. Up to 1940 there were still only 16 nurse-attendants, but 15 years later there were 48.

Following a detailed report by Lloyd Still, medical superintendent of the hospital in Barbados, the local superintendent, Bierzynski, brought about a dramatic change in patient care. There were about 40 fewer patients at the end of 1961 in the hospital, marked increase in admissions and discharges, and a significant drop in the death rate. ECT, modified insulin, and chlorpromazine replaced paraldehyde and bromides. Some out-patient care at the hospital was provided and a Mental Health Association was begun.

Since 1968, under Mahy, up-to-date programs have been adopted. Most of the seclusion rooms have been closed, resulting in a major part of the hospital being locked off.

St. Lucia

The mental hospital at La Toc, St. Lucia is also situated in an old fort. No general hospital psychiatry exists as yet, but praiseworthy attempts have been made in recent years to rehabilitate their chronic patients. An active Mental Health Association, assisted by the Junior Chamber of Commerce, has built a halfway house and a sheltered workshop, and efforts are being made to provide treatment for alcoholics.

St. Vincent

There is as yet no psychiatrist in St. Vincent, but the Pan American Health Organization (PAHO/WHO) and the University of the West Indies carried out a project in 1969, 1970, and 1971 to train public health nurses and inspectors in the follow-up care of patients discharged from the mental hospital (31).

Dominica

Not until 1971 did the first trained Dominican psychiatrist become available. There is now a small psychiatric unit at the general hospital and a community mental health program is beginning to be implemented.

6

THE LEEWARD ISLANDS

The Leeward Islands consist of an arc of islands encompassing the northern group of the Lesser Antilles from the Virgin Islands to Montserrat. Written records of their history exist only from the time of their discovery by Columbus in his voyages at the end of the 15th century. The European colonizing powers—Spanish, French, Dutch, English and Danish—settled and fought for these islands between the 16th and 19th centuries.

In the Leeward Islands Antigua, because of its position at the easternmost tip of this chain of islands, and because of its good and protected harbors like Parham, English Harbour, and St. John's, and suitable soil for sugar cane plantation, became an important shipping and trading center. From the 17th century when it was colonized by the British, it remained constantly under British rule. Because of its hurricane-safe natural anchorage at English Harbour protected by hills, the British built fortifications there and made it the headquarters of their West Indies Fleet.

The first institution caring for the physically and mentally ill was established on the "Ridge" in the 18th century. This was originally a military establishment. At that time there were up to 3,000 Royal Marines stationed at the heights surrounding the English Harbour Navy Base.

In 1828 the Daily Meal Society was established. The original purpose of this institution was "to supply the sick and needy of St. John's [the Capital City of Antigua] and its neighborhood with a daily meal." According to Mrs. Lanaghan, a chronicler of that time, five small houses were erected where "the medical gentlemen of St. John's offered to attend gratuitously the cry of the unfortunate people." This was gradually enlarged and renamed the "Lazaretto"; it also cared for lepers. The first "lunatic asylum" for the mentally ill was built in 1841 where "such inmates of the institution as have shown symptoms of aberration of mind" were transferred.

In 1871 the Leeward Islands were federated into one colony. This Leeward Islands Colony comprised the British Virgin Islands, St. Kitts, Nevis, Anguilla, Antigua, Barbuda, Montserrat, and Dominica. Mental patients, including the "criminally insane" were gradually brought from these territories for treatment or custody to Antigua, to the mental hospital, which was renamed Central Lunatic Asylum. In 1907 the mental patients were transferred to a group of buildings at Skerritts, about two miles from St. John's, which up to then was used as a closed training school for juvenile delinquents. Records of the early days of the Central Lunatic Asylum are scarce. In May 1909 there were 113 patients. Essex, an Englishman, was superintendent of the mental hospital and also of the public works department of Antigua. The buildings of the boys' training school were of wood. It was under Essex's supervision that new buildings, mostly of stone and concrete, replaced the old ones. A Canadian, T. B. Macauley, gave much financial assistance and the female dormitories were named after him.

In 1939 Dominica left the Leeward Islands Federation and joined the Windward Islands. In 1956 the Leeward Island Federation was dissolved. However the Antigua Mental Hospital still cares for the mentally ill from approximately 300,000 inhabitants from the geographical area of this chain of islands, including some from Dominica.

During the 1960's the emphasis shifted from custodial care to intensive treatment. In this way from about 270 patients in 1966, the hospital population decreased to 170 on January 1, 1970, and, though there were 239 admissions during 1970, the hospital population on December 31, 1970 was further reduced to 163. Of 163 patients 75 were from Antigua and Barbuda, 20 from St. Kitts-Nevis, Anguilla, 23 from Dominica, 27 from Montserrat, and 18 from the British Virgin Islands.

The removal of mental patients from these scattered islands to Antigua created difficulties for their rehabilitation. They were isolated from their communities and deprived of contact with their families and friends. Though many recovered within a month or two of admission they had to be kept longer in hospital than the Antiguans who could be discharged on parole and for out-patient follow-up. The other territories paid the Antigua government E.C. $1.56 (6 shillings and 6 pence) per patient per diem for full board, drugs, and treatment; yet sometimes an acutely disturbed patient would be transferred from the British Virgin Islands by chartered plane at a cost of about U.S. $300.00 per flight, the equivalent of his maintenance in Antigua for a full year.

For the past 15 years the Antigua Mental Hospital under Dr. Zoltan Wisinger has been mainly an "open door" one, but one ward on each of the male and female sides has remained closed for disturbed patients. Less than 10 patients per day on the average are on these closed wards.

The arrival of the phenothiazines in the 1950's helped to reduce the hospital population. Fluphenazine enanthate when introduced in 1967 proved to be particularly effective and was largely responsible for the dramatic fall in the hospital population from 270 to 170 in 1970. L. R. Wynter, C.B.E., an Antiguan doctor, performed the first prefrontal leucotomies in the West Indies at the Antigua Mental Hospital in 1950 (35).

Recently a start has been made at introducing psychiatry at the general hospital, patients being transferred to the mental hospital only for long-term care.

7

REGIONAL COOPERATION

A meeting in 1956 between J. R. Rees, President of the World Federation for Mental Health, and Robert Turfboer, a young medical practitioner in the Netherlands Antilles, led to the holding of the First Caribbean Conference for Mental Health in Aruba in 1957. This conference brought together for the first time psychiatrists and other mental health workers, both lay and professional, from the British, American, Dutch, French and independent islands of the Caribbean.

From then on biennial meetings were held regularly in St. Thomas (1959); Jamaica (1961); Curacao (1963); Martinique (1965); Barbados (1967); Trinidad (1969); and Surinam (1971). At the St. Thomas meeting in 1959 the Caribbean Federation for Mental Health was formed, and L. F. E. Lewis was elected its first president. The British Commonwealth Caribbean played a leading role in the first decade, providing all the presidents up to 1971. The CFMH improved inter-island communication and created an increased awareness of the need for better treatment facilities for the mentally ill, and of the need for multidisciplinary collaboration and lay involvement in prevention of mental illness.

During the first six years of its existence the federation was assisted by an American psychiatrist, Bertram Schaffner, who created an organization in New York, the Caribbean Federation for Mental Health of New York, Inc. This organization raised funds and sent psychiatrists, psychologists, social workers, and other professionals in their vacation months to the Caribbean for periods of voluntary service, awakening public interest in mental health (6, 10, 27).

The 1961 conference in Jamaica drew attention to the lack of adequate teaching of psychiatry at the University of the West Indies, and a grant was obtained from the Foundation's Fund for Research in Psychiatry which made possible the creation of a chair and department of psychiatry at the medical school in Jamaica. Michael H. Beaubrun, then President of the CFMH, became the first Professor of Psychiatry in January, 1965.

The new department of psychiatry was faced with the task of upgrading the image of psychiatry which had for so long been stigmatized by association with overcrowded and understaffed mental hospitals. Psychiatric beds were obtained at the University Teaching Hospital. Undergraduate teaching hours were increased and postgraduate training started, and despite stringent budgetary limitations, a considerable improvement in recruitment to the ranks of psychiatry resulted.

The department emphasized the importance of general hospital psychiatry and sought to develop and test models of comprehensive community care with the general hospital psychiatric unit as the main base (7, 14, 25).

The Caribbean Psychiatric Association was started in 1968. The foundation president, Michael Beaubrun, was succeeded by Christiaan M. Winkel of Curacao in 1971. This association covers the whole Caribbean Archipelago including British, Dutch, French, and U.S. possessions as well as independent countries, with the exception thus far of Cuba. Puerto Rico, with some 120 psychiatrists, forms the largest national section of membership.

A joint meeting of the Caribbean Psychiatric Association and the American Psychiatric Association held at Ocho Rios, Jamaica in 1969 gave impetus to the new association. Since then the publication of a regular quarterly newsletter has improved communication among psychiatrists of the region and has begun to stimulate the production of scientific papers.

In retrospect it is clear that the mental health movement played a significant part in advancing West Indian psychiatry in the years from 1957 to 1971.

REFERENCES

1. Annual Reports on the Jamaican Lunatic Asylum o/c Mental Hospital o/c Bellevue Hospital; from 1864 to 1969. Jamaica Govt. Printery.
2. Annual Reports of the Superintending Medical Officer, St. Ann's Hospital, Trinidad: 1958, 1959 and 1960—61.
3. ASPINALL, *West Indian Tales of Old*.
4. AUGIER, R., GORDON, S. C., HALL, D. G. AND RECKORD, M. (1960): *The Making of the West Indies*. Longmans (Caribbean).
5. BEAUBRUN, M. H. (1964): A review of ten years progress in the care of the mentally retarded in Trinidad. In: *Report of Conference on Child Care in Trinidad and Tobago*. Trinidad & Tobago: P. O. S., Govt. Printery.
6. BEAUBRUN, M. H. (1964): The Caribbean. In: *A Mental Health Association: Its Structure and Role*. W. F. M. H. Geneoa: Courier de Geneve.
7. BEAUBRUN, M. H. (1966): Psychiatric education for the Caribbean. *W. Indian Med. J.*, XV, 1, 52-62.
8. BEAUBRUN, M. H. (1967): The treatment of alcoholism in Trinidad and Tobago 1956-1965. *Brit. J. Psychiat.*, 113, 643-658.
9. BEAUBRUN, M. H. (1968): A pilot project for the West Indies. In: R. Williams and L. Ozarin (eds), *Community Mental Health—An International Perspective*. San Francisco: Jossey-Bass.
10. BEAUBRUN, M. H. (1970): Foreign medical training and the brain drain—The viewpoint of the developing world. *Newsletter Carib. Psychiat. Ass.*, 1, 4 and *Psychiatry*, 34, 3, 247-251, 1971.
11. BEAUBRUN, M. H. (1972): The role of mental health associations in social change. *Proc. 24th Annual Meeting of W.F.M.H.*, Hong Kong, Nov. 1971.
12. CRATON, M., AND WALVIN, J. (1970): *A Jamaican Plantation*. London & New York: W. H. Allen & Co. Ltd.
13. DEERR, NOEL (1949): *The History of Sugar*. London.
14. DE SOUZA, JOAN AND BEAUBRUN, M. H. (1967): An evalutation of the U.W.I. programme of community psychiatry. *Proc. of 6th Carib Conference for Mental Health*, Barbados.
15. GEORKE, HEINZ (1956): The life and scientific works of Dr. John Quier. *W. Indian Med. J.*, V, xviii, 22-7.
16. LANAGHAN, MRS. A. (1844): *Antigua and the Antiguans*. London: Saunders and Ottley.
17. LAS CASAS, FR. BARTOLOMEO DE: *Historia de Las Indias*, II, vi.
18. LEWIS, L. F. E. (1956): The use of chlorpromazine and serpasil in the treatment of psychotic patients. *Carib. Med. J.*, XVIII, 1-2, 51.
19. LEWIS, L. F. E. (1965): Ten Years of Progress at St. Ann's Hospital 1955-1964. Memorandum of Mrs. Isabel Teshea, Minister of Health, Trinidad & Tobago (Unpublished).
20. MADA RIAGA, SALVADOR (1933): *Letters and Reports of Early Settlers*. Oxford: Oxford Univ. Press.
21. *Medical and Sanitary Reports of the Department of Medical Services Trinidad & Tobago for the years 1945-58*. Trinidad: Govt. Printing Office.
22. *Official Reports of Commissions of Enquiry into Conditions at the Kingston Public Hospital and the Lunatic Asylum (1857-1859)*. Jamaica Govt. Printers.
23. PARRY, J. A. AND SHERLOCK, P. M. (1966): *A Short History of the West Indies*. London: Macmillan.
24. QUIER, DR. JOHN (1774): *Letters and Essays*.
25. RADIN, R. V. (1972): The U.W.I. programme of community psychiatric care: A current re-evaluation. *Newsletter Carib. Psychiat. Ass.*, 3, 1.
26. REECE, E. A. (1942): A study on bromide therapy and intoxication on psychotic patients. *Carib. Med. J.*, IV, 3, 104.
27. REES, JOHN R. (1967): *Reflections*. New York: W.F.M.H. Publications.

28. RICHMAN, ALEX (1965): *A National Plan for the Development of Comprehensive Community Mental Health in Jamaica.*

29. SEHEULT, R. (1948): *A Survey of the Trinidad Medical Services 1814-1944.*

30. SIMPSON, G. E. (1965): *The Shango Cult in Trinidad.* Puerto Rico. Caribbean Monograph Series No. 2.

31. THESIGER, C. (1972): *The Development of a Community Mental Health Programme in St. Vincent,* P.A.H.O. Report, publication pending.

32. VERE, OLIVER: *A History of Antigua.*

33. WATERMAN, J. A. (1971): Personal communication.

34. WISEMAN, M. V. (1950): *History of the British West Indies.* U. of London Press.

35. WYNTER, L. R. AND BOYD, A. I. (1951): Prefrontal lobotomy with a report on eight cases. *Carib. Med. J.,* XII, 3-4, 83.

22

ISRAEL AND THE JEWS

Louis Miller, M.D., Ch.B.

Chief National Psychiatrist, Mental Health Services,
Ministry of Health, Jerusalem, Israel

1

MENTAL HEALTH IN THE BIBLE

References to states of mental disturbance are frequently found in the Bible. *Deuteronomy* 28:23, 34 views madness as punishment for disobeying the commandments. The tragedy of Saul's last years is ascribed to an evil spirit that troubled Saul when the Lord departed from him. Saul's paranoidal fears and jealousy of David could not be assuaged by David's attempts to help and reassure him by playing the harp (I *Sam.* 16:14-23; 18:10*ff.*; 19:9-10). Later, David himself, in order to escape from Achish, simulated insanity, "scribbling on the doors of the gate and letting his spittle fall upon his beard" (21:11-16). The Bible does not speak of treatment of mental illness or recognize insanity as illness. On the contrary, it was enjoined that the person who was seen to be possessed by spirits should be stoned to death (Lev. 20:27); yet the Bible abounds in counsel for mental health, usually with an ethical intention. In *Proverbs* it is held that understanding is "a wellspring of life" (16:22) and that "a merry heart doeth good like medicine" (17:22).

2

TALMUDIC (POST-BIBLICAL) TIMES

In the Talmud mention of mental illness is generally of a legal nature. The episodic nature of mental illness is taken into account on several occasions and there are references to periods when the person is of lucid or of unsound mind. There are also suggestions of a possible classification of mental illness such as a mental defect, confusion, acute and cyclical psychoses, and those which result from physical illness. The Talmud recognizes mental illness and is chary of accepting popular definitions such as: "He who goes out alone at night, who sleeps in the cemetery, and tears his clothes" (*Tosef.*, Ter. 1:3, and *cf.* Hag 3b). The word *shoteh,* which contains the idea of walking to and fro without purpose, is used to describe the mentally ill. The legal and social implications of insanity are frequently referred to in the Talmud. The mentally ill are not responsible for the damage they cause and those who injure them must bear the responsibility; the insane are not responsible for the shame they cause. They may not marry but, contrary to Greek concepts, in periods of lucidity the individual is considered healthy and capable from every other point of view. The Talmud sets very little store by magical medicines and cures for mental illness which were then current among the nations and were frequently found among Jews in the Middle Ages. It prefers to admit frankly the lack of effective treatment.

3

THE MEDIEVAL PERIOD

In the Middle Ages Jewish physicians no less than others were dependent on the humoral theories of Greek and Roman medicine (Hippocrates and Galen). Some Jewish physicians made original discoveries and contributions. Asaph, the earliest Jewish physician known by name who lived apparently in the 6th or 7th century, felt that the heart is the seat of the soul and vital spirit. In his work, *The Book of Medicines,* he refers to the disturbed behavior of epileptics and to psychosis-phreneticus. Shabbetai Donnolo, who lived in the 10th century, wrote in one of his medical books an analysis of the psychiatric conditions of melancholia and of nightmare. His description of mania contains a complex of conditions and undoubtedly included schizophrenia. Donnolo's psychiatric views while avoiding the magical element are derivative from the humoral theory of the Greeks. Nevertheless, though some of his explanations could be termed psychological his tratment was almost purely medicinal.

Maimonides (Plate CII) in the 12th century added to the genius of his exegetical and philosophic work the brilliant practice of medicine and the exposition of it. His work *Pirkei Moshe* ("The Book of Medicines") distinguishes clearly between motor and sensory nerves and voluntary and automatic activity. This book also deals with the

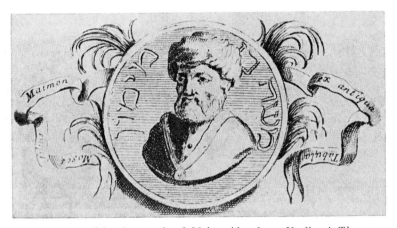

PLATE CII. Traditional portrait of Maimonides from Ugolinus' *Thesaurus Antiquitatum Sacrarum*, Venice, 1744.

anatomy of the brain and organic conditions such as epilepsy, weakness, contractions, and tremor. Maimonides' view of the influence of emotion on bodily function, in producing illness and retarding cure, was unique in his time. He was thus the father of psychosomatic medicine. In *Hanhagat ha-Beriut* ("The Regimen of Health") he sets out these views and instructions for attention to and the mitigation of the emotional state of the patient. He does, however, recognize the limitations of psychiatric care. *Sefer ha-Nimza*, which deals with mental illness, is questionably attributed to him. The *Sefer Madda* in Maimonides' Code sets out clearly his views on the promotion of individual mental health. His orientation to it is, of course, profoundly ethical, yet he relates mental health no less to the pragmatic functioning of the body and its appetites and affects. In essence his view recommends the middle road between indulgence and asceticism. He abjures all magical procedures.

The medieval flowering of Jewish medicine was followed by a prolonged period of folk medicine practiced by peripatetic healers. They acquired a reputation for healing as wonder-workers through incantations, amulets, etc. They treated mental patients as if they were afflicted by spirits, devils, and impure influences. The founder of the hassidic movement, Israel ben Eliezer, in the 18th century, acquired his medical reputation by a rapid cure of a mental case. After him there ensued a further period of decadence in which the healers encouraged and exploited superstition.

4

THE MODERN PERIOD

The reconstruction of psychiatry as a moral practice and a rational system after medieval times was accomplished in Europe only after a prolonged struggle against the demonological beliefs of the Church and the people. Phillipe Pinel's work in France after the Revolution was a turning point. The 19th century saw the progressive definition and classification of mental illness, of the psychoses and the neuroses, and the humanization of treatment in hospital. The first Jewish medical psychologist to join this European movement was Cesare Lombroso who in 1864 published *Genius and Insanity*. He described the delinquent personality carefully and related it to anatomical phenomena and genetic causes rather than moral factors. He thus became a pioneer in human and rational corrective measures for criminal behavior. His work also contributed much to the promotion of scientific thought and methods in psychiatry. Hippolyte Bernheim's name is linked with the investigation of the neuroses which took precedence in the last two decades of the century. Although a careful observer, his interest was not in theory, but in the cure of the patient. He was the first psychologist to advocate the principle of the "irresistible impulse" in legal medicine.

In 1889 Sigmund Freud was a spectator of Bernheim's astonishing experiments in the treatment by hypnosis of mental hospital patients. Freud decided to use hypnosis in the treatment of neurotic patients and was associated in this task with Josepf Breuer, a practitioner in Vienna. In 1895 their epoch-making book, *Studien ueber Hysterie,* appeared. This work embodied the discovery of the unconscious. Freud soon found that he could dispense with hypnosis by letting the patient talk at random and obtained better therapeutic results. This new method Freud called free association. With the publication in 1900 of his *Interpretation of Dreams,* Freud invaded the field of normal psychology, and the borderland between abnormal and normal psychology began to disappear. Freud's theory and technique of psychoanalysis, after much resistance, not only revolutionized psychiatric therapy but was the final and decisive medium in which education, child care, and the treatment of criminals were humanized and made rational.

Alfred Adler challenged the validity of Freud's concepts of basic sexual drives and repression as prerequisites for neurotic symptom formation. In 1912 he coined the term "individual psychology." He reduced the significance of childhood sexual factors to a minimum. For the school which developed around Adler, neurosis stems from childhood experience of over-protection or neglect, or a mixture of both. This leads to a neurotic striving for superiority. His intuitive thinking may subsequently have been confirmed by thinkers who have defined the interaction between the goals of the individual and his social group and environment. Sandor Ferenczi made a singular contribution to psychoanalysis which has been considered second only to that of Freud, with whom he was associated. He attempted to correlate biological and psychological phenomena in his scientific method—bioanalysis. Karl Abraham, one of the founders of psychoanalysis, contributed greatly through his researches to the clinical understanding of the neuroses and the psychoses especially of manic-depressive insanity. A. A. Brill was responsible for the introduction of psychoanalysis into the United States and into the practice of psychiatry there. Max Eitingon founded the first psychoanalytic training institute and polyclinic in Berlin in 1920. This became the model for all psychoanalytic training. He settled in Palestine in 1933, where he founded the psychoanalytic society and institute. Freud's inner circle, or "Committee," by 1919 comprised Ferenczi, Abraham, Eitingon, Otto Rank, Hans Sachs, and the only non-Jew among them, Ernest Jones. Jones has commented on the effect of Freud's Jewishness on the evolution of his ideas and work; he attributed the firmness with which Freud maintained his convictions, undeterred by the prevailing opposition to them, to the "inherited" capacity of Jews to stand their ground in the face of opposition and hostility. That also held true for his mostly Jewish followers. Freud believed that the opposition to the inevitably startling discoveries of psychoanalysis was considerably aggravated by anti-Semitism. Early signs of anti-Semitism appeared in the Swiss analytic group. Freud felt that it was easier for Abraham to follow his thought than for Jung, because Jung, as a

Christian and the son of a pastor, could only find his way to Freud through great inner resistance. Hans Sachs joined Freud in 1909. He abandoned law for the practice of psychoanalysis. Sachs was an editor and trained analyst whose main work was in the application of psychoanalysis to understanding the creative personality.

There were several other Jewish psychiatrists and lay psychoanalysts associated with the earlier phases of the development of psychoanalysis. Among them was Paul Federn, who met Freud in 1902 and was the fourth physician to become an analyst. Theodor Reik was associated with Freud from 1910. Probably his major theoretical contribution was in the field of masochism. Helene Deutsch, as a psychiatrist and analyst, made the pioneer exploration of the emotional life of women and constructed a comprehensive psychology of their life cycle. Melanie Klein and Anna Freud, both lay analysts, were originators of the psychoanalytical treatment of children, which they carried from the Continent to England.

In the United States, Erik Homberger Erikson developed concepts of the development of the identity of the individual and his effort to maintain its continuity while seeking solidarity with group ideals and group identity. Margaret Mahler added to the understanding of normal development in earliest infancy, describing the separation process from the mother. Perhaps the greatest contribution to child psychiatry was made in the United States by Leo Kanner, who, in 1934, first described and named the infantile psychosis, "early infantile autism." Lauretta Bender believed that genetic factors determine the infants' vulnerability to a schizophrenic type of disorder and further related the onset of the psychosis to a biological crisis. Her visual Motor Gestalt Test was widely used to reveal organically based problems. Moritz Tramer, the Swiss child psychiatrist, maintained that childhood schizophrenia exists as a hereditary entity in childhood and runs its course into the adult form. The psychoanalyst Paul Schilder's dynamic concept of the "body image" contributed much to psychological thinking in the study of schizophrenia, especially in children. Beata Rank, while stressing the hereditary and constitutional factors in atypical emotional development, in therapy treated the early parent-child relationship. Rene Spitz, a psychoanalyst, made important contributions in his studies of emotionally deprived infants and those separated from their mothers.

The Jewish National Home (1882-1948)

Prior to 1948 a small number of mental hospital beds were available. There were two mental hospitals founded by Jewish initiative—

one in 1895 in Jerusalem by the Ezrat Nashim Women's Society, and the other (Gehah Hospital near Tel Aviv) in 1942 by the Histadrut Workers' Sick Fund. Two mental hospitals, one for men and one for women, were set up by the British authorities towards the end of the Mandate (Bat Yam and Bethlehem). A number of small private institutions, mostly substandard, with a total bed-strength of 780 beds, existed before the establishment of the State. Chronic cases were sent to these institutions from the four larger mental hospitals. In January, 1949, the total bed-strength was 1,197 beds, of which 208 were governmental, giving a ratio of 1.32 per 1,000 of population.

In the early 1930's the Histadrut Sick Fund established a neuro-psychiatric clinic; other public agencies did the same in general hospitals. The clinics offered diagnostic services and treatment which were essentially symptom and medically oriented.

Psychoanalysis was brought to Palestine from Europe by Eitingon and other pupils of Freud. The Israel Society and Institute of Psycho-analysis was founded in 1934. Its mental health impact was on professionals and child careworkers in education, youth immigration, and communal settlements. Its influence on clinical psychiatry was delayed for a later period.

After the establishment of the state in 1948, the history of psychiatry in Israel may be viewed over three decades: 1948-1958; 1958-1968; and 1968, on.

The First Decade (1948-1958)

Hospital Services. From August, 1948, during the War of Independence, psychiatric installations of several types were established for soldiers within the Army framework. These services provided care in ambulant and in-patient forms for servicemen, especially those who had suffered from battle stress. As a part of this program, two psychiatric wards were set up in general hospitals in the North and the South. A special center for milder reactions was established in Yafo. At the end of the fighting, these institutions were transferred from the Army to the Ministry of Health and became the cornerstone of the state psychiatric and mental health services for the whole population. In 1950, the Histadrut Sick Fund opened a hospital (Talbieh) in Jerusalem for active treatment. This has been affiliated to the Medical School of the Hebrew University.

Thus Israel's psychiatric services developed from three sources: a) the civic effort to provide services within the Jewish National Home before statehood; b) the Mandatory establishments, and c) the military psychiatric institutions developed immediately after statehood was gained.

During the years 1949-1954, these rudimentary services were expanded and reorganized by the Division of Mental Health to meet the urgent needs arising from the inordinately swift growth of the population from immigration. Immigration was not selective, and brought many psychotic and defective individuals. Often, these patients had been neglected in hospitals and other situations for years. But, in every case, they came from a context to which they were adjusted in a certain sense. Therefore, they showed reactions and disturbances in Israel, consequent on their displacement, as well as the deterioration following neglect.

From their inception the state hospital services were based upon definite principles of psychiatric practice; early diagnosis and continuity of care, if possible in the community, and an interdisciplinary "team" approach to the problems of the patient and his family. In the early program of regionalization of the state hospital facilities, each region was to be provided with an interlocking range of functionally distinct facilities, comprising: psychiatric wards in general hospitals, psychiatric hospitals (for short-term care); work villages (for long-term rehabilitation); rehabilitation centers (for the treatment of neurotic patients); custodial services; geriatric services; and services for child psychiatry.

The implementation of this plan for psychiatric hospital facilities was accompanied by a very serious shortage of beds in overcrowded, makeshift structures, patient neglect at times, and marked tensions in the patients' families and new communities, as well as among professional personnel. There was inadequate coordination because of these pressures between the psychiatric services and between them and community facilities. In spite of this, staff was trained and organized, and facilities were founded in such a way as not to crowd out altogether the basic principles of modern community psychiatry. This was supported by the administration's readiness to maintain staffing rates unusually high for the time and to keep hospitals small.

Psychiatric wards in general hospitals. These were established during the decade 1950-1960 in the government hospitals in Haifa (Rambam) and near Tel Aviv (Tel Hashomer). These wards with a total of 90 beds provided short-term intensive treatment, using a high concentration of staff. They admitted patients with early psychoses, especially of the passingly depressive type, and serious neurotic and psychosomatic reactions. The out-patient and after-care facilities attached to these words soon became a feature of the care, and the wards were so managed as to treat an increased number of more serious cases.

In the second decade a small department was opened in the Hadassah-University hospital in Jerusalem, and consultation services in other larger general hospitals, where a limited number of beds are being developed.

The psychiatric wards contributed considerably to the integration of mental health principles in general medicine and to the reduction of professional and popular prejudices and the development of communication between the psychiatrist and the community.

Psychiatric hospitals. While an attempt was made to place the psychiatric hospital as close as possible to the main concentrations of population, this was not possible in most cases because of the lack of available and suitable buildings in the towns. The first such hospitals were at Bat Yam, Be'er Ya'akov, and Akko. They provided emergency services especially during the strained days of mass immigration. They were small (300 to 400 beds) short-stay hospitals, rehabilitating relatively large numbers of patients. Rehabilitation of patients was at first an uphill struggle, because of the condition of the hospital and because the communities themselves were unsettled or not yet formed. In spite of these pressures, the hospitals retained their essential humanity and group spirit and even much of an "open" quality. With the growth of Israel's new communities, an increasingly positive relation developed between them and the hospitals.

Work villages. The accumulation of long-standing and often deteriorated cases of chronic psychotics coming in with the waves of immigration or inherited from the pre-state period, focussed special attention on their needs. Since institutions were being established without any particular tradition it was possible to consider a special type of approach to the hospital care of the chronic psychotic, which took the form of the "work village." As early as 1950, the Ministry opened its first work village, Kfar Sha'ul (Plate CIII), in an abandoned village on the outskirts of Jerusalem. The second, Mazra, was established in 1952 in the North, near Akko.

The work village was designed in the belief that even the most passive chronic psychotic is capable of some personal and social regeneration, if the path to him can be found. It employed every method of social retraining. It attempted to stimulate the personal initiative of the patient, and promote his capacity for social contact and cooperation by enriching his daily experience under therapeutic direction. It relied heavily on the processes at work in the small guided group to deepen the emotional participation of the individual patient. Group situations of this sort were promoted at all times: in the patient's accommodation, vocational training, daily occupations, and leisure.

Patients were housed in small individual units of about 15 persons. At work, small groups were trained in various occupations, such as carpentry, metal work, dressmaking, gardening, and weaving. As their skill increased patients joined small work groups, guided by skilled craftsmen, occupational therapists, and nursing personnel. Commu-

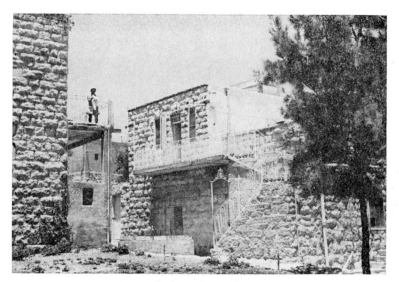

PLATE CIII. A work village in Israel, Kfar Shaul.

nity influences in the village were employed to stimulate the patient's will to social activity and leadership of larger social groups in the community. In leisure hours, hobbies of all kinds and physical and cultural recreation were encouraged. Folk dancing and choir work, so typical of Israel, were particularly popular. Drama, literary, and recreational groups played a distinctive part in the village life, because of the opportunity they give patients to share in them, and the rich material they offer to therapists. The many festivals of an Israeli community, the eve of Sabbath, the week of Passover, and so on, were celebrated in the village and had much significance for the patient. These activities were sometimes initiated and organized by the patients themselves. Staff and visitors, particularly from other institutions, also joined in. Such a therapeutic milieu called for the collective participation of all hospital staff.

The community atmosphere of the work village became the model for institutional care in all in-patient facilities, especially those of the Ministry.

Rehabilitation centers. The quick growth of the country and the stresses on the family, as a result of immigration and culture change, made great demands on psychiatry. A disturbed person within a family subject to immigration stress proved invariably too great a burden. Two open institutions were established for the care of the neurotic and borderline psychotic: Shalvata, of the Histadrut Sick Fund, and Nes Ziona, of the Ministry, with about 100 patients in each of them.

These rehabilitation centers—like the general hospitals—admitted primarily younger adult neurotics and incipient psychotics, who left their backgrounds in *kibbutzim,* the Army, or private homes to remain for several months in these open but sheltered communities. Sometimes they were transferred there after treatment in psychiatric hospitals. In Shalvata the accent was placed on intensive analytic psychotherapy; in Nes Ziona, on group and community living, with staff and therapists employing techniques of occupational reeducation and intensive social work for rehabilitation. There the employment of group and cooperative methods in patient care was a reflection of the social philosophy of Israeli society.

Custodial care. These institutions developed from the small private institutions, substandard homes of, at times, deplorably low quality. Several were shut down and some raised to at least a tolerable standard by the vigorous action of a special team.

Geriatric psychiatric services. Immigration to the National Home before 1948 was drawn in the main from younger age groups. Consequently, in 1948, the population was relatively young (3.8% over the age of 65 years). Subsequent waves of immigration caused a rapid demographic shift in the direction of the older age groups, and with the rising health and social standards, the population began to assume an age-distribution associated with Western countries (5.8% over 65 years of age in 1964). Understandably, in the pre-state period, services for the aged were relatively underdeveloped, and geriatric experience was lacking. Therefore, after 1948, there was little to build on to meet the needs of the larger group of aged citizens, whose problems were more in evidence.

Older people from European countries came to Israel, often alone and deprived of their families, and found great difficulty in re-establishing themselves. Older people from Eastern communities suffered loss of status, because of their inability to earn or to learn new ways of life. Their situation and role in their large families altered. The social change for the aged immigrants from Islamic countries made for great personal stress.

Initially villages for the immigrant aged were established by the services of Malben (AJDC) which provided the requirements of daily living, occupation, entertainments, and social interests. Near one of its villages for the aged, Shaar Menashe, Malben put up a general hospital for the aged, including a ward for geriatric cases that revealed emotional or other psychiatric disturbances. In association with the Ministry, this ward became, in the second decade, the center for a country-wide geriatric-psychiatric program which extended into homes for the aged and into community facilities. A second geriatric unit was later opened in the Tel Aviv region (Neve On).

Child psychiatry. There were no psychiatric facilities of the inpatient type for children until the mid-1950's, when two psychiatric wards for children (a total of 70 beds) were established. They were attached to existing psychiatric hospitals for adults. These settings provided sensitive therapeutically oriented care and educational facilities for children before the age of puberty, who were psychotic or had marked behavior problems.

Before their advent child psychiatry had been confined to consultation, to guidance clinics, special kindergartens, and to professionals at school. Therapy for children developed during the first decade, youth immigration and kibbutz movements participating with their own facilities. Child psychiatry began to take root only with the growth of the hospital based in-patient and ambulant services.

Community Services

Adult mental health centers. These were also essentially an outgrowth of the psychiatric developments in the Israel Army. From 1950 to 1952, the Division of Mental Health in the Ministry established adult mental health centers in the three major cities. They were based on the interdisciplinary team and were to provide a broad diagnosis of the situation of the case, therapy for the individual, and case work and assistance for the family. They also supplied consultation to all other services for the adult, such as probation and court, social welfare, rehabilitation, immigrants' absorption, and health.

The centers were thus favorably placed to introduce mental health principles into the work of health, social and other agencies, by educating workers in conferences and seminars which discussed actual cases. The therapeutic case load was restricted, to give more time for training and counseling of this kind.

On the whole the centers integrated well with other community services, although they in no sense had any impact on community life. The continuity of care between hospital and center left much to be desired.

Child guidance centers. These were set up in the three major cities by the Ministry of Social Welfare. Taken over by the Ministry of Health in 1958, they functioned like the adult centers and in line with traditional methods of child guidance. In 1957, the neuropsychiatric clinic of the Sick Fund was reorganized in two sections, of which one became a mental health clinic. This provided diagnostic, counseling, and therapeutic services. A rising proportion of the work of the clinic became its counseling of family physicians and teachers.

Professional Personnel

Israel had a prolonged period of shortages of professional psychiatric staff of all kinds. This was the result of an unusual rate of expansion of services upon the pre-state background which lacked, almost totally, psychiatrically trained staff and training facilities. Paradoxically there were high expectations of, and demands for service because of the social dislocation and growth. This added to the tensions prevailing in the service.

In the early 1950's continuous in-service training of all categories of workers, qualified or not, became the order of the day, but in most spheres, formal training as well was not neglected.

The first steps to train practical nurses were taken when the hospitals were opened. Selected candidates, with a minimum standard of schooling, were put through theoretical and practical courses of 18 months' duration, at schools attached to the three major psychiatric hospitals.

A small group of registered general nurses took over the nursing direction of the hospitals as they were opened. A 12-month intensive seminar in patient care and human relations in nursing, held in 1954 with the help of a U.S. Technical Assistance consultant, confirmed the status of the fully qualified nurse in psychiatry. Courses of six months for registered nurses specializing in psychiatry continued each year thereafter, becoming the base for the present one-year program for general and public health nurses.

The qualified occupational therapist soon became a member of the psychiatric team. Students of the occupational therapy school were assigned to field work in psychiatry during their three-year course, and many joined mental hospitals. So did a number of skilled craftsmen, who provided several types of vocational training and played an important part in the therapeutic atmosphere of the hospitals. Ministry of Labor vocational courses were held regularly for patients.

Psychiatric social workers had been in the vanguard of development in mental health centers and hospitals, doing much to enhance the hospital-community relationship. Originally, most of those serving in mental hospitals had graduated from the two-year courses of the Ministry of Social Welfare. Academically trained personnel of that sort came at first from schools in the United States and Great Britain. These were followed in the next decade by graduates of the Hebrew University School of Social Work, who in many instances did much of their supervised field work training in mental health settings in Israel. Later still, social work students from Bar Ilan and Tel Aviv Universities joined them.

Clinical psychologists were, from the beginning, also a part of the psychiatric team. They did diagnosis and therapy and helped in training personnel. Fully qualified clinical psychologists of M.A. and Ph.D. standard were employed. Fellowships for post-graduate in-service training, awarded by the Trusteeship Fund of the Ministry and Malben, added considerably, in the second decade, to the number of staff available. The fellowships went in the main to immigrant psychologists who had not been trained in Western methods of diagnosis and therapy.

As services were expanding, senior psychiatrists long resident in Israel, at times trained by the Psychoanalytic Institute, came forward to take responsible positions in public psychiatry. But the dearth of psychiatrists remained very serious. The gravest problem was the profession's inability to attract young physicians to psychiatry.

Mental Health Legislation

Rules for hospitalization of mental patients came into almost spontaneous being, replacing mandatory provisions out of accord with developing psychiatric services. Psychotics could now get hospital care with a minimum of legal or bureaucratic involvement and yet with reasonable safeguards of their own and their families' interests. The rules were duly embodied in the Mental Treatment Law, 1955, which expresses the spirit of psychiatric rather than custodial care.

In each of the three regions, Ministry services were represented by a regional psychiatrist. Administratively, he coordinated government hospitalization. He was empowered by the law to direct hospitalization of a person and to enter mental hospitals and homes and examine treatment of psychiatric cases. He investigated complaints and was generally to be responsible for supervising all mental hospitals in his region.

In each region there was established a regional psychiatric board of three members, including a lawyer: its functions are to parole or discharge patients hospitalized by court order and hear applications by patients and their kin in respect to discharge; in law, it also has the same powers as the regional psychiatrist.

The Second Decade (1958-1968)

In 1959, programs were drawn up to intensify the content of the services and plan a physical reconstruction of facilities. It was at this point that Malben (AJDC) offered its financial and professional support to carry out the new design.

Among the underlying principles and practices of the new programs the following may be pointed out: The community approach of the mental hospitals should be encouraged. Out-patient services were introduced at several community psychiatric hospitals, directed not only to continuing care of the discharged patient but also to early care of ambulant patients and home visits. The swift rise in the number of out-patients began at once to better opportunities for continuity of care and for overcoming the defects and burdens resulting from loss of contact with the patients. Out-patient teams, too, were to mobilize community and service resources for patient care and rehabilitation to a greater degree.

It was determined that the community psychiatric hospital should be no larger than 250 beds, with a variety of community facilities that would, *inter alia,* care for about 50 day patients (this for a population of 250,000). Day care for adults has been developed by the ministry at two hospitals.

With the improvement of community attitudes to the psychiatric hospital, the psychiatric ward in the general hospital ceased to be predominant in early hospitalization. It was suggested that the facility should see itself as an extramural community service, rather than as chiefly in-patient. Work at the general hospital was fostered in two directions: out-patient and, increasingly, day care, consultation, and liaison in the hospital, especially the medical and pediatric wards. It was planned that, with the decentralization of the geriatric services, the general hospital should assume functions in early geriatric ambulant and in-patient care.

The work village, which had performed such an important task in hospitalization of chronic psychotics among immigrants and in charting the paths to rehabilitation, had become freer to accept other responsibilities. A cardinal one was retreatment of psychotic cases who regressed in the community after discharge. The work village thus developed a relation to a progressively larger group of patients in the community, who saw it as the focus for their retreatment and rehabilitation.

As a part of the new design two hospitals were established, in Tel Aviv and in Jerusalem. They were half-way houses for patients not requiring admission to a psychiatric hospital or in process of discharge to the community.

There was also a notable development of services for children during the decade. Forty beds were set up in Nes Ziona for youth, in addition to the existing children's beds. In 1965, a day hospital for 20 children, with a small 24-hour observation unit, was opened in Jerusalem. An experimental nursery school for disturbed younger children was opened in cooperation with the Ministry of Education and Culture and the local authority in Nethanya.

The number of beds in all mental hospitals in 1967 was 6,200, a ratio of about 2.4 per 1,000 of population; 3,000 beds in government hospitals, 400 of the Histadrut Sick Fund, 2,200 in private hospitals, and the remainder in public sponsored institutions.

The mental health centers developed both in number and intensity of penetration into the communities and their problems. Of special significance were the smaller ones in the development towns, often based largely on a visiting team which cooperated with the local education, welfare, and public health agencies. Much of the groundwork for this approach to the services and the community had been laid by community organizers' activity in the locality.

A new type of mental health center of the Ministry combined adult mental health and child guidance in one community and family mental health center. This type, established in conjunction with a municipality, provides, as well, wherever possible on a family basis, supervision and consultation to the school and youth psychological services of the city. A community organizer for mental health linked it with neighborhood public health activity and community organization. In this way, it began to contribute to a mitigation of unfavorable social forces in urban areas, especially where immigrants in the throes of adjustment were living.

An essential part of the plan was the training of psychiatric and allied personnel. A number of public health nurses took a specialization in mental health and psychiatry, and now work in mental health centers and in out-patient departments. Courses in social psychiatry were provided for graduate community organizers, public health nurses, clinical psychologists, and psychiatrists in training. Under-

TABLE 1

Professional Workers in Psychiatric and Mental Health Fields,
Employed in all Institutions and in Those
of the Ministry of Health, 1965

Profession	Employed in	
	All Institutions	Institutions of Ministry of Health
Psychiatrists, including residents in psychiatric hospitals	170	100
Clinical psychologists	60	38
Psychiatric social workers	100	80
Psychiatric nurses, registered	87	72
Psychiatric nurses, practical	100	600
Occupational therapists, registered	151	28
Occupational therapists, practical		79

graduate courses in social psychiatry for medical students were begun.

The rapid growth of child psychiatry vigorously accented the impact of psychiatry on the community and promoted the orientation of pediatricians and other child care workers, for example, those in *kibbutzim* and special schools, probation officers, and those caring for retarded children.

The Third Decade (1968-   )

Before the close of the second decade therefore, Israeli psychiatry had already undergone marked changes. Models for new elements of community service had been established, and were to become the basis of a reconstructed national comprehensive community mental health and community psychiatric plan.

These models had included a comprehensive community mental health program for youth in Tel Aviv based upon a walk-in clinic;

a comprehensive child and family community mental health program in Haifa, based upon a day center in a public health facility; and limited but integrated community psychiatric and hospital care programs for particular geographic areas (Ashkelon, and more recently Jaffa and the Jerusalem Corridor).

A most important early precursor of community psychiatry had been the promotion of community organization and its techniques in the neighborhoods, at the mental health centers, in the housing authority, and in public health service. This had contributed to the possibility of these services becoming more forceful in approaching pervasive mental health needs that have resulted from problems in groups and families undergoing socio-cultural change and urbanization. These social and mental health issues had arisen predominantly, but not exclusively, from the resettlement of immigrants, especially of Oriental origin.

An earlier national plan for the second decade had proposed a simple extension, especially of hospital services, as they had been conceived essentially in the first decade. However that plan did not approach the problems of coordination of services locally nor did it assure continuing, intensive, and comprehensive care through penetration into and responsibility for a given community as had been modeled by the projects of the second decade.

A new plan for the third decade has been evolved and elaborated. This present psychiatric plan for Israel divides the country into geographical areas of about 150,000 in population. Each area will be the sole and total psychiatric and mental health responsibility of one integrated mental health center. This center includes all of the spectrum of functions for all ages—mental health education; home, indirect, out-patient and day care; short and long-term hospitalization—as the responsibility of one single professional organism. However, community organization and community participation in the work of this mental health center is emphasized.

The national program for comprehensive centers is being implemented now on the basis of existing services, so that particular wards in existing mental and general hospitals are being linked through existing or new community clinics to defined populations. Of cardinal importance in this development will be the adaptation of the overall plan to local needs through local planning involving community services and community representatives.

An important feature of the new plan is its preliminary quantitative elaboration of professional staff standards. Staff standards have, since statehood, been relatively reasonable but are now being improved further in the light of the extension of mental health goals, the intensification of community care and of indirect responsibility for community mental health and social action.

REFERENCES

1. KLEIN, H. (1968): Problems in the psychotherapeutic treatment of Israeli survivors of the holocaust. In: Krystal, H. (ed.), *Massive Psychic Trauma*. New York: International Universities Press.
2. KLEIN, H. AND REINHARZ, S. (1972): Community psychiatry in a multi-ethnic Israeli town. In: Miller, L. (ed.), *Mental Health in Rapid Social Change*. Jerusalem: Academic Press.
3. MILLER, L. (1967): The social psychiatry and epidemiology of mental ill health in Israel. *Top. Probl. Psychiat. Neurol.*, VI.
4. MILLER, L. (1969): The Israel Mental Treatment Act. *Israel Ann. Psychiat.*, 7, 1, April.
5. MILLER, L. (1969): Child-rearing in the kibbutz. In: Howells, J. G. (ed.), *Modern Perspectives in International Child Psychiatry*. Edinburgh: Oliver & Boyd.
6. MILLER, L. (1970): Mental health of immigrants. In: Jarus, A. *et al.* (eds.), *The Child and Family in Israel*. New York: Gordon & Breach.
7. MILLER, L. (1972): Mental illness. In: *Encyclopaedia Judaica*. Jerusalem.
8. PALGI, P. (1972): Family types in Israel. In: Miller, L. (ed.), *Mental Health in Rapid Social Change*. Jerusalem: Academic Press.

23

THE ARAB COUNTRIES

TAHA BAASHER, M.D.

Former Senior Psychiatrist, Democratic Republic of the Sudan

1

INTRODUCTION

At present the Arab countries which lie in North Africa, the Middle East, and the Arabian Peninsula form a uniform "cultural continent." The history of psychiatry, as part of this cultural heritage, has passed through many phases.

The Islamic Kingdoms, which extended from India to Andalucia (Spain), came in contact with various cultures and the Arab centers of knowledge moved from one capital to another. Similarly, psychiatric contributions by reputable Arab physicians who lived at one time or another at Jondisapur, Damascus, Baghdad, Cairo, and Cordova have to be sought in a number of general classical bibliograpies (15, 31), which deal mainly with "classes" of doctors more than with the art of medicine. On the other hand, some of the rare medical manuscripts which are kept in the national museums of ancient books in Madrid, Tunis, Istanbul, Cairo and in various libraries are priceless historical treasures, which still await thorough studies and organized research. Recent work by Iskander (33) on cataloging Arabic medical manuscripts in the Wellcome Historical Medical Library is a good effort which needs to be pursued further.

Again, in compiling a history of psychiatry, one has to bear in mind that the difference between modern concepts of psychiatry and ancient views on abnormal behavior and the subsequent healing practices of mentally ill persons, though very interesting, may raise certain difficulties. It is possible to set well defined boundaries for present day psychiatry with its relatively clear nosology, but when the boundaries of psychiatry overlap those of religion, magic, theology, philosophy, and folk practices, the task becomes more complicated.

There are several well known classical books dealing with the history of Arab medicine in general (11, 13) but there are no similar publications on the history of psychological medicine. Indeed there is no all round comprehensive chapter in any foreign language on the history of psychiatry in Arab medicine. However, the *Concept of Mental Health in Ancient Cultures* (19) is a worthy beginning in this respect.

2

THE ROOTS OF PSYCHIATRY IN ARAB COUNTRIES

In the Nile Valley and Mesopotamia, the land between the Tigris and the Euphrates rivers, one sees the beginning of human civilization and the first stages of antiquity. Fortunately there are a number of sources for recorded history of healing practices in these ancient Arab lands. Apart from monuments, *stelae,* etc., the ancient Egyptian *papyri* provide a unique source of information. For later periods, the historical writings of Herodotus and Diodorus Siculus are other important sources of knowledge. The Kahun, Edwin Smith, Ebers, Hearst, London, and Berlin *papyri* remain the best known (35, 43). The Ebers *papyrus,* for example, goes back to the 16th century B.C.; it lists various categories of diseases, and refers to several hundred ancient remedies. This important historical document includes a number of incantations recited by ancient Egyptian priests as part of their curative methods.

Incantations as a psychotherapeutic technique are still a popular practice in traditional treatment in some Arab countries. Of major significance is the fact that the Kahun *papyrus* included more than 30 prescriptions for a variety of diseases attributed to changes in the womb (19). Consequently, the author concludes that the ancient Egyptians anticipated by ten centuries the Hippocratic teachings on the pathogenesis of hysteria. Although it is known that Hippocrates visited Egypt towards the end of the 5th century B.C., when Alexandria was the great center of knowledge, it is difficult to say how far Hippocrates was influenced by ancient Egyptian thinking in formulating his theory of hysteria. The similarity between some of the ethical precepts of ancient Egyptian physicians and the Hippocratic Oath shows the close connection of the origin between pre-Hippocratic medicine in Greece and Egyptian medicine (27).

The Nile Valley

In ancient Egypt, the central philosophy of life and death revolved around the idea that they are part of a continuous cycle—hence the belief in life after death, which demanded elaborate funeral ceremonies and complex magico-religious rituals in preparation for it. Within this belief much attention was given to the psychology of the dead and the personality in the hereafter. The individual was conceived to be composed of three integral parts: the *Khat,* the *Ka,* and the *Ba;* the *Khat* represented the body, and the *Ka* and *Ba* two differentiated types of souls. The *Ka,* which was known as the double, was symbolized by uplifted arms, and its main function was to protect the diseased body; in some circumstances it may have had other meanings as well. The *Ba,* which was depicted as a flying bird carrying the key of eternity, was believed to leave the body after death and reside in heaven, periodically visiting the burial place of the mummified body. It was suggested by Budge (12) that probably the concept of ghosts was developed from this belief.

In the pre-Islamic era, the soul *(hama)* was still thought of by the Arabs as a bird, which leaves the body after death, but continues to visit the burial place. A wide range of superstitions and folk beliefs, like transmigration of spirits and the immortality of the soul, developed from these concepts. Apparently the necromantic theory had a similar origin. It assumed that the soul through magical powers might be forced to re-enter the body and speak through the lips of the dead. However, the idea that the ancient Egyptians believed in the immortality of the soul was disputed by some authors (10). As much as the ancient Egyptians cared for the spirits of the dead, they feared them. It was thought that diseases were either due to evil spirits or to the wrath of the gods. Hence the art of healing was part of ancient religious practices.

One of the interesting psychotherapeutic methods of ancient Egypt was the "incubation," or "temple sleep." This method was associated with the name of Imhotep, the earliest known physician in history (30). *I-em-hotep* (he who comes in peace) was the physician vizier of the Pharaoh Zoser (2980-2900 B.C.). Later he became a patron saint and a god of medicine. He was worshipped at Memphis and a temple was constructed in his honor on the Island of Philae. The temples of Imhotep were busy centers for incubation or sleep therapy, and "shrine sleep" is still encountered in some parts of Africa and the Middle East. The many shrines of holy men in some Arab countries are highly venerated for their power of spiritual healing.

Under the influence of incantations, and through the performance of religious rituals, sick persons were psychologically prepared for such therapeutic procedures. The course of treatment depended greatly on the manifestations and contents of dreams, which were, of course, highly affected by the psycho-religious climate of the temples, on the full confidence in supernatural powers of the deity, and on the suggestive procedures carried out by the divine healers.

Mesopotamia

Another Arab country where ancient roots of psychiatry can be traced is Mesopotamia. Here we find early history recorded on cuneiform inscriptions, some of which contain significant attempts to understand the mental life of individuals.

Oppenheim (40), in his documented studies on the Assyrian book of dreams, pointed out three types of dream interpretations recognized in ancient Mesopotamia. In ancient Babylon, medicine was part of magic, and this practice was so far-reaching that some remnants of it are still seen in Arab culture. Based on Chaldean and Babylonian astrology, certain numerals came to be known for their divine or ominous effects. For example, the number seven, or one of its multiples, was believed to be related to supernatural powers. Complicated sets of mystical numbers were developed as part of magical formulae, which had their various use in human affairs (Plate CIV).

The Period of Ignorance

The inception of Islam brought about radical changes in the behavior of the Arab people. The pre-Islamic era is commonly known as the period of ignorance; it was a dark period in Arab history. Political and economic forces partially caused the fall of ancient Arab kingdoms. In addition, the old Arab civilization which had existed for more than two millenniums and had extended into Assyrian-Babylonian times was lost and forgotten. Ancient poetry, legends, and folklore provide the only source of information on socio-medical matters of this period. The southern trade route was the main line of communication with the external world. Small communities in places like Mecca and Yathrib (old Medina) could lead a settled life, but most Bedouin tribes were constantly on the move in search of pasture or because of socio-political conflicts. Several gods were worshipped, and many cults were practiced. It is because of this that the period is sometimes referred to as the Days of Idolatry.

Beliefs in supernatural forces influenced the attitude of the people towards diseases, and consequently the art of healing. Two things dominated the supernatural field: the gods and the invisible *jinns*. The gods granted occasional oracles, and offerings were made in their names. The oracles were communicated by a diviner (*kahin*), who

4	9	2
3	5	7
8	1	6

PLATE CIV. Mystical numbers from Babylonian culture used in magical healing practices.

interpreted them, explained occult phenomena, and predicted the future.

Of course, Arab physicians at that time were influenced by other cultures, notably by the Indians and the Persians, with whom they came in contact. Though physical causes were recognized, sickness, like other misfortunes in life, was attributed to supernatural forces. Mental illness in particular was thought to be due to evil spirits and *jinns*. Indeed the generic term for madness is *jinn* (*pl. jenun*), for it was believed that in case of madness the person was possessed by the *jinn*. Hence treatment was based on magico-religious practices. Prophylactic devices in the form of amulets and charms were also used.

Arab physicians of that period prescribed a variety of herbal drugs and used cautery, blood letting (*fesada*), and cupping (*hegama*) in the general management of diseases. It is not quite clear whether they applied similar remedies for psychiatric disorders. However, cautery was used at later periods by traditional healers in the treatment of epilepsy and psychotic disturbances.

Mental Health and the Koran

The *Koran* contains the holy scriptures of the Muslims, and describes the revelations made to the Prophet Mohammed by God. These revelations, communicated by Mohammed to his followers, were memorized by the faithful and written on various materials (skins, stones, pots, bones). They were later collected in their final form, in 114 chapters (*suras*), by the third *caliph,* Othman.

The *Koran,* as a new religious code, led the Muslims into a new way of life, which radically replaced the cultural style of the previous period. The psychological effect of the new and dynamic religion was clearly demonstrated by the behavior of Mohammed's followers, who found great values, high hopes, and forceful drives in the meaningful revelations. Obviously the *Koran* is not a medical text, and should not be measured by modern academic standards. Nevertheless, it contains references of psychiatric interest, and provides a valuable source of information about the religious principles that influenced the Arab people's attitude to mental health 14 centuries ago. From the psychiatric point of view the passage of the *Koran* which includes Joseph's interpretations of the pharaoh's dreams of the seven fat and seven lean cows is of great historical significance. Probably this stimulated some of the Arab thinkers to develop an elaborate system of dream interpretation, as will be discussed later.

The *Koran* is precise and firm about psychiatric problems like suicide. It states clearly: "Do not kill yourself, for God was merciful to you." This has been found of great importance in the prevention of suicide. Some of the Muslim patients seen by the author had entertained suicidal ideas, but had stopped short of taking their own lives for fear of acting against the will of God.

In Arab countries there is a low incidence of alcoholism; there is no doubt that one of the deterring factors in this respect is the Islamic influence. The *Koran* includes various passages dealing with wine prohibition that have been the subject of analysis by Islamic theologians. Significantly, the prohibition of wine in the *Koran* was introduced gradually. The first passage states "come not to pray when you are drunk." This was followed by the proclamation that wine drinking is a detestable act of Satan. Finally, it was prohibited as a disgusting way of behavior. Together with wine, gambling was also prohibited. Emphasis was laid on the fact that drinking and gambling bring about "enmity and hatred" between people, and distract from prayer. The prohibition of wine was later extended to other intoxicants and to narcotics. The general rule in Islamic principles is that any beverage or drug which clouds the mind should be prohibited.

Unbelievers who disagreed with the revelations accused the Prophet of being a storyteller and a soothsayer possessed by the *jinn;* this was strongly repudiated in the *Koran* and consequently the old soothsayer, the divine healer *(kahin)* of the Days of Idolatry, was discredited and fell into disrepute.

The expressions Satan and *Iblis* appear several times in the *Koran.* They corresponded to the Christian devil, and were regarded as evil forces that harmed people and interfered with normal behavior. To overcome the influence of these evil spirits, an appeal was made to the divine power in some verses of the *Koran.*

The *Koran* as a "guide and enlightenment" includes a variety of historical events and stories of ancestral figures and prophets. The aim was to encourage people to lead a healthier life by drawing lessons from past events and other human experiences. The eloquent dialogue between the Prophet Lut and his people is an example of exacting endeavors to combat indulgence in homosexuality. It was a serious reminder for the Muslim communities to beware of the gloomy fate of such sexual disorders, and a deterrent to deviant behavior.

There are quite a number of other topics related to mental health which will be mentioned briefly. Several statements in the *Koran* refer to marriage, divorce, family care, adoption, orphans, women, adultery, prostitution, good manners, virtue, cooperation, love, mercy, truthfulness, justice, fraternity, modesty, personal responsibilities, and several other topics that include well-defined principles on moral and civic duties governing human relationship; these had tremendous effects upon the establishment of a strong basis for a more integrated and stable society.

The following passage, which Muslims learn by heart, indicates very well the prescribed belief and the code of behavior: "Piety does not consist in turning your faces to the East, or to the West; but piety consists in believing in God, the Last Day, the angels, the Book, the Prophets, in giving your possessions, while loving him, to your neighbor, to the orphans, the unfortunate, the travelers, the beggars, and to captives; in performing the duty of prayer, in paying the alms-tax, in carrying out your undertakings, in remaining patient in adversity, suffering, and danger."

The teachings expressed in the revelations and compiled in the holy book were supplemented by the traditions *(sunna)* and sayings (*hadith*) of the Prophet. From the medical point of view, a number of these sayings and traditions, as well as being religious regulations, constituted guidelines for remedies. Later the sayings pertaining to medical problems were collected separately, and came to be known as "the medicine of the Prophet" (El Zahaby 1274-1347 A.D.) (22). An attempt was made to focus on the psycho-medical aspects of the Prophet's teaching.

As the sayings are answers by the Prophet to questions asked, or directions on treatment for specific diseases, their historical significance needs no emphasis. Generally speaking, they point out early Islamic concepts, and outline the basis of religious therapy, which has influenced traditional healing to the present day.

As a fundamental principle, the Prophet stressed to his followers that "for every disease there is a cure." Similar meaningful statements were reiterated in due course. The importance of such sayings can be gathered by the fact that Bedouin believers who referred to the Prophet were often undecided whether to resort to treatment or to become resigned to their fate. His precepts gave strong psychological impetus for a greater hope for recovery, and persuaded the people to seek treatment.

When old physicians of the "Ignorant Period" had audiences with the Prophet, one of his more important proclamations to them was to abandon magical practices. The reason for this was that in magical healing occult supernatural powers are invoked, and this was condemned, because it involved polytheistic beliefs.

Of particular importance was the emphasis laid by the Prophet on the relationship between psychological factors and somatic diseases. This was demonstrated clearly in his saying that "He who is overcome by worries, will have a sick body." Such teaching had great influence. Expounding on this, El Kahal (650-750 A.D.) pointed out that fear, sadness, and their like, diminish bodily energies, accentuate diseases, should they be present; and lead to them, if they are absent (17). The same author added that anxiety and unhappiness were among the most severe psychiatric symptoms and both were greatly damaging to the body. Traditionally the cause of death of Abu Baker El Siddig, the first caliph, was attributed to his sorrow over the death of the Prophet.

Epileptic patients also were said to have appealed to the Prophet for treatment. For instance, an epileptic woman (*Masroa'*—convulsed) told the Prophet about her affliction, and asked him to pray for her, which he did. It is difficult to find out how psychosis was regarded and treated during the Prophet's time, but probably it was treated like epileptic manifestations and similar disorders. Traditional religious healers commonly group epilepsy with psychiatric disturbances.

The *Koran,* honey, and cautery were the main remedies generally advocated by the Prophet. In clear words the Prophet proclaimed the usefulness of the honey and the *Koran.* Muslim theologians believe that in this statement the Prophet combined medicine with divine healing, physical treatment with psychological medicine, and secular treatment with heavenly remedy. Obviously the whole *Koran* is endowed with sacred blessing (*baraka*), but there are certain passages or chapters which are more concerned with healing holiness. The passage in the first chapter which states "to thee we worship and into ye we take refuge" is of central importance in incantation and treatment in general, because of its particular submission to God. References are also found to the prophet's consideration of the emotional side of treatment. Muslims were urged to relieve patients of their emotional tensions when visiting them.

Mohammed died in 632 A.D., but his teachings left behind a new spirit in old Arabia. Within a century, the revelations and his sayings engaged the minds of the people from China to the Pyrenees. At the same time the Arabs came into close contact with new cultures, and with other civilizations.

Cultural Influences on Arab Medicine

Prior to the Islamic advance into North Africa and Spain, Greek and Roman influences came to the Near East from an opposite direction. The Nestorian monks who were teaching medicine at Odessa, because of opposition, migrated to Persia, where, towards the end of the 5th century, they established a medical school at Jondisapur. It was through this school that early Arab physicians gained access to Greek and Roman medicine.

By the time of the Abbasides Caliphate (750-1258 A.D.), Baghdad was an important center of learning and science. The era of great caliphs—Al-mansur (754-775), Harun Al Rashid (786-802), and Al Mamoun (813-833)—witnessed genuine efforts to promote scientific knowledge and assimilate other cultures. There was a tireless search for manuscripts. Scholars were busy translating into Arabic the works of Hippocrates, Galen, Dioscorides, and other Greek writers. The Syrian family of Musue contributed tremendously to the translation and the advancement of medical knowledge. As another example, Honain Ibu Ishac (809-873), the Nestorian scholar, became a leading medical authority in Baghdad, and translated the works of Hippocrates, Galen, Oribasius, and Paul Aegina. Among the outstanding physicians of the

Eastern (Abbasides) Caliphate, were Rhazes (860-932), Haly Abbas (died 994), and Avicenna (980-1036).

Cultural and medical activities flourished also in the Western (Cordova) Caliphate (755-1236). Here too, one finds a group of leading philosophers, thinkers, and physicians like Averroes (1126-1198) and Maimonides (1135-1204), who contributed to the understanding of human behavior.

The prosperity of the Eastern and Western Caliphates enabled physicians to grasp ancient Egyptian, Indian, and Greek cultures, and assimilate non-Islamic knowledge consistent with Mohammedism into a more advanced system of medical practice. However, some basic medical doctrines from other cultures influenced Arab medicine more than others, and for this reason deserve to be discussed in more detail. Humoral pathology was one of these.

Blood, phlegm, and yellow and black bile constituted the basis of the humoral theory. Parallel to these humors were the four elements, earth, air, fire, and water, together with the corresponding qualities of dry, cold, heat, and moist. Health and disease depended on the balance or imbalance of these factors. The action of drugs was similarly related to the complex system of humoral pathology. The theory of humoral pathology was one of the few doctrines which was incorporated almost totally into Arab medicine. Unfortunately, this deterred Arab physicians from looking into other pathological causes. Psychiatry suffered because of this theory, which dominated medical thinking for many centuries. The term melancholy, for example, which was borrowed from Greek medicine, became part of Arab terminology, and even today severe depression in called *sawdawi* (black disease), a clear indication of its etymological derivation from black bile.

Psychological Approach

Medical education is a major factor in shaping the future attitude of aspiring health workers. It is therefore interesting to look into the basis of training in early Arab medicine. Medicine was not a specialized subject, and physicians were instructed in a variety of arts (*funun*), and were versed in a number of disciplines (*ulum*). Besides medicine, these disciplines included philosophy, astrology, law, theology, music, and other arts and sciences. Tritton (49) gives several interesting examples of various jobs in which certain physicians were engaged, and of their educational background. Probably this multi-disciplinary approach enabled Arab physicians to develop a global attitude to medical problems, and to the study of human behavior.

The great physician El Tabari (18, 19), for example, divided the medical practitioners of his day into physician-philosophers and non-philosophers, and advocated a philosophical approach in the art of medicine. Similar philosophical and psychological approaches are detected in the handling of medical problems in the works of distinguished physicians like Rhazes and Avicenna. Despite the paucity of recorded clinical material, there are a few references of historic interest.

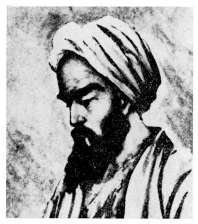

PLATE CV. The great clinician Rhazes (860-932).

An often quoted example is the story of Harun el Rashid's maid, who developed what appeared to be a state of hysterical conversion, involving her right upper limb. The maid lifted her hand up and could not bring it down. Massage and other physical treatments were of no avail. Gabriel (Gibreel Ibn Bakhta Yashue), the court physician, in the presence of the Caliph and his entourage, pinched the maid from behind, and unconsciously the up-lifted arm dropped down. Though the explanation given by Gabriel was based on humoral pathology, his therapeutic approach was obviously psychological.

The teaching of the great clinician Rhazes had a profound influence on Arab as well as European medicine. Rhazes (Plate CV) (860-932) lived at a time when European medicine after Galen (131-201 A.D.) and Vesalius had remained at the same level for many centuries. The two most important books of Rhazes are the *Mansuri* and the *Al-Hawi*. The first, consisting of ten chapters, includes the definition and nature of temperaments, the dominant humors, and a comprehensive guide to physiognomy. *Al-Hawi,* or *Continens,* is the greatest medical encyclopedia produced by a Moslem physician; it was translated into Latin by Farragut (Farag Ibn Salim) in 1279 for King Charles d'Anjou, and was later printed in Brescia, in northern Italy in 1486. On discussing the etiological aspects of disease, Rhazes referred to the influence of "psychic events" on the physical state of the body. Clinically, he emphasized that "a deteriorated intellect is an ominous sign in all diseases," and that "sound intellect may not indicate safety for the patient." His firm belief in a psychological approach in treatment is well demonstrated in his aphorism that "the doctor should always instill a healthy outlook in his patient, and give him hope for recovery, even if he is not sure of it; for the body temperament is disposed to the psychic behavior." Medical historians were so impressed by Rhazes' original clinical work and therapeutic experiments that they ranked him with great clinicians like Hippocrates and Sydenham.

The *Canon of Medicine* by Avicenna (Plate CVI), which superseded another remarkable work, the *Royal Book* (*El maleki* or *Liber Regius*) by Haly Abbas, constitutes, like the *Continens,* a monumental work on the theory and practice of medicine. To measure the concepts, methods, and clinical material portrayed in Avicenna's book by modern standards is superfluous. However, his views on the psychology of emotion, and its therapeutic implications are of great historical significance (29). Within the limited medical techniques available in his day, Avicenna managed to develop, for example, a system for associating changes in the pulse rate with inner feelings. Through the pulse rate he systematically observed the psychosomatic reactions of his patients. His original clinical records included lists of questions relevant to diagnosis, the changes in the pulse rate that they caused, and the conclusions reached. The technique is rather reminiscent of the word-association test of Jung. On the other hand he conceived of psychology generally in terms of faculties.

Besides general medical problems, the nature of the "psyche" and the hidden spiritual forces of life stirred the thinking of a number of Arab physicians, and this was reflected in many of their writings. Certain difficulties are encountered in the terminology. The word *psyche,* which denotes in Greek the "breath" of life (44), seems to conceptualize to some extent similar meaning in Arab culture (*nafs* and *rouh*). In contradistinction to the physical constitution of the human body, the psyche was viewed as a spiritual force, which was

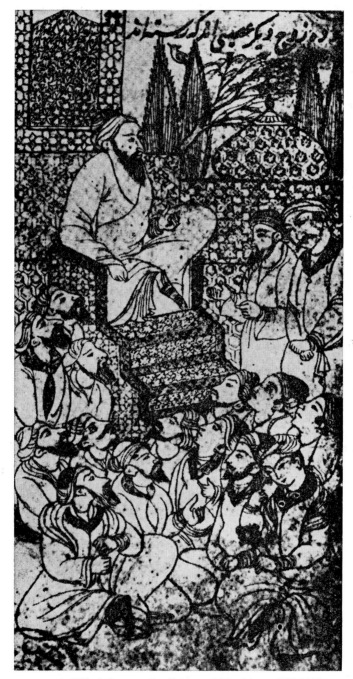

PLATE CVI. Avicenna, the Prince of Physicians (980-1036).

supposed to be the prime mover in life. Differentiation was sometimes also made between the "heavenly" or spiritual and the material or physical aspects of human life. This is clearly seen in Avicenna's *Ode to the Soul*, where he stated, "It descended upon thee from out of the region above." The understanding of the inner-self and the overcoming of its weaknesses was one of the great aims of Muslim thinkers. Mohammedan teachings had stimulated them in this direction. In more than one statement the Prophet declared that "he who knew himself better knew his God best." Some Arab physician-philosophers, like Averroes, considered that the study of anatomy, for example, leads to better understanding of God.

In the field of psychiatry, the *Disease of Melancholy*, by Omran Ibn Ishac, written in the 9th century, is one of the earliest treatises in history (45).

3

THE MIDDLE PERIOD OF ARAB PSYCHIATRY

Arab Folk Psychiatry in the 10th Century and After

Behavioral problems have often attracted the attention of non-medical workers, and folk psychiatry is finding a growing interest. Some cultural concepts of mental illness in Arabic literature can be traced to approximately ten centuries ago. An unusual treatise in this field is *The Sane Insane,* by the Arab scholar Nasaboury (died 1014), published by Kaylani (36). Nasaboury maintained that chapters on the same subject could be found in books by El Hafiz, Ibn Abe-dounia, Loghman, and Baghdadi, and claimed that his work was complete, inclusive, and probably the first of its kind. This work and others offer an outline of the definitions, terms, classifications, and clinical descriptions of mental disorders, hence they are of great historical significance.

The word *jenun* which in Arabic is equivalent to "madness," literally means screened or hidden, and there are more than 25 terms to denote a "mad" person. Nasaboury divided the mentally ill into five categories, apparently classified on an etiological basis:

1. *Matouh*: those who are born mentally ill;
2. *Mamrur*: those disturbed by burnt bile (humoral pathology);
3. *Mamsus*: those touched by the *jinn* and Satan;

4. *Ashig*: those overcome by passionate love to the degree of madness (erotic madness);
5. *Akhrag*: (Syn. *Habanag, Ahmag, Anwak,* etc.). This category includes a group of "sane insane" with defective judgment, incompetence in management, and disturbances of temperament. The group also includes mental defectiveness (*Khabal*).

It is interesting to note that conditions like alcoholism, and what was referred to as "abnormal behavior of youth," were excluded from these categories.

The Sane Insane is a purely literary work, yet its 100 recorded cases gave an overall picture of the social state and behavior of disturbed persons in that early period, and as such are of great psychiatric interest. Clinically, if the group which is referred to as erotic madness is excluded, the remaining individuals manifested either schizophrenic reactions with frank auditory hallucinations or manic depressive states. The story of Bajja is most informative; she was a female patient, who was mentally ill for 20 years and had a spontaneous recovery. Her recovery was associated with a vivid dream, where she was given the choice to continue in her sufferings and eventually go to paradise, or become cured. Then she saw the first two caliphs, Abu Baker and Omer, who prayed for her. On waking, she found herself cured and related her experience to her older brother. It is clear from this and other stories that the community attitude towards mental patients was tolerant and humane. Indeed the love poetry of the so-called "sane insane," like *Majnoun Layla,* was very popular, and probably helped towards the acceptance of mental illness by society. Furthermore, it was believed that some of the mentally ill were endowed with divine powers and could bring about miracles. Hence they were socially accepted, and were often engaged in conversation in order to find out their secrets and their views on future events. The same records indicate that as early as the 10th century some mentally ill patients were kept in Basra hospital. But the majority of them seem to have either been kept at home or left to wander in the marketplace, the mosques, or in lonely places, like the graveyards.

Interpretation of Dreams

In Arab culture the interpretation of dreams is very popular, and the literature on this subject is extensive. Reference has already been made to the psychological importance attached to dreams in ancient Egypt and Mesopotamia. During the "Period of Ignorance," the magicians (*kuhan*) were keen interpreters of dreams. From the very beginning of the Islamic era visions and dreams were highly regarded phenomena. Thus the experiences of the Prophet were remarkable episodes. It is believed that prior to the revelations he had several "holy dreams" during his night sleep. The time of the dream is significant, for it was believed that the diurnal dream was more important than the nocturnal one. It seems that the sayings of the Prophet on dreams, the experiences of other Prophets as revealed in the *Koran,* and their interpretations had great influence on Arab thinkers and philosophers, who were stimulated to study further the psychic nature of dreams. This is indicated by the fact that even in the first century after the Hiegra (Mohammedan year) significant material was produced by famous scholars like Ibn Serein (32), who was the earliest specialist in dream interpretations. The monumental works of El Zahry (23) (15th century) and El Naboulsy (21) (17th century), for example, are of great historical value. Some of the material in these early writings seems modern even by present day standards. They contain a significant list of references, and draw from a wide range of material.

Though references were made to the divine and demoniac sources of dreams, Arab interpreters gave due emphasis to psycho-social factors. They realized the psychological importance of the hidden (*maknun*) part of the dream. Their concepts are remarkably similar to Freudian psychology regarding the latent content of the dream (24). Another interesting feature is that they stressed the cultural influence on the content and form of dreams. An interpreter, to have deep insight into the nature of dreams, had to be well versed in the *Koran,* the traditions and sayings of the Prophet, current literature, proverbs, folklore, etc. Moreover, the personality of the dreamer, his occupation, religion, marital status, and other relevant information were taken into consideration.

Symbolism in dreams was of great interest to Arab interpreters, whose views eventually crystalized into voluminous material. Some of the views given to explain symbols were not unlike those of Freud (24), and the collective unconscious of Jung. Again, that some dreams were explained as wish-fulfillment was commonly accepted.

The lore of symbols included a variety of objects and covered many aspects of human life and natural phenomena. Though it was possible to explain straightforward dreams by standard formulas, the emotional, cultural, and social side of the dream content was often emphasized by leading Arab interpreters. The views of the dreamer were sometimes sought about his dream experience.

Institutional Care

Promotion of social services, including the care of the sick, usually goes hand in hand with socioeconomic progress and political stability. Hence, with the stabilization of Islamic rule, new patterns of medical care developed, and, as early as 707, the Umayyad Caliph El Walid established a hospital at Damascus. It is difficult to say how much care was given to the mentally ill in these early hospitals. On the whole the Umayyad period (661-750) is the least documented in Islamic history. However, in the hospitals which were later built by the Abbasid caliphs at Baghdad and other cities, one can trace the beginning of intramural care for mentally disturbed patients. These hospitals became the centers for training and clinical practice. Due emphasis was laid on the practical side of medical care. This is well illustrated in Rhazes' teaching: "The healing art, as it is described in books, is far inferior to the practical experience of a skillful and thoughtful physician."

As in Baghdad, medical practice flourished in other cities like Damascus, Cairo, and Cordova. By the 11th century medicine was well advanced in Syria. More progress was made under the rule of the great leader Saladin, *Salah El Din El Ayoubi* (1137-1193), who founded the Nasry Hospital in 1171 A.D. His son, Nour El Din, built the Noury Hospital at Damascus, which became a highly regarded medical training center and attracted medical students from all Islamic countries. Moses ben Maimoun, called Moses Maimonides (1135-1204), after he left Cordova and settled in Cairo, became the court physician to Saladin, and in this capacity attended Saladin's son, who was suffering from a depressive (*sawdawi*) state. His book on health care and management written for the Sultan was probably the most original work of the time and exceedingly important. It contained a chapter on psychological health, besides general advice on physical health and diet.

Garrison (27) has given an interesting description of the great Al-Mansur Hospital in Cairo, with its separate wards for important diseases and where "the sleepless were provided with soft music or, as in *The Arabian Nights*, with accomplished tellers of tales."

In the Western Caliphate too, all historical records point to a humanistic attitude towards the mentally ill. In discussing hospital care of mental patients in Spain, Mora (39) has stressed the influence of the Arabs on the Spaniards. He has also pointed out the similarities between the Spanish mental hospitals of the 15th and the 16th centuries in the Old and New World, and the Arab institutions, such as the one built by Mohamed V in Granada in 1365.

The 14th century Kalawoun Hospital in Cairo is extremely interesting in regard to psychiatric care. It had four separate sections for surgical, ophthalmological, medical, and mental diseases. The generous contributions to hospital funds by the wealthy of Cairo allowed a high standard of medical care and provided for the patients during convalescence until they were gainfully occupied. Two features are striking—the care of mental patients in a general hospital, which anticipated modern trends by approximately six centuries, and the involvement of the community in the welfare of the patients.

Unfortunately, the good start which the Kalawoun Hospital enjoyed did not continue for long. Gradually the services were neglected, and the in-patient population was reduced to the mentally ill. At the beginning of the 19th century the mental patients were moved out and accommodated at Azbakeya general hospital. A few years later, they were again transferred to another building in the Boulag area, and from there, in 1880, to Abbasia where a royal palace, damaged by fire, was provided to house mental patients. In the process of renovation, the house was painted yellow and until very recently it has been known as the yellow palace. Further reference will be made to the evolution of mental institutions when discussing the history of modern psychiatric services.

Drug Therapy

The history of drugs reveals in many ways the cultural development of mankind and its continuous striving to overcome discomfort and attain happiness. In ancient Egypt and Babylon drug therapy was part of magical practices and the inherent therapeutic power was attributed to supernatural forces, which were believed to control the destiny of man. The same animistic belief dominated Arab thinking during the "Period of Idolatry."

With the rise of Islamic civilization and the accumulation of therapeutic knowledge remarkable progress was made in the field of drug treatment. Arab scientists became the forerunners of alchemy and the originators of a variety of pharmaceutical preparations. For example the discovery of nitric acid, *aqua regia,* the chemical methods of distillation, filtering, sublimation, and hydrotherapy were all attributed to Gabir Ibn Hayan (702-765). The *Jami,* in which Ibn El Baitar in the 13th century listed 1,400 drugs, is indicative of the therapeutic advances achieved by Arab scientists, whose works became the standard authority through the Middle Ages. Again, a number of drugs introduced by them still have Arabic names, like alcohol, aldehyde, camphor, senna, etc.

It may not be widely known that Avicenna, "the Prince of Physicians," used *rauwolfia serpentina* in the treatment of acute mental symptoms (20). Other references to drugs commonly used for neuropsychiatric conditions in the 9th century are found, for instance, in *Al Dakhira* (46). In this interesting medical book, written by Thabit Ibn Qura (825-900 A.D.) for his son, Sennan, are included a number of diseases, like migraine, apoplexy, hemiplegia, facial palsy, epilepsy, stupor, and melancholia, as well as some physical disorders. The rationale of drug therapy was mainly based on humoral pathology. The long list of remedies for melancholia could be broadly divided into two categories: one for combating the humoral disturbances, consisting of drugs like *myroblan* (*ihlelig*) and *stoechas* (a purgative), which aimed at "purifying the body"; and the other dealing with disturbed thinking, fear, and worry. The latter part of the treatment was particularly aimed at correcting the abnormal "heart mood."

The history of psychoactive drugs, notably *catha edulis Forskal* (*khat*) and *cannabis indica* (*hashish*), in Arab culture is worthy of note. The earliest reference to *khat* was made by Nageeb el Din of Samarkand (died 1220) in a prescription in his rare manuscript of compound drugs or apothecary (*kitab el Akrabazin*) (20). It was used for "euphorizing purposes, the relief of melancholia, and depressive symptoms." Al Magrizi (1341-1442) also described the action of *khat* leaves and drew attention to its stimulant effects. *Khat* is still commonly used in Yemen. Extracted by chewing the leaves and sucking its juices, it contains three alkaloids: cathine (*d-nor-isophedrine*), cathedine, and cathenine. Though its stimulant action has been confirmed, its mode of action is not yet understood.

For several centuries hashish has been mentioned by Arab physicians, travelers, and historians. The historian Ibn Iyas in his Chronicle, *Wonderful Flowers in the History of Ages* (*Badai el Zuhur fi Wakaii el Duhur*) mentioned that in the year 922 the governor, seeing the failure of the Nile to rise in time, made an appeal to the people to invoke divine mercy through prayers and by refraining from hashish and wine for three days. The result was gratifying, for the Nile did rise after the third day.

The psychoactive effects of *khat* and hashish created much interest. The attainment of states of rapture and ecstasy had been sought, though differently, by the mystics, and *khat* and hashish were found to be effective agents. The ensuing psychological reactions were regarded as abnormal, and hence were attributed to divine powers. Similarly the legendary stories of these plants centered mainly on their divine secrets.

The history of the evolution of ideas regarding habit formation or dependence on psychoactive drugs is also interesting, for it was not recognized, and probably not known, in the past. The concept of drug addiction is of recent origin. Most likely it first came into official recognition after the International Opium Convention of The Hague in 1911. Incidently the first Dangerous Drug Act was passed in the United Kingdom in 1920. The prohibition of wine and narcotic drugs in Arab history stems from the *Koran,* as stated above.

Leading Arab physicians attached great importance to the inherent psychological effects of drugs. Rhazes' aphorism stated: "Make haste and use new drugs while they are still effective."

Recent research on the psychological effects of drugs administered as placebos in controlled studies seems to agree with the view expressed by Rhazes more than 11 centuries ago.

Traditional Psychotherapeutic Practices

Social changes in the Islamic world in time led to the development of new ideas and concepts. New cults, such as *sufism,* found their way into the communities. It was suggested that the suffering brought about by repeated wars and invasions caused many to choose the mystic path and find comfort in the attitude of resignation (1). There were, of course, other factors as well. The orthodox Islamic teachings were affected by the decline in the socio-political state of the Muslim communities. As pointed out by Meyerhof (38), "with the beginning of the 14th century, magical and superstitious practices began to creep into the medical works of the Muslim writers." Furthermore, cross fertilization of the Islamic culture with cultures in Africa and Asia had its effects on the development of psychotherapeutic techniques.

The cult of saints, which was not known in the early days of Islam, was closely connected with the spread of religious healing. The significance of this cult lies in the community relationship it creates and in the emergence of the religious healer as a leader. *Sufism* and its mystic path (*Tariga*) were intimately related to the cult of saints. Mysticism opened new avenues for emotional and psychological satisfaction, and the mystical doctrine of *sufism* developed from a mere religious practice into a complex theosophical system, which required training and guidance. Hence disciples grouped around famous saints, and formed new types of religious communities with special centers, which played a considerable role in the dissemination of traditional teachings. They were known in the Sudan as *khalwas, zawias,* and *maseeds.* The *khanka* was commonly known in the Near East, and the *rabat* was famous in the Maghrib. Some of the mentally ill took shelter in these religious houses.

In Muslim countries, traditional healers could be classified as: religiously oriented healers, who make use of religious techniques; and non-religious healers, who utilize magico-religious practices. The traditional Mohammedan healer is known by several names: the *feki*, the *fageer*, the *waly*, the *shareif*, the *sayed*, and the *sheikh*. The terms denote holiness, or socio-religious superiority. The religious healer usually grows up within a "professional" circle, and since early life learns the traditional techniques from his master. There is no system of prescribed courses of learning. The future healer gains the required experience through active participation in therapy with the *sheikh*. When there is any formal teaching, it is limited to the learning of the *Koran*, the sayings and traditions of the Prophet, and formulations and maxims of the *sheikhs*. By listening to the elders, the disciples become familiar with miraculous cures, which are attributed to the divine powers of the dead *sheikhs*. Deifalla (19th century) (14) gave many examples of miraculous cures by venerated Sudanese *sheikhs*. However, all these stories are a legacy of the past.

Traditional religious healers commonly believe that there are three causes of disease: the evil eye; evil-doing (*amal*); and demoniacal possession.

The evil eye as a causative factor in the pathogenesis of disease is firmly established in Muslim countries. Basically, belief in the malignant influence conveyed by it seems to be similar in various religions, except that of the ancient Egyptian (28).

In evil-doing, disease is caused by the presence of certain objects or substances in the body. The underlying magical part of this concept is noticeable here. This concept has no roots in Islamic philosophy. Even those religious healers who believe in evil machinations do not resort to shamanistic practices against them, but employ religious techniques instead. Some traditional healers' practices are covered under a religious cloak, but essentially they lean on witchcraft.

Religious Techniques

Since the dawn of history, the power of certain concepts and the drive behind vital ideas have often shaped human institutions. Religious healers believe firmly in what they do, and this sense of conviction is equally shared and reciprocated by the sick who seek their help. Thus in certain traditional communities and within cultural norms, strong rapport could be established between the healer and the patient. The personality and ability of the healer, together with his reputation, determine to a great extent the outcome of treatment. Whatever techniques are used, the most successful healers are those who can induce heightening of their clients' emotional state, which is followed by the release of inner tension. The patient will often describe this as a strange feeling, which is not infrequently associated with psychological components such as fear of the mysterious and the occult on the one hand, and an unbound faith in recovery by the "will of Allah" and his intermediaries on the other. Certain "vehicles" are used to facilitate suggestion and augment the psychological effects of therapy.

The forms of religious therapy vary greatly, but on the whole the focal point of treatment is the invocation made to God in order to bring a cure. This is aided by the performance of special practices directed against the underlying cause.

Treatment is commonly carried out as individual or group therapy, and the methods used are either prophylactic or curative. Devices or means frequently used were: charms (*hegab, waraga, kilab, hirz, hafeza*, etc.); incantations (*azema, taweza*); fumigation (*bakhour*); and purification (*mehaya*).

The universality of charms used against the evil eye are too well known to be mentioned here. The shape and material of certain charms, and the contents of writings, depend on the scholastic and cultural background of the healer. Numerous examples could be quoted from popular books like the *Shams el marif el kubra* (*The Great Sun of Knowledge*) by El Bowny (b. 1225) (16).

In a simple session of incantation the religious healer puts his first three fingers over the patient's forehead and then draws them together, while reciting specific verses from the *Koran*. The "verse of the throne" is especially selected, for it includes a well-defined appeal to God for mercy and a clear invocation for help.

In Arab tradition, the fumes of substances like alum, benzion, mastic, and so on, are believed to have power against evil spirits. But by far the most potent remedy against evil is believed to be the word of God. Hence verses from the *Koran* are written on pieces of paper and, according to the severity of the disease, the patient burns a number of them and inhales the fumes.

Purification with holy water is a universal practice, called *mehaya* among certain traditional Arab communities. In a specially-designed board (*loah*), the religious healer writes certain symbols, signs, Koranic verses, names of angels, and healing invocations which are traditionally known for their divine power (Plate CVII). The origin of

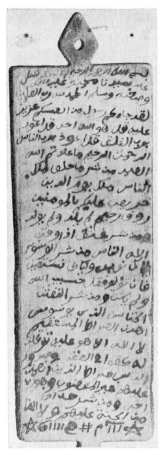

PLATE CVII. Writing board from the Sudan with its religious writing and ancient symbols.

these symbols and signs can be traced to the *Bible* and the *Koran*. The writings on the *loah* are then washed off, the liquid is collected, and the patient either drinks it or washes his body with it.

It is not uncommon to find that well-established healing centers develop their own system of treatment. Apart from receiving individual therapy, the patient becomes an active member of a therapeutic community. Life in these centers is based on communal welfare. Besides having his regular doses of *mehaya* and observing all religious rites, the patient participates fully in all activities and is assigned a specific job in the fields; he may draw the water, cut the wood, cultivate the land, or look after the animals.

The Healing Cult of Zar

Plowden (41), British Consul in Ethiopia in the late 1800's, was the first writer to refer to the popular healing cult of *Zar*. Since then other scholars have shown interest in the same cult and have contributed to its literature. Kahle (34) reviewed some of the literature on *Zar* and made a special study of its musical notes; Trimingham (47, 48) has dealt with certain aspects of its theological and social background.

The origin of *Zar* goes far back into the Ethiopian cultural heritage. Among the Agao tribe the sky god was known as Zar, which with cultural changes degenerated into an evil spirit. Later on, the Galla Muslims absorbed the Agao Zar rite, and from there it found its way into the Sudan, Egypt, Saudi Arabia, and Kuwait.

The *Zar* practice is now a dying art, but is occasionally seen among pre-literate communities. When a sick person consults a *Zar* practitioner, the first visit is mainly diagnostic and an exploratory session is often conducted. Though the techniques are the same, much depends on the cultural background, the originality, and the creativity of the *Zar* practitioner. In communities where such practices are found, the pagan concept of the *Zar* performance has been transformed to fit the cultural matrix of traditional society.

The *Zar* ceremony is usually a big festivity in which old clients, relatives, neighbors, and friends participate. The patient sits on one side and the group assembles nearby. The *Zar* healer and his assistants sit in front. When the aroma of the burning incense fills the air and the place is all ready, the healer leads the crowd by singing calls for the various *Zar* and spirit masters (*asyad* and *mashayekh*), and is followed by the chorus from the "enchanted" group. Every spirit is called by its particular "line" of singing, and special dress is worn for it. The list of masters and spirits is long, and depends on the locality and the culture. The most commonly invoked Muslim *sheikhs* are Abdel Gadir El Geilani (1077-1166) and Ahmed El Badawi (d. 1276). It is probably true to say that the admixture of so many cultural elements in the *Zar* cult has made the addition of new names and terms acceptable.

During a *Zar* performance the beating of the drums continues for hours on end and for fixed days. The rhythm gets faster and faster and the singing of songs becomes louder and louder until the patient becomes emotionally stimulated, and feels the impulse to move and dance. With the heightening of excitement, the patient manifests various behavioral reactions, which are partly influenced by traditional beliefs, and partly by the healers, but mainly reflect the patient's inner conflicts. A state of psychological dissociation may take place and the patient may pass into a trance-like state. During a trance, it is not uncommon to see the dramatization of unconscious wishes, and the acting out of pent-up emotions. The abreaction through which the patient passes usually brings about dramatic results, especially in psychoneurotic patients.

The technical psychotherapeutic features of the healing cult of *Zar* can be summarized as follows:

1. Good initial preparation of the patient for therapeutic techniques;
2. the full confidence of the clients in treatment;
3. the masterly ability of the practitioner and his unwavering faith in the *Zar* practice;
4. the continuous group involvement;
5. the full use of all modalities of sensation, especially auditory (musical stimulation) to the point of dissociation and even collapse;
6. identification with saints and personality cults;
7. use of mystical notions as vehicles for suggestion and persuasion;
8. dramatization and enactment;
9. unloading of emotional feelings;
10. the meaningful utterances during the dissociative phase, which indicate the patient's conflicts, are carefully noted and the patient's needs are duly catered to.

4

RECENT HISTORY OF PSYCHIATRY

General

The influence of European education in the 19th century has caused a major shift in Arab medicine. While under political domination, particularly British and French, medical disciplines, based on the newly developed sciences, found their way into Arab countries. The first European-style medical school was founded in Cairo in 1876, and was followed by others inside and outside Egypt. In Kuwait, Saudi Arabia, and Libya medical schools are still in the making. Academic mental health and psychiatric departments were created rather late.

The first chair of psychiatry was founded in Cairo University at Kasr El-Aini Faculty of Medicine, followed in 1965 by the French Medical Faculty in Beirut and in Ain Shams in Egypt, and by Khartoum University in 1968.

The undergraduate teaching of psychiatry varies tremendously, and much still remains to be done to promote it to the level recommended by the World Health Organization (51). Postgraduate training for a diploma in psychological medicine and neurology and an M.D. in psychiatry were started in Egypt in 1941. But most of the practicing psychiatrists in other Arab countries had their training in the United Kingdom, France, or Switzerland. A few have recently qualified from socialist countries.

The recent history of psychiatry in Arab medicine is characterized by certain features. First, it has lagged behind general medicine. Second, early psychiatric institutions built at the turn of the century copied the European model of mental hospitals. Third, under the effect of accelerating socioeconomic changes in the last decade psychiatric services have increasingly progressed.

Warnock (50), with his long experience as Director of the Lunacy Division, Ministry of the Interior, Egypt, and Director of the Abbasia Hospital, has given a revealing account of the poor state of psychiatry at the beginning of the 20th century. Ford-Robertson (25, 26), who was once the director of the Lebanon Hospital for Psychological and Nervous Disorders, better known as Asfurieh, reviewed the history of the hospital and suggested plans for future developments. The history of treatment of mental disorders in the Sudan by the author (4) includes statements on recent trends in psychiatric services. *Psychiatry in the Arab East* (42), with its detailed, annotated bibliography, offers useful information on present day psychiatry in this important area.

Analyses of general trends of psychiatry in Arab countries vary greatly from one country to another. Psychiatric services range from the repressive custodial and the restrictive legal, to the voluntary, open units in general hospitals, and to out-patient clinics.

In some countries, like Egypt and the Sudan, psychiatric services have become part of the national health plans, while in others they suffer from an absence of progress. In terms of manpower, it is also significant to find adequate and well-qualified personnel in a country like Kuwait, whereas in other places there is no staff to run even a rudimentary mental health service. Shortage in qualified psychiatric nurses, social workers, and clinical psychologists seems to be generally more acute than the shortage of psychiatrists.

Psychiatric treatment in general has been influenced by the orientational background, the available number of psychiatrically trained personnel, the overwhelming conditions of the mentally ill, the great advances in psychopharmacology, and the cultural milieu. Physical methods of treatment are generally used. The phenothiazine group of drugs, haloperidol, lithium, anti-depressants, etc., are commonly administered with good results. The drugs seem to overshadow psychotherapeutic treatment. Orthodox psychoanalysis is rarely practiced. The keenness for psychoanalysis, which was demonstrated, for example, in the *Egyptian Journal of Psychology* (published in Arabic, first issued in 1945 and later discontinued), seems to have fallen out of vogue now. Occupational therapy and activities outside the hospital are receiving increasing attention in recent years.

Clinical material gathered from various sources indicates that the basic psychological disorders seen among Arab communities are not unlike the findings elsewhere. The difference, if any, lies within the context of cultural manifestations (5). It is not uncommon to find that emotional disturbances masquerade as folk beliefs, or become intricately disguised in the cultural jargon. However, it is true to say that certain manifestations, like self-reproach in depressive states, are conspicuously uncommon among some communities, and this, too, can be explained on a cultural basis. In regard to the incidence of psychiatric disorders, it would be improper to make hurried conclusions and common generalizations. Indeed, epidemiological investigations show that the incidence of mental illness not only varies from one country to another, but also from one locality to another in the same country (3, 6). The complacency in the past about the low incidence of mental diseases in developing countries should no longer be accepted. For it is not only scientifically incorrect, it is misleading and detracting from proper assessment of mental health needs, and may give low priority to planning of psychiatric services.

Psychiatric Hospitals

Reference has already been made to the evolution of psychiatric care in Egypt until the time of the establishment of the Abbasia Mental Hospital in 1880, which still remains the oldest and largest mental hospital in the Arab countries, at present accommodating more than 2,500 patients. Though much improvement has recently been accomplished with the view to changing it into a more active therapeutic community, it probably needs further radical changes in its structural set-up in order to play a more effective role in the advancement of psychiatric services. The new program for the training of nurses is very promising, and is a major step towards the promotion of psychiatric care and towards meeting the shortage of qualified personnel.

The Khanka Hospital, which was built in 1912, resembles Abbasia in its large size, and accommodates about 3,000 patients, with a special section for forensic psychiatry. Its general layout, construction, and location (30 kilometers north of Cairo) are other features of a mental hospital built at the turn of the century of a type which was also found outside the Arab countries.

Both the Abbasia and Khanka hospitals are now under the Mental Health Division of the Ministry of Health. In the last decade, and under the leadership of Wagdi, a former director of the Abbasia hospital, tremendous impetus has been given to psychiatric services in Egypt. Within the two five-year national development plans, the key policy has been the decentralization of psychiatric services by the establishment of provincial mental hospitals, of psychiatric units in general hospitals, and of country-wide out-patient clinics. There is no doubt that the new policy with the growing number of qualified personnel is having profound effects on psychiatry in Egypt.

Apart from the state mental hospitals, units, and clinics, there are four privately owned psychiatric institutions in Egypt. The Behman Hospital at Halwan, south of Cairo, is the best known. It was established in 1940 by Behman, an Egyptian psychiatrist. It is a good example of a small hospital of 120 beds with an adequate staff-patient ratio. Hilmiet El-Zeitun, Mustashfa El Nil, and St. Charles Hospital at Maadi, closed down in 1964, are other small hospitals.

The Lebanon Hospital for Mental and Nervous Disorders (Asfurih) is a reputable institution. Situated near Beirut, it was built at the turn of this century by T. Waldmeier, a Swiss Quaker missionary. Its 450 beds are occupied by various categories of mental patients, including medico-legal cases. One of the important features of this hospital is its training program for psychiatric auxiliary workers. Again its affiliation to the Medical School of the University of Beirut has been a significant development in its history.

From an asylum for senile and mentally ill priests, the Hospital of the Cross (Deir El-Saleeb) has developed in the last two decades into a group of institutions which include care for general psychiatric disorders, and for mentally retarded children, an orphanage and a school. As such, it is the largest psychiatric institution in the Republic of Lebanon. It is affiliated to the French Faculty of Medicine, and most of its psychiatrists were trained in French centers.

Similar to the Deir El-Saleeb, the Islamic Neuro-Psychiatric Hospital, which was established in 1959, has a socio-religious background, and is supported by public funds. It has 400 beds, and caters to general psychiatric conditions, as well as to mentally retarded children.

Psychiatry in Lebanon is at a disadvantage because of lack of central organization. The present mental hospitals are handicapped by inadequate extramural facilities (7). However, in the last decade there has been a growing interest in the care of retarded children, and special schools have been built for them. Despite all efforts to overcome chronicity, mental hospitals in Lebanon have a high proportion of chronic patients (2).

The Ibn Sena (Avicenna) Hospital outside Damascus and Dwerrini Hospital near Aleppo are the two state mental hospitals in Syria. The former, with 500 beds, was established in 1929, and the latter, which is smaller, was built in 1956.

The care of juvenile delinquents is attracting increasing public interest in Syria, and the work of voluntary organizations in this field is the finest in Arab countries.

After the closing of Dar El Shifa (House of Treatment) in 1959, Shamaeeyah Mental Hospital, founded in 1953, became the main psychiatric institution in Iraq. It is located 15 miles outside Baghdad, in an isolated area. Overcrowding, shortage of trained auxiliary personnel, and lack of facilities for community care, follow-up, and rehabilitations, are among the important factors which seem to prevent this institution from fulfilling its therapeutic functions effectively (9).

Dar El Rashed, a small private unit in Baghdad, was established in 1943. There is also an active out-patient psychiatric clinic affiliated to the Medical Faculty of the University of Baghdad.

The establishment of psychiatric services in the Sudan is an interesting experiment in a developing country. Prior to World War II there were hardly any organized psychiatric services for the care of mental patients. By 1950 the Clinic for Nervous Disorders, Khartoum-North, was well established, and the Kober Institution was built to cater for 120 forensic psychiatric patients. This was followed by the establishment of four psychiatric units in provincial capitals, at Wad Medani, Port Sudan, El Obeid, and Atbara. In 1964, a 30-bed psychiatric ward was built in Khartoum general hospital (8). Finally, in 1971, plans were laid to start work in Omdurman Psychiatric Hospital, the first of its kind in the history of the Sudan. The underlying policy was first to establish psychiatric units with close links with medical institutions and broad connections with community agencies. After laying this basic foundation, the plan is to develop mental hospitals, if the need arises. Essentially this strategy is the reverse of that in some other countries, where psychiatric care began by the building of huge mental hospitals, to the exclusion of extramural facilities. The Sudan psychiatric model proved to be flexible, made it possible for psychiatric boundaries to expand into various activities, and gave initial coverage to remote areas in a vast country.

Different patterns of psychiatric care are seen in Kuwait, Saudi Arabia, Bahrain, Libya, and other oil-rich countries. Kuwait, for example, managed to attract excellent psychiatrists from the beginning. The story of the improvement of the old dilapidated mental asylum (Malga El Maganeen) in 1955 and the move to the newly built 250-bed Kuwait Hospital for Nervous and Psychological Disorders shows two striking features—first, the dramatic changes in medical services which have taken place within a very short period; and second, the importance of leadership and the availability of an adequate number of qualified staff.

In Saudi Arabia, the inception of modern psychiatry was associated with the construction of Shahar Hospital at Taif in 1962. An extensive plan for a countrywide network of psychiatric out-patient services and in-patient care units in general hospitals is now under way.

It is interesting to note that in Qatar, psychiatric care was initiated as part of Doha General Hospital, where an in-patient unit was organized, and in 1971 an out-patient clinic was established for the first time.

After an initial shortage of qualified manpower, Bahrain managed to establish efficient in-patient and out-patient psychiatric services at its hospital, Manama.

Present plans focus on the training of personnel, improving the quality of psychiatric care, and extending the mental health services into the community.

Similar to other Gulf States, the United Arab Emirates are showing keen interest in mental health work, and plans are under way for establishing psychiatric services on a modern basis.

The Mental Disease Hospital in Tripoli, with its 1,022 beds and the two institutes for mentally retarded children at Tripoli and Jebel Akhdar, form the core of psychiatric facilities in Libya.

In Tunisia psychiatric care is centered round the old Manouba Hospital. Great efforts have been made to decentralize the services and move into the community.

Psychiatry today is more and more recognized in Arab medicine and its whole future depends on the quality and number of qualified personnel who will have the imagination and competence to make effective use of all available resources and develop its services in harmony with the social context and cultural heritage.

REFERENCES

1. AFNAN, S. M. (1958): *Avicenna/His Life and Works*. London: Allen and Unwin.
2. Annual Reports (1963, 1964, 1965): Republic of Lebanon: Ministry of Health.
3. BAASHER, T. (1961): Survey of mental illness in Wadi Halfa. *World Mental Health*: 13, No. 4, November.
4. BAASHER, T. (1962): Some aspects of the history of the treatment of mental disorders in the Sudan. *Sudan Med. J.*, No. 1, 44.
5. BAASHER, T. (1963): The influence of culture on psychiatric manifestations. *Transcultural Psych. Review and Newsletter*, No. 15, 51, October.
6. BAASHER, T. (1965): Treatment and prevention of psychosomatic diseases. Psychosomatic diseases in East Africa. *Amer. J. Psychiat.*, 121, 1095.
7. BAASHER, T. (1966): *Mental Health Activities in Rural Health Units in Iraq and Lebanon*. W.H.O. M.H./68.8.
8. BAASHER, T. AND A/RAHIM, S. I. (1967): The psychiatric ward. *Sudan Med. J.*, 5, No. 3.
9. BAZZOUI, W. I. AND AL-ISSA, I. (1966): Psychiatry in Iraq. *Brit. J. Psychiat.*, 112, 827.
10. BREASTED, J. H. (1959): *Development of Religion and Thought in Ancient Egypt*. New York: Harper & Row.
11. BROWNE, E. G. (1921): *Arabian Medicine*. Cambridge: Cambridge University Press.
12. BUDGE, W. (1899): *Egyptian Magic*. Evanston & New York: University Books.
13. CAMPBELL, D. (1926): *Arabian Medicine*. London: Kegan Paul.
14. DEIFALLA, M. W. (1930): *Kitab el tabagat fi khusus el awlia wa el salheen, wa el olama wa el shoara fi el Sudan*. (Classes of saints, holymen, scholars and poets in the Sudan.) Cairo: Mohmoudia Trading Press.
15. EISA, A. (1942): *Mugam el Atiba*. (Bibliography of doctors.) Cairo: Fathalla Noury & Sons Press.
16. EL BOWNY, A. (1951): *Manabi isoul el hikma*. (The sources of origin of wisdom.) Cairo: El Baby el Halaby Press.
17. EL KAHAL, A. (1955): *El Ahkam el Nabawia fii el sinna el tebia*. (The Prophet rulings on the art of medicine.) Cairo: El Baby el Halaby Press.
18. EL MAHI, TIGANY (1955): *Mugadima fi tareekh el tib el Arabi*. (An introduction to the history of Arab medicine.) Matbaa't Misr (Sudan) Ltd.
19. EL MAHI, TIGANY (1960): *Mafhoum el siha el aglia fi el tareekh*. (The concept of mental health in the ancient cultures of the Middle East.) *Egyptian Historical Society Review*. Cairo: Costa Tsounas Press.
20. EL MAHI, TIGANY (1962): *The use and abuse of drugs*. EM/RC 12/6. Alexandria: W.H.O. Regional Office for the Eastern Mediterranean.
21. EL NABOULSY, A. (1940): *Tateer el anam fi tafseer el ahlam*. (World fragrance with dream interpretation.) Cairo: El Baby el Halaby Press.
22. EL ZAHABY, A. (1948): *El tib el nabawi*. (The medicine of the Prophet). Cairo: Republican Library.
23. EL ZAHRY, K. S. (1940): *El isharat fi elm el ibarat*. (Symbols and their concepts.) Cairo: El Baby el Halaby Press.
24. FREUD, S. (1952): *On Dreams*. Trans. by James Strachey. London: The Hogarth Press.
25. FORD-ROBERTSON, W. (1952): Some problems concerning the approach to a Middle East Psychiatric service. *J. Méd. Liban*, 5, 2.
26. FORD-ROBERTSON, W. (1953): The concept of the mental hospital as a therapeutic community. *J. Méd. Liban.*, 7, 89.

27. GARRISON, F. H. (1914): *An Introduction to the History of Medicine*. Philadelphia and London: W. B. Saunders Company.
28. GLIFFORD, E. S. (1958): *The Evil Eye*. New York: Macmillan.
29. GRUNER, O. C. (1930): *A Treatise on the Canon of Medicine of Avicenna*. London: Luzac & Co.
30. HURRY, J. M. (1938): *Imhotep, the Vizier and Physician to King Zoser*. London: Oxford University Press.
31. IBN ABY AUSAYBAA, M. (1882): *Eyoun el anaba fi tabgat el atiba*. (Sources of information on classes of doctors.) Cairo: Wahbey Press.
32. IBN SEREIN, M. (1957): *Montakab el kalam fi tafseer el ahlam*. (Selected prose in the interpretation of dreams.) Cairo: Istigama Press.
33. ISKANDER, A. Z. (1967): *A Catalogue of Arabic Manuscripts on Medicine and Science*. London: The Wellcome Historical Medical Library.
34. KAHLE, P. (1912): *Zar Beschworungen In Egyptian*, Der Islam, iii.
35. KAMAL, H. (1922): *The Book on Ancient Egyptian Medicine*. Cairo.
36. KAYLANI, W. F. (1924): *Ogala el maganeen by Naysaboury*. (The sane insane.) Cairo: Egyptian Arabic Press.
37. LA BEAUME, J. (1969): *La Koran Analyse*. Remis en arab per M. F. Abdel Baqui. Beirut: Dar Al-Kitab Al Arabi.
38. MEYERHOF, M. (1931): *Science and Medicine in the Legacy of Islam*. Oxford: Clarendon Press.
39. MORA, G. (1967): History of Psychiatry. In: *Comprehensive Textbook of Psychiatry*. Baltimore: William and Wilkins Co.
40. OPPENHEIM, L. (1956): The interpretation of dreams in the ancient far east. *Trans. Amer. Philos. Soc.*, 46, 179.
41. PLOWDEN, W. C. (1868): *Travels in Abyssinia and the Gala Country*. London: Longmans, Green.
42. RACY, J. (1970): Psychiatry in the Arab East. *Acta psychiat. scand.*, Suppl. No. 211.
43. REISNER, G. A. (1909): *The Hearst Medical Papyrus*. California: University of California Publications.
44. ROBERTS, F. (1959): *Medical Terms*. London: William Heinemann Medical Books Ltd.
45. SAYYID, F. (1955): *Les generation des medicins et des sages* (Tabaqat al-atiba wel-hukama). Ecrit compose en 377 H. Par Abu Dawud Suleiman Ibn Hassan Ibn Gulgul al-Andalusi. Edition Critique. Le Cairo, Inst. Fr. D'arch. Orient.
46. SOBHY, G. (1928): *The Book of Al Dakhira*. Cairo Government Press.
47. TRIMINGHAM, J. S. (1949): *Islam in the Sudan*. London: Oxford University Press.
48. TRIMINGHAM, J. S. (1952): *Islam in Ethiopia*. London: Oxford University Press.
49. TRITTON, A. S. (1957): *Materials on Muslim Education in the Middle Ages*. London: Luzac & Co. Ltd.
50. WARNOCK, J. (1924): Twenty-eight years lunacy experience in Egypt. *J. Ment. Sci.*, 70, Parts I, II & III.
51. W. H. O. (1970): *Seminar on the place of psychiatry in medical education*. EM/SEM. MENT/15 EMRO 0112. Alexandria.

24

MID AND WEST AFRICA

T. Adeoye Lambo, O.B.E., M.D.

Deputy Director-General, World Health Organization,
Geneva, Switzerland

1

INTRODUCTION

Africa, the second largest continent on the globe, covering one quarter of the world's land surface, is a true representative of developing countries. This huge but largely underdeveloped continent claims well over 50 of the 125 political units on the globe; it has a rate of progress—political, social, and economic—almost unparalleled in history, and shows a remarkable diversity of ethnic grouping, culture, and potential resources.

Disease, which is older than man, is one of the basic problems which faces every human society, and every society has been known to develop institutionalized methods of coping with it. It has also been found that disease may be of great concern to an African society, without reference to its virulence or epidemiological proportion. Many tribes were known to have spent a considerable part of their productive time in ritualistic ceremonials, most of which were concerned with disease or its prevention. Harley (10) informs us that disease, its healing, and its prevention play a preponderant role in the religion of the Manos of Liberia.

Ackerknecht (1) has warned that "Our medicine is not the medicine nor our religion the religion, and there is not one medicine but numerous and quite different medicines in different parts of the world and in the past, present and future. Measuring everything by

579

our everyday standards, we will never understand either the past or the future." Psychiatry in Mid and West Africa is by historical and evolutionary necessity inextricably interwoven with the history of general health care in Africa. In any case, it would seem historically naïve to look at the content of a part of the culture (e.g. religious ideas), without examining religious institutions and other related institutionalized practices and their interrelatedness.

For practical purposes the history of psychiatry in Mid and West Africa can be divided into three periods: traditional, transitional, and contemporary. The traditional period was essentially tribal and had all the features of communal and folk medicine. It was the precursor of Western medicine. The transitional period was characterized by the combined influence of the Christian medical missions and alien custodial practices of the colonial (metropolitan) powers. The contemporary period has been marked by many features of imaginative, innovative, and eclectic philosophies and practices. It is also in the process of creating a conceptual model which would blend with the socio-economic and cultural goals of the new and emergent societies in Africa.

It should be mentioned at the outset that the three periods—the traditional, which is largely pre-historic (often erroneously termed pre-logical), transitional, which is recent, and modern, which is current—exist side by side, partly in happy syncretism, partly with deep suspicion, and sometimes in fierce confrontation. They overlap and form a historic continuum. This is one of the outstanding characteristics of social change in Africa. In 1961 I observed, "In most African countries today there exist side by side pagan sanctuaries and Christian shrines." This form of symbiosis of European and traditional African cultures is evident in many African countries, especially in Nigeria. Cunyngham Brown (6) observed, "In consequence it may be truly said that Nigeria today furnishes examples of almost every chapter in the long and doleful history of the insane of all countries, from its first recorded beginnings in the days of antiquity up to modern times, with the exception as yet of late 19th and 20th century developments."

2

THE TRADITIONAL PERIOD

Psychological medicine, like any other traditional indigenous institution, nowhere follows its own motivation; its character, impact, and dynamism depend on the place it takes within the general philosophy of the society, its frame of reference to, and its compatibility with, other cultural institutions. The institutionalization of traditional medicine was an important part of the historical evolution of many aspects of traditional cultures in Africa and, in fact, derived from the general development of many socio-cultural institutions throughout the ages.

Tribal medicine, which was usually ritualistic and communal in its operation, tells the history of a nation, its struggles, seasons of excitement and recklessness, religious feeling, modes of thought, intellectual movements, hopes, passions, and fears. It contains within its scope and in a concentrated form the archetype that "expresses premordial ideas, needs, and aspirations of the whole tribe" (15). Galdston (8) has aptly observed: "Individual man, the infinite being, is an 'accident' in time—but he is also the issue of a long past, that is, of historic and collective man. To understand the individual, the infinite person, we need to know a great deal about the extended past of the collective historical man. . . ."

The devotion of the tribal ancestors was chiefly connected with storms and pestilences, famine and death, which were regarded as penal inflictions, and which consequently created an almost maddening terror. Thus the concept of "public health" and prevention of disease in the communities became more broadly interpreted and practiced. Periodic collective group psychotherapeutic practices (e.g. possession, dancing, confession) were common. They constituted powerful psychotherapeutic measures and psychological safety valves through which excessive psychic pressure could be released. Possession, for example, can be induced and is so frequent an occurrence that it can be expected at most tribal ceremonies (Plate CVIII).

"Secret tribal societies in Africa have always engaged in 'collective therapy.' The N'jayei society of the Mende in Sierra Leone, to mention one, concerns itself solely with the treatment of mental disorders, serving a similar purpose as the Yassi society of the Sherbro in the same country, or the Zar cults of Ethiopia and the Sudan" (11).

Through rituals, a capacity for wider group participation was initiated. This provided a basis for the growth of social attitudes and moral development, for not only were the tribes constantly expiating to rid themselves of their collective guilt, they were constantly promoting positive mental health through many culture bound and culturally prescribed practices of an emotional kind. Thus, many institutionalized practices, including magico-religious rituals, enhance the sources of religious emotion through their functional association with the cults of ancestors, cults of major deities, funeral rites, agricultural rites, and many other situations in which the groups freely participate (for example, the institution of sacrifice by communion—the oldest form of sacrifice—"in which the sacrifice of a divine object imparts divinity to all that eat of it") (16). Sacrifice was an exotic sacrament

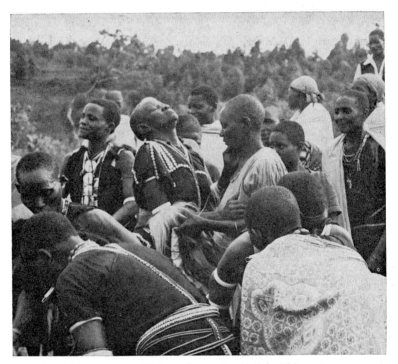

PLATE CVIII. Group possession in East Africa.

resorted to in supreme moments of distress or peril to the clan, tribe, or community.

There is, in many of these cultures, a bewildering array of vast and complicated systems of rituals and magico-religious practices which, in spite of their diversity, emphasize that reality consists of the relation not of men with things, but of men with other men, and of all men with spirits. A thorough and analytical study of these African cultures shows that in many established traditional cults men and spirits were brought together in mystic and emotional relationship "in a joint endeavor to conserve and promote good mental health by a ritual technique as the link with the providential sources of life . . ." (15).

At the most primitive culture levels, man has been found to share with animals and with his fellow man for technological cultures certain instinctive (and perhaps empirical) ways of relief from physical discomfort. These include, *inter alia,* cooling a heated body, applying heat to an infected part, rubbing or pressing for local irritation or pain, raising, resting, or mobilizing an injured limb, cooling and wrapping an injury or a wound. These approaches, in addition to a thorough familiarity with plants, animals, and rocks of man's environment, provide and equip man with a rich diversity of empirical remedies, surgical and other manipulative techniques and instruments to apply them. In many parts of the continent, trepanation of the skull by the medicine-men in cases of serious illness was not infrequent. Margetts (18) presented a detailed account of this procedure among East Africans. In most parts of West and Central Africa plant and animal medicines are taken internally in the form of decoctions, or are applied externally as fomentations or ointments, or as adjuncts to psychotherapy.

The attitude towards disease in general and mental illness in particular and the methods of fighting it vary from tribe to tribe in Central and West Africa. But when analyzed closely, the concepts of health and disease in African cultures can be regarded as constituting a continuous transition with almost imperceptible gradations. Burstein (3), writing on public health and prevention of disease in primitive communities, notes: "Medicine, in our sense, at primitive culture levels, is only one phase of a set of processes to promote human well being: averting the wrath of gods or spirits, making rain, purifying streams or habitations, improving sex potency or fecundity or the fertility of fields and crops—in short, it is bound up with the whole interpretation of life."

Traditional psychotherapy and other forms of prevention healing in Africa, which occupy such a vital part of the whole system of thought, should not be regarded as an absurd system of thought which came into existence through chance, subjective experiences, or superstitions, but one which has been found to be a dynamic and meaningful part of a living culture, quite able to survive changes in spite of the basic differences from the pattern posed by Western culture. Thus Ackerknecht (1) stresses the point that the institution of medicine has more clearly a function of the culture than of environmental conditions. The relevance to, and importance of, the basic African philosophy is to emphasize the close interrelationship between social structure and culture on the one hand and patterns of health care on the other, since it is within a particular socio-cultural framework that man derives his perception of health and disease.

The African Concept of the Causation of Psychiatric Disorders

In many parts of West and Central Africa nearly all forms of mental illness, disease, personal and communal catastrophes, are attributed to machinations of the enemy and malicious influence of spirits that inhabit the world around us. Among some of the tribes, the spirits of the ancestors which have been offended are also believed to cause mental disturbances. On the other hand, many of the tribes are equally aware of the concept of natural causations such as micro-organisms and parasites. The idea of natural causation has been observed to reach its peak among the Masai of East Africa, who seldom attribute disease to spiritual agency and only very rarely to human interventions. Many other tribes (the Shona of Central Africa), also believe that any disease, including mental disorder, may be due to natural causes.

We know that the African culture is far from being homogeneous and that there are distinct and characteristic configurations of culture in Africa. The great diversity of tribes and cultures makes any examination of their social institutions peculiarly difficult, and the task is not rendered easier by the almost complete ignorance about some of the customs and practices in the smaller tribes.

The African culture, if one may be permitted to speak of an African culture, manifests, in common with most non-literate cultures, a sense of an intensely realized perception of supernatural presence, with a kind of adolescent impetuousness, and a fatuous, almost fanatical, faith in the magic of certain symbols to produce certain results. In most African cultures, for example, if a man finds a hair or a nail belonging to, or even a piece of material which has been worn by, an enemy, he believes he has only to "use" them in order to bring about his enemy's death or to injure him. In this mode of thinking, there may be said to be a magical or mystical denial of the concept of causality and of the reality of their spatial and temporal relations.

In many parts of Africa where traditional tribal customs still flourish in considerable strength the style of life and modes of thought have become a great archetype, a center around which countless congenial beliefs are formed. There is no doubt that the Africans have held traditional beliefs similar to those which occupied a noble place among the speculations of antiquity.

The practice of psychological medicines in tribal Africa is based largely upon the belief that there are dynamic processes by which man can compel, placate, cajole, or expel these spirits or mysterious powers, and manipulate them. In these cultures the determinants of health and disease are conceptualized holistically. Thus, causation is multifactorial; causal factors are interconnected; and the manifestations are multifaceted.

Attitudes towards Mental Illness

Social attitudes to mental disorder vary a great deal, but on the whole in Africa there is very little social stigma, if any, attached to mental illness. It has been shown that people of different social classes, from different parts of Africa, of different ethnic groups, and different religious affiliations, differ in attitudes to mental illness and the way to manage it. On the whole, community attitudes permitted the bulk of African mentally ill persons with varying grades of social insufficiency to live as tolerated members of the community in simple, rural, and unadulterated cultures. Consequently, many African psychotics were (and still are) able to keep themselves at some sort of functioning level.

This high level of tolerance made it possible to institute community-oriented therapy, enabling psychotics to be treated among their families and in their homes even when shackled to a log in the traditional manner. Tooth (22), during his survey in Ghana, observed that "the madman is seldom alone for long, is well fed, and enjoys the company of his children and friends." He continues, "This tolerant attitude accounts for the number of harmless lunatics at large; most earn a living as professional beggars but some exploit their eccentricity as buffoons and entertainers."

In large towns and the coastal areas of Africa, however, mental illness was regarded with horror, as a disgrace—something which crippled social activities of the families of the sick and reduced their chances and opportunities. For example, it would be almost impossible to find a husband for a girl who was known to have a mentally ill relative. In the forest zone, especially in Ashanti, the mentally sick were feared and identified with evil.

Diagnosis and Treatment

The psychiatric disorders that were managed by the native healers were schizophrenia, affective states, neurosis, organic states (especially trypanosomiasis, epilepsy, and cerebral arteriosclerosis), and many un-

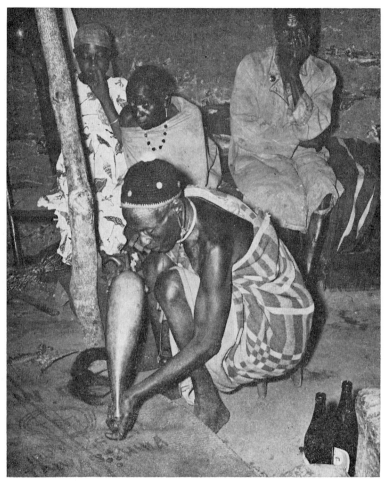

PLATE CIX. A traditional healer in diagnostic and therapeutic session. The woman patient is sitting between two members of her family.

classified (and unclassifiable) amorphous clinical syndromes. The traditional healers achieved outstanding success in the management of various types of anxiety syndromes, some of which border on psychosis (e.g. malignant anxiety, and frenzied anxiety, also known as *bouffée confusionnelle*) (Plate CIX).

Many of the tribes in West and Central Africa have a sound idea of what psychosis constitutes. Madness has always been defined as "loss of insight, irrelevant and peculiar utterances, and foolish actions, with or without violent behavior." They define a person as being mad when he talks nonsense, performs foolishly and irresponsibly, and is unable to look after himself or his family without realizing what he is doing. In addition, minor to major disturbances of a psychological nature are recognized and treated purely by psychological methods. This recognition of the differences between neurosis and psychosis reaches its height among the Yoruba on the West Coast of Africa.

In 1967, Gelfand (9) wrote: "The Shona understand mental backwardness in a child, but often do not recognize the differences between the congenital form and that developed by a normal infant or child after a brain infection, such as meningitis. All forms of idiocy and mental retardation are included in the term *rema,* which is attributed to the action of a witch upon the fetus. Most *nganga* inform me that nothing can be done for this form of mental disorder."

The diagnosis of mental illness in tribal Africa involves many complicated processes. In these and related cultures the patient is usually the center of a whole system of social and interpersonal tensions. The entire management of the patient—treatment (and prevention of future attacks)—is, as a result, dictated by diagnosis which hopes to unravel the immediate cause of the illness: physical devitalization, spiritual possession of an adverse kind; the remote cause: the ancestor spirit or gods offended, the violation of a taboo, the human agent employing magic or invoking malignant spirits to take revenge of an offense, a curse, bewitchment, sorcery; and the form of therapy that should be followed: expiatory sacrifice and/or other psychotherapeutic techniques, usually involving the practitioner, the patient, his family, and his community.

Diagnosis takes many forms. Through the analysis of dreams, projective techniques (e.g. Ifa divination), possession, trances, and communion with gods or spirits, and through the omnipotent power of words, the traditional healer is able to define the psychodynamics and to gain some insight into the total management of the patient.

The *Odus* among the Yoruba tribe of West Africa have a lot in common with the Rorschach test, but are more complicated in parts and certainly more attractive, being structured in a poetic language of their own. Ifa divination is a combined diagnostic and therapeutic procedure. The *Odus* contain some of the most potent power-words ever used in divination. In some instances, the power lies in the way in which the words are used, the order in which they are arranged, or the stark sincerity with which they express a deep and powerful feeling. Although Ifa, through the power of words (e.g. incantations) may be used for the purpose of gaining deep insight, sensitive perception, superhuman knowledge, and guidance in the conduct of everyday life, its great therapeutic use lies in its function of "interpreting signs and omens, dreams and movements of gods, proclaiming oracles, and making known revelations, in the belief that the gods employed inspire men to communicate their will and power to mankind. . . ." This procedure tends to stimulate abreaction in the patient and his accompanying relatives.

I have already referred to the employment by the traditional healers of their empirical knowledge of the properties of herbs for the purpose of curing psychiatric disorder, and that they attained, in this respect, a skill which is hardly equaled by the regular practitioners. Here, I will, therefore, lay emphasis on the various forms of psychotherapy that were practiced—many of which could be termed mystical doctrines, exercising an extraordinary fascination over many minds. These methods seem to have comprised many traditions that have been long current among many African tribes, mixed with many of the old doctrines of rituals, and with a large measure of pure naturalism.

In dealing with the traditional psychotherapeutic practices, I would like to deal specifically with the triad phenomena of rituals, supernaturalism, and ancestor worship, the role of these factors in the psychological functioning of the African, and, lastly, to analyze the habits of thought which make their various doctrines appear probable, harmonious, and consistent.

Most non-literate cultures are at many points especially conducive to states of morbid fear and anxiety. Rituals involving sacrifice, which may connote life-taking (actual or symbolical), are a logical outcome. Sacrifice is the crucial psychological point of all cults, the essential bond between man and deity. It is among the earliest popular traditions of man. Plato did more than any other ancient philosopher to develop the notion of expiation.

Reik (20), in his psychoanalytical studies of ritual, regards the mythological world of the primitives as "older than religion," and, according to him, "it is one of the oldest wish-compensations of mankind in his eternal struggle with external and internal forces." He considers the mythological approach as "of the highest importance for our understanding of the first psychological conflicts of primitive people." In my experience, of all human materials, there is perhaps none that presents to the historian of the human mind a deeper interest than African mythologies, and there is certainly none that tells a better tale of the frustration of human efforts and the futility of human hopes.

In any comprehensive and detailed study (15) of the traditional healers (commonly known in the Western world as witch-doctors), many have proved to be neither imposters nor enthusiasts; their methods are neither the work of a designing intellect nor of an overheated imagination. A good many of them who have come under our observation for long periods displayed extraordinary qualities of mind—common sense, great eloquence, boldness, and dexterity. Generous sentiments, disinterested virtue, reverential faith, and sublime speculations are some of the features and attributes often displayed. By professing to hold communion with and control supernatural beings, the traditional healer can exercise an almost boundless influence over those about him. They are usually greatly respected within the community as men who, through self-denial, dedication, prolonged meditation, and training, have discovered the secrets of the healing art and its magic. They possess mystical characteristics, charisma, and a rather charming eccentricity.

According to Gelfand (9), a *nganga's* (witch-doctor) role is indispensable "in a patient's recovery from a mental breakdown, especially when an external or exciting factor is largely responsible for it." The *nganga*, in his highly colorful dress, creates a deep impression. He stands out as one endowed with a special mystical or supernatural power which his family has inherited for untold generations. He understands his own people in a way that no European, however skilled, can ever hope to equal.

There is no doubt that the *nganga* instills more confidence among the Africans who still constitute the majority on the Continent, than the Western doctor when the complaint is one of a neurosis or an anxiety state. He can achieve far more by pure suggestion, as he is a link with the ancestral spirits of any patient. Through his own divining or healing spirit he is able, it is believed, to contact these spirits and reveal which of them is responsible for the psychological breakdown.

In some tribes, a psychotic patient is usually physically restrained, and heavily sedated with herbs. His head may be shaved and some incisions made in the scalp to facilitate quick and easy absorption into the circulation. The average traditional healer is a trained botanist with an expert knowledge of plants, roots, and trees whose chemistry and pharmacological actions have been empirically established. For the potency of the herb or drug to be achieved and its intrinsic power utilized, the method of its preparation is of great importance. It is usually ritualized through invocation of the spirits of certain ancestors or gods by incantation and of the secret name of the tree or herb or its spirit. In his explanation of the phenomenon of "ego quality" for the purpose of achieving mastery over them, Fenichel (7) writes:

> He who knows a word for a thing, masters the thing. This is the core of the "magic of names," which plays such an important part in magic in general.

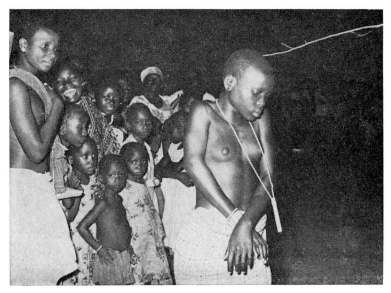

PLATE CX. Dancing as a therapeutic process.

The important and essential psychological function of supernatural-ism, confession, sacrifice, dreams, visions, possession, free emotionality, dances, trances, and the spoken word (e.g. incantation) is that of a buffer by preventing depression and the accumulation of other psychic stresses (Plate CX). The cultures are rich in a variety of abreactive techniques and provisions. The development of psychiatric care in the tribal period was an indivisible part of the total care of the indi-vidual and his community—prevention and cure. In spite of the associated religious tone and deep moral and social implications, primitive medicine "is not a queer collection of errors and supersti-tions, but a number of living unities in living cultural patterns, quite able to function through the centuries in spite of their fundamental differences" from the Western pattern (1).

Experience in various parts of Africa has shown that even in tribal societies, with their own pre-literate causal formulations, the greater the confidence of the community in the nature and form of therapy they could obtain and the people who would treat them, the more readily they would come forward for treatment or encourage their mentally ill relatives to do so.

In summary, traditional medicine, as applied to psychiatry in Africa, employs the concepts of the "family" or "community" doctor in contradistinction to the concept of institutionalization. The traditional medicine-man has supreme confidence in himself, enjoys the same degree of confidence from his client, takes his pastoral duties and obligations seriously, has a deep knowledge of his people and the culture, and is exceptionally mature in handling social problems. Traditional tribal psychiatry operates within the concept of the whole man—physical and spiritual. It recognizes confession of sin (real or imaginary) as vital to the resolution of, and freedom from, conflict. In the treatment of psychological disorders, group therapy is *sine qua non;* the whole extended family is often involved in and actively participates in therapy—singing, dancing, group confession, etc. Until today the African medicine-man's (the traditional healer's) handling of (as well as his total management of) neurosis, psychosomatic disorders, and incipient but troublesome personality problems remains unrivalled. This supremacy is recognized and accepted by Africans of all social classes, sub-cultures, and affiliations.

3

THE TRANSITIONAL PERIOD

Our observations in Africa have shown that indigenous African culture has not yet accepted Western methods of approach to illness in their present form. The African seeks medical help with a considerable degree of ambivalence, but paradoxically with such a degree of dependence, and often a despair of resignation, that increases both the effectiveness and the difficulties of the physician, to the point where he may earn undue credit or undue blame. The realization of this fact has caused me (and my late Sudanese colleague, Tigani El Mahi) to recognize the part played by indigenous psychotherapeutic measures in the total management of the African patient, irrespective of socio-economic level, without any lowering of standard of medical practice. Even though by Western standards this approach would seem to be

indefensible, and though some of these indigenous, culturally acceptable measures may be caricatured as primitive and archaic, they
are nevertheless emotionally reinforced and, as an historical and
traditional legacy, psychiatrists working in the African cultural setting
must be sensitive to their implications and reckon with them.

Swanz (21), writing on traditional medicine in Tanzania, observes:
"The psychosomatic understanding of the illness which the *waganga*
have might be closer to the essence of the nature of illness than the
dominant approach in the modern medicine when the psychic is
separated from the physical, and it is believed that one pill can do
the trick."

Central and West Africa have had sporadic contact with Europe
since the 15th century—explorers, mercenaries, European trading
companies, missionaries and the European imperial powers as colonizers. In the records of early missionaries, of the doctors attached to
trading companies, and others, were found some references "to the
scarcity and rarity of mental illness among the natives on the coastal
belt" (12). In the same year a British army doctor on the West Coast
of Africa observed that he did not think that mental patients were
killed, but confirmed the observation that "insanity" was rare (12).
In 1888 the infamous Adeola case took place "in which the Colonial
Surgeon was accused of negligence" (2), and, going through the files,
it would seem that the woman involved might have been one of the
vagrant psychotics. In some parts of West and Central Africa the
mentally sick with overt aggressive homicidal tendencies and unpredictable behavior were killed by the community, especially if it was
established that they were possessed by evil spirits.

As the British, Germans, French, Belgian, and Portuguese colonized
many of these countries and took over total administrative and political responsibilities, a variety of legal systems were instituted and
criminal laws of the European metropolitan powers were introduced.
Prisons were built and parts were set aside for "lunatics" (Plate CXI).
Here, patients—usually vagrant psychotics, criminals with demon-
strable mental disorders—were locked up and restricted by handcuffs
and ankle shackles. They were kept there to ensure public safety.
Between 1890 and 1900, the annual reports of many of the colonial
territories in Central and West Africa included references to lunacy.

It is important to recognize that the introduction into Africa of the
European concept of mental disorder and its treatment came as part
and parcel of the colonization process, and this was marked by the
imposition of many alien institutions—Christianization, trade, political, administrative, and educational systems, organization of health

services, etc. While the African cultures, including the traditional healers and witch-doctors, recognized the distinction between mental illness and criminality, the European concept at that time still confused the two issues. The asylum sections of the prisons in many of these places soon become overcrowded and a source of sporadic epidemics which claimed a high death toll from the patients.

In the latter part of the 19th century to the early part of the 20th century, when the Public Health Ordinances were established, the

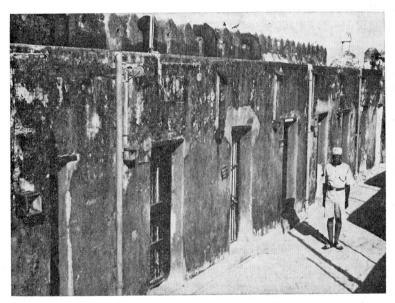

PLATE CXI. An old asylum in East Africa.

responsibility for non-criminal lunatics was transferred to the health department. In many cases asylums were built purely for custodial purposes; there was no organized or scientific medical care for the patients. The first asylum in the British West African colonies was built in Sierra Leone. The British were the only metropolitan powers in Africa to plan some institutional measures for the care of the mentally ill. These were the dark periods; the history of psychiatry in Central and West Africa ran parallel to the history of psychiatry in Europe.

In spite of the appalling conditions, annual admissions to these custodial institutions increased. Health conditions were bad and general

facilities were poor; in many of these countries mortality and morbidity figures were high, especially from communicable diseases. Although the responsibility for the care of psychiatric patients lay with
the health department, very little was done in terms of scientific
psychiatric care. General practitioners, colonial surgeons, and medical
officers were occasionally assigned to these asylums, not infrequently
on a part-time basis.

Local staff members—largely untrained—were recruited and designated lunatic asylum attendants. These people, some of whom held
inferior educational and social status within the community, formed
the core of the staff who later became the psychiatric nurses in the
new mental hospitals. Since, generally speaking, the morale of the
staff of any hospital is inextricably connected with the morale of
the patients, the morale of the staff of these asylums was terribly
low, thereby having an adverse effect on the morale of the patients.

The Role of the Church and the Problem of Spiritual Healing

The medical missions in Central and West Africa did very little in
the field of psychiatric care until very recently, when the subject was
beginning to merit some discussion. However, the extensive and, on
occasion, the comprehensive general health care program, especially
for the vast semi-rural and rural areas of Africa, must have contributed significantly to the prevention of those conditions which were
contributory to poor mental health (infections, malnutrition, anemia,
and injuries).

The Christian churches, especially their medical missions, failed in
promoting and integrating spiritual healing as a non-expendable part
of their medical resources. They succeeded in creating the impression
that they were either helplessly impotent or lamentably unconvinced,
and, as a result, they were unable to mobilize and utilize one of the
most potent and therapeutically powerful resources. By undue concentration on purely materialistic and mechanistic aspects of Western
medicine, and by separating the spiritual dimension, they caused and
sustained a profound degree of scepticism in the minds of many
Africans.

Christianity aligned and identified with scientific medicine. It insisted on order, regularity, predictability, and simplicity—all the
qualities that are usually associated with the world of things in
Western industrial societies but which are frequently absent in the
dynamics of human interactions and relations. Unlike the native
healer or medicine-man, the Christian medical mission failed to em-

phasize the need to approach traditional religious theories of the social causation of psychological disorder with respect, especially since it is now known that the empirical basis of the once accepted theories of Western psychiatry is rather insecure, and these grand theories are probably not as culture-free as one would imagine.

A revolution of rising expectations, the continuing failure of Christian medical missions to meet the basic metaphysical cravings, the consequent realization that Christianity in its present form is an alien religion, totally inadequate for and inappropriate to their needs —all these attempts to secularize medical practice combined and led to the birth of many forms of syncretic religions in Africa, religions which were later found to play a major role in the treatment and prevention of psychiatric disorders in the African in transition.

In many parts of Central and West Africa, new syncretic religions, e.g. the Christ Apostolic Church and Sacred Cherubim and Seraphim Societies, have sprung up in response to new social, spiritual, and ideological needs. The new religions have gained many converts and would seem to succeed largely in therapeutic methodology, especially in the cure of severe emotional disorders.

They have taken notice of the traditional and present-day value systems of the African. The approach to illness, especially the prevention of diseases, is so designed as not to separate worship from healing. According to Peel (19), in his unpublished study on the *Two Aladura Churches of Yorubaland,* these syncretic religions "have welded an answer to these mundane needs as well as the moral and theological aspects of Christianity into a very powerful and attractive synthesis."

The most dramatic and compelling characteristic of African society today is rapid change. The societies are in transition and in a state of crisis. In addition to the familiar and predictable strains of urbanization and detribalization, there are factors of acculturation from within, generated by waves of nationalism. The syncretic religions (the Christ Apostolic Church and the Seraphim Society), constitute a powerful cultural mechanism that is being used to ameliorate the adverse psychological impact of social change on individuals and the community. They employ a similar channel of expression to that of the traditional culture for promoting group catharsis, as formulated by Aristotle in his *Politics* and his *Tragedy.*

The Mohammedian influence is not of great historical significance. There were many Mohammedian "doctors" who made use of talismans containing verses from the *Koran. Washins* from wood or slate on which excerpts from the *Koran* have been written were used as potent remedies. In many countries there were well-developed Muslim states with a well-defined philosophy and ideology within which the concept of mental illness was formulated. Cunyngham Brown (6) observes: ". . . although insanity is resignedly accepted by Mohammedians as the Will of Allah, idiocy, imbecility, and other forms of congenital defects are recognized as originating at birth. . . ."

4

CONTEMPORARY PERIOD

This historical epoch was ushered in by reports of special studies by two great British psychiatrists, commissioned by the British Government. These were *Report III,* on the *Care and Treatment of Lunatics in the British West African Colonies,* by R. Cunyngham Brown (6), and the famous *Studies in Mental Illness in the Gold Coast,* by Geoffrey Tooth (22). These two studies are of great historical significance since they both covered enormous ground and are unusually penetrating, imaginative, and thorough. The two British psychiatrists were sensitive to many socio-cultural, sociological and environmental factors at a time when such factors had not yet gained academic and clinical prominence and significance in psychiatry in Europe. Their approaches to the local psychiatric problems were eclectic and known for their common sense. It was the first time in the history of psychiatry in Central and West Africa that attempts were made to stress the value of epidemiological data and approach in general for evaluation and planning services. This was a very advanced and rather sophisticated approach for the period. In the observation of Cunyngham Brown,

> The disparity between the officially known and the actual number of the insane is well brought out by my experience in one very large native town. Here only one lunatic was officially known at Government headquarters, though, of course, all were aware that there existed a floating number of what were commonly referred to as "village idiots" haunting the market places. Actually, the sprinkling of vagrant lunatics of this kind, to be encountered in every town, are only occasionally idiots or imbeciles, but are composed mainly of the subjects of chronic mental disorders of all kinds, harmless as a rule, but sometimes potentially dangerous. . . . These examples may serve to illustrate two of the many difficulties which confront the compilation of statistics aiming at a true ascertainment of the incidence of mental derangement in this country. . . .

Tooth, in addition to his rather succinct and comprehensive epidemiological studies, made some attempts at classifying the psychiatric disorders occurring in the Gold Coast. In this regard, he concluded with an air of finality:

> One is therefore forced to the conclusion that there are real differences in the quality of the psychotic reactions of individuals with different racial and cultural backgrounds, differences which make it impossible to fit them into the accepted nosological framework.

Both psychiatrists tried to assess critically the effects of Western culture, especially rapid evolution, on the incidence and prevalence of mental disorder. In this connection, Tooth aptly observes: "No part of the population is entirely unaffected by these changes but the speed of evolution has varied greatly in different sections; this unequal growth has had the effect of producing strains both in group and individual life."

One of the important areas to which both investigators paid a lot of attention was the attitudes to mental disorder and towards services available in the community, and Tooth, as well as Cunyngham Brown, noticed a wide difference in different parts of British West African colonies and in different parts of the same country, depending on socio-cultural, religious, and socio-economic backgrounds. Tooth then concluded: "This variation in the public attitude to lunacy from North to South exemplifies in one country and at a single period of time the stages in the evolution of attitude on this subject which have taken place throughout the world with the advance of civilization."

As far as attitudes towards services available in the community were concerned, Tooth strongly recommended:

> It will be objected that a plan of this kind relegates to a lay Authority what is properly a medical responsibility, but a visit to the Gold Coast Asylum should convince an impartial observer that the African's lack of confidence in the European management of this branch of medicine is well founded. Moreover, it seems unlikely that an alien psychiatrist could ever succeed in assimilating the complexities of the West African background in time to make an appreciable contribution in this field. So that, until African psychiatrists can be trained, it would seem better to allow the care of the majority of the insane to remain in lay hands.

These and other important studies, e.g. Laubscher (17), and Carothers (4) laid the foundation for modern scientific psychiatry in Africa and by stressing the need for extra-institutional provisions, especially family care, emphasized the positive role of community resources as an important part of therapy. Cunyngham Brown in his final recommendation stated, with precision, conviction, and a sense of imagination and innovation: "The asylum is not the only, nor is it always the best, form of treatment of the insane. . . . Recognition of this fact has led to the adoption, as a large supplement to asylum care and treatment, of the *family care* . . ." (Plate CXII).

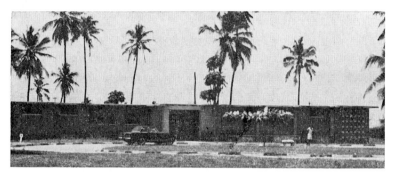

PLATE CXII. A modern provincial psychiatric clinic in West Africa, part of basic health services.

Sixteen years later, Lambo (13) instituted the first village system (ARO, *Abeokuta*) as a therapeutic strategy, utilizing the viewpoints of sociology, psychology, psychiatry, and social anthropology and using the family and the community as the strategic focus.

It is now known that the African family and the community, as at present structured, constitute an ideally strategic orientation for developing a comprehensive therapeutic approach that is meaningful, economical, and methodologically feasible. This approach has allowed for systematic empirical studies; it has become a flexible system which guarantees the free participation of the community and non-professional personnel. It is a reliable and valid instrument of research as well as a focus for education and training of young African psychiatrists and general practitioners.

5

CONCLUSION

Africa has been the recipient of many cultural, political, economic, and social experiences and models. It has had to pose the major question: imitation or innovation? The contemporary trends seem to be that Africa will have to innovate rapidly with a sense of urgency, imagination, and relevance. There is no doubt that not being shackled by heavy tradition and not being committed to any foreign ideology, Africa should be able to evolve a pattern of health care which will have the unique feature of blending the traditional as well as the modern into a happy syncretism; a system in which the total care of the mentally ill will be a prominent feature.

REFERENCES

1. ACKERKNECHT, E. H. (1942): Problems of primitive medicine. *Bull. Hist. Med.,* XI, 501-521.
2. BOROFFKA, A. (1970): *Brief history of the association of psychiatrists in Nigeria.* Unpublished paper.
3. BURSTEIN, S. R. (1952): Public health and prevention of disease in primitive communities. *Advanc. Sci.,* IX, 75-81.
4. CAROTHERS, J. C. (1947): *J. Ment. Sci.,* 93, 548.
5. CAROTHERS, J. C. (1953): *Wld. Hlth. Org. Monogr. Ser.,* No. 17.
6. CUNYNGHAM BROWN, R. E. (1938): *Report III.* Care and treatment of lunatics in the British West African Colonies (Nigeria). London.
7. FENICHEL, O. (1945): *The Psychoanalytical Theory of Neurosis.* New York: Morton.
8. GALDSTON, I. (1969): In: *Proceedings of Symposium, "Medicine and Cuture."* F. N. L. Poynter (ed.). London: Wellcome Institute of the History of Medicine.
9. GELFAND, M. (1967): Psychiatric disorders as recognized by the Shona. *Cent. Afr. J. Med.,* 13, 39.
10. HARLEY, G. W. (1941): *Native African Medicine/with Special Reference to Its Practice in the Mano Tribe of Liberia.* Cambridge, Mass.: Harvard University Press.
11. JILEK, W. G. (1967): Mental health and magic beliefs in changing Africa. *Top. Probl. Psychiat. Neurol.,* 6, 138-154. Basel/New York: Karger.
12. Lagos Public Health Department (1845): Annual Report, Lagos.
13. LAMBO, T. A. (1956): *Brit. Med. J.,* 2, 1388.
14. LAMBO, T. A. (1962): Malignant anxiety. A syndrome associated with criminal conduct in Africans. *J. Ment. Sci.,* 108, 256-264.
15. LAMBO, T. A. (1963): *African Traditional Beliefs, Concepts of Health and Medical Practice.* Ibadan: Ibadan University Press.
16. LAMBO, T. A. (1971): The African mind in contemporary conflict. *WHO Chron.,* 25.8.
17. LAUBSCHER, B. J. F. (1937): *Sex, Custom, and Psychopathology.* London: Routledge.
18. MARGETTS, E. L. (1968): African ethnopsychiatry in the field. *Canad. Psychiat. Ass. J.,* 5, 65-79.
19. PEEL, J. D. Y.: Two Aladura churches of Yorubaland. Unpublished papers. Ibadan: University of Ibadan Library.
20. REIK, T. (1931): *Ritual: Psychoanalytic Studies.* London: Hogarth Press.
21. SWANZ, J. L. W.: Unpublished papers.
22. TOOTH, G. (1950): *Studies in Mental Illness in the Gold Coast.* London: Colonial Research Publications, No. 6.

25

SOUTH AFRICA

Lewis A. Hurst, M.D., Ph.D., F.R.C. Psych.

*Professor of Psychological Medicine, University of
the Witwatersrand, Johannesburg, South Africa*

AND

Mary B. Lucas, B.A.

*Assistant Librarian-in-Charge, Medical School,
University of the Witwatersrand,
Johannesburg, South Africa*

1

THE CAPE OF GOOD HOPE SETTLEMENT

The Cape of Good Hope settlement was established in the 17th century to provide a refreshment station for the crews of the vessels of the Dutch East India Company. Jan van Riebeeck arrived at the Cape in 1652 with instructions to build "a little defensive fort," to lay out a garden, to obtain sheep and cattle by bartering with the natives, and, in short, to establish a settlement so that the company's ships could "refresh themselves with vegetables, meat, water, and other necessities by which means the sick on board may be restored to health" (12).

It is important to realize that in no sense did the Council of the supreme authority of the Dutch East India Company intend to found a colony. Shrewd businessmen that they were, they postulated that the Cape had been established for the benefit of the company, and

600

that it should cost the company as little as possible. Its aim was frankly rehabilitative: the sick were taken off the outgoing fleet; their places were taken by the recovered; on the return voyage from Batavia, sailors who needed hospitalization were landed and replaced by patients recently discharged from hospital. Searle (21) emphasizes that the hospital at the Cape differed from many European institutions because its aims were commercial, while many of the hospitals elsewhere were motivated by the religious view that it is a virtue to help the sick. Van Riebeeck's hospital could perhaps be regarded as an early, and fairly successful, example of occupational medicine.

Psychiatry as a science did not exist in the 17th century, and this was particularly true at the Cape. The company recruited its surgeons from the surgeons' guilds (4); physicians were university graduates or doctors, and were not usually appointed to ships as their salaries were too high (4); the salaries of the upper and lower surgeons ranked between that of the chief carpenter and the boatswain.

The incidence of mental disease at the Cape must have been high. Mentzel (17) gives an account of how the Dutch East India Company recruited its men. They came from the dregs of society, were poorly paid and poorly clad, and were always in debt to the company. People with military experience were preferred and many of these recruits suffered from what was euphemistically called "soldiers' diseases" (21). Drunkenness was common, and became even more widespread when wine-growing was introduced at the Cape. The innkeepers at the Cape were notorious. The voyage to the East Indies was a long and hard one, and the isolation of the Cape in the 17th and 18th centuries was almost complete. Contact with the outside world was maintained only through the incoming and outgoing fleets. Although the company tried to keep the Cape as an outpost of its own, "free burghers" were granted farms in 1657. There was some immigration in the later years of the 17th century, but after the recall of Willem Adriaan van der Stel in 1706, the "17" decided that no more "free burghers" should be sent to the Cape. The *trekboers,* descendants of these "free burghers," multiplied by natural increase and during the 17th, 18th, and the early part of the 19th centuries, lived in almost unbelievable seclusion. Until the coming of the British settlers in 1820, Cape Town was the only town of any size at the Cape.

Lichtenstein's description (13) of the kind of person the *trekboer* was, and Barrow's account (1) of a day in the life of a young Dutch girl give some idea of the remoteness and isolation of rural life. Then there was always a feeling of insecurity. In the early days Robben Island was regarded as a place of refuge to which the whites could retire if the Hottentots gave trouble (6). As the farmers penetrated further into the interior, so the danger from attacks by Bushmen, Hottentots, and Bantu increased. Burrows (4) summarized it thus:

> The pattern of disease in the Cape settlement—hypovitaminosis, alcoholism, infection, exhaustion, and venereal disease—was one which might predispose to mental illness and the records make sporadic mention of the incidence of such cases.

Psychiatry had not yet emerged as a separate medical discipline, hence many things which would today be regarded as primarily the concern of the psychiatrist, were given little importance. Suicide, for instance, was lightly passed over. Van Riebeeck recorded in his Diary that when the ship *Hoff van Zeelandt* arrived at the Cape, it was reported that there had been 37 deaths on the outward voyage. "Two others had jumped overboard in desperation but the rest of the men are mostly healthy" (29).

On December 24, 1705, Adam Tas reported "a singular affair" in his Diary:

> They tell me this day that the Governor's wife had, in a fit of despondency, tried to drown herself by jumping into the fountain behind the house at the Cape; however Mrs. Berg was on the spot, and ran to help her, pulling her out of the water, to whom the Governor's wife lamented bitterly that her life had become one of terror for her on account of the many scandalous acts she must daily hear and witness (23).

The Governor was the notorious Willem Adriaan van der Stel, at whose hands Adam Tas himself was to suffer so severely. Leo Fouché, the editor of the *Diary,* had this to say of him:

> His nature was at once weak and domineering. So soon as he encountered the slightest opposition he was seized by fits of almost maniacal fury. . . . Still worse is his colossal campaign of fraud by means of which he seeks to establish his innocence. Upon his instructions false depositions are drafted by the dozen, and attested as genuine; even the resolutions of the Council of Policy are falsified and confirmed by perjury. . . . His private life was no less reminiscent of his extraction. He was grossly immoral, to such a degree, that he forbade the reading of the Ten Command- ments at any service held in his presence (23).

Fouché attributed the violence of Willem Adriaan van der Stel's disposition to the fact that he was of Eurasian descent (23). Be that as it may, a study of Van der Stel's behavior at the Cape is of interest to a psychiatrist, and in reading of the struggle between the "free burghers" and the Governor we are made aware of the frustrating sense of isolation which affected everyone at the Cape. The only contact with the outside world was through the fleet. According to De Kock (5), whenever the return fleet sailed into Table Bay, complete uproar followed. Sailors ashore habitually got drunk. On one occasion

> ... there were not yet even two hundred souls living at the Cape, we read of the visitors calling along the streets: "What are you doing in this cursed country—this land of famine? Come with us. . . . Whoever likes to go; let him get into the boat: Amsterdam, Zeeland, Rotterdam, Hoorn, Delft, Enckhuysen. . . . Fall in for the Fatherland; the ships are ready to sail" (5).

These roisterers damaged a great deal of property, stole livestock, threw a pole at the Provost and his soldiers, and "merrily ended a busy and boisterious day by setting upon the settlement's one and only policeman and chasing that discomfited official from house to house," while many of the Capetonians took refuge in the ships.

Such escapades occurred often in seaports and there is evidence that the shore-dwellers drank heavily too. As Barrow implies, what else was there to do for the "African peasant" who "was unwilling to work and unable to think?"

> The boor [sic] notwithstanding has his enjoyments. . . . His pipe scarcely ever quits his mouth, from the moment he rises till he retires to rest, except to give him time to swallow his *sopie* or a glass of strong ardent spirit, to eat his meals and to take his nap after dinner (1).

Barrow did not like the Boers; Lichtenstein, who liked the Dutch, refuted much of what he said:

> In their conversation they are lively, even sometimes witty; especially at table, and that without being in the least elevated with wine. Indeed, the African colonists are a remarkably sober race. Out of ten colonists we may be pretty well assured that three at least will not drink either wine or spirits; and the rest will drink very moderately. One of them intoxicated is a very rare sight. Whatever Mr. Barrow may say of the *Soopje* as the favorite drink of the colonists, I can very safely affirm, that I never, during the whole time of my residence in the country, saw three Africans born, in liquor. The Europeans who live among them as schoolmasters or servants, and who were probably formerly matrosses or soldiers, may be very probably guilty of excess in this way; for it is an incontrovertible fact that the lower class of people in our

quarter of the globe are far below the African peasants, in a true sense of decorum as to their moral conduct (13).

Lichtenstein even attributes the great prevalence of "the stone" among men to "bad water and the want of spirituous liquors." He says that, "In those districts where vines are cultivated or where wine is to be had cheap, the evil does not exist" (13).

Other writers do not share Lichtenstein's opinion. Adam Tas is regarded as the South African Pepys, and one of the charms of his *Diary* are the anecdotes about people like Mr. Greeff who "was merry, loudly singing several tunes, but he was full with sweet wine" (23). One night, Tas himself, after spending a pleasant evening with friends, "walked straight home as if I was being drawn with a line, but when I came to a standstill in the house, I discovered that I had it not of hearsay, but that I had spoken to Father Bacchus himself." The next morning was a dull morning and "I felt not at all well this morning and was not myself."

Perhaps the first alcoholic whose case was recorded in South African history was Eva, the first Hottentot to be converted to Christianity. She was brought up in van Riebeeck's house and acted as an interpreter. She married a surgeon, Pieter van Meerhoff, who in 1665 was made Superintendent of Robben Island. In 1667, while on an expedition in Madagascar he was killed and Eva and her children returned to Cape Town, where she disgraced herself by drinking too much. Her behavior caused her to be imprisoned and her children had to be looked after by the church wardens. It was thought that she might reform if she were sent back to Robben Island, but unhappily, after a brief improvement, she had to be returned to Robben Island for a second time (3). Nearly two centuries later a hospital for the insane was established on Robben Island.

Among the factors which Burrows (4) mentioned as predisposing to mental illness was venereal disease. Lichtenstein (13) stated that it was not very frequent among the white people, but that "when they are afflicted with it, from their total ignorance of the manner in which it ought to be treated, it commonly gets to a formidable height."

Both Barrow and Lichtenstein remarked that the Dutch women were both hysterical and fecund. Barrow attributes both to the fact that they had nothing better to do:

> To the cold phlegmatic temper and inactive way of life may perhaps be owing the prolific tendency of all the African peasantry; six or seven children in a family is considered very few; from a dozen to 20 are not uncommon.

Lichtenstein's explanation (13) was more ingenious and was in keeping with the scientific beliefs of the day. We are reminded that the term "hysteria" is derived from the Greek word *husterikos,* which means "of the womb," and that, by definition, only women could be hysterical.

> A very remarkable effect of the climate of Africa and of the modes of living among the women there, is the facility with which they bear their children. A woman dying in childbed is a thing almost unheard of; on the contrary by the fourth day they generally begin to return to their household affairs and by the seventh or eighth leave the house and are perfectly recovered; and this not only among the hard working women in the country but among the ladies in the town, though in many respects they are delicate enough. Perhaps, however, this facility may be a principal cause of their propensity towards growing so extremely corpulent and of *that disposition to hysterical affections which has been mentioned and therefore may be balanced by its concomitant evils.**

Earlier in his book, Lichtenstein described an encounter with a farmer named Therron (*sic*) who had taken his wife to the hot springs at Elephant's River "but to no purpose." Lichtenstein, who was a doctor, gave the woman, who was in hysterics, a "little glass of naphtha" and promised to visit her later when he passed the farm. This he did, and "found her still very ill and left her with the medicines I had promised, with some directions for managing herself, particularly with regard to diet."

It is Lichtenstein too, who tells us about the widow Liewenberg who

> . . . had the terrible misfortune of having three daughters idiots: the young women were grown up and not ill-formed, but according to the information of the neighbours, this imbecility was a family disease: traces of it were to be found in some other of the poor woman's nearest relations (13).

The reading of Barrow's and Lichtenstein's accounts makes one thing clear to us. By the end of the 18th century, the "free burghers" had trekked many hundreds of miles into the interior and the Cape, while still not a colony in the accepted usage of the word, was a great deal more than a refreshment station for passing ships. The sick from the interior could not be treated in the company's hospital in Cape Town. That was for the company's employees only; and Charlotte Searle (21) reminds us that it was not the practice in the

---

* The authors have added the italics.

17th and 18th centuries for ordinary people to be treated in hospitals. Hospitals were for the poor and homeless; other people were cared for at home. If they were not dangerous, the insane, too, were looked after by their own families, an outside room being often built specially for them. This was in keeping with Roman-Dutch law which stated that the insane were the responsibility of their own families.

The Church looked after the indigent chronic sick and those mentally ill who could not be cared for by their families were often boarded out by the Diakonie of the Dutch Reformed Church (21).

And what of the dangerous insane? Cape Town was the only town of any size, but the hospital there was only for the employees of the Dutch East India Company. According to Searle, quite commonly they became deranged because of the prevalence of pellagra and were then given free accommodation in the hospital, where they were allowed to wander at will, and even go into the town. Violent cases were locked in a small windowless room and the barber-surgeons treated them. Blood-letting, opiates, and restraint were the methods employed. Searle reported that: "Chains were never used. In the equipment lists of the hospital of that period one finds reference to leather belts, wrist straps, and canvas restraints" (21). Dangerous lunatics were sent to Robben Island, where there was a penal settlement. For instance, in 1718 a patient in the hospital ran amok, killed one patient, and wounded ten others. He was sent to Robben Island (4). Again according to Burrows, "there is a record of a dangerous lunatic being confined in a small room in the Company's Slave Lodge." This, however, was not a unique occurrence, as Searle implies that the Slave Lodge was used for this purpose on more than one occasion.

2

THE 19TH CENTURY AND THE BRITISH OCCUPATION

In 1795 the British occupied the Cape for the first time. The Dutch East India Company had gone bankrupt and, in 1795, most medical services came under the control of the military; from then lunatic asylums were administered by the State, setting the pattern of present day developments. During the 19th century the population increased vastly; new territory was developed, and South Africa was increasingly drawn into the affairs of the rest of the world. This had psychiatric

implications; with greater urban development, provision for the
mentally afflicted increased.

Robben Island

In 1818 Samuel Bailey established the first civilian hospital at the
Cape, later to be known as the Old Somerset Hospital (Plate CXIII);
it provided accommodation for lunatics as well as for other patients.
In 1821 Bailey, being bankrupt, was forced to sell the hospital to the
Burgher Senate. In later years the mismanagement of this hospital
became the subject of a great deal of criticism from James Barry—the

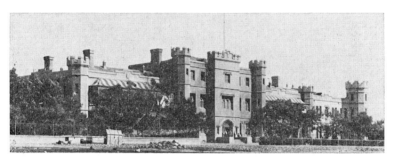

PLATE CXIII. Somerset Hospital, 1900.

military doctor who, after death, was discovered to have been a woman.
In 1824, Barry found that five out of the 15 lunatics in the hospital
were quite sane, and that the wards were as dirty as the patients (4).
The case of the seaman Abel Smith, whom Barry considered sane
because "the absence of vinous and spirituous liquors was sufficient
to restore him to his senses, such as they are" (20) caused a flutter
in governmental circles because Barry's forthrightness was not in
accord with protocol. Besides being the colonial medical inspector,
Barry was also inspector of lepers and of prisons, and she did her
best to alleviate the suffering of all unfortunate people.

In 1826, Wehr reported to the Supreme Medical Committee that
John Honey and an attendant named Gaches had ill-treated two
lunatics at the Somerset Hospital. Gaches had flogged a patient called
Hartwick, who was a mason by trade, with a horsechase because he had
scraped off some plaster from his cell wall. Honey had flogged a
female Hottentot patient while she was held down by two men because she had been noisy. Honey said that he had seen other eminent
physicians apply the same treatment with beneficial results. The

Committee considered that flogging mental patients was reprehensible for "it was highly discreditable to the respectability of character and the propriety and decorum of conduct to be expected from the different members of the medical profession" (21).

The Old Somerset Hospital became the Lunatic Asylum for the whole of the Cape Colony, for there was no other institution for the insane. It was evident that it was becoming increasingly inadequate and, in 1843, John Montagu, the secretary to the government, a member of the Legislative Council and chairman of the Central Board of

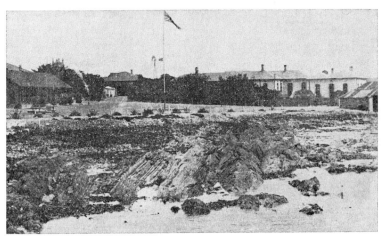

PLATE CXIV. Robben Island, c. 1900 (the Mental Hospital is on the right).

Commissioners of Public Roads, found a solution (6). As he had an ambitious road-building plan for the Colony for which he needed labor, he decided to bring the convicts from the penal settlement at Robben Island to the mainland and set them to work building roads. Lepers from Hemel-en-Aarde and chronic sick and lunatics from the Old Somerset Hospital could be sent to Robben Island. A new hospital could easily be built at Robben Island and the Old Somerset Hospital could be sold at a profit (Plate CXIV). The government adopted his plan, but did not sell the Old Somerset Hospital. It was felt that the existing buildings on the island would be sufficient. The Old Somerset Hospital continued to be used mainly as a shelter for patients awaiting transit to Robben Island.

From the beginning Robben Island was an unsuitable place. The boat journey to the Island was a frightening experience for patients

who were unused to sea voyages. The island was a remote spot and
many patients never saw their friends or relatives again. Minde (18)
tells us that "In the early days the only means of communication
between the Island and the mainland was by boat or Pigeon Post, so
that in stormy weather it was often cut off for many days on end. In
1894 the heliograph was introduced and in 1900 Robben Island was
linked to Cape Town by telephone. The lighting remained the primitive oil lamp throughout." There was no jetty, and male mental patients were often called out at night to take passengers and cargo
from the boats. The buildings were comfortless and ill-adapted. The
mental patients were the most inadequately housed, since their quarters were in the convicts' prison. In 1852, when the storekeeper preferred charges against John Birtwhistle, the surgeon-superintendent,
the government decided that a commission of inquiry should be appointed to inquire into the state of affairs at Robben Island (4). The
commission found that supervision was lax, that violent and tranquil patients were housed together, that there was no separation of
the sexes, and that some female patients had become pregnant. There
was a public outcry in Cape Town; in 1855, Birtwhistle was dismissed and succeeded by J. C. Minto.

Minto introduced many reforms. Knives, forks, and spoons were
provided for patients who could use them; basket and mat making
was introduced as a form of occupational therapy (4). The government encouraged visitors to the island in the hope of alleviating the
terrible isolation. But despite this it was repeatedly urged that an
asylum should be built on the mainland.

Grahamstown

Elsewhere, accommodation shortage was acute and many mental
patients were housed in jails, until they could be transferred to
Robben Island. J. W. Matthews, one of the first doctors to practice in
Kimberley, gives this account (16):

> It is a painful thought, that among the poorer patients, who from
> the ills of life suffer mental alienation . . . that these, all suffering
> from diseases that might have been stayed, should be thrust into
> jails without attendants, simply put in irons if violent, and almost
> compelled through sheer inhumanity and neglect to suffer the
> misery of incurable lunacy. As I have just said, in all colonial
> towns except two . . . the jail is the receptacle of the lunatic.
> Kimberley with its wealth . . . is no exception. What tales the
> walls of its jail could tell! One poor black, to my certain knowl-
> edge, has been locked within its gates for twelve long years, and

there you can see him—tomorrow if you like—bemoaning his fate, and cursing the government in the same breath! A poor white girl, the daughter of a man whom old residents remember well in the palmy days of the Diamond News, has day after day, and *every* day since 1876, paced like a caged tigress up and down a small court yard, panting for freedom, and growling in despair! One poor girl, black her skin may be, is handcuffed, so I learnt, for days together, to prevent her from stripping herself of all she wears. Two women I saw there myself, not three days ago, clad simply in nature's garb, as naked as when born.

Cape Town, of course, was one of the exceptional "colonial" towns mentioned by Matthews as having special accommodation for mental patients; the other town was Grahamstown where an asylum had been established in 1875 with Robert Hullah as superintendent. The need for such an establishment had long been felt in the Eastern Cape and the famous William Guybon Atherstone persuaded the premier, Molteno, that an asylum should be established in Grahamstown. Atherstone went on a visit to England to study mental institutions. His experiences were of great importance to the development of mental services in South Africa, for Atherstone chose an English superintendent, and the English custom of separating mental hospitals from general hospitals was followed (21). This has been the practice ever since, so that today general hospitals are administered by the provincial administrations, while the mental hospitals are administered by the central government.

In the 19th century it was appreciated that, if the insane were to receive adequate treatment, special hospitals would have to be provided for them, but, because of financial difficulties, existing buildings had to be converted for this purpose. In some cases, buildings were taken over from the military. In Grahamstown, Fort England was thus adapted. Fort Napier in Natal was once a barracks; and the practice continued into the 20th century—the predecessor of the Tara H. Moross Hospital was the 134 Military Hospital of the Union Defense Force.

Legislation

A significant 19th century contribution was the development of legislation for the protection of the insane. Ordinances of 1833, 1837, 1879, and 1891 culminated in the Mental Disorders Act, 1916 (Act. No. 38 of 1916) of the Union of South Africa, as amended by the Mental Disorders Amendment Act (Act No. 7 of 1944) and Regulations (28).

Section 6 of this Act prescribes the standard certification procedure for commitment to a mental hospital or institution for the mentally defective. There is a sworn application and two medical certificates which, if satisfactory to a magistrate, result in his issuing his reception order. These, together with the medical superintendent's report, are scrutinized by a judge in chambers before the final order for detention is issued. Even after this order, the onus is on the medical superintendent to discharge the patient on recovery, or to send him on leave of absence on improvement of his condition. As well as by the elaborate certification procedure, the rights of the patient are safeguarded by the Mental Disorders Act in many other ways. If dissatisfied with the medical superintendent's decision regarding further detention, patients and their relatives can appeal to a visiting board appointed by the state-president, who must visit the mental hospital at least once in two months. Furhtermore, a judicial enquiry, entailing the visit of two judges to the mental hospital concerned, may be instituted should the appeal to the visiting board fail. There is, moreover, a regulation providing for the forwarding, unopened, of patients' letters to certain prescribed authorities. On admission to a mental hospital, the patient automatically receives a *curator-ad-litem* in the person of the attorney-general of the province in which he is resident and, as *curator bonis,* the master of the supreme court acts unless the assets of the patient are of an order to warrant the appointment of an individual curator.

Where admission of the patient is so urgent, in virtue of suicidal or homicidal propensities or need of immediate care, that the two or three days normally required for the certification procedure cannot be contemplated, Section 9 of the Act provides for admission on the basis of a sworn application and one medical certificate only. In this case the second medical certificate and the magistrate's reception order are issued retrospectively after admission, the further procedure for the judge's detention order thereafter remaining identical with that for Section 6 cases.

Section 44 provides for the admission of voluntary boarders, who are not certifiable and who apply for admission on their own free will for periods varying from one day to a year. Whatever period has been contracted for, the patient reserves the right of giving seven days notice at any time, and from his side the medical superintendent retains the right to dismiss a voluntary boarder for failure to comply with the rules governing the hospital.

The Amendment of 1944 provided for two new categories of patient, the temporary patient and the inebriate. Temporary patients are admitted under Section 49 on a sworn application and two medical statements (advisedly called statements and not certificates to get away from that emotionally colored word "certification"). No magistrate's reception order is issued in these cases, the period of detection is limited to six months, with a maximum of two three-month extensions, and the applicant retains the right of removing the patient from hospital even against the advice of the medical superintendent. This form of commitment with its permissiveness in so many directions, in comparison with the standard certification procedure, was devised in an era when detention in a mental hospital had become therapeutic, instead of being purely custodial. Its aim was to encourage relatives to admit mentally affected persons for treatment by the wide variety of methods, psychological, social, and physical, that had become available.

Section 52, for inebriate patients, was devised for both alcoholics and drug-dependent persons who were prepared to seek voluntary admission to a mental hospital for a period of six months, with the knowledge that this period could be reduced subsequently only by the visiting mental hospital board or by the commissioner for mental health. These voluntary applications differ from those made by the ordinary voluntary boarder in this greater restrictiveness in the matter of release from hospital, in comparison with the seven days notice too often invoked by the voluntary boarder. The longer period laid down by the new inebriate category is clearly advantageous from the point of view of having time for attempting fundamental therapy and cure.

Apart from the civil admission procedures described above, the Mental Disorders Act provides for medico-legal cases. Sections 27 and 28 provide for periods of observation in mental hospitals on the basis of which the medical superintendent, or his deputy, issues a certificate for the consideration of the Court, and where necessary appears in court to defend or elaborate it. The question of criminal responsibility in relation to mental disorder at the time of the crime, and the patient's fitness to plead are central themes in these cases.

In South African law (10) the M'Naghten Rules supplemented by the defense of irresistible impulse hold sway in the sphere of mental disorder in relation to criminal responsibility. The extended concept, long accepted in Scotland, of partial (or graded) responsibility, and the psychiatrically more acceptable Durham Decision of the United States which, by implication, takes into account aspects of the personality other than the purely cognitive ones enshrined in the M'Naghten Rules, have not as yet gained currency in South Africa, although the Rumpff Commission of Enquiry into the Criminal Responsibility of Mentally Disturbed Persons contains in it the seed of such liberalization of the law (22).

Patients under observation, found to be mentally disordered, if accused of minor offenses, have the charges against them withdrawn and are then certified in the ordinary way under Section 6. In the case of more serious offenses, the individuals are declared state-president's decision cases (Sections 29 and 30 of the Act). Discharge of such patients, after recovery, is generally subject to a period of observation, more or less prolonged, to confirm that sustained recovery has been achieved, in the interests of public safety. When discharge is finally recommended through the visiting board to the minister for health via the commissioner for mental health, certain conditions are commonly imposed, often involving periodical reports from the custodian and the district surgeon, before discharge becomes complete. Section 34 makes provision for the detention and treatment in a mental hospital of a prisoner who becomes mentally disordered, while serving a sentence in jail.

Turning to the civil rights of mentally disordered patients, the role of the attorney general as *curator-ad-litem* and the master of the supreme court as *curator bonis* has already been pointed out. Divorce is another area provided for in the Act as follows. The patient must have been detained continuously for a period of seven years under the provisions of the Mental Disorders Act, and must have been declared incurable by three medical witnesses, two of whom must be registered psychiatrists. Moreover, in the case of a woman, the husband must not have been responsible for mental disorder, for example, he must not be the cause of her alcoholism and subsequent progressive alcoholic psychosis.

At certain times, and in different parts of South Africa, attempts have been made to extend the use of the voluntary boarder category to match liberal trends overseas. If this policy is pressed too far, the patients may lose the protection of their interests so carefully planned in the Mental Disorders Act.

Further Institutions

As the country became more densely populated, more institutions developed. The Institution on Robben Island, already referred to, was a leper colony as well as an institution for the mentally disordered; it was established on March, 1846 and its medical superintendent assumed his duties exactly a year later.

The achievement of responsible government by the Cape Colony in 1872 was followed by an active period in the provision of mental hospital facilities on the mainland resulting in the establishment of institutions at Grahamstown, in 1875, Port Alfred in 1889, Cape Town in 1891, and Fort Beaufort in 1894.

In Natal the pre-Union mental hospital services are synonymous with the Town Hill Hospital at Pietermaritzburg, which commenced as a "temporary lunatic asylum" in 1868, with 24 inmates maintained at the expense of the colonial treasury. In 1882 the first full-time resident medical superintendent was appointed in the person of James Hyslop.

In the Transvaal, one hospital, the mental hospital at Pretoria, now known as Weskoppies Hospital, provided the only mental health services available. In 1891 the Volksraad authorized the construction of a lunatic asylum and appointed a *College van Curatoren* to supervise the administration of the institution, which came into being in 1892. Prior to its opening the mentally ill were kept in gaols. In February, 1892, there were still 25 lunatics in various gaols. By the end of 1892, the new hospital housed 15 white and 14 non-white patients. The medical officer, Messum, attended part-time only, at a salary of £50 per annum, and it was not until May, 1895, that a full-time physician superintendent (*geneesheer-directeur*) assumed duty.

In the Orange Free State, the mental hospital at Bloemfontein, now known as the Oranje Hospital, came into being in 1884. Before its foundation, the president was empowered to convey mental patients requiring care from outlying districts to Bloemfontein to a government building hired for the purpose. Shortly after Union in 1910, the part-time medical officer, Dr. Kellner, was replaced by a full-time physician-superintendent, E. W. D. Swift.

To summarize the position in the year of Union, the statistics on January 1, 1910, are as follows:

TABLE 1

Province	Hospital	NUMBER OF PATIENTS		
		European	Non-European	Total
Cape	Valkenburg	428	—	428
	Robben Island	56	399	455
	Grahamstown	403	—	403
	Port Alfred	79	204	283
	Fort Beaufort	—	480	480
Orange Free State	Bloemfontein	116	157	273
Natal	Pietermaritzburg	255	334	589
Transvaal	Pretoria	355	358	713
	TOTAL	1,692	1,932	3,624

3

THE 20TH CENTURY AND THE UNION
OF SOUTH AFRICA

When the Union of South Africa came into being on May 31, 1910,
"all the laws affecting the insane and all the institutions established
for their treatment in the four Provinces were placed under the administration of the Minister of the Interior."

John T. Dunston

John Thomas Dunston, who became the first Commissioner for
Mental Hygiene of the Union of South Africa, received his medical
education at Guy's Hospital, achieving a London M.D. at the age of
24. He became first assistant medical officer at the Pretoria Lunatic
Asylum on August 3, 1905, and on October 18, 1908, he was promoted
to the position of Medical Superintendent. He made a major contribution to the drafting of the Mental Disorders Act of 1916, and
was appointed commissioner for mentally disordered persons as laid
down in that Act. His title was changed to Commissioner for Mental
Hygiene in 1922. Dunston played an important role also in influencing
the provision of the Act for the certification, care, and supervision of
mentally defective persons.

The Mental Defectives

Concern for the care of the mentally defective had resulted in the
formation, in 1913, of a National Society for the Care of the Feebleminded which later widened its terms of reference to become the
National Council for Mental Hygiene with local branches (19). At the
first annual meeting of the Cape Town Society, held on July 23,
1914, the Chief Justice, Sir James Rose-Innes, presided. Resolutions
were passed relating to the adequate and efficient treatment of the
feebleminded and to the need for a Mental Deficiency Act. These
resolutions were proposed and seconded by figures of national importance: J. X. Merriman, former Prime Minister of the Cape Colony,
and Patrick Duncan, a future Governor-General of the Union of South
Africa.

Fick, a Potchefstroom boy, educated at the South African College
(now the University of Cape Town) and later at Harvard, where he
obtained a doctorate in education, played a leading role in the assessment, measurement, and epidemiology of feeblemindedness in South

Africa (7), and conducted surveys in various parts of the country. The founding in quick succession of two institutions for mental defectives, the Alexandra at Maitland, Cape, in 1921, and the Witrand Institution at Potchefstroom, Transvaal, in 1923, was largely due to him.

Dunston himself, C. Louis Leipoldt, a poet, pediatrician and inspector of schools, and J. Marius Moll, the earliest practicing psychiatrist in Johannesburg and also consultant in nervous and mental diseases to the Transvaal Education Department, also had important roles in the field of mental deficiency. Leipoldt and Moll cooperated in standardizing the first intelligence tests for South African children. Dunston's first report as commissioner (24) records the surveys on the incidence of mental defect in orphanages, industries, schools, reformatories, and rescue homes. Later surveys were conducted by K. Gillis, psychiatrist in the South African Mental Service, and L. van Schalkwyk, organizing inspector for the Union Education Department (11).

In 1926 the number of mental defectives in South Africa was estimated at 300,000. When in 1927 the president of the Carnegie Corporation visited South Africa, the Dutch Reformed Church requested his assistance in investigating the matter. The Carnegie Corporation gave substantial financial assistance and provided the services of C. W. Coulter and K. L. Butterfield to assist in research.

The government commission appointed to investigate the problem was one of multidisciplinary experts, with R. W. Wilcocks of Stellenbosch University as psychologist. The five-volume report that appeared in 1932 described the extensive intelligence testing of schoolchildren between the ages of 10 and 13, and analyzed factors determining the lower scores of "the poor white" (30).

Investigation of the intelligence of the non-European has claimed the attention of C. T. Loram (14), M. L. Fick (8), and S. Biesheuvel (2). Biesheuvel's work *African Intelligence*, published in 1943, adduces environmental differences in explaining the difference in test intelligence between whites and non-whites, which Fick had considered innate. He also discusses the merits of devising culture-free tests in assessing African intelligence.

The 1929 Interdepartmental Committee on Mental Deficiency (Union of South Africa, Education Department) (27) consolidated many theoretical issues and assisted in implementing practical programs.

The three main institutions for mental defectives in South Africa are the Alexandra Institution, Maitland, Cape, opened in 1921; the Witrand Institution, Potchefstroom, opened in 1923; and the Umgeni Waterfalls Institution, Howick, Natal, opened in 1949. There is a smaller institution at Westlake at the Cape. A private institution, worthy of mention because of its progressive methods, is the Selwyn Segal Hostel, Johannesburg. Table 2 below, modified from the most recent annual report of the Commissioner for Mental Health (25), shows the amount of accommodation available in the four state institutions for the mental defectives.

The present position in regard to the population of mental hospitals is best seen by reference to Table 3 (25).

TABLE 2

Patients Accommodation, December 31, 1969

Institutions for Mental Defectives	Total	Whites		Non-Whites	
		Male	Female	Male	Female
Alexandra	879	353	526	—	—
Umgeni Waterfall	445	357	88	—	—
Westlake	487	—	—	232	255
Witrand	2,143	729	893	521	—

TABLE 3

Patients Accommodation—December 31, 1969

Hospital or Institution	Total	Whites		Non-Whites	
		Male	Female	Male	Female
Bophelong	2,500	—	—	1,583	917
Fort England	798	289	238	271	—
Fort Napier	876	198	130	244	304
Komani	1,498	241	329	521	407
Kowie	530	—	—	261	269
Madadeni	1,488	—	—	1,010	478
Nelspoort	174	—	—	111	63
Oranje	1,636	296	215	752	373
Sterkfontein	2,016	384	267	676	689
Stikland	1,197	491	453	253	—
Tower	1,539	—	—	753	786
Town Hill	909	155	157	483	114
Valkenberg	1,911	238	283	862	528
Weskoppies	2,122	472	422	989	420

National Societies

Passing reference has already been made to the role played by the National Society for the Care of the Feebleminded in the case of mental defect or subnormality. The mental health movement originated in the United States, and came out of the experience of Clifford

Beers. As a result of his endeavors in this direction, the National Committee for Mental Hygiene of the United States came into being on February 19, 1909, followed by the creation of local bodies in various cities, a pattern followed in South Africa and many other countries.

The settings in which the impact of the movement reached the shores of South Africa were a Baby Week Exhibition under the auspices of the Child Life Protection Society, in May, 1912, in which our mental health shortcomings were set forth in a leaflet, and a drawing room meeting, held on June 24, 1913, under the chairmanship of Sir John Graham, which resulted in the formation of the National Society for the Care of the Feebleminded. It was out of this concern for the feebleminded that the scope of the work broadened out until the care of the feeblmeinded was one only of its many activities in the field of mental health. It was not until September 22, 1920, that the National Council for Mental Hygiene and for the Care of the Feebleminded was duly constituted, with G. W. Cook, B.Sc., F.G.S., of Potchefstroom, as its first president, and J. T. Dunston, the Commissioner for Mental Hygiene, as an *ex officio* member. At that time there were 11 societies, including child welfare societies, doing mental hygiene work. Two bulletins on mental hygiene had been issued during the previous year. In 1946, the name of the national body was changed to the National Council for Mental Health. In 1948, this National Council joined the World Federation for Mental Health as a foundation member, and in 1950 it began publication of a magazine entitled *Mental Health*.

Minde (18), in evaluating the work of the National Council, comments as follows:

> We have now surveyed the career of the National Council for Mental Health since its early beginning in 1912 and have followed its vicissitudes. We have seen it has achieved successes but has also had to acknowledge failures. The question arises—has it been worthwhile?
> One feels that this question must be answered in the affirmative when a balance sheet is drawn up. When one compares the situation in 1952 with that of 1912 there is no doubt that there has been a marked advance in mental health fields over these 40 years, an advance for which the National Council may legitimately claim a commendable portion of the credit.

The local Mental Health Societies in the large cities such as Johannesburg serve a number of functions. Their clinics, staffed by psychiatrists, psychologists, and social workers, are active in the early diagnosis and treatment of psychiatric conditions and in case work supervision of patients discharged from the mental hospitals. They also have an educational program, for instance, through such media as films, about the early recognition and treatment of mental disturbance both in the child and in the adult.

Psychopathology in relation to urbanization and industrialization of the rural African is an important concern of mental health, and is reflected in the practice not only of mental hospitals, but also of mental health societies and general hospitals in South Africa.

Fisher and Hurst (9) have conducted an investigation into the attitudes towards mental health in a sample drawn from the general wards of South Africa's largest general hospital serving Bantu-speaking people, namely Baragwanath Hospital, Johannesburg. The findings show that, rather than a decrease, there is an increase in the popularity of witchdoctors in the urban area of Johannesburg and the Reef.

The Universities

Psychiatric education at university level is available in all South African medical schools, as is postgraduate education at the Universities of the Witwatersrand, Johannesburg, Cape Town, and Pretoria.

The University of Cape Town is the oldest medical school in the Republic of South Africa. Its history has recently been written by J. H. Louw (15). Undergraduate teaching of psychiatry commenced in 1922 at Valkenburg Mental Hospital, the lecturers being the successive physician superintendents, G. C. Cassidy, E. W. D. Swift, G. J. Key, and D. S. Huskisson. This teaching was supplemented within the general hospitals at first at the New Somerset Hospital and later at the Groote Schuur Hospital. F. N. Kooy became the first lecturer in the general hospital department in 1923 and was succeeded by S. Berman in 1952 as head of the department of neurology and psychiatry. The department of psychiatry achieved the status that goes with a full time chair only when L. S. Gillis was appointed to this position in 1968, after a tutelage of six years as head of psychiatry at a sub-department of medicine. This department is based upon the general hospital, with separate facilities for day patients in a large house adjoining the hospital and a special unit for the treatment of alcoholics by up-to-date methods, including group psychotherapy at the William Slater Hospital in Rondebosch, a mile or two away. In addition to undergraduate training, a two-year course for the diploma in psychological medicine is also offered. The main emphasis of this department is on a psychodynamic approach and community psychiatry in the field of alcoholism.

The University of the Witwatersrand Medical School began teaching psychiatry in 1924, when J. T. Dunston, Commissioner for Mental Health, was appointed clinical lecturer in psychiatry. Dunston was honorary professor of psychiatry from 1927 until his retirement from the mental hospital service in 1932. He was succeeded both as Commissioner and honorary professor of psychiatry by William Russell. The part-time professorship was then held by J. Twomey of Sterkfontein Hospital, Krugersdorp, serving Johannesburg. This appointment ended in 1952 when he retired on reaching the age limit. By this time the University had decided that, in the light of the widening scope of contemporary psychiatry including a shift of emphasis from the mental hospital to the general hospital, the chair should become a full time appointment; this was achieved in 1959 with the appointment of Professor L. A. Hurst.

The tradition of the Department of Psychiatry and Mental Hygiene at the University of the Witwatersrand, Johannesburg, is ideologically eclectic, giving free scope for psychoanalytic, behaviorist and existential approaches. It stresses teamwork between psychiatrists and members of the paramedical disciplines and has an active orientation in community psychiatry, emanating from both Johannesburg Hospital and Tara, the H. Moross Center. Psychological and social disciplines are not cultivated at the expense of the biological field; thus teaching and research in genetics and biochemistry are prominent endeavors.

Pretoria University has been teaching psychiatry only since 1946, with part-time professors, and the department has been based primarily on the mental hospital (Weskoppies Hospital) with some extension into the general hospital (The H. F. Verwoerd Hospital, Pretoria). The first professor, P. G. de Vos, appointed in 1946, and his successors, I. R. Vermooten and A. M. Lamont, held the positions of physician superintendent of Weskoppies Hospital and Commissioner for Mental Hygiene. During this period psychiatric education was essentially at the undergraduate level. With the appointment of A. J. van Wyk in 1966, despite the part-time nature of his appointment, psychiatric education entered its postgraduate phase. The language at Pretoria University is Afrikaans.

There are two other Afrikaans medical schools, where the development of psychiatric education is at an earlier stage than at Pretoria. At the University of Stellenbosch, Paul Cluver, formerly a part-time lecturer, became full-time professor for the last two years of his career. The University of the Orange Free State at Bloemfontein has been extending its undergraduate medical course annually and, in anticipation of reaching the stage at which psychiatry will be taught, has advertised a professorship with a view to systematic advanced planning.

The University of Natal Medical School, which serves exclusively for the education of non-whites, has R. W. S. Cheetham as head of the department of psychiatry. The medical school has been established entirely for African, colored, and Indian medical students and is the only one of its kind in the Republic. It was established in 1951 when the first students, totaling 35 in number, enrolled for a seven-year course.

Professional Bodies

One other channel for obtaining a qualification recognized for registration in the Speciality of Psychiatry in the South African Mental and Dental Council is the College of Medicine, formerly the College of Physicians, Surgeons, and Gynecologists of South Africa, a national body which holds postgraduate examinations twice yearly in all recognized medical disciplines. Hitherto the examinations have been held in Cape Town during the first half and in Johannesburg during the second half of the year. The qualification offered in psychiatry is the fellowship of the faculty of psychiatry—F. F. Psych (S.A.). It is roughly equivalent to the diploma in psychological medicine of the universities of Cape Town and of the Witwatersrand. This fellowship meets the specialization needs in psychiatry for doctors who, for geographical or other reasons, are unable to attend the D.P.M. courses offered by the universities in Cape Town and in Johannesburg.

4

CONCLUSION

South African psychiatry is starting at the crossroads of its administrative and governmental setting. As we have indicated, psychiatry in this country developed in the mental hospitals under the control of the Central Government. Lately, however, at Johannesburg and at Cape Town, with Durban well on the way, academic departments in the contemporary tradition have developed in the general hospital. Two government commissions, the Schumann and the Van Wyk Commissions (reports as yet unpublished), have declared in favor of the contemporary model based on the general hospital under the provincial administrators. On the other hand a Draft Bill (26) currently before Parliament may be paving the way to the central government taking over of all medical and hospital services. Psychiatric services at a third level—the municipal level—have just begun in the Colored and Bantu townships in the vicinity of Johannesburg.

With three variables, in the guise of the three layers of government in South Africa—central government, the four provincial governments, and the municipalities—the destiny of the organizational framework of psychiatry in the Republic of South Africa is difficult to predict.

REFERENCES

1. BARROW, SIR JOHN (1806): *Travels into the Interior of Southern Africa in Which Are Described the Character of the Dutch Colonists of the Cape of Good Hope and of the Several Tribes of Natives beyond Its Limits.* London: Ptd. by Cadell and Davies. 2v.

2. BIESHEUVEL, S. (1943): *African Intelligence.* Johannesburg: South African Institute of Race Relations.

3. BOSMAN, D. B. (1942): Die biografie van 'n Hottentotten, 'n eksperiment in beskawing. *Huisgenoot* July 1942 *quoted by* De Villiers, Simon A. (1971). *Op. cit.*

4. BURROWS, EDMUND H. (1958): *A History of Medicine in South Africa up to the End of the Nineteenth Century.* Cape Town: Balkema.

5. DE KOCK, VICTOR (1950): *Those in Bondage: An Account of the Life of the Slave at the Cape in the Days of the Dutch East India Company.* London: Allen & Unwin.

6. DE VILLIERS, SIMON (1971): *Robben Island: Out of Reach, Out of Mind: A History of Robben Island.* Cape Town: Struik.

7. FICK, M. L. (1938): *An Individual Scale of General Intelligence for South Africa.* Pretoria: S. A. Council for Educational and Social Research.

8. FICK, M. L. (1939): *The Educatability of the South African Native.* Pretoria: South African Council for Educational and Social Research.

9. FISHER, C. & HURST, L. A. (1967): Attitudes to mental health in a sample of Bantu-speaking patients at Baragwanath Hospital, Johannesburg. *Topical Probl. Psychiat. Neurol.,* 5, 179-204.

10. GARDINER, FREDERICK GEORGE & LANSDOWN, CHARLES WILLIAM HENRY (1946): *South African Criminal Law and Procedure.* Cape Town: Juta. 5th ed. 2 v.

11. GILLIS, K. (1953): Personal communication to M. Minde (1953) *Op. cit.*

12. LEIBBRANDT, H. C. V. (1898): Precis of the Archives of the Cape of Good Hope: Letters received, 1649-1662. Cape Town. 2v. *Quoted by* Fouché, L. (1963) Foundations of the Cape Colony; 1652-1708 In: *Cambridge History of the British Empire.* v. 8: *South Africa, Rhodesia and the High Commission Territories.* 2nd ed. Cambridge University Press.

13. LICHTENSTEIN, HENRY (1928): *Travels in Southern Africa in the Years 1803, 1804, 1805 and 1806.* A reprint of the translation from the original German. Van Riebeeck Society. 2v.

14. LORAM, C. T. (1917): *The Education of the South African Native.* London: Longmans.

15. LOUW, J. H. (1969): *In the Shadow of Table Mountain: A History of the University of Cape Town Medical School.* Cape Town: Struik.

16. MATTHEWS, J. W. (1887): *Incwadi yami; or, Twenty Years Personal Experience in South Africa.* London: Sampson Low.

17. MENTZEL, O. F. (1920): *The Cape in the Mid-Eighteenth Century; Being the Biography of Rudolf Siegfried Allemann, Captain of the Military Forces and Commander of the Castle in the Service of the Dutch East India Company at the Cape of Good Hope*. Trans. by Margaret Greenlees. Cape Town: Maskew Miller.

18. MINDE, M. (1953): *Mental health services in South Africa, 1652-1952*. Unpublished work. 2v. Copies in the Library of the Commissioner for Mental Health, P.O. Box 386, Pretoria.

19. Proposed National Society for the care of the feebleminded (1913): Pamphlet issued in Cape Town, August 1913. Copy in Minutes of the National Council for Mental Health, Johannesburg.

20. RAE, ISOBEL (1958): *The Strange Story of Dr. James Barry*. London: Longmans.

21. SEARLE, CHARLOTTE (1965): *The History of the Development of Nursing in South Africa, 1652-1960*. Cape Town: Struik.

22. South Africa (Republic) *Kommissie van ondersoek na die toerekening vatbaarheid van geestelik versteurde persone en aanverwante aangeleenthede*, 1967. Verslag. Pretoria. Government Printer. R.P. 69/1967.

23. TAS, ADAM (1970): *The Diary of Adam Tas, 1706-1709*, ed. by Leo Fouché and rev. by A. J. Boeksen. English trans. by J. Smuts. Cape Town: Van Riebeeck Society.

24. Union of South Africa 1924: *Commissioner for Mental Hygiene*. Report of the Commissioner for Mental Hygiene, 1922-1923. Pretoria: Government Printer.

25. South Africa (Republic) (1971): *Commissioner for Mental Hygiene*. Annual report for the year ended December 1969. Pretoria: Government Printer.

26. South Africa (Republic) (1972): Health Bill. As read a first time; introduced by the Minister of Health. Pretoria: Government Printer.

27. Union of South Africa (1929): *Education Department*. Report on the interdepartmental Committee on Mental Deficiency. Pretoria: Government Printer.

28. Union of South Africa (1945): Mental disorders act, 1916 (Act No. 38 of 1916) as amended by Mental Disorders Amendment Act (Act No. 7 of 1944) and regulations. Pretoria: Government Printer.

29. VAN RIEBEECK, JAN (1952-1958): *Journal of Jan van Riebeeck*, ed. with an introduction by H. B. Thom. Cape Town: Balkema. 2v.

30. WILCOCKS, R. F. (1932): The poor white problem in South Africa. In: *Carnegie Commission Report*. Stellenbosch: Pro Ecclesia Press. v.2.

26

INDIA

A. Venkoba Rao, M.D., Ph.D. D.P.M.,
F.R.C. Psych.

*Professor of Psychiatry, Madurai Medical College,
Department of Psychiatry, Erskine Hospital
Madurai, India*

1

INTRODUCTION

The history of psychiatry in India dates back to the prehistoric period and the period preceding the Indus valley civilization. The art and science of psychiatry have been the accumulated result of contributions from such sources as folklore, Vedas, Upanishads, many philosophical systems of India, the great epics Ramayana and Mahabharata and a number of ancient medical schools, among which the *Ayurveda* is of great importance. All these factors are relevant to the development of psychiatric and psychological thought in India. It is interesting that there was no Sanskrit equivalent for the terms "psychology" and "psychiatry," although the words *manas* and *unmād* were freely used to indicate mind and insanity respectively. Psychiatry does not appear to have received the status of a separate discipline in ancient Indian medicine, although the division of medical sciences into surgery, diseases of the head, treatment of ordinary diseases, pediatrics, demonology, and toxicology was recognized. However, in his compendium, Caraka, an ancient Indian physician, devotes a separate chapter to the etiology, symptomatology, pathogenesis, management, and prognosis of insanity (2-11). This reflects the early recognition that treatment of

624

insanity was the concern of the physician. Varma (38) believes that psychiatry was known as a speciality in ancient India.

The history of Indian medicine can be conveniently divided into four phases: Pre-Vedic, Vedic, Post-Vedic, and Modern. The same delineation can also be applied to psychiatry.

2

THE PRE-VEDIC ERA

This period extends from the paleolithic and neolithic age through the Indus valley civilization to the time of the Aryan invasion of India (Harappa civilization), i.e., up to 1500 B.C. During these centuries, the inhabitants of the subcontinent of India were guided by an animistic religion, worship of animals, trees, and snakes, reverence for the deified souls of departed ancestors, and a strong belief in the supernatural. To them, disease, physical or mental, was an act of possession by a demon or divine agents, or revenge by the spirit of the dead. Remedy lay in prayers, incantations, amulets, and talismans. Such magico-religious notions about disease and its cure in ancient India were consistent with those of contemporary Egyptian, Mesopotamian, and Cretan civilizations. The ancient Egyptians believed that sickness resulted from an intrusion of a spirit, soul of the dead, or god into the body of a person and that treatment consisted in discovering the type of agent from the underworld and driving it out by magic. Religious techniques took precedence over any medicine, however powerful. Incantation and divination were practiced by Mesopotamians to bring relief from disease, which they believed was caused by the conspiracy of hostile and evil spirits or demons, or by the influence of heavenly bodies. Temple medicine was prevalent in ancient Crete. At this distance of time, it is difficult to assess to what extent medical and psychological ideas were interchanged from one to the other of these great civilizations. It is likely that similar beliefs and practices in different lands were due to simultaneous but independent projection of similar mental attitudes of their people. Atharva Veda is believed to belong to this period and deals extensively with demonology—an outcome of the religious and medical beliefs of the times. Though called the last among the four Vedas, it is considered to have preceded the other Vedas.

3

THE PSYCHIATRY OF THE VEDIC PERIOD

The Vedas are four in number: *Rig, Yajur, Sama,* and *Atharva.* According to Max Muller, the great German Indologist, the Vedas are the oldest books in the library of mankind (30). The main contribution to medicine and psychiatry during this age comes from the *Atharva Veda,* although some material is found also in the *Rig Veda. Atharva Veda,* also called the *Brahma Veda,* deals exclusively with "goblins and ghosts, magic and sorcery, spells and curses, diseases and cures" (27). It is a massive compendium on demonology. "When a man falls ill, a magician and not the physician is sent for. The wizard is greater than gods. His herbs and amulets are sovereign remedies" (22). Even now in modern India, prayers, amulets, incantations, and charms are employed for "treatment" of diseases—physical and mental, "for never, probably, in the history of India was there any time when people did not take to charms and incantations for curing diseases or repelling calamities and injuring enemies" (13) (Plate CXV).

There were hundreds of demons, as well as techniques and methods for incantations. "The powers of an amulet are equal to thousands of medicines given by thousands of medical practitioners," says Ayurveda. Atharvanic charms were used among the host of other things for quickening intelligence, or preventing bad dreams, epileptic fits, and possession by different species of evil spirits. At the time of *Atharva Veda,* rational medicine was also gradually but definitely emerging. The diseases were classified as those due to supernatural agents and those due to dietetic factors. Treatment for the former was by charms, the latter were tackled with drugs. Although several drugs are mentioned in Vedic writings, their chemical actions were not clear and it was thought that they depended for their benefit upon the supernatural powers. The "drug acted as an internal amulet" (18). Thus one finds a gradual but definite shift from magico-religious pre-Vedic medicine towards an empirico-rational medicine during the Vedic era of Indian history.

4

PSYCHIATRY OF THE POST-VEDIC PERIOD

During the post-Vedic era, several systems of philosophy developed and reached eminence in India; the 6th century B.C. saw the beginning of scientific medicine, and from this time up to the 2nd century of the Christian era Indian medical schools enjoyed their most creative period. With the advent of philosophical systems, medicine left religion and magic and slowly aligned itself with philosophy. Caraka, Susrutha, and Bhela brought out their compendia during this period. Caraka (literally "wanderer"), believed to have lived sometime between the 1st and 2nd centuries, is essentially identified with ancient Indian medicine (Plate CXVI). He was the court physician to King

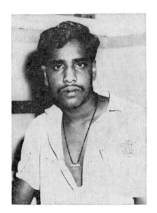

PLATE CXV. Patient wearing talisman and amulets.

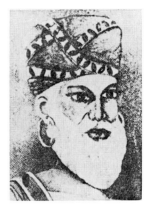

PLATE CXVI. Caraka, ancient Indian physician.

Kanishka in Purushapur (modern Peshawar in Pakistan). Susrutha's contribution was mainly to Indian surgery. Caraka's compendium deals with several aspects of insanity and will be discussed later. Both Caraka and Susrutha developed their medical and surgical concepts on the bases of the then prevailing Indian philosophic systems, *Nyaya,* *Vaiseshika,* and *Sankhya.* The Nyaya school was founded by Gautama, according to whom the world of matter was constituted by five elements—earth, fire, water, air, and sky or ether. Kanada developed the Vaiseshika school, which upheld the doctrine that the world originated from atoms. Kapila, exponent of the Sankhya school, propounded the dualistic theory of matter and soul. He theorized that evolution proceeded from the undefined to the defined (30). The modern phase in the history of Indian psychiatry is marked by the introduction of mental hospitals and will be considered in a later section.

Mind—Its Nature and Seat

The speculations and concepts in respect of the nature of the mind and its location have been as many as the number of systems of philosophy and schools of medicine. At no time did there exist a system of empirical psychology in ancient India. "Indian psychology is based on metaphysics; the psychological accounts of some problems, e.g., perception of the self, perception of the universe, etc., are unintelligible without consideration of metaphysical foundation" (31). Indian psychology is based to a greater extent on such techniques as introspection and observation, and much less on experimentation. Although mind has been considered as equivalent to soul, there is ample evidence to suggest that it was referred to as a psychological instrument and one of the organs of senses. In ancient Indian writings, mind was given the status of the sixth sense organ. In the *Rig Veda,* mind (*manas*) was regarded as the seat of thought, with emotion dwelling within the heart (13). However, the *Atharva Veda* lists mind and consciousness (*citta*) as different organs; mind is considered as an inner organ, and *citta* represents thought. The *Atharva Veda* also accords to the heart the importance of being the seat of mind. A verse in the *Atharva Veda* says: "O Mitra and Varuna, take away the thinking power from the heart of this woman, and making her incapable of judgement, bring her under my control."

Several systems of Indian philosophy regard the mind as one of the sense organs. For example, *Nyaya-Vaisesika* holds that mind is an inner instrument for perception. According to the *Sankhyan* school, mind, ego, and intellect together form an "internal organ" whose chief function is to receive impressions from the external environment and respond to them suitably. This equipment has sensory and motor organs as accessories. "This whole apparatus, consisting of the internal organ, and its several accessories, may be taken as roughly corresponding to the brain and the nervous mechanisms associated with its function, according to modern psychology" (16).

Among the ancient medical thinkers, the views of Caraka, Susrutha, and Bhela on the seat of mind merit attention. Caraka thought that the mind resided in the heart, together with pleasure, pain, and cognition; however, he qualified his statement by saying that the heart is not the place where these faculties stay, but that they depend upon it for their proper functioning. "If the heart is wrong, they also go wrong; if the heart is well, they also work well. Just as rafters are supported by the pillars, so are they all supported by the heart" (13). The heart has attained a prominent place in the Carakian system;

it is considered as the center of the currents of physical and psychological activities. To Susrutha, the heart, "the lotus with nine gates," is the seat of the mind. In his writings he declares, "The body consisting of the limbs, knowledge, the senses, the five objects of the senses, the soul as invested with attributes, the mind and thoughts are all established in the heart. Heart is the center of sensations, consciousness, and mind" (13). Caraka's and Susrutha's views are similar to those of Aristotle on the subject.

On the other hand, Bhela, probably as old as Caraka, remarkably considers the brain to be the center of mind—"a view unique in Sanskrit literature" (13). This corresponds to the Hippocratic view and the modern concepts. "*Manas,* which is the highest of all senses, has its seat between the head and the palate; being situated there, it knows all the sense objects, and tastes that come near it" (13). Bhela distinguishes between *manas, citta,* and *buddhi. Manas* is connected with cognitions and is situated in the brain. *Citta* controls various feelings and is located within the heart. Homer's concept of *noos* and *thymos* seems to find a parallel in Bhela's thinking. Bhela explained the origin of insanity thus: "the *doshas* (morbid humors) in the brain affect the mind and consequently involve the heart; from the affection of the latter, the understanding is impaired and this leads to madness" (13).

The Vedic literature includes metaphysical treatises referred to as *upanishads.* In *upanishadic* literature, the heart is spoken of as the central point of mental functions—for example, the *Taittiriya upanishad* places the "mini-person" in the heart; it is the converging point of many channels. (The different dimensions of personality in the *upanishadic* system are dealt with under another section). The *Aitereya upanishad* has a verse that denotes that heart is the seat of mind. "The heart sprang up: from the heart proceeded the mind; and from the mind moon." The ancient Indian views that the heart is the abode of the mind (with the possible exception of Bhela's view) is similar to those of the ancient Egyptians, the Chinese, and Aristotle.

In the Indian Tantric system of anatomy, which is different from the Ayurvedic school, nerve plexuses are described in detail. One of the plexuses is described as being situated between the eyebrows (mind plexus). To this is attributed the function of the sense, knowledge, and dream knowledge. The school holds that the upper cerebrum is the seat of the soul and describes a connecting structure—*jnana nadi*—between the mind and the soul (13). Throughout time, the heart and the brain have in turn claimed to be the proud lodgers and controllers of the mysterious faculties of mind. Some of the ancient concepts on the seat of the mind have been discussed by the author elsewhere (42).

Homeostasis—Philosophical and Psychological Concepts

The quest for man's mental poise and his physical and social well-being has been the endeavor of the philosophies of all lands—from the spiritually oriented Vedas and *upanishads* to the materialistic schools of European Epicureanism and Indian *Lokayata*. *Ataraxy, shanti*, and *sthithaprajna*—although terms from different schools of philosophy, have a common meaning indicating tranquillity. Vedic saints, perhaps the most ancient of thinkers, perceived an order in nature which they called *rita*. Worshippers of nature, they named a multitude of divinities that presided over every aspect of the universe. The deity who controlled the cosmic order was called *Varuna*. "He was the custodian and chief executor of this eternal Law *Rita*: this was at first the Law that established and maintained stars in their course; gradually it became also the Law of right, the cosmic and moral rhythm, which every man must follow if he would not go astray and get destroyed" (23). It would be a myopic vision of history if we were to content ourselves with the names of Claude Bernard, Sigmund Freud, and Walter Cannon while discussing any aspect of physical and mental homeostasis.

The diary of mankind is not without entries of what Sorokin preferred to call the "Columbus complex," meaning that each new discovery is in fact a rediscovery. The belief that a law of constancy or orderliness rules the animate and inanimate worlds has come down to us from the beginning of human cognition. Vedic seers, like the early Greeks, saw a parallel between the universe and man. They found in man the same order which they perceived in nature. To them man was universe in miniature while the universe was a magnified man. They discerned elements of both dynamic and static states in nature and man. *Rupa* and *nama* in man correspond to *sthitham* and *yat* in nature. These are akin to the *morphae* and *eidon* of Plato's system. While the Vedic men were analysts and admirers of nature and divined gods in every aspect of nature, the *upanishadic* were philosophers who turned their searching eyes inward to understand man's "inner breezes," to Alexis Carrel's "man the unknown." This *upanishadic* doctrine was echoed by Alexander Pope who expressed the view that the proper study of mankind is man. "*Dehasthya sarva vidya*," says one of the Indian Tantric books.

The *upanishadic* writings conceive personality as consisting of several dimensions which, while collectively functioning, aim at its equilibrium. Whether such ideas represent the concrete coverings of the human *soma,* or metaphysical or psychological abstractions, they clearly portend the later emerging concepts on homeostasis. The *upanishads* conceive the physical body as *annamaya kosha,* since it is derived from food—*anna.* Next is the layer called *pranamaya,* which literally means animation with sensation. The third layer is the mind called *manomaya,* whose functions comprise perception, cognition, and memory; this layer marks the transition from the concrete to the abstract. *Vignana kosha* is the next stratum that subserves "consciousness," which forms the basis of life. Finally there is the state of bliss, represented in the sector called *anandamaya kosha* which is the ultimate goal, tranquility (28). A harmonious functioning of these so-called sheaths contributes to an equilibratory state and their functioning extends along a spectrum going from materialism to spiritualism. Such an *upanishadic* concept of personality homeostasis was much advanced by a concise treatise called *mandukya upanishad,* which is wholly devoted to the exposition of different states of consciousness. It describes man's waking, sleeping, dreaming, and blissful states. The restorative or re-equilibratory purpose of dreaming is implied in the *upanishadic* aphorism: "He who desires, dreams; he who does not desire does not dream." Modern research has pointed out that dreaming is a biological necessity, and that dream deprivation causes psychopathological phenomena. It may be recalled at this point that *upanishadic* thinkers realized that dreamers should not be disturbed. They realized too the need for dreaming: "In the waking state one gets troubled owing to manifold activities of the body and the organs; he gets some relief by discarding them in dreams." Samkara (Plate CXVII), the well known interpreter of the *upanishads* and the founder of a non-dualistic school of philosophy, commented thus on dreams: "It is an instinctive attempt to avoid misery and to obtain pleasure" (26). Caraka, too, has alluded to the effects of loss of sleep (5). A comparison between the *upanishadic* and the psychoanalytical concepts of dreaming has been attempted by Venkoba Rao (40).

The Sankhyan school of philosophy compares life, or even personality, to a field (*kshetra*) within which forces (*gunas*) are always at work. These forces are of three types, physical (*tamas*), physiological (*rajas*), and psychological (*sattva*). They maintain a balance —in fact life is described in Sankhya as "the web of *gunas*" (*gunajala*). The homely example of the lamp is offered by the Sankhyans to illustrate the contribution of these triple forces to any process: the wick, the oil, and the flame represent respectively the *tamas* (physical), *rajas* (physiological), and *sattvic* (psychological) aspects. Disturbance can result if any one of the three *gunas* grows out of proportion, at the expense of the other two (16).

Caraka defines man as an aggregate of mind, spirit, and body. "The mind, spirit, and body are together, as it were the tripod: The world endures by reason of cohesion; and on that are all things established" (4). Ayurveda upholds the doctrine of *Tridosha*—humoral trinity— which implies that the three constituents, *vata* (wind), *pitta* (bile),

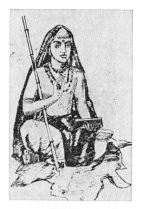

PLATE CXVII. Samkara (A.D. 788-820). The Indian saint and philosopher who propounded the non-dualistic school of Indian philosophy.

and *kapha* (phlegm), always exist in right measure and support a state of equilibrium during health—a state of *"dhatu samya."* *Dhatu vaisamya,* a sign of disease, results when there is a disturbance in the quantity and distribution of these constituents. Hence, the aim of Ayurveda is the maintenance of a state of *dhatu samya* by prescribing diet, medicine, and a suggested code of behavior (13). "Just as it is necessary that religious duties, wealth, and desires should all be attended to equally, or just as the three seasons of winter, summer, and rains all go in a definite order, so all the three—*vata, pitta,* and *kapha*—when they are in their natural state of equilibrium, contribute to the efficiency of all the sense organs, the strength, color, and health of the body, and endow a man with long life. But when they are disturbed, they produce opposite results, and ultimately break the balance of the system and destroy it" (2). The concepts of homeostasis from Indian psychological and philosophical schools have been discussed by Venkoba Rao (43).

5

PSYCHIATRY IN AYURVEDA

Ayurveda (*Ayur*: life, *Veda*: knowledge) is the ancient Indian system of medicine whose earlier origin is shrouded in obscurity. It is ascribed to a divine revelation. However its relation to Atharvaveda is established and the compendia of Caraka, Susrutha, and Bhela among others constitute the important sources of knowledge on Ayurveda. The period between the 6th century B.C. and the 2nd century A.D. has been described as the golden era in Indian medicine. The contribution of Ayurvedic medical authorities in regard to the seat of the mind has already been mentioned. Ayurveda recognized the importance of mental diseases when it classified the human ills into three categories: exogenous, endogenous, and psychic. The doctrine of *Tridosha* (three humors described above as *vata, pitta,* and *kapha*) plays a pivotal role in the consideration of etiology, pathology, diagnosis, and therapeutics in this system of Indian medicine.

In the *Atharva Veda* one also finds the diseases classified into *abhraja* (wind), *vataja* (bile), and *sleshma* (phlegm) types, corresponding to the malfunction of *vata, pitta,* and *kapha* humors. That wind, bile, and phlegm form the constituents of the human body and by their decay cause diseases has been brought out in the Indian epic *Mahabharata*. It is likely that Ayurvedic doctrine developed out of this concept from the *Mahabharata* and the *Atharva Veda*. Some historians believe that the Greeks were the originators of this humoral theory, and that India borrowed from them. Kutumbiah (18) has effectively countered this view. These humors (*doshas*) according to Ayurvedic concepts, become pathogenic only when played upon by certain precursors, or predisposing factors called *nidanas*. These conditions, or the excited *doshas*, act upon the basic constituent system, called *dhatu complex*, and lead to its disequilibrium, resulting in disease.

Caraka classified *vata, pitta* and *kapha* as somatic *doshas*; *rajas* and *tamas* are the mental *doshas* which are of etiologic significance for psychological maladies. Caraka has outlined the etiological mechanism of insanity: "The mind being afflicted and the understanding disturbed, the mental *doshas* are provoked; reaching the heart and obstructing the ducts through which the mind operates, they initiate insanity" (10). Bhela's theory of insanity has already been referred to. The psychological and temperamental characteristics of individuals were believed to be largely dependent upon and determined by the overwhelming action of one *dosha* on the other. Several types of personality were described that had their counterparts in Greek terminology—*apoplecticus, pthisicus, phlegmatic, melancholic,* etc. Caraka offered the following classification of insanity (*unmād*):

TABLE 1

I. *Endogenous Group*:
  A) Insanity produced by "bodily humors"
      a) *Vatonmād*
      b) *Pittonmād*
      c) *Kaphonmād*
      d) *Sannipathonmād*

  B) Insanity produced by "mental humors"
      a) *Rajasonmād*
      b) *Tamasonmād*

  C) Insanity produced by a combination of factors in A and B.

II. *Exogenous Group*:
      a) *Adhijonmād*
      b) *Vishajonmād*

The etiological factors in this group include possession or punishment by gods, sages, demons and the *manes,* and failure to perform duties in this or a previous life. The humoral disturbances play little or no role in this variety.

Insanity, to Caraka (9), is "the unsettled condition of the mind, understanding, consciousness, perception, memory, inclination, character, behavior, and conduct." Discussing the general etiological factors, Caraka mentions faulty diet, disrespect towards the gods, teachers, and the twice-born, mental shock resulting from excess of fear or joy, and faulty bodily activities. Among the premonitory symptoms of endogenous insanity Caraka lists "feeling of voidness in the head, noises in the ears, hurried respiration, anorexia, cardiac spasm, misplaced mental absorption, anxiety, horripilation, intoxicated condition of the mind, frequently dreaming of roving, moving, of sitting on the wheel of the oil press, of being churned as it were by whirlwinds, of sinking in whirlpools of tinged waters." Among the general symptoms he lists (19): "confusion of intellect, extreme fickleness of mind, agitation of the eyes, unsteadiness, incoherence of speech, mental vacuity. Needless to say, he knows no mental ease. Deprived of memory, understanding and his wits, he keeps his mind wavering restlessly." Among the exogenous types (*aganthunmād*), Caraka describes the etiology and symptomatology of some eight types—all resulting from "possession." Among the general symptoms of this type are included "superhuman strength, energy, capacity, grasp, memory, understanding, speech, and knowledge."

The specific symptoms of some types of insanity as described by Caraka are offered below:

TABLE 2

I. *Endogenous type*:
   a) *Vata* variety — Constant wandering; jerking of eyelids, brows, lips and other parts of the body; incoherent talk; laughing; dancing; singing; loudly imitating the sounds of the lute, flute, conch; adorning with queer and unornamental objects; hankering after unobtainable viands; emaciation; swelling; redness of the eyes.
   b) *Pitta* variety — Irritability, anger, excitement in the wrong place, striking oneself or others with weapons, sticks or fists; nudity, craving for shade, cold water and food; prolonged attacks of anguish; coppery, green, yellow and furious look of the eyes.
   c) *Kapha* variety — Rooted to one spot; silence: no inclination for movement; dribbling of saliva; lack of desire for food; love of solitude; constant somnolence; whiteness and fixity of eyes.

II. *Exogenous type*:
   Superhuman strength; energy, capacity; grasp, memory, understanding, speech, and knowledge.

Caraka holds that insanity resulting from the discordance of all the three humors (*Tridoshonmād*) is dreadful and is to be given up as incurable.

The therapeutic measures for insanities in Caraka's compendium vary from "words of sympathy and comfort" to "terrorizing by means of snakes," from purgation to venesection. He recommended purification procedure by emetics and diaphoretics. If these were of no avail, ocular and nasal instillations with medicated *ghee* (melted butter) were recommended. The drugs used include colocynth, pepper, valerian, turmeric, Indian sarsaparilla, cardomom, pomegranate, cinnamon leaf, sandalwood, garlic, *jejube,* radish, ginger and asafetida; goat's and cow's urine, and ox or jackal bile were used as vehicles. In some instances of disoriented mind such measures as anointing with mustard oil, exposure to sunlight, branding with hot irons, or scourging with a whip were recommended. Terrorizing by snakes whose fangs are removed, or by trained elephants or lions, or by men dressed as bandits or men with weapons, and intimidation with threats of immediate execution, were employed when all other measures had failed on the plea that "threat to life is more potent than fear of bodily injury" (6).

There are elements of psychotherapy or even psychopharmacology in the statement of Caraka (7): "As regards the mental derangement resulting from an excess of desire, grief, delight, envy, or greed, it should be allayed by bringing the influence of its opposite passion to bear on the prevailing one and neutralize it." *Ghee* has attained a celebrated status in ancient Indian therapeutics. Of *ghee* preserved for over 100 years it has been said that "there is no disorder which it cannot cure." "Even the sight, smell, or touch of this substance is curative of all kinds of spirit possessions." For insanity resulting from exogenous causes, charms and privations, worship, sacrifices, incantations, propitiatory rites and ceremonies, and pilgrimages to sacred places are the suggested measures. There is a vague suggestion of preventive psychiatry in Caraka's writing, "The man of strong mind, who abstains from flesh and alcohol, observes a wholesome diet and is always dutiful and pure, will never fall a victim to insanity, whether exogenous or endogenous."

Caraka recognized also an incurable type of insanity caused by the "spirit desirous of avenging itself." He also commented on the signs of improvement in mental illness. In his treatise, however, there is no mention of asylums, or social or legal provisions for the insane.

Rawolfia serpentina was a popular drug for insanity in ancient India. Known as *sarpagandha* in Sanskrit, it was used in treating a variety of diseases and symptoms ranging from constipation to insanity. The following verses describing the plant and its medicinal use are taken from an ancient Indian text (29):

> The flowers appear in the summer season and the petals are bluish brown and reddish in colors; in rainy season it yields fruits of bluish and reddish color; the root is thick and of yellowish white color and circular inside; this white plant is famous and is known as *Chandra* (moon) the odor of which is that of serpent. This plant known as *sarpagandha* is rough, bitter, pungent, produces heat in the body. It stimulates good appetite, digestion, assimilation, helps in the evacuation of bowels, clears phlegm and excessive wind from the body. It is effective in giving sound sleep and peace of mind. It eradicates stomachache, fever, germs,

sleeplessness, lunacy, passion, misapprehensions, or delusions, indigestion, poison, giddiness, loss of appetite, excessive gastric troubles, epilepsy and high blood pressure.

6

SUICIDE IN ANCIENT INDIA

Suicide has been known in India from the beginning of her history. *Vedic* and *upanishadic* literature contain several references to this form of self-destructive behavior. The early *Vedic* period, literally an era of rituals, sanctioned suicide as a religious ritual. There are several *Vedic* hymns that indicate that suicide was a prized sacrifice of the times. On the other hand, there was a revolt against suicide during the *upanishadic* period. It was called "irreligious and foolish" by the *upanishadic* seers—Yagnavalkya, Videha, Janaka and others. "Those who take their lives reach after death the sunless regions, covered by impenetrable darkness," declared the *Isavasya Upanishad*. However, a concession was made in a later minor *upanishad* to "the *Sanyasin* who has acquired full insight and who may enter upon a great journey, or choose death by voluntary starvation, by drowning, by fire or by a hero's fate."

The great epics of India also offer instances of suicide. Rama, hero of *Ramayana*, gave up his life in the waters of the river Sarayu after learning that his brother Lakshmana had killed himself. The news of the death of these brothers depressed and shocked the citizens of the capital city of Ayodhya and there followed an epidemic of suicide. In *Raghuvamsa*, a sanskrit drama by Kalidasa, whose theme deals with the genealogy of the Ikshvaku dynasty, one finds that depressive illness affected several royal personages. King Aja became depressed following the death of his wife Indumathi, and starved himself to death. King Dasaratha, father of Rama, suffered from three episodes of acute depression, the last one proving fatal. In the *Yoga Vasishta*, it is recorded that the young prince Rama suffered from depression in his 18th year and was treated by a discourse of the royal priest Vasishta. In another Indian epic, *Mahabharata*, Madri, the queen of Pandu, gave up her life after the death of her husband. Kautilya, the famous law-giver of ancient India, condemned suicidal deaths and prescribed harsh treatment for the bodies of suicides. The bodies were to be drawn on public roads and were denied funeral rites. Even a relative who performed the funeral rites of suicides was denied the rites for his own funeral and was deprived of his property and abandoned by the people. The bodies of suicides of either sex were exposed to indignities and public insults.

However, the religious authorities of India permitted suicide under certain special situations:

1. *Sati*: Self-immolation of a woman during or after the cremation of her husband (Plate CXVIII).
2. Suicide by drowning at places of religious pilgrimages or at the confluence of sacred rivers.
3. Suicide as an escape from suffering due to incurable disease, or from old age incapacitating an individual to such an extent as to prevent him from discharging religious duties.
4. Suicide by ascetics.
5. A long journey during the final stage of one's life, with suicidal intention.

Sati and *Jauhar* are the two types of suicide that have been an important factor in Indian history. *Sati,* a form of widow-burning, was an ancient religious suicide. This practice was not peculiar to India, but "owes its origin to the oldest religious views and superstitious practice of mankind in general." It was believed to be prevalent in ancient Greece, Germany, and among the Egyptians and the Slavs. It was known in China until the present century. *Sati* monuments (Plates CXIX and CXX), with inscriptions on sculptured stones, are found in many parts of India. *Sati* is not practiced in modern times, although an occasional news item suggests that it still occurs sporadically. It was during the viceroyalty of Lord Bentinck that legislation was enacted, in 1829, to declare all those who encouraged *sati* as guilty of culpable homicide.

Jauhar was a type of mass suicide resorted to by women of Rajasthan (Western India) in the event of an invasion to escape sexual dishonor and captivity by the victors. The earliest *jauhar* occurred when Alexander invaded Punjab. A similar epidemic took place when Akbar conquered Marwar.

In ancient India, *sati* and *jauhar* embodied the noble sentiments of marital love and patriotism respectively. During recent times, hunger strike as a form of *satyagraha* has become increasingly common. It was originally suggested and practiced by Gandhi as a weapon to fight the British rule in India. The first fatal result was the death of one Jatin Das, a revolutionary leader of Bengal who fasted for 61 days in jail. The death of Potti Sriramulu in Madras, after fasting for 51 days, triggered the formation of linguistic states in India. There have been many deaths from fasting; the most recent was that of a man called

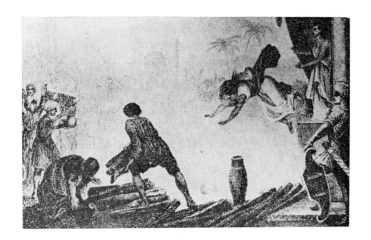

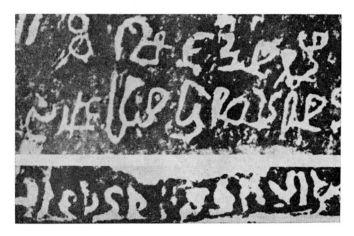

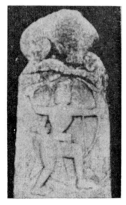

PLATE CXVIII (top). Sati showing the
leaping of the widow and the funeral pyre
of her husband. PLATE CXIX (center). Sati
inscription installed at the side of the act
of sati as a commemoration. PLATE CXX
(left). Sati memorial stone.

Pheruman, over the demand for inclusion of Chandigarh into the state of Punjab. These deaths, caused by denying oneself food and water, although politically motivated, have a religious fervor about them. Among the Jains of India, death by starvation prevailed and this method was called *sallekhana*. It was permitted only for the Jaina ascetics, who regarded quick methods of suicide as evil and vulgar. "Renouncing all food and death, I patiently wait for my end" (33). These types of suicide have become extinct now. Several aspects of the history of suicide in India have been discussed by Thakur (33).

7

PERSONALITY THEORY—INTEGRATION AND BREAK-UP

In several ancient Indian writings, one comes across concepts relating to personality and recommended paths for its healthy growth and the ways in which it breaks down. For example, *Sankhya* philosophy and the *Bhagavad Gita* dwell at length on the so called *gunas*, or psychological characteristics. *Sattva, rajas,* and *tamas* are the modes that are present in all human beings, although one predominates over the other two. Men are said to be *sattvic* (good), *rajasic* (passionate), or *tamasic* (dull) depending upon the trait that predominates. The psychological effects of these different *gunas* are brought out in an interesting verse in the *Gita* (24): "Those who are established in goodness rise upwards; the passionate remain in the middle; the dull steeped in the lower occurrences of the modes sink downwards." The Indian trinity of gods reflects the dominance of these three *gunas—sattva* in Vishnu, *rajas* in Brahma, and *tamas* in Siva; they represent respectively the functions of protection, creation, and destruction. The *Gita* also sets out the path of the decline of personality, ultimately resulting in deterioration.

> A man thinking of objects of senses becomes attached to them; attachment causes longing; from longing grows anger, from anger arises delusions; from delusions arise a loss of memory; from the loss of memory arises a ruin of discrimination and from this loss of discrimination, he ultimately perishes (32).

The *yoga* system of philosophy, first propounded by Patanjali, lays down a course of rigorous discipline for an integrated personality. The method comprises eight practical stages arranged in sequence. Hence, these aspects of the yoga are called *Ashtanga* (eight limbed). The first two consist of restraint (*yama*), and discipline (*niyama*). Together, these help the individual toward self-regulation and temperance. The third stage consists of body posturing (*asanas*). It is believed that a steadying of the body prepares man for steadiness of mind. Interdependence between mind and body have been stressed in *mahabharata*, too. The next stage is the control of breathing (*pranayama*). This is a precursor of a state of contemplation. The second set of four exercises is concerned with the psychological dimensions of the personality and includes withdrawal (*pratyahara*), fixed attention (*dharna*), contemplation (*dhyana*), and a state of complete tranquility (*samadhi*), which *yoga* philosophy calls the *summum bonum* of life. These yogic practices are in vogue in India even today. Modern work has given a neurophysiological basis to *yogic* phenomena. The use of *yoga* in psychiatric therapy has been reported by Vahia, Vinekar, and Doongaji (34). The *Gita* recommends that a tranquil mind should be like a "lamp sheltered in a windless place." The concept of personality as held in *upanishadic* writings has been mentioned earlier under the section on homeostasis.

There are ancient Indian parallels to the modern description of personality types such as asthenic (cerebrotonic), pyknic (gastrotonic), and athletic (musculotonic). The important and popular characters of Mahabharata typify these: *Yudhistira*—a keen intellectual, physically lean, sensitive to wrong actions, an upholder of righteousness; the corpulent *Bhima*—a man of action, emotionally unstable; and the muscular *Arjuna*—a warrior whose instinct is to fight. Some ancient Indian concepts of mind, insanity, and mental hygiene have been dealt with by Venkoba Rao (39).

Personality in Ayurveda

Basically three personalities are recognized in *Ayurveda*, namely the pure (*sattvic*), passionate (*rajas*), and ignorant (*tamas*). "The pure mind is considered to be without any taint as it represents the beneficent aspect of the intelligence; the passionate mind is tainted as it represents the violent aspects; the ignorant mind also is tainted on account of its representing the deluded past."

Several variations of personality types are possible due to several varieties of body type. Caraka (8) describes 16 personality types: 7 belong to the *sattvic* type; 5 to the *rajas* type, and 4 to the *tamas* type.

Sattvic Personality

Brahma type. He is impartial, pure, devoted to truth, self-controlled, endowed with knowledge, understanding, and power of exposition and reply, possessed of good memory, free from greed, conceit, desire, infatuation, intolerance. He is capable of scientific, philosophical and religious discourses. The name *Brahma* is derived from one of the Indian trinity responsible for creation.

Rishi Type. He is devoted to sacrifice, study, vows, celibacy; he is hospitable, devoid of pride, and endowed with genius, eloquence, and retentive power. *Rishi* is one who is devoted to contemplation and is a bachelor.

Indra Type. He is brave, energetic, authoritative of speech; endowed with splendor; possesses foresight, and is given to pursuits of wealth, virtue, and sensual pleasures. He is blameless in his work. *Indra* was known as the king of gods.

Yama Type. His conduct is governed by considerations of propriety, authority; he is free from passions, attachment, is unassailable, is constantly up and about, and has a good memory. *Yama* is the god into whose realm the souls enter after the death of the body.

Varuna Type. He is valiant, courageous, intolerant of uncleanliness; devoted to the performance of sacrifices, fond of aquatic sports, and his anger and favor are well placed. As indicated earlier, *Varuna* is the deity who presides over the cosmic order.

Kubera Type. He commands status, honor, luxuries and attendants; is given to pleasures of recreation, and his anger and favor are patent. *Kubera* is known for his wealth.

Gandharva Type. He is fond of dancing, song, music, and praise, and is well versed in history, poetry, and stories; though addicted to the pleasures of fragrant unguents, garlands, women, and recreation, he is free from envy. *Gandharva* denotes a celestial dancer living among the trees.

Among the seven types described above, the *Brahma* type is considered the most desirable since the "beneficent aspect of the mind is represented in it" (8). Nevertheless all the personalities are beneficial to the society in which they live.

Rajas Personality Types

Asura Type. He is valiant, despotic, possessed of authority, terrifying, pitiless, and fond of self-adulation. *Asura* is an enemy of God.

Rakshasa Type. He is cruel, gluttonous, intolerant, and full of hate—fond of flesh foods, somnolent, and of indolent disposition. He is capable of biding time and striking. *Rakshasa* is a demon with evil designs.

Pisaca Type. He eats voraciously, is fond of secret company with women, hates cleanliness, and is given to abnormal recreations and food. *Pisaca* is a demon who loves luxury and women.

Sarpa (Snake) *Type.* He is brave, touchy, of indolent disposition, arouses fear in the beholder, and is addicted to pleasures of food and recreation.

Preta Type. He is fond of food; his character, pastimes, and conduct are of painful description; he is envious, covetous, and disinclined to work. He lacks power of discrimination. *Pretas* haunt the burial ground and live on human corpses.

Sakuna (Bird) *Type.* He is constantly devoted to eating and sports; he is fickle, intolerant, and unacquisitive.

Tamas Personality Types

Pasva (Animal) *Type.* He is mentally deficient, disgusting in his behavior and dietetic habits, abandoned to sexual pleasures, and given to somnolent habits.

Matsya (Fish) *Type.* He too is poorly endowed, cowardly, gluttonous, fickle, prone to anger and sensuality. He loves water and is of itinerant habits.

Vanaspatya (Plant) *Type.* He is lazy, and exclusively devoted to the business of eating. He is of subnormal intellect.

It may be seen that the Ayurvedic writers conceived personality as comprising the important dimensions: intellectual, social, emotional, spiritual, and moral. The *sattvic* and *rajasic* represent the intellectual and emotional types respectively. The *tamasic* group broadly represent the intellectually deficient ones. The descriptive types of mentally deficient as animal, fish, and plant varieties is interesting (38).

8

REFERENCES TO PSYCHIATRIC SYNDROMES IN INDIAN EPICS

References to suicide in Indian epics have already been alluded to in an earlier section. There are references to depression in *Ramayana* and *Mahabharata*.

In *Ramayana*, the father of the hero Rama suffers from three depressive episodes. The first was precipitated by his accidentally causing the death of a son of blind parents by his arrow; the second was triggered by separation from his dear children, when the latter were taken away by the sage Viswamitra; the final one was ushered in when his son Rama, accompanied by his wife Sita and his brother Lakshmana, left for the forest abode in fulfillment of a vow of his father to his stepmother. The king Dasaratha was overwhelmed by a grief that proved fatal. Dasaratha's father Aja too suffers from depression for eight years following the death of his wife Indumathi; he ultimately starves himself to death. "In his haste to follow his beloved, Aja looked upon even that cause which was sure to terminate his life and which was incurable as a gain." The depressive illness in the Ikshvaku dynasty has been described by Kalidasa and is an example of a dominantly inherited illness. *Yoga Vasishta* (21), another ancient Indian treatise, narrates the depressive symptoms of Rama. In his 15th year Rama's "once radiant body became all at once emaciated like the river floods going down in summer; his red cool face with long eyes became wan like a white lotus; and he ever seated himself in a Padma posture with his hands resting on his chin and his young feet tinkling with bells; wholly absorbed in pensive thought, he forgot to perform the daily allotted duties of life and his mind grew despondent. His followers, noticing the ever static-like position their master had assumed, fell at his feet and asked him of the cause of his moody temper, to which Rama merely replied by performing his daily duties with such a depressed mind and dejected face as affected all those who saw it." Explaining the "delusion" that had affected Rama, the royal priest Vasishta remarked "the great delusion that has now arisen in him is unlike any that springs out of disappointment as to any desired object or out of any accident but is only a stepping stone to the acquisition of divine wisdom through indifference to worldly objects and true discrimination" (21). Herein one can discern the exogenous and endogenous varieties of psychological experiences.

The background of the story of *Mahabharata* is a family feud between two related dynasties—the Pandavas and the Kauravas. The battle scene in Kurukshetra is a spectacular event in the epic. The opposing forces are arranged on the battlefield and the Pandava hero Arjuna's mind is stricken with grief over the enormity of the sin that is about to be committed by slaying his relations. Krishna, in the role of the charioteer and guide, offers counseling. The dialogue between Krishna and Arjuna forms the central theme of the *Gita,* which is an inset into the *Mahabharata.* The first chapter of the *Gita,* which has 18 chapters in all, deals with, and is called, "Arjuna's Grief." Being struck with depression and unable to fight, he expresses his physical and psychological feelings thus:

My limbs quail, my mouth goes dry,
my body shakes and my hair stands on end.
The bow gandiva slips from my hand
and my skin is burning all over;
I am not able to stand steady
and my mind is reeling.

—*Gita* 1, 28-30 (24)

The rest of the *Gita* deals with psychotherapy offered by Krishna with the result that Arjuna's grief and anxiety are dispelled. He surrenders with the declaration "I stand firm with my doubts dispelled, I shall act according to Thy word." I have reported on the reference to depression in Indian epics elsewhere (41).

Hindu philosophy holds that life in its broadest sense does not end with death, which only opens the door to the next life whose quality is determined by the way the preceding one was utilized. This is the law of *Karma,* or cosmic justice, that occupies the central place in the Vedantic philosophy. The attitude towards death, which colors the symptoms of psychiatric illness and of suicidal attempts and suicide, was expressed in an interesting manner in the *Mahabharata*. In the chapter entitled "Enchanted pool" answering the voice of his divine father, who commanded him to say what the greatest wonder in the world was, Yudhistira, the eldest of the Pandavas, replied, "Every day men see creatures depart to *yama*'s [the god of death] abode and yet those who remain seek to live forever. This verily is the greatest wonder" (25). This same thought was echoed by Sigmund Freud (15) in the 20th century: "Our own death is indeed unimaginable and whenever we make the attempt to imagine it we can conceive that we really survive as spectators. Hence, the psychoanalytical school could venture on the assertion that at bottom no one believes in his own death, or to put the thing in another way, in the unconscious, everyone of us is convinced of his own immortality."

9

MENTAL HOSPITALS AND LEGISLATION

Mental Hospitals

No specific mention has been made in ancient Indian medical writings of mental hospitals. None is mentioned by Caraka. However, a mental hospital was believed to have been in existence near Mandu

(Bihar) around 1,000 A.D., although particulars of it are not available (38).

Attempts were first made to segregate the mentally ill towards the middle and the latter part of the 19th century. Forsaken stables, barracks and prisons were freely used and, whenever necessary, high walls were raised around dilapidated buildings which were used to house the patients. They were left to the care of the keepers and rods, confined by straight jackets, locked up in cells, and treated with morphia, opium, hot baths, and leeches. Until 1905 all the asylums were under the charge of a civil surgeon; in that year "alienists" were appointed to look after the insane. This provision was the result of the efforts of Lord Morley, the then Secretary of State for India. Although in general the conditions of the asylums were very unsatisfactory and the "achievements of the psychiatrists, barring a few notable exceptions, have been practically nil (36)" there have been instances of psychiatrists who did outstanding work.

"The history of psychiatry in this country is the history of establishment of mental hospitals and then increasing their accommodations from time to time as the exigencies of time demanded" (36). This stage corresponds to the recent or the modern phase of Indian psychiatry.

The earliest asylum in India existed around 1787 in Calcutta, to take care of the Europeans who fell mentally ill while in India; the asylum was reported to be under the charge of a surgeon named Kenderdine. Subsequently several asylums were constructed in different parts of the country, the important ones being in Bengal, Bombay, Madras, Bihar, and Orissa. The year 1912 marks an important milestone in the history of India and its psychiatry. The capital of the country was shifted from Calcutta to Delhi and the Lunacy Act was passed by the legislature in that year. Another landmark was in 1922, when "lunatic asylums" began to be called "mental hospitals."

Varma (36, 37) has described the staff and conditions prevailing in all mental hospitals in India. There are some instances of pioneering efforts by the psychiatrists of those times. For example, John Martin Honigberger, a court physician to Maharaja Ranjit Singh, treated his patients with "cleanliness, some physic, douche bath, decent dress, good food, amusements, occupations, presents, and promises. . . ." All this suggests that kind treatment could scarcely fail to bring some improvement. "I never beat them, never ill-treat them, but I prevent them doing any mischief to others or to themselves." The names of Berkeley Hill, Lodge Patch, Honigberger, Valentine Conolly, and Dhunjibhoy stand out prominently in the history of

psychiatry during the British rule in India. The details of their contribution have been dealt with by Varma (36, 37) and Lodge Patch
(19). The conditions of the Indian mental hospital towards the close
of the British rule were described by Taylor (37) as "disgraceful and
have the makings of a major public scandal." He said that "the majority of the mental hospitals are quite out of date and are designed for
detention and safe custody without regard to curative treatment."

The first psychiatry department in a general hospital in India
started in Bombay in its Jamsettjee Jeejibhoy Hospital by K. R.
Masani in 1938. J. C. Marfatia was his first houseman and joined him
in 1941. The psychiatric department in the King Edward VII Memorial Hospital, Bombay, was organized by N. S. Vahia in 1947. The
first child guidance clinic in Bombay was also started by K. R. Masani
at Nagpada in 1939 (35).

Legislation

The bulk of the law relating to the custody of lunatics and the management of their estates in India was contained in various legal acts
passed in 1858. These acts were based in great measure on the English
Lunacy Regulation Act of 1853 and the English Lunatic Act of 1853.
They were subsequently replaced by the Lunacy Act of 1890, and
amended by the Lunacy Act of 1891.

The Indian Lunacy Act of 1912 defines a lunatic as an idiot or a
person of unsound mind (Section 3 (5)). However the words "idiot"
or a "person of unsound mind" were not defined. Both these terms
are used to indicate an abnormal state of mind as distinguished from
weakness of mind or senility. A man of weak mental strength cannot
be called an idiot or a man of unsound mind. The act was not intended to protect dull-witted persons, but only those who suffer from
mental illness. There are provisions in the act for reception, care, and
treatment of the mentally ill, their discharge from asylums and management of their estates. "Criminal lunatics" and the establishment
of asylums are also covered by the same act. There is provision to
receive voluntary boarders into an asylum based on similar provisions
in the English and Scottish law (supreme court rules). The procedure
prescribed for the issue of reception orders is based on the English
Lunacy Act of 1890 (1).

Indian Psychiatric Society and Its Official Journal

The Indian Psychiatric Society came into being in 1947 by the un-
ceasing energy and initiative of R. B. Davis and N. N. De. Before the

organization of this society, psychiatric interests rested with the Indian branch of the Royal Medico-Psychological Association, which had a membership of about 40. Unfortunately it did not remain active—for four years the branch held no meetings. Its last president was Banarasidas, a former superintendent of Agra Mental Hospital. Attempts to revive it having failed, the Indian Psychiatric Society, an independent association, was organized (14). Its first meeting was held in 1947 in Delhi under the presidency of J. E. Dhunjibhoy, in conjunction with the Annual Conference of the Indian Science Congress. It was reported that 13 members attended this conference. R. B. Davis was the first secretary and treasurer of the Society. The first annual conference was held at Patna in 1948 under the presidency of N. N. De. The official journal of the Society was started in 1949 under the editorship of N. N. De, who subsequently resigned on grounds of ill health. L. P. Varma was entrusted with the editorship in the council meeting of the Indian Psychiatric Society held on January 3, 1951 (17). The journal, initially called the *Indian Journal of Neurology and Psychiatry,* later became the *Indian Journal of Psychiatry,* published quarterly.

REFERENCES

1. All India Reporter Manual (1961): *The Indian Lunacy Act, 1912,* 2nd Ed., Vol. 10, (Eds.) V. V. Chitaley and S. Appu Rao. Bombay: The All India Reporter Ltd.
2. CARAKA SAMHITA (1949): *Cikitsasthana,* Vol. 1, 12, 13. Jamnagar, India: Shree Guleb Kunverba Ayurvedic Society.
3. CARAKA SAMHITA (1949): *Cikitsasthana,* Vol. 5, Chap. 9, Verse 7.
4. CARAKA SAMHITA (1949): Vol. 5 Chap. 1, Verse 46.
5. CARAKA SAMHITA (1949): Vol. 5, Chap. 7, Verse 23.
6. CARAKA SAMHITA (1949): *Cikitsasthana,* Vol. 5, Chap. 9, Verse 82-83.
7. CARAKA SAMHITA (1949): *Cikitsasthana,* Vol. 5, Chap. 9, Verse 86.
8. CARAKA SAMHITA (1949): *Sarirasthana,* Chap. 4, Verses 36-46.
9. CARAKA SAMHITA (1949): *Nidanasthana,* Vol. 5, Chap. 7, Verse 5.
10. CARAKA SAMHITA (1949): *Nidanasthana,* Vol. 5, Chap. 7, Verse 9.
11. CARAKA SAMHITA (1949): *Nidanasthana,* Vol. 5, Chap. 7, Verse 7.
12. DAS GUPTA, S. N. (1951): *A History of Indian Philosophy,* Vol. 1. Cambridge: Cambridge University Press.
13. DAS GUPTA, S. N. (1952): *A History of Indian Philosophy* 2, p. 273-436, Cambridge: Cambridge University Press.
14. DUBEY, K. C. (1953): *Psychiatry in distress,* Presidential address, Annual Conference of the Indian Psychiatric Society. *Indian J. Neurol. Psychiat.,* 4, 101.
15. FREUD, S. (1915): Thoughts for the times on war and death. In: *Collected Papers,* Trans. by J. Riviera. Vol. 4, pp. 288-317. London: Hogarth.
16. HIRIYANNA, M. (1960): *The Essentials of Indian Philosophy,* p. 106-128. London: Allen & Unwin.
17. Indian Psychiatric Society (1951): Minutes of the meeting of the Council. *Indian J. Neurol. Psychiat.,* 3, 94.
18. KUTUMBIAH, P. (1969): *Ancient Indian Medicine.* Madras: Orient Longmans.

19. Lodge Patch, C. J. (1939): *J. Ment. Sci.*, 85, 391.
20. MACDONELL: quoted by Das Gupta.
21. NARAYANASWAMI AIYAR, K. (1914): *Yoga Vasishta* (Laghu), 2nd Ed. Adyar, India: Theosophical Society.
22. RADHAKRISHNAN, S . (1923): *Indian Philosophy*, Vol. 1, p. 119. London: Allen & Unwin Ltd.
23. RADHAKRISHNAN, S. (1927): *Indian Philosophy*, Vol. 2. London: Allen & Unwin.
24. RADHAKRISHNAN, S. (1949): *The Bhagavad Gita,* Chap. 14. London: Allen & Unwin.
25. RAJAGOPALACHARI, C. (1958): *Mahabharata* (Eds.) K. M. Munshi and R. R. Diwakar. Bombay: Bhavan University, Bharatiya Vidya Bhavan.
26. RAMACHANDRA RAO, S. K. (1960): *Samkara, A Psychological Study.* Mysore, India: Kavyalaya Publishers.
27. RAMACHANDRA RAO, S. K. (1962): *Development of Psychological Thought in India.* Mysore, India: Kavyalaya Publishers.
28. SARMA, D. S. (1961): *An Anthology of Upanishads* (Eds.) K. M. Munshi and R. R. Diwakar. Bombay: Bhavan University, Bharatiya Vidya Bhavan.
29. SHARMA, P. (1968): *Dravyaguna Vijnan,* Vol. 2. Benares, India: Chowkamba Vidya Bhavan.
30. SIDDHANTALANKAR, S. (1969): *Heritage of Vedic Culture.* Bombay: Taraporevala & Sons.
31. SINHA, J. (1958, 1961): *Indian Psychology,* Vols. 1 & 2. Calcutta: Sinha Publishing House.
32. SWARUPANANDA SWAMI (1909): *The Bhagavad Gita,* Chap. 11, Verses 62-63. Mayavati, Himalayas: Advaita Ashram.
33. THAKUR, U. (1963): *The History of Suicide in India.* Delhi: Munshiram Manoharlal.
34. VAHIA, N. S., VINEKAR, S. L., & DOONGAJI, D. R. (1966): Some ancient Indian concepts in the treatment of psychiatric disorders. *Brit. J. Psychiat.,* 112, 1080.
35. VAHIA, N. S. (1971): Personal communication.
36. VARMA, L. P. (1953): History of psychiatry in India and Pakistan. *Indian J. Neurol. Psychiat.,* 4, 26.
37. VARMA, L. P. (1953): History of psychiatry in India and Pakistan. *Indian J. Neurol. Psychiat.,* 4, 138.
38. VARMA, L. P. (1965): Psychiatry in Ayurveda. *Indian J. Psychiat.,* 7, 292.
39. VENKOBA, RAO, A. (1964): Some ancient Indian concepts of mind, insanity and mental hygiene. *Indian J. Hist. Med.,* 9, 13.
40. VENKOBA RAO, A. (1966): Dreams—some gleanings from Upanishads. *Indian J. Hist. Med.,* 11, 13.
41. VENKOBA RAO, A. (1969): History of depression—some aspects. *Indian J. Hist. Med.,* 14, 46.
42. VENKOBA RAO, A. (1971): The seat of mind—some ancient considerations. *Indian J. Hist. Med.,* 16, 1.
43. VENKOBA RAO, A. (1971): Homeostasis—some Indian philosophical and psychological concepts. In: *Walter Cannon Centenary Commemorative Volume.* Published and edited by S. Parvathi Devi and A. Venkoba Rao, Madurai.

27

THAILAND

PHON SANGSINGKEO, M.D.

Special Consultant to the Director,
SEATO Medical Research Laboratory,
Bangkok, Thailand

1

INTRODUCTION

The history of psychiatry has had a long evolution, as had other branches of medical science. Psychiatry existed from the creation of the earth. When there is more than one man, opinions differ. When emotions are disturbed, symptoms of disease may appear. When these symptoms cannot be understood, they become a mystery.

In antiquity, mental illness was attributed to the intervention of gods, angels, ghosts, and spirits, who took control of the lives of men. When anyone was affected by mental illness, it was said that he or she was in the power of these forces and was possessed by a ghost or spirit. Protection was sought through sacred rituals and objects such as holy cloth and other materials. These superstitions still exist in parts of Thailand today.

In the North and North-Eastern provinces, people believe in *phii pob,* a spirit that can take the form of any human being. It is supposed to be the cause of illnesses similar to the effects of the "prescribed poison" found in the Southern provinces. Particular people are believed to be *phii pobs* and are regarded with fear and dislike. *Phii bah* (crazy ghost) is another term used for certain people who are obviously lunatic. They are so called because they are believed to be possessed by ghosts. When they have recovered from their mental illness they are believed to have expelled the spirits from their bodies, and they are then allowed to live normally in the community without being avoided by other people. This belief that the convalescent patient is now free from spirit possession makes people willing to accept them and helps the patients psychologically by enabling them to live a normal life. The conception of *phii pob* and *phii bah* is also useful in relieving people of the burden to try to explain phenomena beyond their understanding.

Treatment in the old days was carried out according to local belief. Some people preferred to pray at their sacred temples, some preferred the witch doctors to perform ceremonies to drive away spirits, whereas others would drink water from holy wells. Holy wells in central Thailand still exist today. An example of them is Phran Boon Larng Nuer, near Saraburi province. The legend is that, at the time when Sri Ayudhya was the capital city, Phran Boon (a hunter by the name of Boon) went hunting for deer with bow and arrow. He wounded a deer with an arrow but it managed to run away into a deep forest. When it reappeared it was again fresh and strong. The hunter explored the forest and discovered a well full of clear water. It was believed that the deer drank that water and thereby recovered from its wound. This belief was so widespread that the well came to be considered holy. People suffering from mental illness or nervous disease often went there to bathe and drink the holy water. If the patient still had not recovered from his insanity after these mild ministrations, he would then be chained. If he remained hysterical, he might be beaten unconscious. For a long time it was customary to chain patients; since relatives did not know of any other way to restrain a patient, they put him in chains to prevent him from doing them any harm. This practice is now gradually disappearing.

2

THE BUILDING OF MENTAL HOSPITALS

The First Asylum

When misconceptions faded and more humanitarian treatment of the mentally ill was adopted, the era of hospital-building emerged. The first mental hospital in Thailand was established in 1889 at Klong Sarn, Dhonburi, a sister city of Bangkok. This oldest establishment for mental patients was not a "hospital," as we understand it today, but an asylum. The original building, situated on the west side of the Chaophya River at Klong Sarn, was founded during the reign of the fifth king of the present dynasty: King Chulalongkorn. Other hospitals were built during the same period (Siriraj Hospital, Burapa Hospital, and Bangrak Hospital). The mental hospital was a building originally owned by a businessman, Phra Bhakdi, who donated it to the king. When first opened, on November 1, 1889, it had 30 patients, the administration was under the control of the ministry of education, and the original intention was limited to confining mental patients, because they were unable to live together with patients in other hospitals. Therefore imprisonment and chaining took the place of treatment. Occasionally there was some treatment in the form of herbs and "magic."

European Influence

Late in the year 1905, Thai medical science advanced into a new phase. A medical health unit was established in the local ministry which included a hospital for mental patients known as Pak Klong Sarn Mental Hospital. The supervisor of this hospital had a rather primitive medical education, but the administration was under the control of an Englishman, a government official, H. Campbell Hyed, head of the medical health unit during that period, and he was consequently the first doctor to administer the original Pak Klong Sarn Mental Hospital. Unfortunately, he had very little time to supervise the hospital personally, because his position as head of the medical health unit burdened him with many other duties. He could visit the hospital only once in several months, or even in a year.

According to the records of 1910 there were 296 mental patients admitted to the hospital, a much higher figure than before. But supervision was still shamefully neglected. In the report of Hyed dated September 14, 1910, he said ". . . there are 264 male patients and 32 female. Out of these 54 patients are dangerous and may attack at any time. These are kept separately. But due to shortage of room some of them have to be kept together and often fight each other. Some are chained to the floor like fierce animals. Some of the rooms need repairs badly and cannot be kept clean. This accounts for the diarrhea and dysentery suffered by the patients. This hospital is shamefully falling apart. It is quite apparent that the government should do something to improve it. I myself cannot find stronger words to show how humiliated and disgusted I am." This report gave a picture of conditions similar to those deplored by Phillipe Pinel in France, and by many others during these early times, when negligence and ill treatment eventually gave place to the unchaining of patients and the improving of hospitals in the name of humanity.

In Thailand, at the beginning of this century, the government decided in favor of building a new mental hospital on the site of the present Somdej Chaophya Hospital. The land totalled 17 acres, and was located less than a kilometer north of the original Klong Sarn. It was purchased from the families of Somdej Chaophya and others. The building was completed and opened in September, 1912. Treatment changed from the old methods of imprisonment and primitive medicine to those of modern medicine. Food and accommodations were improved, chaining was abolished, and the staff tried to run it as any other hospital, despite the fact that some wooden buildings were fitted with bars and patients had to sleep on the floor.

The building of the present Somdej Chaophya Mental Hospital, known as Hospital for the Insane in 1912, was under the care of M. Cathew, who was Hyed's direct subordinate.

Cathew, the English doctor who took over the directorship of the hospital, was the first chief of the new mental hospital. He was not a psychiatrist. His task was to keep patients from endangering the public and at the same time treat their physical ailments. Patients' rooms resembled cells in a prison and were surrounded with bars, but they were also bright and comfortable thanks to Thailand's hot climate. The buildings had no windows, but had red roofs similar to buildings commonly seen in England. The structure of the building was changed later, during and after World War II (Plate CXXI).

Since Cathew was the first true physician-administrator of the newly built hospital and personally supervised patients, a number of documents describing his work have been preserved. His character is well depicted by the Chinese and Thai saying, ". . . holding a whip in the right hand and a money bag in the left." Although he was not a psychiatrist, he was well versed in psychiatric theories. He was much influenced in his practice by the English way of thinking and the methods of Conolly, who advocated "treatment without chains." Not only did he participate in planning the hospital, but he also created a masterpiece by designing the green and peaceful orchard. The many kinds of trees seen there today reflect Cathew's conception. He insisted that at least part of the orchard be preserved because it was a symbol of release and peace of mind. Cathew was later given the rank of Phraya Aryuravej Vichak—an honor similar to a knighthood—which was bestowed on him by the King.

The next director of the mental hospital was R. Mandelson, well known personal surgeon to King Vajiravudh. He was simultaneously the director of the Central Hospital and assistant chief of the Medical Health Unit in Bangkok. With so many responsibilities, there was not much evidence of his work at the mental hospital. However, he arranged for Thai doctors who had graduated in modern medicine to

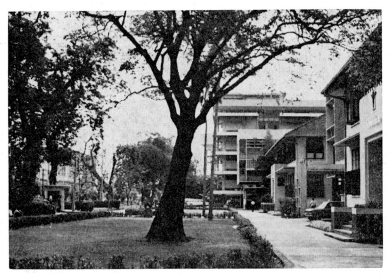

PLATE CXXI. Somdej Chaophya Mental Hospital today.

take turns in supervising the hospital; they were then called "doctors in charge." Six doctors undertook this task in 1922.

Takeover by Thai Physicians

Supervision continued in this way until 1925, when all the European doctors were discharged. The first Thai director was Luang Vichien (Plate CXXII). He greatly changed the administration of mental hospitals, and also changed the name of the hospital from "Hospital for Insane" to "Mental Hospital." In 1929, he became the first Thai medical doctor to study in the United States, where he underwent postgraduate training in psychiatry. When Luang Vichien returned, in 1931, he concentrated on developing the hospital, its welfare, and especially hospital discipline. He began lectures in psychiatry at the medical college and lectures on mental health for teachers and for the public.

In 1918, when a public health department was established within

the ministry of the interior, the hospital was transferred to the jurisdiction of the public health department. The number of patients
treated was steadily increasing. In 1926, there were 721 patients, although the hospital was designed to hold only 430 patients. The
situation was very unsatisfactory and necessitated the discharge of

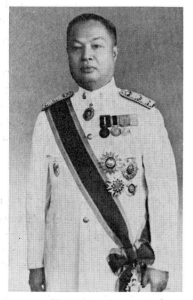

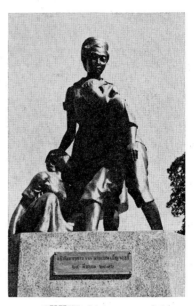

PLATE CXXII. Dr. Luang Vichien, the first Thai Director, Somdej Chaophya Hospital.

PLATE CXXIII. Monument of Sympathy, Somdej Chaophya Hospital.

Chinese patients, who had immigrated from China and were now
returned to their native country. Later, however, many of them came
back. Two more buildings were erected to accommodate 100 patients,
but space was still insufficient. In 1929 the "Convicts' Ward," was
constructed in cooperation with the penitentiary department. This
ward was used for patients who were convicted of serious crimes; it
accommodated up to 50 patients. In 1936 V. Teek Pao donated a sum
for building a hospital ward, the first to be built by public donation;
it accommodated 40 patients.

In order to relieve the crowding of patients at Dhonburi, and dis-
tribute them more evenly throughout the country, another mental
hospital was built in 1937 in the southern part of Thailand, in the

Surath province. In 1938, another mental hospital was built in the northern part of Thailand, in the Lampang province, and was later removed to the Chiang Mai province.

It is interesting to note that, although hospitals were built in different parts of the country, the number of mental patients at Dhonburi did not decrease. Records show that, in 1940, there were still 1,100 patients there. It was therefore necessary to transfer some of the patients to a new hospital in Nondhaburi, a suburb of Bangkok, which was built in 1941. This hospital was built to serve Central Thailand; in addition to treatment it offered rehabilitation of patients by industrial and agricultural training.

Phon Sangsingkeo, who was trained in psychiatry in the United States and had been the previous assistant to the director, was appointed director of Dhonburi Hospital in 1942. He devoted his time and energy not only to the construction of a hospital of the open-ward type but also to the training of personnel and the revising of curricula for medical undergraduates and other professional groups.

Establishment of a Ministry of Public Health

On March 10, 1942, the Ministry of Public Health was established, including a Medical Services Department. The mental hospitals were then transferred to the jurisdiction of the Medical Services Department, which is now responsible for all hospitals in the kingdom. The mental hospitals division is responsible for all mental hospitals and for all mental health services.

The year 1943 marked the beginning of a drastic reorganization of both the administration and the technical aspects of the hospital in Dhonburi, with the aim of establishing a clinic equal to the best international standards and a determination to destroy misconceptions about mental hospitals and mental patients. By sympathy and kindness and within the limits of personnel and funds available the hospital was greatly improved. The bars installed in 1912 were demolished and living quarters were rebuilt and furnished with new beds; a new system of sewage disposal was installed. Doctors, nurses, and other officials were reoriented to modern medical practice. The educational system, in cooperation with the university school of medicine, was improved and expanded to international standards. All these changes were made possible by government budget allocations and public donations. In 1943 and 1944, during World War II, the price of iron rose, so the hospital disposed of iron bars and built wooden wards instead. Income from the sale of iron was utilized in building a new ward at Nondhaburi. Two hundred patients were then transferred there to work in the rice paddies as occupational therapy.

In 1943 King Rama VIII, Ananta Mahidol, graciously donated his private income for the rebuilding of the male section ward at Dhonburi.

The amount of treatment and the number of consultations provided for out-patients increased year by year due to the greater number of patients and the better results of in-patient treatment. Therefore, in 1948, after five years of effort, a grant was obtained to build a new out-patient section, a reinforced concrete and brick structure. This ward included offices for the doctors and other administrative officials. The modern buildings helped raise the status of the mental hospital to the same level as other good hospitals. The public began to regard the hospital with more interest and less prejudice.

Misconceptions, fear, and contempt for mental patients are hard to dispel, especially when the public has no firsthand experience of mental hospitals. A well-to-do merchant whose son was sent to a mental hospital provides an example of how public opinion changes. This merchant could not bring himself to visit his son, fearing that he would have to see his son being hurt. But one day he could not resist the longing for his son, and he asked for permission to visit him. When he got to the hospital, things were not as he expected; he saw no torture, no imprisonment. What he did see was kindness. Patients were allowed to walk around, and his son was improving amazingly. The merchant was so impressed by what he saw that he asked for permission to build a memorial in front of the male section of the hospital. It was named "Monument of Sympathy" and represents a nurse, standing with a male and female patient on each side, showing love and pleasure. The monument stands today (Plate CXXIII).

Other patients' relatives began to be interested and to trust the hospital. In 1949, Lady Jotika Rajsethi expressed her wish to build a new solid brick ward. The hospital took this opportunity to hold its annual fair. Money received was used to buy medical equipment and beds for the patients.

For the sake of decentralization and service to the people of the North-Eastern region of Thailand, another psychiatric hospital with all out-patient facilities was built at Ubol province late in 1946. For the first two years, a rota of psychiatrists from Dhonburi was assigned to take charge of Ubol Hospital.

The Naming of Hospitals

We now call all the hospitals by their individual names, and not "mental hospitals." This helps people to regard mental illness as any other disease and promotes better feelings among the patients and their relatives. It also helps to destroy misconceptions among the public regarding mental hospitals. A hospital may be named after the locality in which it is situated, or after an ancestor who was highly respected, or a sacred figure in people's faith. Thus, the mental hospital in Dhonburi is named Somdej Chao Phaya Hospital, after the name of a person and the locality. The mental hospital of Chiang Mai is called Suan Proong after the name of the locality. The mental hospital in the Ubol province is named Phra Sri Mahabhodi after the most sacred possession of that province, the sacred Bhodi tree brought from Ceylon and worshipped by the people. The mental hospital in Nondhaburi was named to enhance the pride of its locality, which produces good rice, and hence the name Srithunya. The naming of the mental hospital in Surath has a charming story. The Hospital is situated on a beautiful small hill that used to be occupied by the regent of the old Surath region, and was often visited by the sixth king who admired the beautiful and fresh terrain. He graciously named the hill *"Suan Sararnrom,"* meaning "happy garden." Later, when a mental hospital was built there, the name Suan Sararnrom was adopted.

3

THE LAST PHASE

The history of the work for promotion of mental health in Thailand began with treatment of patients in the hospital, and only later reached out to the public. Therefore the work and the study of mental health in Thailand began at the psychiatric hospital.

Child psychiatry also has been developed in recent years, with emphasis on the early treatment of mental disorders and the promotion of preventive measures. Study of mental health at day clinics is not adequate, but the necessary facilities for some mentally sick children to be fully cared for day and night do include hospitals that can be true centers for the study of child psychiatry. To this end a hospital for child psychiatry has been built at Samrong. The site of this hospital has been contributed for the public welfare by Luang Vitayes, a senior Thai physician. The hospital was opened to the public in 1965.

In 1953 the medical services department, with the cooperation of the World Health Organization, built a mental health clinic at Somdej Chao Phaya Hospital. Margaret Stepan, a World Health Organization psychologist, joined the staff of the Mental Hygiene Clinic, with Subha Malakul as its first and present chief.

Two years later, the service was extended to patients with neurotic and neurological disorders; these were 30 times as many as the number of strictly psychiatric in-patients. The service was also extended to psychiatric patients who were at an earlier stage of their illness, as it was appreciated that if they were treated at the first indication of mental abnormality, it might be much more beneficial to their health and future than later treatment. Once healthy, they could participate in the economic development of the country. Consequently it was decided to build another neurological hospital at Phaya Thai, Bangkok. This was accomplished through the government budget and public donations. Later, the King donated funds received from benefit performances and other sources to build a neurological research unit, so that more research in this field could be done. The director is Prasop Ratanakorn. Work at the Prasart Hospital advanced rapidly in a very short time and more cooperation with international agencies of study and research has been achieved. This hospital later changed its name to Hospital and Research Institute in Neurology.

Arun Bhaksuwan was the successor of Phon Sangsingkeo as director in 1958. He was also trained in psychiatry in the United States and was the previous assistant to the director. With the support of the government he has changed most of the hospital wooden buildings to concrete and brick structures, recruited more trained staff, and participated more in the education of medical students and professional groups, raising the status of the hospital to that of a teaching center.

King Rama IX, Bhumiphol Adulyadej, donated income from the showing of the film of his visit to southern Thailand to build a ward for special patients which was opened to the public in June, 1960. Through His Majesty's kindness, people themselves became more kind and friendly to patients. Later this hospital was expanded; buildings were added, including some for education and in-service training, and residential quarters for government officials and aides.

In every mental hospital, there are some retarded patients who also suffer from mental illnesses. These people are a serious problem to society, since they cannot help themselves. Therefore, it is imperative that they be treated in a separate institution, and trained to be useful in society and the public in the future. In 1960, a hospital for mentally handicapped people was built at Samsaen, Bangkok; Roschong Tasnanjali is the director.

In 1966, Thanyarak Hospital, with Prayoon Norakanphadung as director, was established to treat patients addicted to drugs; this hospital is situated at Klong Rangsit, north of Bangkok. Since 1959, in Thanyaburi, 12 kilometers east of the present site, there has been a sanatorium with wards for drug addicts. Wards for this category of patients also exist in some provincial hospitals. This is in accordance with the United Nations desire to eradicate opium traffic and addiction.

There is also a need for mental hospitals in North-East Thailand, a surrounding area, which holds one-third of the population of the whole country. Up to the present time there has been only one hospital in that region, in the Ubol Province. The establishment of another hospital in the Khonkaen Province was approved; it was completed in 1971, with Udom Laksanavicharn as its director. This hospital will also serve as an institution for nursing education, and for the training of university students, especially medical students.

The number of mental patients who commit crimes while they are mentally ill has been increasing. Thus far there have been no special places besides mental hospitals where they could receive proper treatment. Hence, the government approved the building of a Forensic Psychiatry Hospital in the Dhonburi Province. This hospital was completed in 1971 with Yanyong Bhotharamic as the director.

Trying to overcome people's fears and getting them to accept the mental patient in their families is very difficult, due to superstition and economic, social, and environmental factors. Nevertheless, in 1946 there was a general effort to organize living quarters for mental patients, enabling them to live and work outside the hospitals. In 1958, the first halfway house was opened in Thailand, supervised by Sritanya Hospital. Convalescent patients are allowed to work at a farming village, and are thus provided with a livelihood. Later, they are discharged to live with their families and society. Day hospitals were also established at Somdej Chao Phya Hospital in 1960.

Since 1933, the old tradition of unity of body and mind has again been recognized in Thailand; thus, the study of psychiatry has been included in the curriculum of medical students. The new government has initiated an enlightened program whereby students do part of their training at mental hospitals and are given the opportunity to undertake postgraduate courses in psychiatry and neurology in Europe and in the United States. Interest in psychiatric training includes the nursing school.

A revision of the curriculum was completed, in 1955, with the cooperation of the Thai government, the World Health Organization and the U.S. AID. Problems of shortage of teaching staff were overcome by cooperation with the Medical College Hospital and a four-year program, amounting to 204 hours, was evolved. The first psychiatric ward in a school of medicine was established in 1962 at Chularlongkorn Hospital and was followed by similar developments, which included a department of psychiatry in each school of medicine. The first of these was opened in 1969 in Siriraj.

Since 1945, a one-year course in psychiatry for nursing aids has been established in Dhonburi by the mental hospital division of the medical department. Postgraduate, residential training courses in psychiatry have also been established since 1954. In the same year, the Thailand Psychiatric Association came into being and was followed, in 1958, by the foundation of the Mental Health Association.

Statistics show that in Thailand there are four mental patients in every 1,000 persons. Therefore, with 35,000,000 people there are 140,000 mental patients, and we have hospitals sufficient to accommodate only 7,000 patients. The remaining 133,000 patients must stay at home or be cared for in other places. Therefore it is preferable to work with the public by promoting community health centers, clinics, and health education.

The present-day trend for psychiatry in the general hospital and for community psychiatry is spreading to Thailand. This will not only increase the number of mental patients who benefit from proper care, but will also improve the quality of the services offered.

28

THE FAR EAST
Reflections on the Psychological Foundations

ILZA VEITH, PH.D.

Professor and Vice-Chairman, Department of the History of Health Sciences, University of California, San Francisco San Francisco, California, U.S.A.

Every sect has its truth, and
Every truth has its sect.
(*Chinese Proverb*)

1

INTRODUCTION

The history of psychiatry in Eastern Asia has never been systematically pursued, which is, in all probability, a reflection of the fact that psychiatry itself has not been systematically practiced in those regions which we have come to describe as the "Far East." Although this description is geographically correct only so far as the European point of view is concerned, it has also become meaningful by usage and connotation to the Americans for whom the *Extrême Orient* is located in the "Far West."

But whether it is the Far West or the Far East, there is implied in the latter expression a notion of great distance and the "ultimate" of the orient, even if its geographic beginning is not perceived in the American continent. Travelers, from the 16th century on, soon became conscious of the fact that their destination was the gate, not to one but to a whole series of vastly different and exotic civilizations,

662

and those who had a professional interest in the nature and composition of civilizations made it their business to pay attention to this change. Among them there were those whose aim in life was to bring about conformity—conformity in religions and mores; in short, the missionaries of all denominations.

What they, rather than historians or sociologists, considered and recorded first and foremost were the deviations from what in their unwavering belief was the norm. Still, the missions were made up not only of the clergy proper but also of adjuvant professions, particularly physicians and nursing personnel. It is this group, less prepossessed perhaps and somewhat scientifically trained, that first furnished palpable evidence, not exclusively of exotic religious beliefs observed, but of the emotional climate in general in the Far East and of the concern with mental aberration. Their reports were complemented by descriptions from merchants in the service of the various East India companies stationed in outposts in China and Japan, the territories that came to be known as the Far East.

Even more than the religious tenets of Judeo-Christian beliefs influenced the emotional climate of the West, have religious considerations guided the behavioral attitude of Far Eastern man toward health and disease. This hardly facilitated the investigation, as most of the early Western observers, whether merchants, scientists, or missionaries, were devout Christians and their attention was first drawn to the differences in the religious practices they witnessed. Moreover, they tended to look down upon the adherents of foreign faiths as heathens, and upon their worship as deviant behavior. The situation, of course, was further complicated by the difficulty of communicating in a common language. Hence the behavior on both sides was open to the most farfetched interpretations.

On the whole, the Western observers soon came to specific conclusions concerning the mental health of the incomprehensible, enigmatically exotic, yet seemingly calm peoples of the Far East. Most impressive were the Chinese, whose apparent passivity and serenity convinced the uncomprehending visitors of the near total absence of mental disease (25).*

In reporting about their impression of the Chinese as self-restrained and even phlegmatic, the Western observers were entirely unaware that notorious episodes of mass hysteria had repeatedly disturbed

---

* A good example for such statements in belletristic literature is the following: "There is almost no insanity among the Chinese now—almost none among those who have stayed at home and have given the treaty ports a wide berth. In the old days there was no insanity in all of China." (13)

the calm of the Middle Kingdom.* Although we have already seen how superficially the belief in Chinese equanimity must have come into being, there is no other evidence to prove or disprove the observations of the early visitors on the relative infrequency of mental disorders among individuals or groups of Chinese.

It is of interest, rather, to see the Chinese and the Japanese as the first Western visitors saw them, and to reconstruct from their reports, and from the religious beliefs and practices of the Orient three or four centuries ago the personality of the Asians as they must have appeared to the emissaries of the West. And, so far as China is concerned, it did seem to the Western visitor that the Chinese, at least, were almost completely free from the scourge of mental disease.

Western psychiatry entered Chinese medical thinking only very recently. The first mental hospital accommodating 30 patients was opened in 1897, in Canton; but although it grew into a 500-bed institution, it had to close its door after only 40 years of existence. The small number of additional mental hospitals founded in succeeding years fared little better, and in the course of the Pacific War in the 1930's and 1940's almost all of them were terminated (24). It was only after the conclusion of that war that psychiatry became a recognized specialty in Chinese medical schools.

2

THE TRADITIONAL PSYCHOLOGICAL FOUNDATIONS

In view of this late and scant acceptance of Western psychiatric endeavors in China it is of interest to study the earlier Chinese medical literature for traces of indigenous thought on mental health and mental healings. It is also of interest to examine the structure of traditional Chinese society for reasons why psychiatry in the Western sense of the word was neither developed in China nor took hold after it was introduced there from the West. The study of Chinese medical literature reveals an early awareness of the mind-body relationship and a profound understanding of what is now called psychosomatic medicine. There is relatively little mention of insanity, although it

---

* See Henri Maspéro: *Melanges posthumes sur les religions et l'histoire de la Chine,* Paris, 1950, pp. 163-169, for a description of the Yellow Turbans (184 A.D.). Other such movements were the T'ai-p'ing rebellion and the Boxer uprising, and to a lesser degree, the uprisings caused by the Red Eyebrows (25 A.D.) and the many other secret societies which were formed after the pattern of the Yellow Turbans.

undoubtedly existed as is indicated by a number of ideographs denoting mental alienations.

One ideograph was: *tien k'uang*, which may be translated in various ways as "mad, deranged, infatuated, insane, delirious, or simply crazy." The expression *tien k'uang*, like the one associated with the ideograph for wind disease, *feng k'uang*, suffers from an even greater vagueness and lack of definition than do such English expressions as madness, insanity, or perturbation. Because of the composition of the character *k'uang*, which makes up part of the above-mentioned terminology, and the character *chiao*, also denoting mental abnormality, we know that consciousness, perception, and comprehension, as well as their disturbances, were always associated with vision (i.e., disturbances of sight). It is difficult, therefore, to determine—even from context—whether these ideographs denote a permanent impairment of the mental faculties or a temporary derangement, possibly caused by fever delirium.

According to the oldest Chinese medical writings any disease, but particularly mental disease, was caused by an imbalance of the two primary forces in man: the *yin* and the *yang*. These two forces which stand for the negative and the positive, the dark and the light, the moon and the sun, the noxious and the beneficial, also denote the female and male elements, both of which are ever-present in man and woman alike. Disease arises when the proportions of the two elements begin to vary from the normal.

This is not the place to go into detail about the fanciful variations that can be achieved by the two hypothetical forces, *yin* and *yang*. For the purpose of this chapter it is important only to realize the strangely penetrating awareness of a bipolarity, a dual force, within every human being, a consciousness that within man there is something female, and something masculine within woman. Of greater significance is the alleged cause for the imbalance of *yin* and *yang*. This imbalance, it was believed, was caused by the patient himself, who had committed a transgression by deviating from the prescribed way of nature and society. It was this concept of the "way," known in Chinese as the *Tao*, which provided the guiding principle of all human conduct.

By means of these seemingly abstract theories, the ancient Chinese arrived at two extremely important conclusions: first, that disease is rarely localized but generally affects the entire human being; and second, that disease is often associated with behavior, i.e., guilt about the infringement of a natural law. The following passages translated from the oldest Chinese medical book illustrate these points (22):

Just as the breath of the blue sky is calm so the will and the heart of those who are pure will be in peace, and the breath of Yang will be stable in those who keep themselves in harmony with nature. Those who fail to preserve good-conduct will [find] . . . the breath of protection lost to them.

Man's fear and apprehension, his passion and his suffering, his motion and his rest, they all cause changes [within the body and the mind].

Those who act contrary to the laws of the four seasons . . . dissipate in their duties and if Yin is not equal to Yang, the pulse become weak and madness results (19).

In spite of their antiquity—or rather because of it—the passages continued to be expressive of what we now term psychiatric thinking throughout the history of Chinese medicine proper and, in large areas of China, even after the arrival of Western psychiatric teaching. In order to appreciate this, we must be aware of the Chinese predilection for ancient authorities which helped to preserve their oldest medical classics as the basis of all subsequent medical thinking. While, as will be shown below, in the more recent centuries demoniacal possession, the spirit of vengeful ancestors, and similar superhuman phenomena have been credited with causing mental disease, this was believed by unlearned and socially inferior persons only. Persons of education and social standing concurred in their theories on the origin of mental disease with the traditional view of the medical writers.

Unlike other cultures, the Chinese never personified a figure of a creator who might demand adoration and obedience and punish transgression. Instead of believing in one all-powerful creator, the Chinese conceived of creation as having been accomplished by *Tao*, an impersonal force, which continued to exist as the physical and spiritual guide of the universe and the individual. In the medical texts the spiritual requirements of the *Tao* were simply life in accord with the laws of nature; or, perhaps somewhat more concretely, the fulfillment of the requirements of the seasons. The philosophers, however, elaborated and specified the *Tao* and built around it an ethical superstructure that provided for all eventualities in life and for all essential types of interpersonal relationships. In doing so they still did not create a watchful and punishing god, but rather achieved a means for society to guide itself and, more important even, for the individual to be the chief guardian and judge of his own conduct (22). Nevertheless, there came to exist with the introduction of Buddhism into China in the 5th century a well-developed system of belief in guilt and sin, salvation and perdition, the latter with a veritable hierarchy of hells of various degrees of severity (7).

All the so-called Confucian classics, including the writings of Mencius, could serve to illustrate this point. I shall, however, restrict myself to a few quotations from the book on *Filial Piety* and the *Analects* (16), for they contain the essential maxims of Chinese conduct.

> Filial piety is the root of all virtues and (the stem) out of which grows (all moral) teaching.

> In filial piety there is nothing greater than the reverential awe of one's father. In the reverential awe shown to one's father there is nothing greater than the making him the correlate of Heaven.

> The service which a filial son does to his parents is as follows: in his general conduct to them, he manifests the utmost reverence; in his nourishing of them, his endeavor is to give them the utmost pleasure; when they are ill, he feels the greatest anxiety; in mourning for them, he exhibits every demonstration of grief; in sacrificing to them, he displays the utmost solemnity.

> Anciently, the intelligent kings served their fathers with filial piety, and therefore they served Heaven with intelligence; they served their mothers with filial piety, and therefore they served Earth with discrimination.

> Therefore even the Son of Heaven [the emperor] must have some whom he honors. . . . In the ancestral temple he manifests the utmost reverence . . . he cultivates his person and is careful of his conduct, fearing lest he should disgrace his predecessors.

In the *Analects* we find the expression of very similar sentiments: "asked what constituted the superior man, the Master [Confucius] said, 'he acts before he speaks, and afterwards speaks according to his actions'" (II: xxiii). Confucius also said: "A youth, when at home, should be filial, and abroad, respectful to his elders. He should be earnest and truthful and cultivate the friendship of the good" (I: iv). "The student of virtue has no contentions" (III: vii) for "filial piety and fraternal submission! Are they not the root of all benevolent actions?" (I: ii).

Confucius also quoted other sages to corroborate his own opinion. Thus it is stated in the *Analects*: "The philosopher Tsang said: 'Let there be a careful attention to the performance of the funeral rites to parents, and let them be followed when long gone with the ceremonies of sacrifice; then the virtue of the people will resume its proper excellence'" (I: ix) (14).

Ancestor worship is certainly not reserved to China and Japan but has been practiced in many other, even Western cultures. An impressive parallel may be found in the history of ancient Rome where the *lares* and *penates,* the ancestral spirits, became the spiritual protectors of the household who were in charge of the well-being of the family and its continuity. If we compare the Roman family with that of China, we find that the former never arrogated unto itself the supremacy that was maintained by the Chinese family. The Roman family, in fact, aimed at nothing so much as at being a building block of the strong and mighty state. Similarly the *lares* and *penates,* the Roman ancestral spirits, were simply household gods and never claimed ascendency over the national deities as they did in China.

As William Haas so cogently explained, the Roman state derived its external power and internal strength from its close relation with the family. In China, however, state and family never merged and they remained strangers to each other; the Chinese family, in fact, "tended to make it difficult for the state to assert its full authority" (9).

Haas also points out that in all advanced civilizations it is the clergy and the military aristocracy that vie with each other for the leading positions in state and society. Only in China, owing to its dependence on agriculture and nature, was it the farmer who maintained the leading position in society. In the general esteem of society the farmer had to compete with the scholar whose social advantage was evident, inasmuch as he must have passed the all-important examination upon the happy outcome of which depended all positions in government and local offices. Thus, not only Chinese society but also the orderly function of the government and its material progress rested on both the farmer and scholar. It is clear that the patriarchal agricultural family was best able to worship its ancestors, as the burial place was located on the family property. In all probability the origins of the ancestor cult can be traced back to the earliest days of animistic religion when the belief in the continued existence and benevolent disposition of the deceased gave reassurance to the surviving members of the family. Interestingly, there existed in China rigid social distinctions in the form of ancestor worship. These distinctions arose from the form in which the emperor conferred nobility upon a family. It was in fact the emperor who designated the number of ancestors a family was permitted to venerate. Advancement in position and rank was expressed by permission to venerate yet another more distant ancestor. Eventually, ancestor worship spread beyond the aristocracy and permeated the entire Chinese society and thus became the essential feature of the Chinese family.

The patriarchal family was the most important factor in Chinese society. While in the aggregate the family, or rather, the many families, gave power and cohesion to the state, they yet remained—each one of the families—a disparate unit and thus a little state within the State.

As has been shown in the preceding discussions and the Confucian writings quoted above, most of the veneration accorded in other cultures to a superhuman being, or beings, was in China devoted to the father, to the family, and, above all, to the ancestors. But this veneration went beyond service, tangible offerings, and prayers; it entailed a moral conduct beyond the reproach of the living and the dead. Needless to say, this rigid, lifelong obedience to the family hierarchy and the family honor must have imposed a severe psychological strain on many individuals. But so long as it was the standard of behavior among the majority of the people, it was accepted without question, especially since the solidarity of the family also conveyed a deep sense of security upon the individual. This is borne out by a study of traditional Chinese literature, prose, poetry, and drama alike, where any deviation from filial piety was treated with horror, shame, and perhaps occasional pity.

The devotion to family and ancestors was accompanied by yet another phenomenon which helped to guard the sanctity of irreprochable personal conduct. It is the concept of the "face" (10, 11), which had arisen as early as the 4th century B.C. Around it there developed a specific terminology, some of which has been assimilated by other languages, though perhaps not with the full weight of the original meaning. In the Western world we are all familiar with expressions such as "to lose face" and to "save face"; but we do not employ such terms as "to lose face for someone else," "to add to one's face," "to pad one's face," "to have no face," and all the other possible variations of this concept.

In the words of Hsien-chin Hu, *mien* or "face" refers to the confidence of society in the moral character of ego. The concept of sin does not figure to any great extent in Chinese culture, but the assumption of human nature as inherently good places on the individual the responsibility of training his character according to his own light and not the demands of his status. *Mien* is both a social sanction for enforcing moral standards and an internalized sanction (11).

It is undoubtedly true that the consistent public supervision of personal conduct has had a significant influence on the behavior pattern of the Chinese people, and it has certainly produced extreme sensitivity in some. The loss of face for the student who fails to pass his examination, and the loss of face of the suitor who fails to win his bride are almost irreparable. These and other defeats have led to extremely serious consequences. They have been contributing factors to acute psychoses (28) and have even led to suicide, which is extremely rare in China, as it is considered offensive to the spirit of ancestral devotion. While students can do little to protect themselves from the trauma of failure in examinations, other situations make possible the employment of middlemen, who sound out the situation and prevent the voicing of a rejecting staetement. For this reason the go-between in courtship, business, diplomacy, and politics is an important figure. On the whole, however, the intricacies of "face" are conducive to highly circumspect behavior; thus in many respects the concept of "face" removes frictions from interpersonal relationships which have grated upon the sensitivities of Western people.

I have described at some length the concepts of the *Tao,* filial piety, and "face," for they constitute the psychological foundation of the traditional Chinese personality. By no means do they negate or confirm the early assumption that insanity is scarce in China, but they do make for an emotional climate that was utterly alien and baffling to the non-Chinese observers who attempted to introduce Western ideas of medicine and psychiatry into that country. Their bafflement was most certainly increased by their lack of familiarity with the Chinese language, which deprived them of direct communication and caused them to miss a great many symptoms. It is true that Western psychiatrists saw in the larger cities a number of raving maniacs who were locked in small cells and chained to the walls (19, 25), it is also true that here and there they observed the wife of a coolie who believed herself transformed into a chicken or haunted by a disgruntled ancestor and gave a vivid presentation of her delusion (20). But although there were rarely ever more than 1,200 psychiatric beds for a population of 500,000,000 Chinese (19), this proportion never looked as blatantly inadequate as it would have in a Western country.

And yet, a number of statistical studies of the 20th century covering small sectors of China disclose that the incidence of mental illness is not negligible by any means.* Again it is the ancient moral and philosophical teachings that furnish the reasons for this seeming incongruity. Without the concept of sin and without the tradition of

---

* Tsung-yi Lin (20) deals with a regional study in Formosa; a study by B. Dai discusses the case histories of 2,400 Peking patients in *Amer. soc. Rev.* (vol. 16, 1941). See also A. Kasamatu: *Ueber die vergleichend psychiatrische Untersuchung in einem Dorfe bei Canton, Psychiat. Neurol. Jap.,* 1942, 46, 188-194; W. LaBarre: *Some observations on character structure in the Orient: the Chinese, parts 1 and 2; Psychiatry,* 1946, 9, 212-237, 375-395.

vengeful deities smiting mortals with the curse of madness, mental disease was never associated with religious guilt (6), nor was it apt to be the cause of family disgrace. Indeed, the Chinese, failing to observe the frequent hereditary factor of this illness, often recommended marriage for therapeutic reasons, a practice also encountered sporadically in the history of Western medicine (23). Thus, unlike his Western counterpart, the Chinese mental patient was never set apart from his accustomed surroundings. These old practices which are rooted in the concept of filial piety and reinforced by the demands of "face" prevailed even after the opening of the Western-type mental institutions; they account for the reluctance of the Chinese to commit family members to institutional care. Actually, filial piety imposes a dual obligation upon the family; above all, the literal one, where the children feel obliged to honor their parents and to care for them, even if senile *dementia* or general paresis have transformed the patriarch into a burdensome and foolish old man. But the filial piety which is lavished upon the head of the household also protects and shelters the youngest and most distant member of the family. This was, of course, made easier by the fact that the traditional Chinese society was more tolerant than the Western world of mental borderline cases, idiocy, or various neurotic manifestations. It could afford this tolerance because the sprawling, one-storied architecture of a Chinese country house permitted easy seclusion of a disturbed family member, and the agricultural society was able to find work even for the retarded and the deficient.

Whether the tremendous security emanating from the closely knit family system of Chinese society reduced the incidence of mental disturbances or simply hid them from view will never be known; nor will it ever be possible to estimate the amount of neuroses that may have been engendered by this concentrated and involved family life. It has been observed, however, that the removal from the family home into distant cities and even foreign countries has made the Chinese more vulnerable to mental disorders; although even there they take with them the precepts of filial piety and the requirements of "face." But the sensitivity engendered by the latter is apt to cause tensions in strange and foreign surroundings, and the absence of an immediate object for filial piety may produce an emotional void and heighten the feeling of loneliness. This is particularly true for temporary residents of Western countries, such as students, whose life is spent in close association and competition with non-Chinese (1, 27). Among the "overseas" Chinese, on the other hand, where the traditional pattern of family and community life is in full operation, the relative percentage of recorded mental disease is appreciably lower than that of any other racial group.*

Of course, these findings may be partly due to the fact that "overseas" Chinese, like those of the mainland, have less sharply defined notions of normal and deviant behavior than those held by peoples of Western extraction, and that the type of mental disease brought to the attention of the physician is only that which cannot possibly be managed in the home. Yet, regardless of the underlying reasons, it becomes clear that the Western observation on the relative stability of Chinese mental health contained more than one grain of truth. But we also see that, far from being the result of specific racial qualities, this apparent stability is closely linked with the ancient ethical and social precepts of the Chinese.

The severe rationality of Confucianism may have stifled much personal initiative and left unsatisfied a great many impulses and desires. To the less enterprising, however, the tight framework of Confucian ethics coupled with the rituals contained in the Chinese social structure must have been eminently comforting. By channeling human conduct along a minutely prescribed "way," by holding up self-respect and equanimity as the most desirable attributes, and by making family ties indissoluble beyond death, social philosophy succeeded in creating a standard of behavior and an emotional climate of such repose and security for the individual that it remained effective for far more than two millennia.

It should become evident from the abovementioned that there was in Chinese thought no clear-cut separation between mind and matter, body and soul, psyche and soma, and that dysfunction of one necessarily brought about the dysfunction of the other. This belief in the unity of health and disease in man was the result of reasoning based upon the classical writers. Hence it became part of the system of thought of the intellectual aristocracy, who were the ones who had access to the learned literature, while the common folk, most of whom were illiterate, operated along other lines of reasoning.

In all these respects Japanese and Chinese medical thought were identical for the longest part of their history, as medicine, philosophy, the science of historiography, and even the art of writing were introduced from China into Japan and were gratefully adapted by the Japanese.

Together with the introduction of these learned, scholarly, and

---

* According to recent registration of mental cases by race, arranged by the Bureau of Mental Hygiene of the Board of Health of Hawaii, for the years 1947, 1948, and 1949, the mental disease rates for whites was double that for the Chinese (9).

philosophical concepts, the Chinese also carried away their systems of folk beliefs and folk medicine, that evidently were remnants, or holdovers, from the original animistic religious beliefs, which also remained active within China itself. And so it was that for centuries the coexistence of two divergent streams of thought could be observed: the learned, philosophical, and strictly medical stream, and the one that led to popular beliefs and practices. As was to be expected, it was the latter that dominated the majority of the populations of each country, and it is particularly the latter to which I now wish to direct my attention.

To summarize briefly, the scholarly explanation for mental disease in China and Japan was the belief in the dyscrasia of *yin* and *yang*, and the patient's past infringement of the precepts of *Tao* (i.e., the laws of nature). Illness could be prevented by strict adherence to *Tao* and the following of ethical precepts; cure could be achieved by return to *Tao*, the "way of righteousness."

The popular theories, on the other hand, relieve man of his own responsibility for his illness and dysfunction, and center around beliefs of superhuman causation that are of a somewhat capricious nature. There is doubtless a superficial similarity between the oriental supernatural powers and those that haunted the minds of the medieval Western world. They did differ in their relative complexity, although the somewhat more exotic permissiveness of Oriental fantasy was not terminated by a scientific awakening such as that experienced by the Renaissance people of the Western world and continued into modern times.

Moreover, no witches were burned, and there followed no self-consciously horrified withdrawal from such practices. There was no turning point heralding an intellectual artistic, and—above all—scientific renaissance.

If we wish to study the popular theories of mental health and dysfunction we cannot find them in scientific treatises of medicine or scholarly works on philosophy. They are, however, contained in folk tales, novels, short stories, travel reports of Orientalists, and anthropologists who published their reports from the 17th to the 19th centuries. From all these writings there emerges a pattern of thought that is internally consistent, though actually worlds apart from the sober, naturalistic, philosophy of classical Chinese and Japanese literature. The pattern that emerges from this literature is built around a nether-world of wizardry, nature spirits, animal demons, and benign and malignant ancestral spirits, were-foxes, each of which can bring madness as well as cure it.

3

POPULAR BELIEFS AND PRACTICES

Before describing in detail the nature of these sinister powers in relation to mental disease, we must return once more to the aforementioned dichotomy between popular and scholarly ideas. The learned,
as was said, held the unchangeable assumption of the indivisibility of
spirit and substance, and of mind and matter, in which assumption
they were guided by the earliest philosophical writings, such as Lao-
Tzu's *Tao Te Ching*.

The popular mind, however, saw body and mind as separate entities; it conceived of a duality of mind and matter, all of which was
corroborated by Buddhism and the latent ideas of the transmigration
of souls with the belief in reincarnation. Sleep, and especially dreams,
were another corroborating factor in the body/soul dichotomy. Thus,
when man dreamed of strange adventures in vaguely familiar or
hitherto unknown landscapes, houses, and castles, what else could that
prove but that his soul was traveling by itself, far away from the body,
or that it was returning to scenes of the dreamer's earlier life?

From that belief there arose the customary need to awaken a sleeper
slowly and gently, in order to give time to the absent soul to return
to its proper body. Since such orderly return of the errant soul was
not always possible, there were countless souls in the universe that
were homeless and turned into independent spirits and hence tended
to cause mischief. This belief and the animistic tradition of ancient
days account for the proverb which held that "Three measures above
man's head begins the spirit world."

But in conformity with ancient beliefs, the spirit world was not
confined to the upper regions. It was everywhere. The spirits were
in the water, in caves, within the branches and the roots of trees, naturally also in the vicinity of graves, and even in houses and on the
highways. The last mentioned were especially dangerous at night, as
that time was governed by *yin,* the element of darkness, and those
who encountered demons on the highway at night were apt to die without any visible injuries. The combination of the belief in the reign
of *yin* in conjunction with the nightly demons makes it evident how
intertwined were the popular and scholarly beliefs in the nature of
the world.

Although the emperor was by the very nature of his position a
personage of faultless filial piety and therefore scarcely prey to revenge

from ancestral spirits, there were other disembodied apparitions that even haunted the Imperial harem, known as the "Forbidden City."

> The Forbidden City was haunted in the *Süen hwo* period (1119-1126) by a being known as *lai,* a lumpish thing without head or eyes. Its hands and feet were covered with hair shining as varnish. When at midnight a thundering noise was heard, the people in the Forbidden City all cried: 'The lai is coming!' and they bolted the doors of all buildings. Sometimes the specter lay down in the bed of a lady of the harem, which was then felt to be warm; and at daybreak it rolled out of the bed and disappeared, nobody knowing where it had gone. And when the ladies of the harem dreamed that they were sleeping with somebody, that somebody was the *lai* (2).

Other apparitions similarly described as hairy, of monstrous height, intent on violating young maidens, and known to cause sudden madness in those who beheld them, were dreaded equally in China and Japan. If we study their descriptions minutely we find that these hairy, monstrously tall apparitions are very similar to the beings the modern world has come to describe as "abominable snowmen." In all probability, indeed, this apparition is a descendant of the much dreaded *lai,* since the persons who first reported seeing the "abominable snowmen" were themselves descendants of those who first beheld and believed in the appearance of the *lai.*

But, in returning from the modern "abominable snowman" to the older apparitions that molded the psyche of Far Eastern man, it is of interest to realize that the fear of these specters, though ever-present, did not lead to precautionary defense measures, but defense was marshalled only at the moment of threat of actual harm. There is an ironical Buddhist proverb that reveals that lack of depth of actual religiosity and the opportunistic approach to religion. "Kiss the feet of Buddha when you are sick; when you are well, you may forget to burn incense."

With the first indication of illness, however, especially when it strangely affected the mind, or, rather, the patient's behavior, specific rituals came into play that had gradually developed for just such occasions. They were carried out by certain priests whose preeminent function it was to counteract and defeat the noxious powers that had caused the illness. It is noteworthy that in their apparent irrational rites there was a faint connecting link between the popular and scholarly views of mental alienation. In their very role as priests, even though they used magical influence, they belonged to the realm of *yang,* i.e., to light, life, and the positive element. Thus they were endowed with an ascendency over disease which was in the realm of *yin* which stood for darkness, death, and all negative attributes.

In this connection it might be of interest to study the composition of the ideograph *I* or *Y,* which stands for healing, medicine, and the physician, and to realize that in its original form the lower part, *wu,* is derived from the early priesthood of animism and might be understood as wizard, witch, and expeller of demons. When disease was thought to be caused by demons, *wu* became almost synonymous with the physician, for his ability to act as a healer was vested in his power to exorcise, a power that was essential in mental disease.

There were male as well as female *wu* in old Far Eastern practice. Their resourcefulness was unlimited and their intricate rites and procedures were logically related to the assumed care of each specific disease. The *wu* used ruses, decoys, force, or incantations, depending on each given situation. Since they were often dealing with violently psychotic patients, the priest-healers frequently were not only in danger themselves, but even tended to endanger their patients with their healing rites. Well known examples are the sword dances of the healer, whereby the *wu* lashed out at the patient with blows of the sword, not without inflicting occasional injury to the defenseless patient. Whether such injury may be termed iatrogenic is a matter of unresolved semantics. More frequently than inflicting injury upon the patient, the priests injured themselves with one or several from their manifold arsenal of instruments which consisted of five swords of different weights and lengths, and spiked iron-prick balls on a chain which the priest swung around himself, occasionally piercing his own skin and flesh. The priest furthermore, frequently stabbed his own tongue with a spear, so as to utter the appropriate sounds, and often he was carried to the patient's home on a litter of nails.

It stands to reason that rites of such strenuousness and discomfort required youth and agility on the part of the priesthood which, like most Oriental priesthoods, was believed to be divinely endowed. The *wu,* the priest-healer, was believed to be divinely endowed with a gift of healing which usually affected the entire family, thus making the priest-healership a family tradition. In keeping with the divine endowment, and the resulting moral obligations, the healers never asked for remuneration, but depended upon their patients' gifts in order to make a living.

In their work of exorcising the spirit from those who were believed to be possessed, the *wu* usually dealt with spirits of ancestors or of others who had died, and who took their revenge for an unjust death or a neglectful funeral. Such spirits were thought to be especially tenacious and required enormous efforts on the part of the exorcisers, most of whom were, in their early years of life, young enough to cope with rituals as strenuous and hazardous as walking across a bed of glowing coals to separate the healer from the pursuing spirits of the dead.

The dead were often believed to steal the souls of the living, especially during sleep, when dreams seemed to transport the dreamer away from his actual surroundings. It was therefore customary to approach a sleeping person cautiously and to awaken him slowly so that the errant soul was given enough time to return to the body of the sleeper. Similarly, daydreams were believed to be caused by wandering of the soul to other regions where it might be snatched and forever hidden by a vengeful ancestral spirit. Easy prey to mischief on the part of ancestral spirits were the unmarried daughters in the family. These unfortunate girls had no place in the family hierarchy; neither being mothers of a new generation, nor serving as daughters-in-law to the previous generation, these hapless old maids tended to become isolated and emotionally unbalanced. In some the delusion eventually led to insanity. According to one author the spirits of the dead took particular delight in tormenting frustrated young women with erotic desire, which, by leading to masturbation, eventuated in madness (5).

The description of this last sequence of events seems hardly plausible in the light of the general Chinese theory that female masturbation was not associated with any dire consequences, and therefore need not be discouraged. This permissive attitude is quite in contrast with that towards masturbation in the male. In men it was believed that the semen carried the essential life force and that, at birth, each male was endowed with a specific quantity. Each ejaculation expended a portion of this vital essence which could never be fully replenished. These theories had much deeper roots than more popular belief. They appear to have been part of the early scholarly Chinese medical writings, which are no longer extant in their original form. They were incorporated however, in a large compendium of Chinese medicine, the *Ishimpō*, which was compiled by the Japanese physician Yasuyori Tamba in the 10th century. Although this book was not printed until the very end of the Tokugawa period (1954), it was frequently copied by hand and became an important textbook for Japanese physicians.*

Because of this intense concern on the part of men with the preservation of semen, an irresistible urge toward masturbation and nocturnal

---

* One of the original manuscript editions is preserved in the Historical Library of the Takeda Pharmaceutical Company in Osaka, Japan.

emissions was usually interpreted as the work of vengeful spirits who took the shape of seductive young women and even pursued their victims in dreams. The consequent psychic disturbances were doubtless often due to fear of the dire effects which followed the irreplaceable loss of vital substance.

Another cause of mental derangement was the ability attributed to the dead to steal the souls of the living. Such catastrophes were believed to happen during sleep, when the soul was occupied with dreams and could easily be lured away. One group of spirits was held to be particularly powerful. This was the *T'ien Ku,* in China, known as the *tengu* in Japan, both of which may be literally translated as "celestial dog." Originally conceived in China as dog-faced comets or meteors, the *tengu* later were regarded as mountain demons and as such became known in Japan. As such, the belief in the *T'ien Ku,* like the belief in *lai,* may very well have found its way into Tibet and the regions near the Himalaya mountains, and may therefore also account for the apparitions known as the "abominable snowmen." In Japan, the *tengu* concept was eventually incorporated into Buddhist beliefs and assumed the role of the ghosts of departed priests who had led dissolute lives and had thus become emissaries of the devil. In this capacity the *tengu* drove people to madness. If they found other evil priests, they led them to the *tengu* road, which was one of the dreaded punishments for vanity and hypocrisy in the Buddhist hell (7). Even in the recent past the *tengu*'s powers were considered limitless and dangerous to all. Guided by sheer whim, they possessed their victims and spoke through them in strange voices, led them astray, and deprived them of their memory. They caused unending anxiety among the parents of young sons, who were thought to be the favorite victims of these evil demons (3).

With this strong implication of the spirit of the dead in all forms of mental alienation, it was reasonable to attempt restoration to sanity by immediate efforts to propitiate the departed. Sometimes unmarried girls found temporary consolation by means of the assumption of being haunted or possessed by one of the various animistic spirits that haunted mankind. Ceremonies and gifts at the graves and ancestral altars and elaborate rituals were devised to recapture the souls of the demented for their rightful owners. Since the supernatural was involved, failure to produce the desired results was not considered the fault of the medical priests who conducted these rites, but was ascribed to the implacable hostility of the dead. Moreover, there was always a chance that other and less easily specific forces might have caused the disease for, actually, any component of the vegetable, mineral, and animal kingdoms was recognized as the potential abode of malign spirits.

This latter belief persisted from China's early religion, animism, which was never completely abandoned but continued to exist side by side with the realistic sophistication of Confucianism. It is interesting that Confucius confined his teachings to the cultivation of character, the art of governing, and personal ethics, and never expressed himself "on extraordinary things, feats of strength, disorders, or spiritual beings." He never even pondered over the mysteries of life and death. Whether by doing so he ignored the myths of his people or accepted them without question is unresolved. His followers preserved silence on these subjects also, and did not voice any opposition when Taoist and Buddhist writers made free use of the old myths and legends to further their own doctrines (8).

Vestiges of animism were distinctly interwoven into the later, more formalized, practices of Taoism, and it was absorbed even more completely in the vast pantheon of Buddhism. This complex religious fabric was further modified and adapted to Japanese thought with the adoption of the Chinese language and culture. The figure of the *tengu* exemplifies the animation of an inanimate object such as a meteor, its change of identity in China, and finally its further transformation in the folklore of Japan. Innumerable other animate and inanimate substances have been equally endowed with spectral potency.

Fox-lore

Although each of these substances has had a place in the popular thought and beliefs of the Far East, no single figure has had as important a role in Chinese and Japanese phantasy as the fox. Indeed, so rich is the lore of this animal's protean powers that a complete survey of all the legends and fairy tales devoted to the fox-spirit are beyond the powers of any one individual. Examination of the fox-lore is further complicated by the fact that it evolved independently in both China and Japan. Here I propose to cite but a small number of tales, selectively drawn from the vast store of such narratives in both the Chinese and Japanese literature, to illustrate their relation to concepts of mental disease. Collectively, they may give an impression of the enormously wide range of attributes and roles of the fox, which has so colored Far Eastern popular thought concerning behavioral aberrations (Plate CXXIV).

In Japan, the fox was originally regarded as the messenger of Inari, the rice-goddess who was believed to have had a vulpine shape,

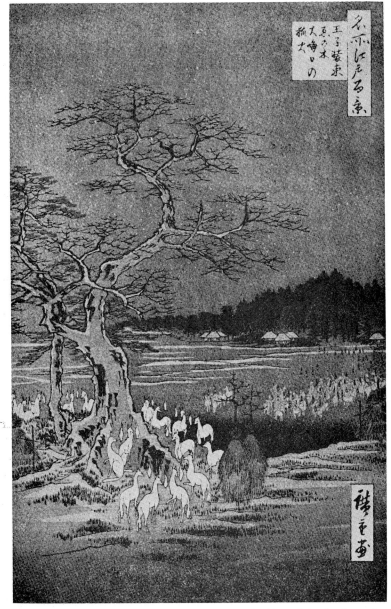

PLATE CXXIV. Assembly of foxes, each preceded by his soul in the form of a flame, known as *Kitsune-bi*, or fox-fire. Wood block print by Hiroshige (1797-1858).

and in this context the fox was a benign creature; vestiges of this aspect are still preserved in Japanese fox-lore. But later, even Japan adopted almost entirely the ancient Chinese belief in the animal's demonic traits and its consummate skill in taking human shape for the purpose of haunting and possessing men.

The earliest known reference to the malign role of the fox is found in the *Book of Odes* (26), where its very appearance on the scene was interpreted as having presaged the collapse of a kingdom. Later, during the Han dynasty (206 B.C.-220 A.D.), the fox assumed a more personal role which affected individuals, singly or in groups, bringing disease, insanity, and death, as well as economic or political misfortune. It is this capacity which has persisted through the centuries, with gradually increasing emphasis on the causation of psychic diseases ranging from minor disturbances to severe psychoses. In achieving these ends, foxes were believed able either to enter human beings and to take possession of their souls, or themselves to assume human appearance in order to exert their influence on others.

To the Western mind the dual role often played by the fox is confusing, especially when he appears as the cause of mental disease, and, at the same time, as a medical impostor who pretends to cure it. A typical example is a story from the *Hsüan-shih-chi* (late 8th century A.D.). It tells of a ten-year-old boy, the son of a minor palace official, who was intelligent, studious, and so well-mannered, that he was beloved by all. An illness, however, began to transform his personality completely. The father was on the point of summoning a doctor of Taoist arts, when a man knocked at the door and identified himself as a healer. Offering to dispel the affliction with charms, he said: "This boy suffers from a sickness which is caused by a fox demon." He thereupon applied his arts, and suddenly the boy rose from his bed and exclaimed with a normal voice that he was cured; and indeed he seemed restored to his old self. The grateful father generously rewarded the "doctor," who took his leave and promised that henceforth he would call every day, because

> . . . though the boy was cured of that disease (still he lacked sufficient quantity of soul, wherefore he uttered every now and then insane talk, and had fits of laughter and wailing, which they could not suppress. At each call of the doctor, the father requested him to attend to this matter too, but the other said: "This boy's vital spirits are kept bound by a specter, and are as yet not restored to him; but in less than ten days he will become quite calm; there is, I am happy to say, no reason to feel concerned about him." And the father believed it.

When the disease dragged on, however, another doctor was called in, and finally a third, and suddenly the three began to fight noisily. When eventually silence ensued, the frightened father returned to the sick room. There he was startled to find ". . . three foxes stretched on the ground, panting and motionless." He then realized that one of the three foxes must have been the first "doctor" and that it was he who had not only caused the disease but had even wilfully prolonged it. Enraged he beat all the foxes until they were dead, and ". . . in the next ten days the boy was cured" (2).

Favorite disguises of the "were-foxes," as they were termed by de Groot in his classic work on *Demonology* (2), were the bodies of lovely young girls who seduced their male victims into sexual, and even marital relationships and caused them forever to lose interest in other women. If the deception was discovered by a priest or relatives of the victim, and the woman, now revealed as a fox, was exorcised, the young man might soon be cured of his obsession. But when the infatuation was arbitrarily terminated by the demons, there often followed long periods of profound mental disturbance, melancholia, and even death or suicide. So well-known was this affliction that it inspired the T'ang poet Po Chü-i to exclaim: "A woman who fawns upon a man like a vixen destroys him at once and forever; for days and months she causes his mind to quiver."

But men were not the only victims of foxes. It was believed that through a series of metamorphoses the same animal could assume successively the images of enchanting females and seductive males, in order alternately to plague their male and female prey. In a widely quoted passage of the *Hsüan-chung-chi,* which was composed in the early centuries of our era, these magic changes are described as follows: "When a fox is 50 years old, it becomes a beautiful female . . . or a grownup man who has sexual intercourse with women. Such beings are able to know things occurring at more than a thousand miles distant; they can poison men by sorcery, or possess them, and bewilder them, so that they lose their memory and knowledge. And when a fox is a thousand years old, it penetrates to heaven, and becomes a celestial fox" (2).

This is further elaborated by an author of the Ming dynasty (3), who, however, exempts women from fox-possession:

> When a fox is a thousand years old, it goes to heaven for the first time and does not haunt people any longer. The purpose of the foxes in enchanting men is to take the vital spirit away from them in order to transfer it to their own bodies. But why do they not enchant women? Because foxes are animals of *Darkness* [like

women they belong to the principle of *yin*], and he who has *light* [the principle *yang*] within himself is liable to be enchanted by them. Even male foxes always take the shape of women to seduce men (4).

The immunity of women to fox-possession, so logically expressed in this quotation, was not accepted by many; and there are innumerable accounts of females who were so beguiled. The following Japanese story, however, is unusual, since it was told by a minister and involved a princess of imperial blood. In keeping with an ancient costume, this young virgin had been sent at the time of the emperor's coronation to the imperial shrine at Ise, where she was to stay throughout his reign. After four years in the temple, she was heard to call out with a loud and strange voice, stating that a god was speaking through her. Those who heard her said she appeared insane. This impression was further confirmed when she ordered two Shinto temples to be built in the vicinity of the shrine and summoned a large group of irreverent people to join her there. These she commanded to perform a sacred dance and then to continue with other wild dances for many days and nights. The evil sorcerers of the capital soon realized that the princess was possessed by a fox and made an image of this animal, which they declared as the chief deity of the Temple of Ise.

Since further information is lacking, it is of course impossible to arrive at a satisfactory opinion as to the cause and nature of the princess' derangement. It seems, however, reasonable to assume that among the contributing factors was the exalted yet exceedingly lonely life as a temple virgin without any knowledge as to its further duration. The absence of any attempt at exorcism or treatment and the freedom given to the patient in permitting her to act out her delusions were probably due to the deference accorded to her noble birth.

Although this is by no means the only fox legend involving royalty, the more frequent subjects are the peasants and villagers of the rural regions. In this setting most tales tell of men's amorous involvement with vixens, and of women seduced by foxes into sexual intercourse which could even result in pregnancy. An interesting example of this latter event was brought about by a fox-impostor who posed as a Buddhist saint. The story takes place during the T'ang dynasty (A.D. 618-906) in the province of Shansi; it has as its chief figure a young girl who lived at home with her widowed mother, while her brother served in the army. One day mother and daughter were visited by one such Bodhisatwa, who appeared riding on a cloud. He announced to the mother that he was pleased with the virtue of her house and that he wished to abide in it, but that neither she nor her neighbors must ever speak of it to anyone:

> . . . They accordingly admonished each other to hold their tongues, and the Bodhisatwa had intercourse with the girl, so that she became pregnant. A year passed by, and the brother came home; but the Bodhisatwa declared that he did not desire to see any male creatures, and prevailed upon the mother to drive her son out. The latter thus being unable to approach the saint, used his money for securing the help of a Taoist doctor, and finally found one who applied his arts on his behalf. They thus discovered that the Bodhisatwa was an old fox; sword in hand, he rushed into the house, and dispatched the brute (2).

According to general belief, the offspring borne from such unions tended to develop like other children and to merge with the human community. They were recognized as fox-children only by others like them and by priests. Doubtless, the existence of such legends was frequently used as a convenient explanation for illegitimate birth. Yet they were invariably taken at face value and most certainly appeared entirely plausible when the mother was feeble-minded or deranged and thus presented conclusive evidence of supernatural mischief.

The fox-lore quoted so far has largely been drawn from the early writings on the subject, since they provided the pattern for the numberless later tales. Before leaving the earlier period, reference must be made to a rather unusual story, some features of which are suggestive of certain aspects of the Oedipus legend. It was included by Yü Pao in Chapter 18 of his collection of marvelous tales, the *Sou-Shen-Chi*, which was written in the early part of the 4th century, and much quoted and altered in the T'ang dynasty (26).

The story is laid during the Tsin dynasty (265-419) in the Chehkiang province. It tells of a farmer and his two sons who were harvesting their field. The father, whose work had taken him away from his sons, returned to them and, without apparent provocation, began to berate and beat them. On reaching their home, the dismayed sons complained to their mother, who asked the father why he had hurt them. The astonished father, unaware that anything out of the ordinary had transpired, declared that it must have been the work of a fox-demon who had impersonated him and sent his sons out into the fields to destroy it. The demon, however, did not reappear, and when the father went to seek his sons in the fear that something evil had befallen them, the young men attacked and killed him, believing him to be the demon. The fox, however, had meanwhile again assumed the shape of their father, and entered their dwelling. When the sons returned and told him of the slaying, the impostor and their mother expressed their joy.

For years the young men remained ignorant of their dreadful deed, until one day a priest revealed to them that their father was known to be an evil person. This conversation was carried back to the father, who exhibited such a fearful rage that the sons fled to warn the priest. But the latter, sustained by his righteousness, bravely entered the house. At first sight of him, the impostor turned back into an old fox and was slain by the sons. Only then did they realize that much earlier they had killed their real father. They tried to atone for their fearful violation of filial piety by burying their father in a proper grave and by mourning him for a long period. Yet life had become altogether unbearable, and shortly afterwards one son killed himself, while the other sank into profound melancholy and died of remorse.

The protagonists of this tragedy appear to be completely innocent targets of a vicious prank. Unlike the ancestral spirits which strike in retribution for insults or neglect, the fox generally prefers harmless, and sometimes even virtuous, victims for his malign play. There are a few exceptions, however, and among them the following story is of particular interest, since it appears to deal with a case of vicarious guilt. Its locale is Yedo (now Tokyo), its period the second decade of the 19th century, and it is told in the *Tōen Shōsetsu* (1825) (4). The victim, a young girl, who lived with her mother, was found to be insane with unmistakable signs of fox-possession. When she was subjected to searching questions, the answers were given by a voice which was recognized as that of a fox. In accounting for the reasons for the girl's abstraction, the fox revealed that ". . . her mother, a widow, had illicit intercourse with a silk merchant who often passed the night in her house." After making these revelations, the fox "went out" of the patient, the silk merchant fled, the widow was sent back to her native village, and the girl, now completely restored, went to the house of relatives.

Viewed in the frame of modern psychology, this case would suggest that the weight of the shameful knowledge of her mother's improper conduct so preyed upon the daughter as to cause her emotional disturbance. Unable, because of considerations of filial piety or fear of loss of face, to speak about this situation, she unconsciously took refuge in the fox-disguise and so achieved her purpose.

During the millennia of recorded fox-lore, speculations were frequently voiced as to any possible common traits among those who were particularly predisposed to fox-possession. A significant comment on this subject was made by Kojima Fukyu in the early 18th century:

The fox is an animal of Darkness to the most degree. Therefore the external evil [in the shape of the fox] enters people whose Light-spirit has diminished. In general, exaggeration of joy, anger, sorrow, pleasure, love, hatred, and greed causes man to lose his original character and to become empty, and only possessed of the spirit of Darkness. How could it happen otherwise on such occasions but that bad demons should enter into him?

The implications of this passage seem so entirely clear that one cannot but wonder whether the author really believed in his supernatural imagery, or whether he used it only because it was the idiom of his day. He points to the early subtle changes of personality which are rarely noticed except in retrospect and describes them as mere exaggerations of normal emotional behavior. They progress at so gradual a pace that the disturbance becomes evident only when the disease is full-blown. "It causes man to be empty and only possessed of the spirit of Darkness." What better characterization could one find of melancholia, of depression, and of all the other forms of alienation, which were, according to Far Eastern thought, but stages of the same process?

Irrespective of whether Kojima Fukyu actually accepted fox-possession or simply pondered the mysteries of the diseased mind, the folk-belief of the Far East almost invariably ascribed preternatural causes to all forms of aberrant behavior, including sexual disturbances such as impotence and frigidity, nymphomania, and satyriasis. Indeed, the association, equally prevalent in China and Japan, of sex and psychological aberrations is frequent in fox-lore and existed also in most other forms of animal and spirit possession. This emphasis seems particularly remarkable in view of the fact that sexual inhibition was generally not a dominant feature in the mores of the Far East. This was particularly true prior to the Ming dynasty when most supernatural beliefs had been crystallized (21). Much additional study will be required to arrive at a full understanding of this phenomenon. Future research might wish to examine the role played by the traditional Oriental desire for numerous male offspring. The fear of failure to fulfill that desire may well have been a contributing factor to this extraordinary sexual preoccupation, which so easily assumed pathological dimensions.

Another conspicuous feature of most Oriental stories relating to mental disease is the apparently sudden onset of the derangement without noticeable premonitory symptoms. No matter whether it was caused by haunting ancestors, *tengu, lai,* foxes, or other specters. Equally prominent are the reports of the abrupt cures, either by exorcism or other violent measures to hasten the departure of the intruding demon. While it is probable that the subtle prodromata which generally preceded the obvious "madness" were not recognized as such, as has been indicated above, the narrators doubtless also made use of poetic license in telescoping the events, so as to render their stories more dramatic.

The most important conclusion to be drawn from the study of Oriental folklore is that inherent in the belief of the spectral origin of mental disease there is a definite assumption of its reversible nature and curability. Each aberration had its specific cause, and a curative magic was directed towards the expulsion of the offending agent. Since many of the ceremonies were associated with violence that may have acted somewhat in the nature of shock treatment and all of them involved an intensive preoccupation with the patient, it is likely that the treatment was often effective. Above all, the belief in demonic powers made the patient an innocent victim and placed the correction of his derangement beyond the influence of rational treatment and into the hands of priests. As a result no stigma was attached to mental disease, and society was ready to receive the patient on pre-illness terms as soon as his behavior became normal.

While the scholarly medical literature in China and Japan was concerned with theoretical and philosophical theories of mental disease and was particularly emphatic in its prophylactic recommendations, these writings were of little practical influence among the general population, few of whom were even able to read. The prevailing ideas, as has been shown from the examples in folklore and popular literature, were concerned with the supernatural. Hence, there developed two psychiatric attitudes, which existed side by side with little interplay, but apparently also without hostility or professional jealousies. Herein lies the greatest difference between the histories of Far Eastern and Occidental thought.

So far, we have spoken of the simple psychotherapy inherent in the scholarly medical attitude, i.e., the emotional modification towards contentment and serenity, as it emanated from the adherence to *Tao,* the "right way of life." We have also spoken of the methods of magic healing in response to the popular beliefs in ancestral spirits, mountain ghosts, and were-foxes, all of whom were held responsible for certain mental aberrations. So far as psychiatry from the Western point of view is concerned, none of these methods of healing appears to be of any truly practical value, nor are the descriptions of psychopathology sufficiently explicit for the Western observer.

Fertility

There is, however, one aspect of the make-up of the Far Eastern psyche which is of great importance in the determination of behavior in sickness and in health. This deals with the beliefs surrounding longevity, fertility, and sexual potency. For the reasons of filial piety, as mentioned above, fertility—the production of ancestor-worshipping offspring—has always been of uppermost importance. Clearly also, fertility and potency, i.e., virility, were generally equated and there arose a vast literature that concentrated upon these essential features. This literary documentation of the interlinking of longevity, fertility, and sexual prowess is most explicitly documented in the famous Indian *Kama Sutra* and in Book 28 of the *Ishimpō,* the earliest Japanese book on the art of healing. In the latter work, it is important to note that knowledge of erotic practices is not only listed in a chapter entitled *"Chamber Arts,"* or *"In the Chamber,"* but also appears in a long section dealing with the maintenance of general health, even including geriatrics. For reasons which were mentioned above, it was considered to be life-preserving for men to expend their semen but sparingly, as they had been endowed from birth with a limited amount only which was to last for their entire lifetime; and hence each seminal emission was believed to bring man closer to his end. Although semen itself could never be replenished, there were ways by which the essence of youth could be absorbed from the partner in the sex act. It was for sexual renewal that Chinese and Japanese men tended to seek very young concubines. While this vicarious rejuvenation was held to be possible on the part of men as derived from young women, no hypothetical provision was made for the reverse exchange, namely of older women extracting youth from younger male partners.

The immense preoccupation with virility and its most important symbol, the creation of male offspring, also gave, and apparently still gives, rise to a psychotic disturbance which deludes the sufferer with the sensation of penile shrinkage and fears of dissolution. This psychosis, which is known as *Koro,* is geographically limited to South China, the region of Canton where it is described as *Suk-Yeong*. According to P. M. Yap (29), who observed *Koro* in South China, it was first described in 1897 by Van Brero in South Celebes. Another Dutch observer, some 40 years later, described a corresponding affliction of women who were convinced of the shrinkage or disappearance of their vulval labia and their breasts. Although Yap never observed this illness in other parts of China, except in the South, including Hong Kong, there are interesting parallels in European psychiatric literature, including the writings of Kraepelin and the most phantastic of all European documents, the *Witches Hammer* (1494) from the pen of two Dominican priests, Heinrich Kramer and James Sprenger. Prominent among the sexual delusions suffered by those who thought themselves to be bewitched was the firm belief in the loss or shrinkage of their primary sex organs.

While in Southern China this terror of the sudden shrinkage or disappearance of the penis was simply a part of a psychotic castration anxiety without any belief in superhuman intervention, the medical world of Christianity felt that such a terrifying occurrence could happen only through witchcraft and the direct influence of the devil. Nevertheless, the priests who were consulted by the terror stricken patients rarely invoked exorcism but proceeded in a manner that resembles an intelligent form of psychotherapy by making the patient himself discover by palpation the "return" of his penis. This seems to have been possible within the short period of one or two visits at the confessional.

Koro, the Chinese form of castration anxiety, on the other hand, required complicated and long-term psychotherapy. According to Yap, the patients were hospitalized and treated with personal therapy, an appropriate mixture of tranquilizing and hypnotic drugs, as well as insulin—and electroshock treatment.

4

RECENT DEVELOPMENTS

Hospitalization

In connection with the hospitalization for *Koro,* it is essential to stress the difference between the hospitalization of Oriental patients from that of the West. Thus in the West where we tend to believe that the home environment is the pathogenic one, hospitalization usually means the strict separation of the patient from all vestiges of his pathogenic background. In the Far East, on the other hand, where contact with the family is absolutely essential for the maintenance of even a vestige of the original personality, it has been customary that at least one family member, the mother or a sister, accompany the patient into the hospital regardless whether it be for physical or mental illness. In the sickroom there is a raised platform, upon which the accompanying relative administers to the patient's needs. His clothes are kept by the accompanying relative, his favorite foods are prepared upon a *hibachi* brought from home. In fact, we hear that in Japan, in cases when a female member is not available, or cannot be spared by the family that remains at home, arrangements are often made to employ a mother surrogate in the form of a private attendant who performs for the patient all the services that would ordinarily be performed by his mother or sisters.

From this it must be evident that the Far Eastern families have learned to give in to the inevitability of hospitalization of a mentally ill patient, and in doing so the Japanese have come through an intermediary period of remarkable fumbling by trial and error. Perhaps the most logical transition from home care to institutionalization was the development of a community totally devoted to the care of mental patients. This village was organized like Geel in Belgium, although it was not influenced by its example. The simultaneous evolution of two communities, at different ends of the world, entirely given over to the care of mental patients is interesting, all the more so because both communities terminated their home-care program at about the same time and for the same reasons. It was, in fact, the national health insurance systems which ended the benevolent care of mental patients in private homes by families who had for generations concentrated upon that effort. The health insurance systems in both countries preferred to see the patients under the care of mental health professionals, rather than in the benevolent custodial care of an experienced village population.

The end of community mental care coincided with the end of a simultaneous and horrifying mode of treatment of mental patients which was practiced in Japan from 1900 to 1950. As described by Kumasaka and Yoshioka, this was based upon the so-called "law of private imprisonment" of the mentally ill.

These laws stipulated the responsibility of the family whose member had become mentally ill, to make provision for that patient's imprisonment at home. It was literally imprisonment and not simple confinement, as the patients had to be housed in specifically constructed cells. In these small cells which apparently resembled nothing as much as animal cages, the patients were left to the care or neglect of the family, which often led to indescribable misery. It is clear that the enforced family responsibility absolved the local and national government and the public from all necessity to make any efforts whatsoever on behalf of the mentally ill, and hence no attempts were made to construct hospitals or to provide for physicians especially trained to care for these mental patients who were housed in their prison-like cells like animals in cages. This neglect of, and actual brutality to, mental patients was directed towards their evident inability to fit their behavior within the framework of a tightly structured and disciplined society. Hence the incarceration took the place of punishment for infractions of the customs and mores of society (19).

The law of imprisonment of psychiatric patients in private cells was in force from 1900 to 1950. The resulting statistics which were gathered by Kumasaka and Yoshioka begin with the year 1906 when the population of Japan numbered approximately 50,000,000. In that year there existed hospitals with about 2,500 psychiatric beds, while 4,658 patients were housed in private cells. In 1957, when the population had risen to 91,500,000, and the law of private imprisonment had receded into history, 57,300 psychiatric beds had gradually become available while the number of cells had shrunk to zero.

The current scene in psychiatric hospitals in Japan is fairly similar to that of the Western world. Especially impressive is the quiet discipline that seems to pervade most mental institutions, and the open-door policy, both of which are made possible by psychotherapy that is reinforced by tranquilizing drugs. Different, however, is the aforementioned presence of a lay attendant in the sick room who, like the patients themselves, is usually clad in colorful kimonos, as white— the Western hospital uniform—is the color of mourning and would be a constant reminder of impending death, especially in a psychologically labile population of a mental hospital.

Morita Therapy

The transition from incarceration in private cells to Western-style hospitalization was naturally not a direct one, but occurred by way of Morita Therapy which is a form of psychotherapy that is unlike any known to the Western world. This form of psychotherapy, which came into being in 1918 and still exists today, was originally based upon Zen Buddhism. It was formulated by a Japanese physician Shōma Morita, of Jikei University, after he had conceived the idea of extracting the essential curative elements from Zen Buddhism and developing from them a specific form of psychotherapy.

While much of the material contained in this chapter pertains to attitudes towards mental health, mental illness, and mental healing in both China and Japan, Morita therapy is of purely Japanese provenance and does not have an exact Chinese counterpart. Morita therapy follows and emphasizes the Japanese devotion to and dependence upon nature, and actually it is nature, or the patient's concentration upon it, that serves as the healer; and the physician is nature's minister.

It is no doubt, true that all religious thought, especially if it led to organized withdrawal from worldliness, has always furnished helpful refuge for many who were emotionally unstable and incapable of coping with the demands of society. It was for these reasons also that Zen monasteries continued to attract inmates who had joined the order not entirely for its rigid demands of discipline and mental concentration, but rather for the feeling of safety and natural protection conveyed by these convents.

To explain why this should be preeminently true for Zen monasteries above and beyond those devoted to other forms of Buddhism would require a treatise by itself. Nevertheless an attempt will be made here to convey such insight into the essential features of Zen Buddhism as is necessary to understand its potentials for the recovery of mental health.

It is important to realize that this sect of Buddhism practices a form of religious meditation which is best known to the West by the Japanese pronunciation *Zen*. Originally stemming from India, it was described in Sanskrit as *dhyāna*; afterwards it migrated eastward into China, where it became known as *ch'an*; and it was from there that Buddhism found its way to Japan, where Zen became the most highly regarded school because of the great importance it gave to meditation. Indeed, meditation in Zen is not only a means for achieving ultimate truth, it is an end in itself—truth in action.

While other Buddhist schools have relied mainly on certain texts of the scriptures, Zen foregoes literary bridges and, rather, transmits teaching "from mind to mind"—that is, from the master directly to his disciple without the intervention of rational argumentation or formulation in conceptual terms. Above all, *ch'an,* or *Zen,* is a religious discipline which requires complete submission to the will of the "master," who alone can guide authoritatively and insure the correct transmission of the "truth." Zen teaches "becoming a Buddha just as you are," believing that "Buddha-nature" is inherent in all human beings and can be seen through meditative introspection. To attain Buddhahood, the great Zen masters advocated "absence of thought" so as to free the mind from the bonds of the external world. They also taught the need to ignore one's feelings, which is so important in the psychotherapy that has evolved from the doctrine.

To make clear the pertinence of a Buddhist sect to medicine, and especially to psychiatry, I wish to stress two major tenets of Zen Buddhism. They are, first, the importance that nature and a life in and with nature play in Oriental society. This is especially so among the Japanese and among the adherents of Zen. Of further importance is the immersion of the individual in the family, the group, or the community to which he belongs. Deviance from these tenets is thought to be not only asocial, but actually neurotic.

It was for this reason that Zen monasteries were long used—or rather, misused—as temporary refuges for psychiatric patients. Naturally, the monks were in no way conversant with any form of psychotherapy, nor were they eager to become therapists; they simply insisted on coercing all inmates, including those who had come as patients, into a strict conformity to all rules of conduct.

As the results often were surprisingly fortunate, Shōma Morita conceived the idea of extracting the essential curative elements from Zen-conduct and constructing from them a form of psychotherapy. Thus it was that Morita therapy was born; an absolutely typical Japanese mode of dealing with neurotic patients which has no correlate or parallel in the Western world. Its first major element in the combatting of the egocentricity which is the most striking symptom of the patient's neurosis. The second element of Morita therapy is the correction of the patient's alienation from nature because dependence upon, and love of, nature characterizes the Japanese in physical and emotional health.

It is remarkable, of course, that there should be a form of therapy that can restore love of nature and abolish egocentricity; and it stands to reason that both these major emotional adjustments can be achieved only with the iron discipline that is practiced in the Zen communities. To illustrate what I mean by "iron discipline," I wish to give you the basic tenets of Morita therapy, which differs so completely from any psychotherapy that has been evolved by Western minds. From my descritpion you will realize that this form of therapy is entirely impossible on an out-patient basis.

Regardless of the age or sex of the patient, Morita therapy follows a specific schedule, or ritual, on which recovery is said to depend. Upon his arrival at the hospital, the neurotic patient—overt psychotics are not accepted—must have complete bed rest for a period up to a week. During this time he is not permitted to associate with anyone else. This initial seclusion in hospital is remindful of the "Rest Cure" of the famous Philadelphia neuropsychiatrist, S. Weir Mitchell (1829-1914). He must not read, write, smoke, telephone, or watch television. The patient is left alone with his illness until he and his illness become one—he has to accept his illness in complete solitude. This initial period of absolute isolation and immobility in bed is by far the most traumatic phase of Morita therapy.

Subsequently, the patient is gradually restored to the world. He is encouraged to engage in work in the garden surrounding the hospital. This, however, is not the occupational therapy known in the hospitals of the Western world; rather, it is intended to encourage the patient's emotional return to nature. Gradually, also, the patient is permitted renewed contact with other persons. Rather late, he also meets with the therapist, not in the intimate setting of the doctor's office, but on a walk through the garden, during a game of table tennis, or during a similar diversion. In short, there is no occasion, or encouragement, for the patient to bare his soul, because that would only serve to reinforce the egocentricity which is the essence of his neurosis. Furthermore, in a subsequent stage of therapy when the patient is given the task of keeping a diary, he is enjoined to refrain from recording anything that relates to his emotions or to his illness; and the physician who checks the daily entries, somewhat in the manner of a severe teacher, applauds the patient if he is able gradually to free himself from the hypochondriacal self-importance that held him in bonds. In fact, it is the physician's explicit task to induce the patient to become once more a part of society, from which he had been alienated.

The patient must learn to associate with his fellow men without friction, and to perform his work as best he can, not by his own estimation but by the standards of healthy society. To be sure, the patient must never in the course of his treatment be permitted to think of himself as an emotional invalid or as different from the rest of the community.

It is clear that this tightly scheduled mode of therapy, a rigid form of re-education, is an outgrowth of a basically different concept of mental health and disorder than the underlying Western therapy, which is derived from the rather loose and undefinable concepts of the psyche, spirit, or soul. None of us—in fact, no one in the West—would now, in the middle of the 20th century, claim positive knowledge as to the actual location of the soul, spirit, or emotions. This has been traditionally different in China and Japan. Thus, in a modern Japanese dictionary (Ross-Innes), we find the character *shin* to mean "core," and in the pronunciation *kokoro* to mean "the heart," that is, the center of sensations and emotions or the "mind." And the word for mental phenomena that would correspond with the prefix psych-, as in psychology or psychoanalysis, is *shinri*, which may literally be translated as the "rules or the principles of the heart."

Despite the appropriateness of Morita therapy for Japanese patients, there is only a limited number of such specialized hospitals. The majority of mental patients come to Western-style psychiatric hospitals where they are looked after by psychiatrists, their personal companions, and hospital personnel. Here they are treated with the neuropsychiatric approach that had become so popular in Japan ever since that country's medical information was derived from the German school of medicine where neuropsychiatry long existed as a cohesive discipline. Most of the actual treatment in these hospitals has consisted of drug therapy and electroshock therapy, combined with a psychotherapy that is somewhat reminiscent of the classificatory approach of Kraepelin.

Psychotherapy

Psychoanalytically oriented psychotherapy has failed to make incisive inroads into the Japanese medical profession or the patient population. Although there is no one definitive argument against psychoanalysis in Japan, numerous reasons may be listed why the psychoanalytic approach fails to be applicable to the traditional Japanese personality. Important among these reasons is the family cohesion which still exists even in modern Japanese society; this involves more than vestiges of the old, unquestioning, filial piety which would make an analytical approach to one's parents difficult, if not entirely impossible. Furthermore, Japanese family life which takes place in houses in which the rooms are divided by walls of paper, does not permit any of the privacy that has long been the basis of family life in Western society—and especially in that society upon which Victorian Freudian doctrines are based.

In the same view, communal bathing, or rather family bathing and relaxation in the very hot water of a large built-in tub, makes for a totally different attitude towards the human body between Japanese parents and their children. This is reinforced by the constant physical closeness between children, especially male children, and their mothers, which often includes sharing the same bed until the first intimations of adolescence make such intimate proximity impractical.

The Stress of Education

As soon as the son advances beyond the earliest years in primary school he begins to be under enormous pressure to do as well as humanly possible, because his entire subsequent career and even the social standing of the family will depend on the extent of advanced education he is able to acquire; and, in order to be considered for admission to the university for any specialized education, such as law or medicine, an almost superhuman effort is required of the applicant who must have high grades at high school graduation and at the university entrance examinations. So intense, in fact, is the competition for the limited number of student vacancies in the various universities that, by the time the applicant has been accepted and begins his studies, he is apt to be so exhausted from the ordeal of admission that he no longer can muster the drive to do well that had sustained him throughout the preparatory years of pre-university schooling. In the lives and careers of many scholars and scientists, there often are discernible traces of this exhaustion during the early years of academic study; this reservoir of exhaustion and incapability of further competition will often lead to discernible neuroses or even transitory psychoses which may harmfully influence the victim's entire career.

By way of illustrating the previous descriptions, I submit the following personal experience: During one of my visits to Japan I was asked to give the commencement address in a medical school. I was told it was to be a "commencement" in the true sense of the word, inasmuch as I was to address myself to the graduating class who were to commence their careers as physicians as well as to the incoming class of new medical students. As a desirable subject for my talk I was advised to select the title *"Students Be Diligent."* It was in this fashion that I became acquainted with the exhaustion syndrome that so often befalls those who have just been accepted into the field of study they so ardently desire to pursue. I am not certain about the quality of the academic address I based upon that bizarre heading, nor do I know how much of my English speech the audience understood, but I do know that I tried to keep it in a light vein and injected a few faintly humorous remarks; when these elicited some audible amusement, I assumed that I had managed to communicate with the audience. The anxiety about university admission and subsequent graduation is shared by the student's entire family, who feel that their social position will either remain static or rise with the son's acquisition of a university degree.

Since earlier reference was made to the Japanese indebtedness to China for its artistic, scholarly, and religious values, we recognize in this emphasis upon education the traditional Chinese examination system which has controlled the careers of untold millions of aspiring Chinese youths. And indeed, as late as 1966, P. M. Yap detected traces of these old traditions in some of the troubled youths of Hong Kong (15):

We find striking examples of traditional Chinese attitude to child upbringing: the excessive insistence on book-learning, bound up as it is (since knowledge has not yet been dehumanized) with moral indoctrination; the anxious emphasis on diligence; and the close parental surveillance—especially of boys, who bear the family's hope of social advancement and who sometimes are over-protected to an extent unimaginable elsewhere. We see the strengths and weaknesses of the traditional family; the semi-parental functions of amahs, intervention by grandparents, the jealousy and rivalry caused by concubines—all of which may sometimes bring health and stability to the child, but more often a confusion of identities, standards and values.

Yap's report does not deal with traditional continental China but with the somewhat Europeanized scene of Hong Kong; he speaks of culture change and conflict, which make themselves felt at home as well as in the institutions of learning. In the over-crowded and over-populated crown colony of Hong Kong, just as in Japan, there is "intense competition for school places and the fear of failing examinations, leading to quite undue demands on the child by parents who, unawed by the 'I.Q.,' hold that industry can overcome all innate weaknesses." Although according to traditional tenets the *pater familias* was solely responsible for the guidance of his healthy, as well as aberrant children, the modernized Chinese of Hong Kong were content to permit the child guidance center of the University to take over the care and treatment of those children who had proved unequal to the pressures of higher education and changing society.

While this development occurred in the Chinese sector of the crown colony, the picture of mental health and healing in the People's Republic of China followed a somewhat different development. The Hong Kong Chinese, whether conscious of it or not, were guided by Confucian thought, which was summarized as follows by Yap:

> Confucius taught a rationalistic ethic without recourse to super-natural sanctions, based on the premise that man was essentially not evil by nature, although he could become evil through the vicissitudes of upbringing. Wrong behaviour was not the result of original sin inherited, but of social and psychological harmony disturbed. He was interested not in theology or metaphysics but in personal relationship, the cultivation of character, the har-monious regulation of the passions, and the attainment of a ma-ture, integrated personality, with the fusion, we might say, of the Super-Ego and Id into the Ego. He did not teach the need for personal salvation through a transcendental agency but insisted that evil was something to be overcome naturally, by recognition of wrong and by assiduous self-cultivation. Virtue was discussed

by psychological terms and departure from this was regarded as something analogous to disease. In keeping with this, different degrees of moral responsibility were recognized.

In his further reflections, Yap speaks of the great stress that was given to the cultivation of the child to the extent that—at times— certain scholars exchanged children so as to give them better education and guidance. But this guidance was customarily the task of the real or the adoptive father, and not of a child guidance center.

Like most ideas and practices that emanated from Chinese Confucianism, the practice of adopting sons for surposes of special education also found its way into Japan. In that country, however, the practice of adoption, while occasionally undertaken for the sake of a particularly promising young boy, was actually most frequently carried out with the intention of founding or extending a family dynasty, all of whose male descendants were to follow the same profession as their predecessors. This was particularly true in the case of some families of physicians whose dynasties often spanned several centuries. It became apparent, even without the corroborating evidence of the surviving family registers, that some of the links in the long dynastic chain were reinforced not by reliance upon the accident of male offspring but by adoption of a suitable heir and successor.

In Hong Kong parents accepted psychiatric assistance fairly readily for children who were evidently mentally disturbed; they were, however, somewhat less inclined to submit to child guidance for those youngsters who had become affected by the rising tide of juvenile delinquency. Child psychiatry was acceptable, as it fell within the wide sphere of pediatric medicine, and it had long been the custom that an ailing child was to be treated by a physician; guidance, however, even of a wayward child was traditionally to emanate from the family. Since now guidance might be offered in a somewhat officious fashion by mental health workers, it was often considered as meddling, and acceptance was somewhat more reluctant.

5

DEVELOPMENTS UNDER COMMUNISM IN CHINA

Community Psychiatry

In China proper, on the other hand, acceptance of guidance or therapy is not left to the whims of the recipient or of his family. In both cases "politics are in command." For political, social, and economic reasons the Chinese have insisted upon a social structure that stresses practically total conformity. Hence, the threshold of tolerance for aberrant behavior has been lowered from what it was in earlier days; equally reduced is the permisiveness towards juvenile abandon and delinquency. But, as in the earlier days the traditional family system provided the individual with emotional and physical security, the present-day Chinese in the People's Republic derive this feeling of protection from the state and society at large. All necessities of life— food, clothing, education, housing, and medical care—are now available as basic essentials. In return for such protection on the part of the state the individual is required to play by the rules of society without exception or deviation.

Community medicine and community psychiatry, which have recently enjoyed such great popularity as apparent innovations in the Western world, are self-understood parts of the medical care of the People's Republic of China. As public health and preventive medicine are the mainstays of modern Chinese medical philosophy, the health workers who are acquainted with their respective patient population visit their districts regularly to sound out the communities, the farms, and even the factories, as to whether any of the fellow workers or fellow citizens show adverse personality changes or appear to be in some personal trouble. In this fashion, by going into the community, the health workers are enabled to institute treatment and to forestall worsening of an existing condition.

Addiction

In the Western mind the Chinese have generally been associated with drug addiction, especially opium addiction, without full realization of the fact that the opium habit was originally forced upon the Chinese by foreign nations whose motive was monetary gain from the opium trade and the weakening of the Chinese political structure. It was therefore the expressed interest of all Chinese governments, ever since the introduction of opium by th Europeans from the 16th to the 19th century (18), to suppress that habit and the resulting addiction. In the 1930's the *Kuomintang* initiated a program of "total suppression of the chronic use of morphine and heroin." For morphine this was to be accomplished within two years; for the total suppression of opium six years were allowed. The program included compulsory treatment to accomplish sudden withdrawal during a period of hospitalization of a few weeks, and a subsequent period of hard labor in the capitals of Peking and Nanking where the addict was given a chance to recondition his deteriorated physical and mental health. As might have been expected this form of "cold turkey" withdrawal was far from permanently effective, but relapses into addiction were met with harsh penal measures, including incarceration and capital punishment. This eventually brought about a nearly complete disappearance of the opium habit from the life of China.

Venereal Disease

Another factor in the picture of mental illness was the wide dissemination of venereal disease. Until the establishment of the People's Republic of China in 1949, prostitution was a long-accepted social institution; but it furthered the spread of venereal disease ever since that scourge had been introduced into China, presumably by European sailors and traders in the early 16th century. Since the takeover by the Communist government, with its emphasis on equal right and dignity for all inhabitants, all houses of prostitution were closed. Sexual promiscuity in general was frowned upon by the new leaders of China. With strong social disapproval of sexual permissiveness and the absolute termination of prostitution, the nearly impossible was achieved, and venereal disease was almost completely eradicated. Nevertheless, the few remaining syphilitic patients with neurological damage, as well as the congenital syphilitics, could be looked after and receive intelligent genetic counseling.

Neuropsychiatry

Under the *Kuomintang* regime, the field of neuropsychiatry, previously confined to a small number of doctors, expanded widely and was supported by the famous Peking Union Medical College—generally referred to as PUMC. The expanding group of neuropsychiatrists also encouraged a proliferation of psychiatric hospitals, and it is reported that the number of psychiatric beds had risen to 20,000 in less than ten years after the Communist takeover. Where formerly Chinese mental patients, like those of Japan, had been severely restrained and even caged, modern methods of treatment by means of occupational therapy, drug therapy, and psychotherapy were introduced and found to be extremely helpful. Electroshock treatment, which had been used during the government of the *Kuomintang*, was discarded after the Cultural Revolution.

As in most countries, the Chinese medical profession found itself avidly interested in the study and research of schizophrenia, which so rarely yielded to any form of treatment. Together with the Western methods of psychotherapy, the Chinese had recourse to their own, established therapeutic methods of acupuncture, moxibustion, meditation, and breathing therapy. The last-mentioned, an outgrowth of the Taoist movement, is closely akin to *yoga* practices, which, as has been learned, can influence not only mental well-being, but also the rate of respiration, indeed even the rate of blood pressure and heart beat.

The Chinese Scene Today

From Ruth Sidel, the wife of one of the recent distinguished American China visitors, we learn much about the current psychiatric scene. One of the most impressive modes of treatment is carried on within the hospitals by the hospital population and is based upon patterns established by the People's Liberation Army, many of whom do in fact join in the task of hospital administration. Following the Army model, the patients are arranged into divisions and groups whose illness shows a similar degree of severity or improvement, with the ultimate aim of forming a "collective fighting group instead of a ward." Thus the patients are encouraged to help each other in their common goal of recovery from mental illness.

The burden of therapy is shared by the physicians with the patients, inasmuch as the latter are urged to study their illness and their symptoms. Treatment and its aim is explained to them, and the patients are requested to observe their own response to treatment and to recognize and prevent possible relapse.

Medication by means of tranquilizers is also practiced in China. Here it is of significance that the original tranquilizing substance was derived from *rauwolfia serpentina,* a plant which originated in the Orient and had long been in use in India. *Rauwolfia* itself was synthesized and formed the point of departure for many derivatives with a similar effect. This widespread use of a substance derived from the ancient Oriental *materia medica* served to reinforce the East Asian faith and pride in the efficacy of ancient indigenous healing practices and inspired renewed confidence in the value of traditional medicine. The collaboration of patient groups of approximately the same level of illness or recovery is somewhat remindful of the group efforts of Western psychiatry; the Chinese psychiatrists' meeting with groups of patients, as an alternative to individual treatment, also is most certainly a parallel to our form of group therapy. The latter form of group therapy takes place not necessarily as a treatment of choice, but rather, because there still are not enough specialists to take care of each individual patient in spite of the proliferation of psychiatry in China. Yet the patients are not lost sight of until they have been reintegrated into their family, their community, and the type of work that they can handle best.

The absolute faith each Chinese now derives from his belief in the all-encompassing power and compassion of Chairman Mao even follows the patient into the obscurity of his mental facilities and into the mental hospital. In the process of treatment and recovery the patients are encouraged to give testimony to Mao Tse-tung's sustaining presence and to their confidence in his help towards their eventual recovery. This belief seems to be retained even by minds that are clouded with the illusions and confusion of schizophrenia, and it is all the more valid, as even hospital life is as rigidly disciplined as the life of the healthy community.

6

NOTE ON SOURCES

In addition to the references and the footnotes listed in the body of this chapter, the sources of information for these reflections on Japanese and Chinese psychotherapy are derived from the author's own observations and publications, the publications of the late William Caudill, Y. Kumasaka, and S. Yoshioko, and contemporary Japanese belletristic literature, such as the novels of Tunezaki, Yukio Mishima, and Tomio Niwa which give graphic insight into the social and family life of modern Japan. These novelists, like Thomas Raucat, the brilliant author of *The Honorable Picnic,* and Lady Chihibu Murasaki, author of the epic *Tales of Genji,* round out what books on history, sociology, and medicine leave unsaid.

For similar background information concerning Chinese social and emotional life of the past we are indebted to such classics as the inimitable *Chin Ping Mei* and the *Dreams of the Red Chamber,* both of which have long existed in excellent translations into Western languages. Information on modern thought in Chinese psychiatry has been furnished by the brilliant Chinese psychiatrist, P. M. Yap, who was associated with the department of psychiatry of the University of Hong Kong, and who combines his psychiatric knowledge with that of sociology and anthropology. Insight into the most recent developments in psychiatry in the People's Republic of China is derived from Ruth Sidel's chapter on "Mental Diseases and their Treatment" in *Medicine and Public Health in the People's Republic of China* (17).

REFERENCES

1. Chou, S. K. & Mi, C. (1937): Relative neurotic tendency in Chinese and American students. *J. Soc. Psychol.*, 8, 155-184.
2. de Groot, J. J. M. (1892-1910): *The Religious System of China*, Vol. V., bk. 2. *On the soul of ancestral worship: Demonology*. Leyden: E. J. Brill.
3. de Visser, M. W. (1908): The Tengu. *Tr. Asiatic Soc. Japan*, 36, 2, 25-99.
4. de Visser, M. W. (1908): The fox and badger in Japanese folklore. *Tr. Asiatic Soc. Japan*, 36, 3, 10.
5. de Zwaan, J. P. K. (1917): *Völkerkundliches und Geschichtliches über die Heilkunde der Chinesen und Japaner. Natuurkundige Verhandelingen van de Hollandsche Maatschappij der Wetenschappen to Haarlem*, derde Versameling, Zevende Deel: Haarlem de Erven Loosjes.
6. Duyvendak, J. J. L. (1951): Review of Henri Maspero's "Mélanges posthumes." *T'oung Pao*, 40, 374.
7. Eberhard, W. (1967): *Guilt and Sin in Traditional China*. Berkeley: University of California Press.
8. Edwards, E. D. (1937): *Chinese Prose Literature of the T'ang Period*, Vol. II. London: Arthur Probsthain.
9. Haas, W. S. (1956): *The Destiny of the Mind, East and West*. New York: Macmillan.
10. Haring, D. G. (1949): *Personal Character and Cultural Milieu*. Syracuse: Syracuse University Press.
11. Hsien-chin Hu (1944): The Chinese concept of face. *Amer. Anthrop.* 46, 45-65.
12. Hsü, F. L. K. (1953): *American and Chinese: Two Ways of Life*. New York:
13. Jordan Miln, L. (1925): *Ruben and Ivy Sên*. New York:
14. Legge, J. (1861): *The Chinese Classics*. Hongkong, London: L. M. Dent & Sons.
15. Li, L. & Wright, A. (1966): *Children with Problems*. Introduction. Child Guidance, Hong Kong University.
16. Müller, F. M. (Ed.) (1899): *The Sacred Books of the East*. Oxford: Oxford University Press.
17. Quinn, J. R. (Ed.) (1972): *Medicine and Public Health in the People's Republic of China*. Washington: Dept. of Health, Education and Welfare.
18. Schadewaldt, H. (1972): Zur Geschichte einiger Rauschdrogen. *Materia Medica Nordmark*, 24, 1-2.
19. Schaltenbrand, G. (1931): Psychiatrie in Peking. *Z. Ges. Nerol. Psychiat.*, 137, 170-175.
20. Tsung-Yi Lin (1953): A study of the incidence of mental disorder in Chinese and other cultures. *Psychiatry*, 16, 322-323.
21. Van Gulik, R. J. (1961): *Sexual life in Ancient China*. Leyden: E. J. Brill.
22. Veith, I. (1970): *The Yellow Emperor's Classic of Internal Medicine*. Berkeley: University of California Press.
23. Veith, I. (1970): *Hysteria: the History of a Disease*. Chicago: University of Chicago Press.
24. Wong, K. C. (1950): A short history of psychiatry and mental hygiene in China. *Chinese Med. J.*, 68, 44-48.
25. Woods, A. (1929): The nervous diseases of the Chinese. *Arch. Neurol. Psychiat.*, 21, 542.
26. Wylie, A. (1968): *Notes on Chinese Literature*. Shanghai: American Presbyterian Mission-Press.
27. Yap, P. M. (1951): Mental diseases peculiar to certain cultures: a survey of comparative psychiatry. *J. Ment. Sci.*, 407, 326.
28. Yap, P. M. (1954): The mental illness of Hsung Hsiu-ch'üan, leader of the Taiping rebellion. *Far East. Quart.*, 13, 287-304.
29. Yap, P. M. (1965): Koro—A culture bound depersonalization syndrome. *Brit. J. Psychiat.*, 111, 43-50.

29

AUSTRALIA AND NEW ZEALAND

E. Cunningham Dax, F.R.C.P., F.A.N.C.P.

Coordinator in Community Health Services, Mental Health Services Commission, Hobart, Tasmania, Australia

1

INTRODUCTION

Notwithstanding the 1,000 miles which separate New Zealand and Australia, some of the earlier explorers visited and discovered both land masses together. In fact, it was as the result of Captain Cook's voyage of 1768, in which he sailed round New Zealand and up the East Coast of Australia, that the first settlement of convicts took place in 1788 at Botany Bay. Thus, in the 200 years since British settlement, the modern history of Australia and New Zealand has evolved while the very different demands of the indigenous Australian aborigines, after 30,000 years, and New Zealand Maoris, after 500 years, have in some part been met.

The history of occupation is short enough for the major social stresses to be seen in comparatively recent perspective and for accompanying psychiatric consequences to be recognized. In Australia, history is easily divided into three nearly equal periods: settlement, between 1788 and 1850; discovery, from 1851 to 1901; and development, since the states achieved federation.

2

AUSTRALIA

Settlement

The English Parliament, under Lord Sydney's advocacy, grasped the opportunity created by Cook's voyage of discovery to dispose of their unwanted criminals to this new land, after transportation to America and Africa ceased. The early records of the settlement show that those making the decisions were almost totally ignorant of the difficulties and privations that would be met or of the suitability of their initial choice as a place of settlement.

The convicts must have been a motley lot; they varied from the most troublesome and violent types, who had lived in hulks on the Thames, to minor pickpockets and children who had stolen for food. These were diluted by a number of political prisoners, usually Irish; by 1848, 58 out of 83 female admissions to the New South Wales lunatic hospital were of Irish extraction.

The first group was dispatched in 1789, and consisted of 550 male and 230 female convicts, and 296 military guards, who constituted the first Australia Corps (the numbers differ slightly in various reports). Of those leaving England, 40 prisoners died on the way, 52 were sick or old and unfit to work, and 78 more died in the first six months after arrival. The second shipment was even less fortunate.

It needs little imagination to picture the privations of these people, closeted together below decks, many in irons, bewildered by their transportation, mixed together indiscriminately and separated, perhaps forever, from their families and friends. The bitter resentment of many undernourished convicts suffering from scurvy, cruelly disciplined, often unjustly transported, and completely uncertain of their future, must have been accompanied by a hopeless despondency, when symptoms of psychotic illness would be an expected response.

There is little literature available which describes mental illness aboard the convict ships. Suicide is never mentioned, although it might be thought of as a reasonable solution, but in periods of extreme suffering, when life is cheap and death is a daily occurrence, suicide ceases to be a protest or to have a meaning. However, in the Boys' Prison at Port Arthur, in 1834, mention is made of a "suicide rock," a print of which is in the Mitchell Library in Sydney, though there is no evidence of deaths actually occurring (16).

Mental illness among those disembarking is more frequently reported and, in some of the original records, which by good fortune are still preserved, notes have been made of people being moved to the jails or lunatic asylums directly after landing from the ships. It was said that the women often suffered from mania and, some 50 years later, in the records of the first Victorian mental hospitals, the association between the journey and insanity was fairly frequently recorded.

Within the next 30 years considerable development took place. There were many free settlers, land was cultivated, and flocks multiplied. But at the same time rum became a major item of barter and often the equivalent of coinage, so that much alcoholism existed. By 1802, the annual consumption of imported drink, apart from that distilled locally, was almost six gallons of rum and three gallons of wine for every man, woman and child of the 5,800 population. It is interesting that the first Sydney hospital was built free of charge by three private individuals in return for a monopoly of the importation of 45,000 gallons of rum. There are frequent references to inebriety and, in 1820, a letter from Governor Bourke said, "A lunatic asylum is an establishment that can no longer be dispensed with. In this Colony the use of ardent spirits induces the disease called *delirium tremens,* which frequently terminates in confirmed insanity."

In the early days the insane were kept in jails, and this practice persisted in some states for over 50 years. In New South Wales, which was the first area to be settled, an asylum was opened in 1811. The *Sydney Gazette* reported a statement of Governor Macquarie: "His Excellency, commiserating the unhappy condition of persons laboring under the affliction of mental derangement, has been pleased to order an asylum to be prepared for their reception . . . and every provision that humanity could suggest has been made for their accommodation and comfort." However, the first report available shows that patients were sleeping in the kitchen due to overcrowding. By 1805, rules had been made governing the estates of the mentally ill and, in 1810, a board was formed from a committee of surgeons for certification and discharge.

Governor Macquarie, in 1814, gave personal instructions to the superintendent. One stated: "You are not to allow the keepers or other persons attending them to exercise any unnecessary severity towards the Lunatics, but see they are at all times treated with mildness, kindness, and humanity." Almost all the keepers were convicts. The rules also stated: "Such of them as are fit for manual labor, are, with the permission of the Surgeon, to be employed in cultivating the garden . . . which will be the means of not only amusing them, but will likewise prove a wholesome exercise highly beneficial to their health."

The next asylum, built in Van Diemen's Land in 1829, was closely associated with convict history. The convicts, who landed in New South Wales, were at various times dispersed to Moreton Bay to the North, to Norfolk Island, 1,000 miles to the East, and to Tasmania, or Van Diemen's Land, as it was called after its settlement in 1803.

There were a number of convict prisons in Tasmania, but the most famous of them was at Port Arthur, to which eventually they were all removed. It opened in 1830, with 68 guards and prisoners who constituted a "sawing gang." At the end of the same year 22 boys were sent there "to learn to become sawyers." So great was the production that within two years the commandant asked for 100 more men (20).

Eventually, 1,000 convicts were kept there; many of them were the more desperate characters who had been removed from New South Wales. When violent they were placed in a model prison and the worst of them were confined in a sound-insulated pitch-black room, where they were almost in sensory isolation. One prisoner after discharge from the "dumb" cell feigned insanity: "He was then taken to the insane depot and douched with three buckets of cold water which made him abandon his pretense." It sounds as if a "shower cabinet" (Plate CXXV) such as was discovered by Brothers at the Kew Mental Hospital may have been used there (14).

In 1842 an asylum was opened at Port Arthur. There were four dormitories, a central hall, 24 cells, and a padded room. One patient spent long periods in a cage. Port Arthur then had an evil reputation, and Britain, in a wave of belated guilt, ordered the penal settlement to be abandoned, so that by 1879 only 64 prisoners, 126 paupers (presumably housed in the invalid block), and 69 lunatics remained. They were called "imperial lunatics"!

Another matter of psychiatric interest at Port Arthur was an adjacent establishment at Point Puer which contained up to 730 delinquent boys, mostly aged 9 to 18. Some were transported for trivial offenses. It appears that Governor Arthur made a real attempt to educate and train them as stonemasons, sawyers, and in other trades. Their re-education on one ship at least would be a model for present day-care. This was due to Alexander Nesbitt, the naval surgeon in charge. The establishment was abandoned in 1848 and they were transferred to Hobart. An interesting book by Hooper (16) gives a brief account of their subsequent history and of their lives in jail.

At Lachlan Park there was both an invalid hospital, where those sick and aged convicts not in Port Arthur were transferred in 1829, and an asylum, built behind the hospital, consisting of 14 male cells and two male wards, 12 female cells and one female ward built for

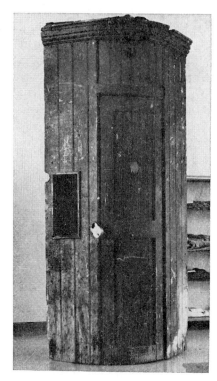

PLATE CXXV. Shower cabinet.

PLATE CXXVI. Shock machine. Old Lachlan Park Hospital.

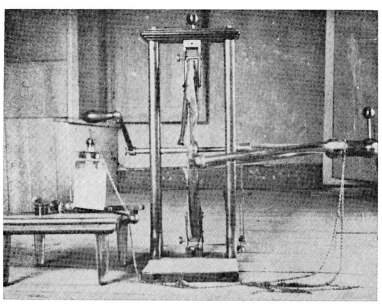

the lunatics. A remarkable electrical machine (Plate CXXVI) was discovered there and records from 1851 onward were kept of patients being frequently shocked. In some cases "an Electrogalvanic current was applied for half an hour daily"; it seems to have been especially used in cases of catatonic stupor and feeding difficulties.

The next psychiatric event in Australia was the opening of the Tarban Creek Asylum in 1838, which also accepted patients from Victoria, who were transferred there by ship from Melbourne. This practice continued until 1848, when the Yarra Bend Asylum was opened. In the first place Yarra Bend was classified as a ward of Tarban Creek, though 600 miles away, since New South Wales included Victoria until 1850.

The considerable frustrations of opening a new asylum at that time are reflected in Bostock's carefully documented account in the *Dawn of Australian Psychiatry* (3). As an example, straw for patients' mattresses was refused, because it would cost 3d. a day. An interesting section is devoted to the surgeon's case notes from 1848-50. Cummins' studies (9) reflect the same difficulties. Governor Gipps, all of whose dealings in this field represent an attitude of miserly obstruction, wrote in 1834: "The lunatic asylum is not a hospital, it therefore is not under the charge of the Deputy Inspector General of Hospitals, though in the management of it, it will often be necessary to have the benefit of his advice"; thus the first possibility of integration was lost.

By 1840, the convicts and ex-convicts represented only one in ten of Sydney's population; there were 27 male and 18 female free patients in the asylum and 28 male and 14 female convicts. In 1841, the first application for voluntary admission was received, without there being any means for the patient's acceptance.

The Dangerous Lunatics Act was promulgated in 1843, and in 1848 55 patients were admitted. Nostalgia was regarded as a physical cause. Almost as many women as men were alcoholics. Flogging was still considered a cause of mental illness, and being lost in the bush and sunstroke were accepted etiological factors. "Bush madness" was referred to in 1905 by Ernest Jones (17) though he had not seen cases of it, but a number of explorers, and convicts who had escaped, were recorded as becoming insane with exhaustion and starvation.

The causes of disorder were divided into moral and physical, a subject which inflamed the controversy between lay and medical administration in the hospitals (1). At this time Bowie, the Victorian Inspector General, referring to the Yarra Bend Asylum, wrote: "In this asylum, as in others, there are divinities, kings, queens, emperors, prophets, poets, millionaires, and speculators, puffed up with pride and strutting about with the greatest self-importance. Patients of this kind are very difficult to manage and their cases, if curable at all, are generally very tedious."

Discovery

Following upon the development of the wool industry from 1830 to 1850, there was a turmoil created by the discovery of gold at Bathurst in New South Wales and at Clunes in Victoria (as it was called when obtaining its independence from New South Wales, in 1850). Men left their homes and jobs, migrants poured in, bushrangers abounded, roads were clogged, grog shops flourished, prices soared and fortunes were made and lost overnight. The combined population of Victoria and New South Wales went up from 265,503 in 1850, to 886,393 in 1860. In five years, from 1851 to 1856, there was an increase of 2,000,000 sheep and 1,000,000 cattle, along with other corresponding developments associated with population growth and newly found wealth.

There could hardly have been a period of more rapid social change and adjustment, or such an opportunity for sociopathic traits to be mobilized. Such was the demand upon the mental hospital services in Victoria that in 1867 two mental hospitals in gold mining areas, at opposite ends of the state, were opened within ten days of one another. A third, at Kew (Plate CXXVII), admitted its first patients only five years later, with the object of relieving Yarra Bend, the first asylum in Melbourne. All three hospitals were modeled upon the patterns of the Colney Hatch and Hanwell asylums in London and the central buildings still stand as magnificent edifices.

As gold mining declined, unemployment increased, and the government embarked on a bold scheme of enormous borrowing to relieve the unemployed and improve the essential services in the state. Speculations in land were rife, there were numerous bankruptcies, a series of strikes and a financial crisis in 1891. When all the excitement was over the usual breakdowns in mental health followed. During these years accommodation for inebriates grew more urgent and an increasing number of people who could afford private mental treatment became ill. This resulted in the first inebriate institutions being opened, and the appearance of private mental hospitals in Sydney, Melbourne, and Adelaide. Up to this time lunatics in Queensland, South Australia, and West Australia had been either put in jail, or in temporary and unsatisfactory accommodation.

In Adelaide, in 1846, a house had been rented on the site of the present psychiatric hospital for £25 per annum called "The Colonial Lunatic Asylum" (Plate CXXVIII). It was to "make provision for the safe custody of and prevention of offenses by persons dangerously insane; and for the care and maintenance of persons of unsound mind." It was an old timber house which, without extensive measures of

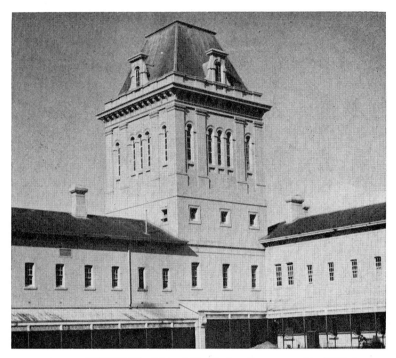

PLATE CXXVII. The Mental Hospital at Kew, opened in 1872.

restraint, could hardly have kept anyone secure. The new asylum at Parkside (Plate CXXIX) was opened in 1870 on the design of the Essex Asylum at Brentwood.

In Western Australia, at Fremantle, a striking building took the place of the Old Gaol as a repository for lunatics (Plate CXXX). Though now partly used as a Maritime Museum, it still retains some interesting features, like the open wooden sewerage channels, and the dark cells for isolation. In one part a bow wall had been blocked across to serve as a room for seclusion, though it would have been impossible to lie down there.

The first patient in Western Australia was a maniacal doctor, who afterwards returned to practice; he was kept in a repaired shipwreck (13).

In Queensland the Woogaroo Asylum (later called Goodna) was built in 1864. Before this, many of the convicts who were mentally ill were looked after in the large Moreton Bay Hospital in the convict settlement. It was at about this time that steps were taken for the segregation of the mental defectives from the mentally ill. It was also during this period that the first signs of a breakaway from cus-

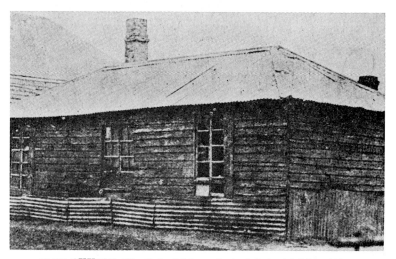

PLATE CXXVIII. The Colonial Lunatic Asylum in Adelaide, 1846.

todial care were shown. In 1838, when Tarban Creek was opened, the superintendent had requisitioned 63 iron bedsteads, six chairs for violent cases, 16 cribs of wood for dirty cases, 12 pairs of leather hobbles of various sizes for males and females, 12 hard belts of strong leather and iron cuffs attached to them with straps, 12 cuffs and belts for the hands in less violent but mischievous cases to fasten with buckle locks, six tick sleeves, etc.

It must be remembered that even chloral hydrate, bromides, and paraldehyde were not in use until after the middle of the century. At that time, drugs did not appear in the yearly costs. Patterson in South Australia commented in 1871: "The new remedial agent chloral hydrate has been used extensively during the year, and has been found to answer well. It has been very serviceable in the restlessness of *gen-*

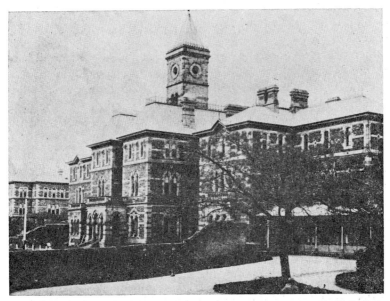

PLATE CXXIX. The Asylum at Parkside, opened in 1870. The "Ha-Ha" ditch is in front of the wall in the foreground.

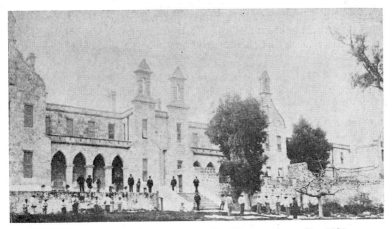

PLATE CXXX. Fremantle Asylum in Western Australia, 1890.

eral paralysis and *senile dementia*. It procures sleep in acute mania better than any other drug I have tried, but except in one case, I do not think it has exerted any favorable influence on the progress of the disease."

Other progressive developments towards the end of the 19th century are evident in the building of better accommodations for the mentally ill and in the introduction of occupational therapy. For instance, in Callan Park in Sydney, which was built in 1878 after the pattern of Chartham Downs in Kent, a cottage of 12 beds was added, and similar cottages were attached to the hospital at Ararat. Provisions were made for occupational therapy and, in 1885, the average cost per patient of materials for occupational purposes was 2¾ to 3 pence per week. In his report the Inspector General of the insane in New South Wales in 1885 says of Paramatta Asylum, which housed 645 male and 355 female patients:

> A fair proportion of the patients have been usefully employed in various occupations such as in the garden and grounds, laundry, woodyard, kitchen, stores, farm and wards. As in former years every attention has been paid to the amusement of the patients— the usual fortnightly dances were held—thanks are due to the lady and gentlemen members of the various dramatic and glee clubs . . . in aiding to make a few hours pass pleasantly for the inmates. Besides the above-mentioned means of amusement a great number occupy themselves with quoits, bowls, draughts, bagatelle, billiards, cards, and cricket. Cricket has charms for a greater number than any other amusement and the ground is used by men at least three times every week.

Another instance of the implementation of arrangements for occupational therapy is the report of the superintendent at Beechworth in Victoria; in 1883 he wrote: "The sewing room and workshops have employed a number of patients and their labor has been reproductive [*sic!*] as well as beneficial to themselves."

In 1882, 2.84 persons per 1,000 of the New South Wales population were in mental hospitals, a proportion identical with that in England at the same time.

At least 40 percent of admissions were reported as recovered, and 11 percent as relieved. The death rate was only 6.5 percent for the total resident population. Overcrowding still remained, but plans were prepared for the separation of the alcoholics and the imbeciles from the insane, since it had become evident that they could not be treated together. For the first time, complaints appeared about the elderly being sent to asylums.

However more attention was being paid to classification and an observation ward at Darlinghurst Prison was built for those patients whose diagnosis was alcoholism or transient lunacy. Of 122 patients received there, in 1878, 12 were of sound mind, 10 were sent to hospitals for the insane and 86 to the police courts. From 1869, five units for lunatic patients were established in district hospitals in Victoria, which had an average of 80 to 90 patients annually.

There is little record of any special treatment other than the usual purging, bleeding, blisters, and setons. The electrical machine at Lachlan Park in Tasmania has already been noted, and an ominous sounding "acid to the spine" was mentioned, but without explanation. The *Vagabond Papers* (first series), published in 1876, give a stimulating account of the conditions existing in the mental hospitals. "Garryowen," the writer of social commentaries in the *Argus,* took a post as an attendant in the Kew Asylum in Victoria to gather first-hand information; he was also for a short time at Yarra Bend.

Throughout the latter half of the century there were a series of committees of enquiry and commissions, often as the result of staff quarrels and accusations. Very early in the century official visitors were first appointed and provisions for them are officially incorporated in the Victorian Lunacy Act of 1843. Their enthusiasm was both variable and unpredictable.

Federation

The third period of the history of Australia is Federation, inaugurated in 1901. During this period comparable changes to those overseas have taken place in the psychiatric services and practices in Australia, but their progress has been both uneven and uncertain. Yet in a number of interesting developments Australia has been ahead of its time. Innovations were often achieved by enthusiastic individuals, but sometimes they were delayed by official obstruction, or impeded by governmental apathy; they make a depressing history as well as a comparatively dull chronicle of achievements and failures.

We can place Beattie-Smith in the category of innovators; he was an irate and explosive man, who became superintendent of Kew Hospital in Victoria, but left the Department of the Insane in 1902 to be one of the first alienists in private practice in Australia. He had already made some progress in teaching and later started a course in psychiatry for medical students, put the nurses in uniform, and advocated nursing training. By 1902, thanks to his efforts, six trained nurses were employed in Victoria, and in the same year some female nurses were for the first time placed in male wards. When Beattie-Smith died in 1922, he left money for a yearly public oration on insanity. In the lectures delivered in 1938 the one-time Inspector-General of the Insane in Victoria, W. Ernest Jones (17), gave an account of the state of the services for the mentally ill in Victoria between the time of his appointment in 1905 and his retirement that reflects the general conditions in Australia at that time.

At the end of the recession of the 1890's, the hospitals were in a poor state and the *Age* in Melbourne published an article which stated that "Very few if any, of our asylums have been kept up to a proper standard of efficiency, and none of them will bear the slightest comparison with hospitals for the insane in New South Wales."

Although new Inspectors came to similar conclusions in both Western Australia and Victoria in the first five years of the century, there was scant government support for the mental health services. There were periodic public outbursts, though often silenced politically by convenient, but unproductive inquiries or commissions.

In his Beattie-Smith Lectures, Ernest Jones said of the conditions in 1905: "The fabric of all buildings was being neglected and funds for repairs were down to zero. There was no system of water-borne sewerage anywhere. The cooking was in the hands of male cooks and patients, and the conditions were more than primitive, they were in fact disgraceful, the wards themselves were ill-lit, badly ventilated, and overcrowded. The airing courts were surrounded by high walls or stockade fences. There was no provision for the isolation of patients with infectious disease . . . phthisis, asylum dysentery and typhoid . . . and the appliances for fighting an out-break of fire were antiquated and inefficient."

These apparently represented the general conditions throughout Australia at about that time. Twenty-five years later things were little better. The *Australian Medical Journal* which in the 1920's published yearly reports of the mental hospitals, including staff salaries, was usually politely restrained in its criticism. However the conditions became so bad as to provoke leading articles (19) in 1939, 1943, and 1947 making "violent protest about the shameful neglect by governmental authorities in New South Wales of the mental hospitals department."

The state of Victorian Medical Hospitals in 1952 was similarly described in *Asylum to Community* (10), which showed that little improvement had occurred.

> The wards were mostly very dirty and little more could be expected from the insanitary state of affairs. Chamber pots were used

.nearly everywhere and frequently stored during the day in the same place as the food was prepared. The smell was abominable because straw mattresses were fairly generally used and only periodically refilled, the filthy straw being turned out onto a heap. The toilets were without seats, frequently broken and were quite insufficient in numbers. There was a considerable amount of mechanical restraint and solitary seclusion used, and the staff must have been in the greatest possible difficulties to know what to do for the patients with no facilities available for their care.

These deplorable conditions were accentuated by an overcrowding of about 1,500 people, many of whom were sleeping on mattresses on the floor. The serving of the food and its preservation were revolting. There were few facilities for occupation and one was confronted by the distressing spectacle of hundreds of ill-dressed people walking up and down staring at the ground within concrete or bare earth airing courts surrounded by railings.

Conditions were almost identical in the other mental hospitals throughout Australia. In 1950 the late Professor Alexander Kennedy made a blistering report on the Victorian Mental Health Services. As a result of this report, newspaper activity, and the possibility of the government falling, a mental health authority was appointed; this was the beginning of a program of remarkable reorganization and modernization of the mental health services throughout Australia in the last 20 years. It has been a very exciting era in mental health development; following these primitive conditions of only a few years ago mental health services can now take their place with the more progressive organizations elsewhere in the world (11).

This reorganization started in 1955, when the commonwealth government invited Alan Stoller to survey the Australian mental hospitals, and as a result of his report made £10,000,000 available, provided the states contributed £20,000,000 for capital works. Thus a vast rebuilding and upgrading program was inaugurated.

A Royal Commission at Callan Park in Sydney took place some years later, with considerable changes to follow, while a series of comparable reorganizations elsewhere resulted in states almost competing one with another to excel in this field.

Further Aspects

Legislation. As the states are individually responsible for their mental health services, there has been no common legislation. Since the beginning of the century a series of uneven acts has been produced largely for the purpose of separating the mentally ill from the intellectually handicapped, for the forensic services, for the licensing of private hospitals, and for the provision of observation wards and early treatment hospitals. Other acts have been passed for dealing with alcoholism and drug addiction, for non-statutory admissions, for the informal reception of patients, and for the formation of new administrative commissions.

Organizational Developments. The opening of the first out-patient psychiatric department in 1911 was followed by others and by the acceptance of voluntary patients, an innovation that in 1914 predated by 16 years similar legislation in England. The Royal Park Hospital in Victoria started to provide, in 1907, treatment for disorders in the early stages and thus stimulated similar facilities in other hospitals, which also offered more advanced techniques of treatment, hydrotherapy, and electroshock therapy.

In 1915, the first Repatriation Hospital, independent of other mental hospitals, was opened for mentally ill ex-servicemen. Voluntary aid in the mental health services was undertaken by a number of people (2,000 in Victoria alone by 1968) who were organized in the Mental Hospital Auxiliary, founded in 1933. The open-door policy, inaugurated in 1932, was followed by hostels in 1936, day hospitals in 1960, and other facilities which aim at using statutory and voluntary services within the community, like industrial rehabilitation, therapeutic social clubs, emergency calls, etc.

Teaching. There was little training in relation to mental illness before the turn of the century. Those in Victoria wishing to take an M.D. had to make 13 visits to one of the asylums; clinical clerks were advocated at that time. The first diploma of psychological medicine was established in Sydney in the mid-1920's, but only for internal students. Other states followed the example later.

The first professor of psychiatry, W. S. Dawson, of *Aids to Psychiatry* fame, was appointed to Sydney in 1922, and, after a long interval, this appointment was followed by that of a research professor in Queensland and six others elsewhere in Australia. The various diplomas of psychological medicine are gradually being replaced by an examination for the membership of the Australian and New Zealand College of Psychiatrists.

The Australasian Association of Psychiatrists was founded in 1946, largely due to the efforts of H. F. Maudsley (a nephew of the founder of the Maudsley Hospital in London). In 1964, it became the Australian and New Zealand College of Psychiatrists housed in Maudsley House in Melbourne (Plate CXXXI). The College has now 770 members and fellows and within it there are sections of forensic psychiatry and child psychiatry. The *Australian and New Zealand Journal of Psychiatry* was published for the first time in March, 1967 and the *Australian Journal of Mental Retardation* in March, 1970.

Treatment. Despite the statement at the 1884 Royal Commission that there was a comparative absence of scientific spirit in the colony,

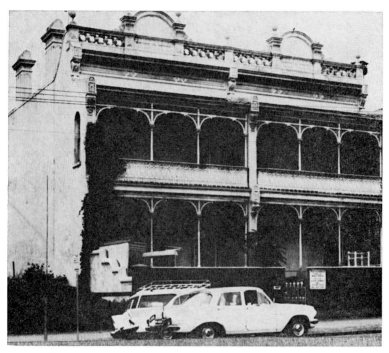

PLATE CXXXI. Maudsley House, Melbourne, the seat of the Australian and New Zealand College of Psychiatrists. The building has now been renovated.

by 1905 (ten years after the first pathologist was appointed to the London County Council) an asylum pathologist was employed in Australia. Thus by 1910 Wasserman tests were carried out on all imbeciles and general paralysis was being vigorously investigated. Pathological laboratories and libraries were set up and scientific papers were read at medical meetings.

These clinical advances led to new forms of treatment, especially for syphilis. By 1913 Salvarsan was in general use, thyroid extract was being used for *dementia praecox,* and in 1914 salvarsanized serum was heroically injected into the lateral ventricles of the brain for general paralysis. Sulphosin was given for schizophrenia, followed by insulin and cardiazol in 1937, and leucotomies were performed in 1943.

Birch, the Director of the mental health services in South Australia, built an ECT machine, without ever having seen another model, and later he built an electroencephalograph. Both of them worked most efficiently.

From 1926 on, malaria therapy, tryparsamide, and finally penicillin were used for GPI. In 1949, Cade published his observations on lithium, and by the 1950's the research units in Melbourne and Sydney had been set up; the former has become particularly well known as a center of epidemiological investigation.

Mental Deficiency. In 1872, recommendations had been made to found a separate institution to care for imbeciles as had been done· ae Leavesden and Caterham near London. A barrack at Newcastle in New South Wales was occupied in 1878 by "Idiots and Weak Minded Children"; 121 males and 76 females were in residence. The Inspector-General's report reads "60 males and 40 females attend divine service. Many of the children have very sweet voices and are trained by members of the Superintendent's family and the nurses."

In 1887, at Kew, in Victoria, three cottages, each with 20 occupants, were opened for the care of idiot children on a family basis. The psychological sections of the medical congress visited there, when the inmates' trade activities were praised as unique, while the cottage system was said to be "second to none."

Among the more interesting features in the mental deficiency field was a day center for imbeciles begun in 1885 by a doctor and his daughters in Melbourne; it continued to function up to his death in 1913.

More recent years have seen three outstanding residential centers for the intellectually handicapped opened in New South Wales, South Australia, and Western Australia, considerable study and teaching in Queensland, and a regional service organized in Victoria. The Australian Group for the Scientific Study of Mental Deficiency is the professional organization, and the Australian Association for the Mentally Retarded the voluntary body, dealing with this branch of mental health in Australia.

Among the more famous names in this field were R. J. Berry, who first applied psychometrics at the Melbourne Children's Hospital in 1921, Stanley Porteus (of *Porteus Maze* fame), who was the first headmaster of a special school in Melbourne in the 1930's, and Sir Norman

Gregg, who discovered the association between rubella and other forms of disability in 1941.

Alcoholism and Forensic Psychiatry. Despite the long history of alcoholism in Australia and the fairly frequent notes on the provisions for alcoholics, the first legislation for their control was enacted in 1872. In 1873 an alcoholics' retreat was opened in Melbourne and a further two in 1889. In one, 19 out of the 46 patients discharged were cured! The history of institutions of this type in all the states was short and unsuccessful, and, with the exception of the development of Alcoholics Anonymous, little happened of note until recent years. The present services for alcoholism and drug addiction were described at the International Congress in Sydney, in 1969 (12).

Despite the long association of the mentally ill with the jails, it was not until the Reception House for the Insane at Darlinghurst was constructed in the 1870's that a service for forensic cases began. There is then a gap until the 1940's, when a psychiatric consultant was appointed to the prisons in Sydney, and until 1960, when in Melbourne a division of Pentridge Gaol was constructed and provided with a full psychiatric staff. It was associated with out-patient facilities for discharged prisoners, for court cases, and for alcoholism.

Native Populations. It is difficult to obtain material relating to the Aborigine's practices for dealing with the mentally ill. Of recent years there has been a good deal of investigation of their difficulties in adjustment in relation to stress. Professor John Cawte of the University of New South Wales, who has been especially concerned in this field, wrote on *Medicine Is the Law: A Source Book of an Aboriginal Society,* published in 1972 (7).

D. G. Burton-Bradley, who has done more work than anyone else on mental health in Papua and New Guinea, has given a very complete account (5, 6) of transcultural psychiatry as far as it is known. A psychiatric service was started there in 1959 "based on clinical and transcultural principles." Since then he has written extensively on present-day findings and developments.

Literature. Australian psychiatry is well documented. Bostock's *The Dawn of Australian Psychiatry* (3), Tucker's *Lunacy in Many Lands* (22), Brothers' *Early Victorian Psychiatry 1835-1905* (4), Crabbe's *History of Lachlan Park Hospital* (8), Kay's *Centenary of Glenside Hospital* (18), Cummins' *Administration of Lunacy and Idiocy in New South Wales* (9), and Dax's *Asylum to Community* (10), all give reports which mark the conditions existing at some particular date and the progress which ha sbeen made over the years. Moreover there is still

a vast amount of material in many relevant papers, some of which are
noted in the list of references to this chapter (13).

The annual reports of those in charge of hospitals and mental health
services are mostly complete, while many of the first admission orders
and of the old record books are still available and give immense opportunities for future study and research.

Much material of all kinds has been accumulated in the Mental
Health Museum of Melbourne, and other museums have commenced
in Auckland and Fremantle.

3

NEW ZEALAND

The history of the psychiatric services in New Zealand must be considered separately, because although there are parallels to the evolution of the services and the stresses met in Australia, they are not close
enough to be described under the same heading. This is partly due
to a different time and method of settlement, the considerable differences between the Maoris and the Australian Aborigines and the fairly
early and complete separation of New Zealand from Australia. The
documentation and understanding of the Maori culture is considerably
more advanced than that of the Australian Aborigines, among other
reasons because they are better integrated with the population, of
which they represent a higher proportion than the Aborigines in
Australia.

Both Blake-Palmer (2) and Gluckman (15) have been especially
active in this field. Gluckman wrote me that he is in the course of
writing a history of insanity in the Maori culture before 1840. Once
more, as in the case of the Aborigines and the natives of Papua-New
Guinea, it is impossible to write any psychiatric history into this chapter as the anthropological work is too diffuse to summarize. What little
is known of the practices and beliefs in regard to mental illness must
be considered against the background and origin of the races concerned (2).

New Zealand was discovered by Tasman in 1642. Afterwards came
Captain Cook's voyage in 1768, concurrently with French, Russian,
American, and Spanish expeditions of discovery. They might have
remained and explored further and earlier had it not been for the
hostility and cannibalism of the Northern Maoris. However, by the
end of the 18th Century some whalers and sealers were established

there, and in 1814, the Reverend Samuel Marsden and his missionaries went to New Zealand from New South Wales and begged the English government to repeat the Australian experiment there, but their request was refused.

Marsden, a notable character, was a considerable landowner. Shaw (21) wrote, "That holy man, the Reverend Samuel Marsden, was interested in his animal flock as well as his human one." He had much political influence and was also concerned with the asylums in Sydney. In 1815 the Sydney *Gazette* stated that "all reports and casualties respecting the Lunatic Asylum at Castle Hill are in future to be made to the resident magistrate at Paramatta, and the Rev. Samuel Marsden will be pleased to give such orders and instructions regarding this department as he may deem advisable for the care and comfort of the lunatics." It appears that he had too many other duties to attend to the wants of the asylum, though he seems to have had the onus of being a trustee of the estates of some of the mentally ill.

New Zealand was annexed to Great Britain by Captain William Hobson in 1841. Certain Maoris ceded New Zealand to the Crown in the Treaty of Waitangi, thus causing the first Maori War in 1845, followed by a second from 1860 to 1865. There was tremendous enmity between the Maoris who supported the Europeans and those who were against them; the remnants of this dissension still exist.

Among the outstanding events which have been major factors as community stresses were the discovery of gold in 1852, the depressions about 1870, and the period from 1880 to 1895 when wool and wheat prices fell. The population increased rapidly with the years of prosperity from 100,000 in 1861 to 490,000 in 1885, and to 770,000 in 1901, with resultant economic and social changes. The discovery of the means of exporting frozen meat in 1901 made an enormous difference to the country's wealth, and by 1956 the population was 2,039,500, including 135,000 Maoris. New Zealand had an advanced early social legislation with old age pensions in 1891, widows' pension in 1911, and family allowances and assistance for the care of the handicapped.

The first recorded case of insanity was in 1841, and in 1844 a pauper lunatic asylum was attached to Wellington Gaol. In 1851, a public subscription was launched to build a lunatic asylum in the grounds of the Auckland Colonial Hospital. The appeal was apparently successful as the buildings opened in 1853.

But the first true, though unsatisfactory, lunatic asylum in New Zealand was that in Wellington, which started functioning in 1854; Sunnyside Asylum in Christchurch and the Dunedin Asylum were both opened nine years later. These were followed in 1867 by another at Whau in Auckland, and a Medical Superintendent was appointed there. In 1878, Seacliff Asylum (Plate CXXXII) was commenced, conveniently surrounded by impenetrable scrub, ultimately to replace the Dunedin Asylum. Only four years later, Ashburn Hall, which has made its name as an outstanding private mental hospital, was also established.

The need for mental hospitals is evident in the report of the Inspector-General of lunatic asylums, Skae, who stated that "the amount of

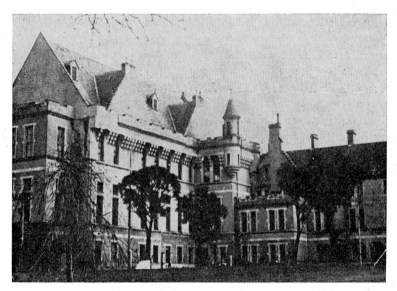

PLATE CXXXII. Seacliff Asylum, New Zealand (now demolished).

insanity is very large—larger than in England, where in 1879 the number of persons who became insane was one in every 1,944 of the population as against one in every 1,282 in New Zealand. This difference is no doubt partly due to the great amount of insanity caused by drink in this colony, but that is an explanation which hardly makes matters any better." Skae was dismissed in that year, after a Royal Commission had studied brutality at the Mount View, Wellington, asylum where there were 146 patients. In his report he speaks of the excess of restraint there, which sounds almost justified as no doubt he meant it to be, when he goes on to say with breathless indignation: "Nothing could be more unreasonable than to expect in a wretchedly constructed building, perched upon a cutting on a hillside where there is not even room to make an airing ground, you can carry out in its entirety the same method of treatment which, amidst immeasurable difficulties, risks and anxieties is pursued in the splendid asylums of England by accomplished and resident physicians with large and highly trained staffs of attendants." In Wellington, Porirua Hospital was opened in 1887.

In 1881 Tucker, who visited New Zealand while collecting the material for his book *Lunacy in Many Lands,* found 1,125 patients, 729 male and 396 female, in seven asylums, though the accommodation was only meant for 893.

Of Mount View, Dr. Tucker said, "In this as in other asylums in New Zealand the attendants are indistinguishable from the patients except by the bunch of keys they have hanging from their waists. . . . The superintendent could give me no information regarding the pay patients, and neither in this nor in the Dunedin Asylum could they supply me with statistics relative to recoveries and deaths." Auckland did not seem to be much better and of it Tucker wrote: "I was not shown the back parts of the asylum, nor any of the airing courts, but I cannot say much for the good order or cleanliness of the parts I did see."

An interesting incident was the passing of the Lunatics Amendment Act in 1894 allowing for the first time women to become official visitors of the asylums. It would be interesting to know how forceful a reformer the first lady appointed became and whether feminine influence was felt during the next 20 years, when observation wards were started, mental defectives segregated, nurses trained, and Oakley and Tokanui hospitals opened.

From 1924 to 1927 Truby King, of infant diet fame, was Inspector General. Malaria therapy began under him in 1924, and by 1925 outpatient clinics and observation wards in general hospitals had been inaugurated.

In the first enthusiasm for physical treatment, insulin was used in 1938, prefrontal leucotomy in 1942, ECT in 1943, and an EEG machine was installed in 1950, while a rehabilitation hostel was opened in 1960 and a day hospital in 1963.

With the amalgamation of the bureaus of mental health and medical services in 1965, the Alcoholism and Drug Addiction Act and the Mental Health and Criminal Justices acts were amended and a new and advanced security unit opened at Lake Alice.

The influence from England and the wish to emulate the improvements there are typified by the museums of Oakley dedicated to Conolly, one of the earliest pioneers of patient freedom in England.

A large silver centerpiece shows Conolly standing like the deity surrounded by patients with loosened chains. It was presented to him when he left Hanwell and, together with a very good portrait, it was found in the basement of the Auckland Museum, from where it was transferred to Oakley.

4

CONCLUSION

Parallel changes in Australia and New Zealand are easily seen. Although both countries were identified over 300 years ago, it was 150 years before Australia and 200 years before New Zealand emerged as clearly defined countries.

Through the period of transition the very different but fairly numerous native inhabitants had lived in small discrete groups, with their own tribal customs and traditions. Absorption and readjustment have proceeded at a slower pace in the more primitive Australian Aborigines than in the Maoris.

By the time New Zealand gained independence, the unhappy period of convict settlement had passed in Australia. But New Zealand had two Maori wars to face with all the bloodshed and tensions, and this was a situation which Australia escaped.

The sudden influx of population with settlement, the gold rush, and rural prosperity were similar in Australia and in New Zealand, as were the financial crises, which, with all the accompanying hardships, followed the periods of prosperity. The New Zealand social services were ahead of those in Australia.

Among other stresses for the settlers were the hazards of the long sea voyage. There was also administrative procrastination from Britain, local abuse of power, and the hard struggle inherent in establishing a foothold in a new country; moreover, in the early days the men greatly outnumbered the women, creating yet another problem. All these stresses may have not in themselves caused mental ill health, but they contributed to the constant demands for increasing the accommodation for the mentally ill.

Throughout the superintendents' reports references are frequently made to the effects of alcohol as a major factor in insanity, and inebriates' institutions flourished for a while, then petered out one after another. Perhaps their closing reflected the failures of treatment and the discouragement which followed the initial enthusiasm. The usual problems of overcrowding of the asylums are stressed in every report. Reluctance of governments to spend money until crises had arisen, the conveniently appointed enquiries and Royal Commissions to play for time and avoid responsibility, and the domestic quarrels and intrigues within the hospitals, make a constant repetitive pattern.

Although the two wars and the long period of neglect, especially of the old buildings in the first half of the 20th century, brought the psychiatric services to a low level, nevertheless, from the 1930's onwards, the new physical measures of treatment were adopted at the same time as in the United Kingdom. Yet Australia and New Zealand were less ready to receive them then than were many of the hospitals overseas. For, in spite of the attempts to separate the mentally defective from the mentally ill before the end of the last century, the classification in the late 1940's was still inadequate. Years of government apathy and lack of public interest had allowed the hospitals to deteriorate, with the consequent neglect of both the staff and buildings. Moreover, a considerable amount of mechanical restraint was still being used. Perhaps these were the reasons why the upsurge of enthusiasm generated by the new physical methods of treatment did not produce until later the same wave of excitement and optimism seen elsewhere.

To redress the balance and correct past neglect, large sums of money were poured into the mental health services with the aim of meeting the needs of the mentally ill. The staff increased enormously, while the number of university teachers and of private psychiatrists grew correspondingly. Old buildings were completely renovated and new units built; clinics were organized in association with the general hospitals; and the regional organization brought the services nearer to people in their widely scattered home towns.

REFERENCES

1. Benn, K. M. (1957): The moral versus medical controversy. *Med. J. Aust.*, 1, 126.
2. Blake-Palmer, G. (1956): Maori attitudes to sickness. *Med. J. Aust.*, 2, 401.
3. Bostock, J. (1968): *The Dawn of Australian Psychiatry*. Mervyn Archdall Medical Monograph. No. 4.
4. Brothers, C. R. D. (1962): *Early Victorian Psychiatry*. Victorian Government Printer.
5. Burton-Bradley, B. G. (1969): The traditional practitioner in Papua and New Guinea. *Aust. N.Z. J. Psychiat.*, 3, 1.
6. Burton-Bradley, B. G. (1969): Papua and New Guinea transcultural psychiatry. *Aust. N.Z. J. Psychiat.*, 3, 124 and 130.
7. Cawte, J. E. (1971): Personal communication.
8. Crabbe, G. M. (1966): *History of Lachlan Park Hospital*. Tasmanian Government Printer.

9. Cummins, C. J. (1968): *The Administration of Lunacy and Idiocy in New South Wales 1788-1855.* University of New South Wales.

10. Dax, E. C. (1961): *Asylum to Community.* Melbourne: F. W. Cheshire.

11. Dax, E. C. (1967): Psychiatry in Australia. *Amer. J. Psychiat.,* 124, 2, 180.

12. Dax, E. C. (1971): *Alcohol and Drug Dependence Treatment Resources in Australia.* 29th International Congress. Sydney: Butterworths (Australia).

13. Ellis, S. A. (1971): A brief history of psychiatry in Western Australia. (Unpublished).

14. Emmerson, R. & Stoller, A. (1968): Shower cabinet in the treatment of the mentally ill in Victoria. *Aust. N. Z. J. Psychiat.,* 2, 101.

15. Gluckman, L. K. (1968): The Maori adolescent in urban society. *Aust. N.Z. J. Psychiat.,* 2, 251.

16. Hooper, F. C. (1967): *Prison Boys of Port Arthur.* Melbourne: F. W. Cheshire.

17. Jones, W. E. (1938): Psychiatry, past, present and future. *Med. J. Aust.,* 1, 249 and 287.

18. Kay, H. T. (1970): *Centenary of Glenside Hospital.* South Australian Government Printer.

19. Medical Journal of Australia. Leading Articles: 1939, 1. 435; 1943, 1, 301; 1947, 1, 373 and 763.

20. Pretyman, E. R. (1966): *Port Arthur 1830-1877.* Tasmanian Museum.

21. Shaw, A. G. L . (1955): *The Story of Australia.* London: Faber.

22. Tucker, G. A. (1887): *Lunacy in Many Lands.* N. S. W. Government Printer.

Author Index

Indexes as prepared by M. Livia Osborn

Subject Index